From The Library Of
Dennis Clum

Second Edition
Medical Management of Radiation Accidents

Second Edition
Medical Management of Radiation Accidents

Edited by
Igor A. Gusev, D. Biol.
Angelina K. Guskova, M.D., PH.D
Fred A. Mettler, Jr., M.D., M.P.H.

CRC Press
Boca Raton   London   New York   Washington, D.C.

Library of Congress Cataloging-in-Publication Data

Medical management of radiation accidents / edited by Igor A. Gusev, Angelina K. Guskova, Fred A. Mettler, Jr.—2nd ed.
    p. cm.
Includes bibliographical references and index.
ISBN 0-8493-7004-3 (alk. paper)
  1. Radiation injuries. 2. Nuclear accidents. I. Guskova, A. K. (Angelina Konstantinovna) II. Mettler, Fred A. (Fred Albert), 1907- III. Title.

RC93 .G87 2001
617.1'24—dc21   00-052909
                                                                                                                                 CIP

This book contains information obtained from authentic and highly regarded sources. Reprinted material is quoted with permission, and sources are indicated. A wide variety of references are listed. Reasonable efforts have been made to publish reliable data and information, but the author and the publisher cannot assume responsibility for the validity of all materials or for the consequences of their use.

Neither this book nor any part may be reproduced or transmitted in any form or by any means, electronic or mechanical, including photocopying, microfilming, and recording, or by any information storage or retrieval system, without prior permission in writing from the publisher.

All rights reserved. Authorization to photocopy items for internal or personal use, or the personal or internal use of specific clients, may be granted by CRC Press LLC, provided that $.50 per page photocopied is paid directly to Copyright Clearance Center, 222 Rosewood Drive, Danvers, MA 01923 USA. The fee code for users of the Transactional Reporting Service is ISBN 0-8493-7004-3/01/$0.00+$.50. The fee is subject to change without notice. For organizations that have been granted a photocopy license by the CCC, a separate system of payment has been arranged.

The consent of CRC Press LLC does not extend to copying for general distribution, for promotion, for creating new works, or for resale. Specific permission must be obtained in writing from CRC Press LLC for such copying.

Direct all inquiries to CRC Press LLC, 2000 N.W. Corporate Blvd., Boca Raton, Florida 33431.

Trademark Notice: Product or corporate names may be trademarks or registered trademarks, and are used only for identification and explanation, without intent to infringe.

Visit the CRC Press Web site at www.crcpress.com

© 2001 by CRC Press LLC

No claim to original U.S. Government works
International Standard Book Number 0-8493-7004-3
Library of Congress Card Number 00-052909
Printed in the United States of America 1 2 3 4 5 6 7 8 9 0
Printed on acid-free paper

Dedication

This book is dedicated to the pioneers in radiation medicine who not only discovered the fundamental principles, but also taught us and others so that there would be a better understanding of the basic mechanisms of radiation medicine, as well as better treatment of radiation accident patients.

Preface

This is the second edition of *Medical Management of Radiation Accidents*. The first edition was published in 1990 and was predominantly concerned with radiation accident experiences in the United States. The second edition is substantially different. It represents an international cooperative effort. The majority of the work is a Russian–American effort; however, there are also authors from Austria, Brazil, Canada, China, France, Japan, and Peru. The material reflects current international approaches and experiences related to the medical management of radiation accidents as we begin a new millennium.

The book is organized into five broad areas. The first area deals with the fundamental aspects of radiation accidents, their medical characteristics, and their classification. The second area is concerned with the fundamental aspects of radiation on the entire body and specific tissues. This will provide a complete reference and, should an accident occur, the reader would not have to refer to additional texts. The third area includes chapters on the history of accidents in various countries throughout the world. The fourth area endeavors to give a general overview of a certain type of accident and to present specific examples, which we feel have major teaching points. Some of the accident examples are historical and others are very recent. We have not included details of accidents that did not possess significant medical teaching points (such as the Three Mile Island Accident in the United States). The fifth area covered in the middle of the book deals with criticality, industrial irradiators, industrial radiography, local radiation injury, radiation therapy, and internal contamination accidents and their management. There are many excellent descriptions of individual accidents in the literature (for example, by the International Atomic Energy Agency) but we hope that, with this text alone, the reader will be able to find an example of virtually any type of radiation accident and use the material as a basis to manage accidents in the future.

The final portion of the book includes a section on the follow-up of persons accidentally exposed to radiation with considerations related to epidemiological studies and a few selected examples. Finally, there are chapters on radiation protection and dosimetry issues, psychological considerations, and accidental exposure of pregnant women.

There are six appendices that include sample hospital protocols, a list of World Health Organization radiation accident centers, conversion and absorbed dose tables, specifics of radionuclides, and a glossary. We hope our readers will find this a useful text.

Igor A. Gusev
Angelina K. Guskova
Fred A. Mettler, Jr.
Editors

Acknowledgments

We would like to acknowledge the extensive editorial assistance of Charlotte Hendrix and the photographic artistry of Joseph Tafoya in the preparation of this manuscript. We also recognize the work of a vast number of our colleagues throughout the world that has resulted in scientific publications that provide the foundation for this text. Finally, the scientific and editorial comments of George Voelz were extremely valuable.

Editors

Igor A. Gusev, D. Biol., is Head of the Health Physics Laboratory, Department of Radiation Medicine at the Institute of Biophysics in Moscow, Russia since 1984. He received his Doctor of Biology degree from the Moscow Engineering Physics Institute in 1984. He also received an IAEA certificate in occupational radiation protection in 1993 from the Argonne National Laboratory.

Dr. Gusev is a member of the International Commission of Radiological Protection, Russian Nuclear Society, Russian Medical Physics Society, and the accidental reaction team of the Ministry of Health of Russia. He has also served as an expert for the International Atomic Energy Agency and on the International Chernobyl Project. Dr. Gusev is the World Health Organization REMPAN liaison executive. He is the author and co-author of 78 publications including those on medical assistance given to personnel of the Chernobyl Nuclear Power Plant after the accident in 1986.

Angelina K. Guskova, M.D., Ph.D., is Professor at the Institute of Biophysics in Moscow, Russia. She graduated with an M.D. degree from the Sverdlovsk Medical Institute in 1946, where she went on to work until 1949. Dr. Guskova has worked in the Medical Facility of Mayak Atomic Weapons Complex, the Institute of Biophysics (Mayak affiliated branch), the Institute for Labor Hygiene and Occupational Diseases, and the Institute of Biophysics (Moscow). During these tenures, Dr. Guskova received her Ph.D. in 1951 and D. Sc. in 1956.

She has authored and co-authored more than 700 publications, including *Radiation Sickness in Man* (1975). Dr. Guskova is a professor for the Associate Member of Russian Academy of Medical Sciences, a commissioner of the International Commission on Radiological Protection, member of the Russian Nuclear Society, and a number of other professional medical and radiation protection agencies.

Dr. Guskova lives in Moscow, Russia and has recently been named the 2000 winner of the Sievert Gold Medal from the Swedish Academy of Sciences.

Fred A. Mettler, Jr., M.D., M.P.H., is Professor and Chairman of the Department of Radiology at the University of New Mexico School of Medicine. He graduated with a B.A. in mathematics from Columbia University, and in 1970 he earned an M.D. degree from Thomas Jefferson University. He performed a rotating internship at the University of Chicago and subsequently completed a Radiology and Nuclear Medicine Residency at Massachusetts General Hospital. He received a Master's degree in Public Health from Harvard University in 1975.

Dr. Mettler has authored more than 270 scientific publications, including 15 books. He holds 4 patents. He is Vice-President of the National Council on Radiation Protection and has chaired two committees for the Institute of Medicine/National Research Council. He is currently the United States Representative to the United Nations for radiation effects and is one of the 13 members of the International Commission on Radiation Protection. He was the Health Effects Team Leader of the International Chernobyl Project and also has served as an expert for the Peace Corps, World Health Organization, the International Atomic Energy Agency, the International Agency on Research on Cancer, and the Japanese Government.

Contributors

Victor Anderson, B.S., CHP
University of California, Davis
Sacramento, California

Anjelika V. Barabanova, M.D., Ph.D.
State Research Center of Russian Federation
Institute of Biophysics
Moscow, Russia

Alexander E. Baranov, M.D., Ph.D.
State Research Center of Russian Federation
Institute of Biophysics
Moscow, Russia

Steven M. Becker, Ph.D.
University of Alabama
Birmingham, Alabama

Mary Ellen Berger, RN, Ed.D.
REAC/Training Site
Oak Ridge Associated Universities
Oak Ridge, Tennessee

Bryce D. Breitenstein, Jr., M.D.
Department of Preventative Medicine
State University of New York
Stony Brook, New York

Jerrold T. Bushberg, Ph.D.
University of California, Davis
Sacramento, California

Hervé Carsin, M.D.
Hospital Percy, Service de Santé Des Armées
Paris, France

Douglas B. Chambers, Ph.D.
Canadian Commission on Nuclear Safety
Richmond Hill
Ontario, Canada

Roxana Ching, M.D.
Hospital San Juan de Dios
San Jose, Costa Rica

Krishna Clough, M.D.
Oncologic Surgery
Institut Curie
Paris, France

Jean-Marc Cosset, M.D.
Radiation Oncology and Radiopathology
  Department
Institut Curie
Paris, France

Thomas Ferguson, M.D., Ph.D.
University of California, Davis
Sacramento, California

Shirley A. Fry, M.D.
Health Programs
Oak Ridge Associated Universities
Oak Ridge, Tennessee

Ivette Garcia, M.D.
Hospital Nacional de Ninos
San Jose, Costa Rica

Ronald E. Goans, M.D., Ph.D.
Oak Ridge Associated Universities
Oak Ridge, Tennessee

Abel J. Gonzalez, Ph.D.
Division of Radiation and Waste Safety
International Atomic Energy Agency
Vienna, Austria

Patrick Gourmelon, M.D.
Institut de Protection et de Sureté
  Nucléaire
Fontenay-aux-Roses, France

Igor A. Gusev, D. Biol.
State Research Center of Russian
  Federation
Institute of Biophysics
Moscow, Russia

Angelina K. Guskova, M.D., Ph.D.
State Research Center of Russian
 Federation
Institute of Biophysics
Moscow, Russia

Elizabeth C. Holloway, R.T.
Oak Ridge Associated Universities
Oak Ridge, Tennessee

Leonid A. Ilyin, M.D., Ph.D.
Institute of Biophysics
State Research Center of Russian
 Federation
Institute of Biophysics
Moscow, Russia

Charles A. Kelsey, Ph.D.
University of New Mexico
Albuquerque, New Mexico

Torsten Landberg, M.D.
Department of Oncology
Malmö University Hospital
Lund University Hospital
Malmö, Sweden

Joyce L. Liptzstein, Ph.D.
Institute for Radiation Protection and
 Dosimetry
National Nuclear Energy Commission
Rio de Janeiro, Brazil

Fernando Medina-Trejos, M.D.
Radiotherapy
Hospital Calderon Guardia
San Jose, Costa Rica

Dunstana R. Melo, Ph.D.
Institute for Radiation Protection and
 Dosimetry
National Nuclear Energy Commission
Rio de Janeiro, Brazil

Fred A. Mettler, Jr., M.D., M.P.H.
Department of Radiology
University of New Mexico
Albuquerque, New Mexico

Natalia M. Nadejina, M.D.
State Research Center of Russian Federation
Institute of Biophysics
Moscow, Russia

Shigenobu Nagataki, M.D.
Radiation Effects Foundation
Hiroshima, Japan

Jean-Claude Nénot, M.D.
Institut de Protection et de Sureté
 Nucléaire
Fontenay-aux-Roses, France

Kazuo Nerishi, M.D.
Radiation Effects Foundation
Hiroshima, Japan

Carlos Nogueira De Oliveira, Ph.D.
Emergency Assistance Services
Division of Radiation and Waste Safety
International Atomic Energy Agency
Vienna, Austria

Pedro Ortiz-Lopez, Ph.D.
International Atomic Energy Agency
Vienna, Austria

H. Earl Palmer, M.S.
Palm Leaf Products, Inc.
Richland, Washington

Vincinio Perez-Ulloa, M.D.
Radiotherapy
Hospital Mexico
San Jose, Costa Rica

Ralf U. Peter, M.D.
Department of Dermatology
University of Ulm
Federal Armed Forces Hospital
Ulm, Germany

Harriet A. Phillips, Ph.D.
Risk Assessment/Toxicology
Canadian Commission on Nuclear
 Safety
Richmond Hill, Ontario, Canada

Ceasar Picon, M.S.
Instituto Nacional de Enfermedades
  Neoplasicas
Lima, Peru

Luis Pinillos-Ashton, M.D., DMRT, FRCR
Jefe de Departmento de Radiologica
  de la UPCH y Medico Asistente
  del Departmento de Radioterapia
  INEN
Instituto Nacional de Enfermedades
  Neoplasticas
Lima, Peru

Robert C. Ricks, Ph.D.
Oak Ridge Associated Universities
Oak Ridge, Tennessee

Chris Sharp, M.D.
Anglian Water Services, Ltd.
Huntington, U.K.

David K. Shelton, M.D.
University of California, Davis
Sacramento, California

Vladimir Soloviev, M.D.
State Research Center of Russian
  Federation
Institute of Biophysics
Moscow, Russia

Mayela Valerio-Hernandez, M.D.
Hospital Calderon Guardia
San Jose, Costa Rica

George L. Voelz, M.D.
Occupational Medicine Group
Los Alamos National Laboratory
Los Alamos, New Mexico

Gerry Westcott, B.S.
University of California, Davis
Sacramento, California

Mayer Zaharia, M.D., FRCR, FACR
Jefe Division de Investigation
Departmento de Radioterapia INEN
Lima, Peru

Pan Ziqiang, Ph.D.
Science and Technology Commission
Beijing, China

Contents

Chapter 1
Fundamentals of Radiation Accidents 1
Fred A. Mettler, Jr. and Charles A. Kelsey

Chapter 2
Medical Characteristics of Different Types of Radiation Accidents 15
Angelina K. Guskova

Chapter 3
Radiation Sickness Classification 23
Angelina K. Guskova

Chapter 4
Acute Radiation Sickness: Underlying Principles and Assessment....................................33
Angelina K. Guskova, Alexander E. Baranov, and Igor A. Gusev

Chapter 5
Treatment of Acute Radiation Sickness 53
Fred A. Mettler, Jr. and Angelina K. Guskova

Chapter 6
Direct Effects of Radiation on Specific Tissues...69
Fred A. Mettler, Jr.

Chapter 7
The Safety of Radiation Sources and the Security of Radioactive Materials 133
Abel J. Gonzalez

Chapter 8
Review of Chinese Nuclear Accidents 149
Pan Ziqiang

Chapter 9
Radiation Accidents in the Former U.S.S.R...157
*Vladimir Soloviev, Leonid A. Ilyin, Alexander E. Baranov, Anjelika V. Barabanova,
Angelina K. Guskova, Natalia M. Nadejina, and Igor A. Gusev*

Chapter 10
Radiation Accidents in the United States...167
Robert C. Ricks, Mary Ellen Berger, Elizabeth C. Holloway, and Ronald E. Goans

Chapter 11
Criticality Accidents..173
Fred A. Mettler, Jr., George L. Voelz, Jean-Claude Nénot, and Igor A. Gusev

Chapter 12
Medical Aspects of the Accident at Chernobyl..195
Angelina K. Guskova and Igor A. Gusev

Chapter 13
Accidents at Industrial Irradiation Facilities 211
Fred A. Mettler, Jr.

Chapter 14
Local Radiation Injury..223
Anjelika V. Barabanova

Chapter 15
Accidental Radiation Injury from Industrial Radiography Sources 241
Fred A. Mettler, Jr. and Jean-Claude Nénot

Chapter 16
Accident Involving Abandoned Radioactive Sources in Georgia, 1997................................259
Ralf U. Peter, Hervé Carsin, Jean-Marc Cosset, Krishna Clough, Patrick Gourmelon, and Jean-Claude Nénot

Chapter 17
Localized Irradiation from an Industrial Radiography Source in San Ramon, Peru 269
Mayer Zaharia, Luis Pinillos-Ashton, Ceasar Picon, and Fred A. Mettler, Jr.

Chapter 18
Exposure Analysis and Medical Evaluation of a Low-Energy X-Ray
Diffraction Accident..277
Jerrold T. Bushberg, Thomas Ferguson, David K. Shelton, Gerry Westcott, Victor Anderson, and Fred A. Mettler, Jr.

Chapter 19
Local Irradiation Injury of the Hands with an Electron Beam Machine 289
Fred A. Mettler, Jr. and Charles A. Kelsey

Chapter 20
Accidents in Radiation Therapy 291
Fred A. Mettler, Jr. and Pedro Ortiz-Lopez

Chapter 21
A 2-Year Medical Follow-Up of the Radiotherapy Accident in Costa Rica..........................299
Fred A. Mettler, Jr., Torsten Landberg, Jean-Claude Nénot, Fernando Medina-Trejos, Roxana Ching, Ivette Garcia, Vincinio Perez-Ulloa, and Mayela Valerio-Hernandez

Chapter 22
Medical Accidents with Local Injury from Use of Medical Fluoroscopy 313
Chris Sharp

Chapter 23
Assessment and Treatment of Internal Contamination: General Principles 319
George L. Voelz

Chapter 24
Lifetime Follow-Up of the 1976 Americium Accident Victim 337
Bryce D. Breitenstein, Jr. and H. Earl Palmer

Chapter 25
Two Los Alamos Plutonium Accidents 345
George L. Voelz

Chapter 26
Internal Contamination in the Goiânia Accident, Brazil, 1987 355
Carlos Nogueira de Oliveira, Dunstana R. Melo, and Joyce L. Liptzstein

Chapter 27
Fatal Accidental Overdose with Radioactive Gold in Wisconsin, U.S.A. 361
Fred A. Mettler, Jr.

Chapter 28
Skin Wounds and Burns Contaminated by Radioactive Substances
(Metabolism, Decontamination, Tactics, and Techniques of Medical Care) 363
Leonid A. Ilyin

Chapter 29
Iridium-192 Acid Skin Burn in Albuquerque, New Mexico, U.S.A. 421
Charles A. Kelsey and Fred A. Mettler, Jr.

Chapter 30
Hospital Preparation for Radiation Accidents 425
Fred A. Mettler, Jr.

Chapter 31
Emergency Room Management of Radiation Accidents 437
Fred A. Mettler, Jr.

Chapter 32
Application of Radiation Protection Principles to Accident Management 449
Fred A. Mettler, Jr.

Chapter 33
Monitoring and Epidemiological Follow-Up of People Accidentally Exposed 453
Shirley A. Fry and Fred A. Mettler, Jr.

Chapter 34
Issues Involved in Long-Term Follow-Up of Persons after Radiation Exposure........................461
Shigenobu Nagataki and Kazuo Nerishi

Chapter 35
Long-Term Follow-Up after Accidental Exposure to Radioactive Fallout
in the Marshall Islands..471
Fred A. Mettler, Jr.

Chapter 36
Manhattan Project Plutonium Workers at Los Alamos..477
George L. Voelz

Chapter 37
Epidemiological Evaluation of Populations Accidentally Exposed
Near the Techa River..485
Angelina K. Guskova

Chapter 38
Instrumentation and Physical Dose Assessment in Radiation Accidents....................................489
Charles A. Kelsey and Fred A. Mettler, Jr.

Chapter 39
Evaluation of Neutron Exposure..501
Fred A. Mettler, Jr. and George Voelz

Chapter 40
The Current Status of Biological Dosimeters..507
Douglas B. Chambers and Harriet A. Phillips

Chapter 41
Psychosocial Effects of Radiation Accidents...519
Steven M. Becker

Chapter 42
Accidental Radiation Exposure during Pregnancy..527
Fred A. Mettler, Jr.

Glossary..541

Appendix 1: Sample Radiation Emergency Plan for a Medical Facility....................................557

Appendix 2: World Health Organization Radiation Accident Coordinating Centers................571

Appendix 3: Conversion Tables for SI and Conventional Units..575

Appendix 4: Absorbed Dose Estimates from Radionuclides...579

Appendix 5: Specific Gamma Ray Constants 587

Appendix 6: Radionuclides Listed Alphabetically 589

Index 593

1 Fundamentals of Radiation Accidents

Fred A. Mettler, Jr. and Charles A. Kelsey

CONTENTS

Introduction 1
Electromagnetic and Particle Radiations 2
    X Rays and Gamma Rays..2
    Particle Radiations 3
Quantities and Units...4
    Exposure 5
    Dose...6
    Equivalent Dose 6
    Effective Dose 6
Radioactivity 7
    General 7
    Nuclear Transformations 7
Biological Response...7
Types of Radiation Accidents 9
Principles of Dose Reduction 10
    Time...10
    Distance...11
    Shielding..11
Dose Limits 12
References 13

INTRODUCTION

Radiation accidents inevitably draw wide attention whenever they occur. Those involved, the first responders and health care providers, and the general public are all concerned. The consequences of every radiation accident are not limited to the biological and physical effects of the accident but include the psychological fallout as well. Everyone responding to a radiation accident will come under the microscope of public scrutiny and the inevitable second guessing of "experts" who were not there. For this reason it is important that any real or potential radiation accident be carefully, methodically, and scientifically assessed.[1-3]

Many radiation accidents combine radiation exposure with physical injury. In such cases initial actions must focus on responding to the physical injuries and stabilizing the victim. Even acute life-threatening radiation exposures do not require medical attention within the first few hours. Evaluation of the radiation exposure and consideration of possible countermeasures should wait until after the victim's urgent physical injuries have been treated.

ELECTROMAGNETIC AND PARTICLE RADIATIONS

Radiation accidents involve either electromagnetic or particle radiations. The electromagnetic spectrum extends from low-energy, long-wavelength radio waves to extremely high-energy, short-wavelength cosmic rays. Figure 1.1 illustrates the electromagnetic spectrum. When dealing with radiation accidents, only the X-ray and gamma-ray portions of the spectrum are of concern because they have high enough energy to penetrate into the body and produce ionization. Ionization is the removal of an electron from an atom to produce an ion and a free electron.

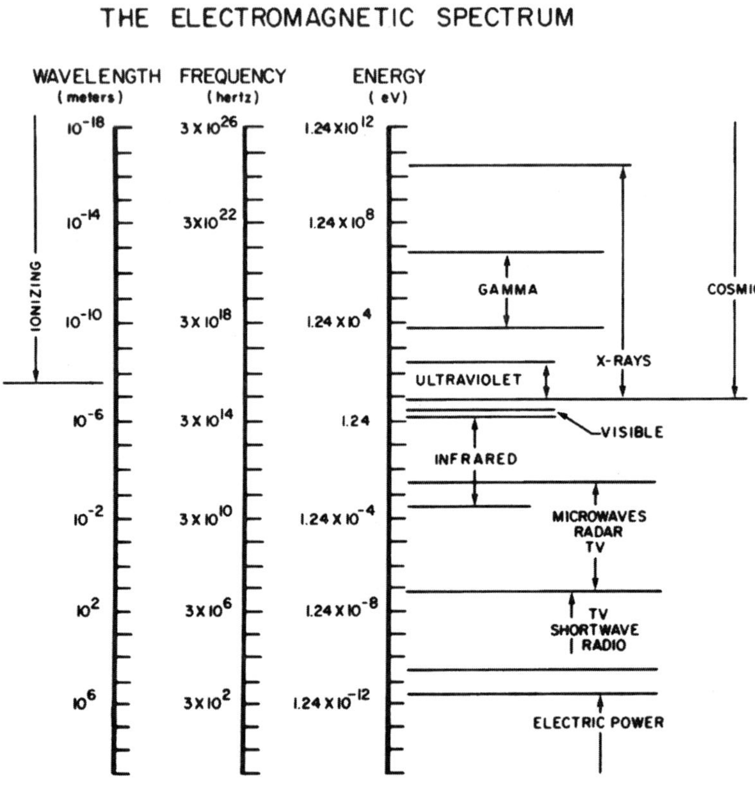

FIGURE 1.1 The electromagnetic spectrum.

X Rays and Gamma Rays

X rays and gamma rays differ only in their origin. X rays are produced in the outer shells of the atom; gamma rays come from within the atomic nucleus. X rays and gamma rays have zero mass and zero charge. One measure of their ability to ionize tissue and other matter is called the linear energy transfer, or LET. The LET measures how much ionization is produced along the radiation track. The amount of ionization is directly related to the amount of energy deposited along the track. X rays and gamma rays are low-LET radiations; that is, they deposit relatively low amounts of energy along their tracks and lose energy slowly as they penetrate into tissue (Figure 1.2). Their penetration in tissue depends on their energy, but can be tens of centimeters or more (Figure 1.3). One measure of penetration is the half-value layer (HVL). The HVL is the thickness of material required to reduce the intensity of the radiation to half its original value. Higher-energy radiations have larger HVLs. Table 1.1 presents the HVL for different energy X and gamma rays.

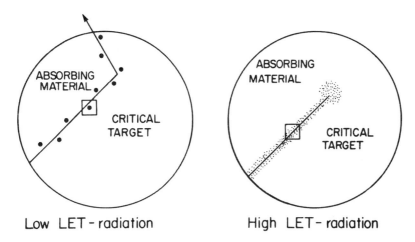

FIGURE 1.2 Deposition of energy in tissue by low- and high-LET radiations.

THE PENETRATING POWER OF RADIATION

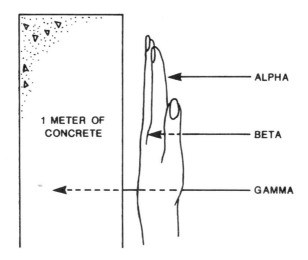

FIGURE 1.3 Schematic presentation of penetration of alpha, beta, and gamma radiations.

PARTICLE RADIATIONS

Radiation accidents may involve either beta particles or alpha particles, or both, in addition to X rays or gamma rays. Particle radiation differs from X rays and gamma rays because it has a definite range rather than an HVL.

Beta particles have a mass of 1/2000 atomic mass units (AMU) and a positive or negative charge. Beta particles are electrons. They are moderately penetrating, a few centimeters in tissue, and have intermediate LET values. Their penetration is about $^1/_2$ cm/MeV (Table 1.2).

Alpha particles are heavy particles with a mass of 4 AMU and a charge of 2. They are high-LET particles, which means they deposit large amounts of energy along their path and have very short (fractions of a mm) penetration in tissue (Table 1.3).

Radiation accidents involving nuclear reactors, nuclear fuel, or nuclear weapons may also include neutron radiation. Neutrons have a mass of 1 AMU and 0 charge. Neutrons are indirectly

TABLE 1.1
Half Value Layers for Different Photon Energies

Photon Energy (MeV)	Tissue (cm)	Concrete (cm)	Lead (cm)
0.1	4.2	1.7	0.015
0.2	5.0	2.3	0.065
0.4	6.5	3.0	0.27
0.6	7.8	3.6	0.5
0.8	8.8	4.0	0.7
1.0	9.6	5.0	0.9
2.0	14.0	7.0	1.3
5.9	23.0	11.0	1.5

TABLE 1.2
Maximum Penetration of Beta Radiation (cm)[a]

Beta Energy (MeV)	Air	Water[b]	Lead
0.1	15	0.015	0.001
0.2	40	0.05	0.004
0.3	65	0.08	0.006
0.4	94	0.12	0.009
0.5	130	0.16	0.013
0.7	200	0.24	0.021
1.0	315	0.40	0.034
2.0	790	0.96	0.081
3.0	1360	1.70	0.144
4.0	2020	2.30	0.210

[a] Beta emitting radionuclides emit a spectrum of energies. Average energy is about $1/3$ of the maximum energy.
[b] A useful rule of thumb is that the range in centimeters in water or tissue is equal to the energy in MeV divided by 2.

ionizing; they produce ionization by collisions with other charged particles. They have intermediate LET values and penetrations similar to low-energy gamma rays. Table 1.4 presents the characteristics of radiations that are commonly involved in radiation accidents.

QUANTITIES AND UNITS

Amounts of radiation can be expressed in several different ways. The number of gamma rays or particles could be counted, the amount of energy deposited could be described, or the effect of the radiation could be measured. Each of these approaches has advantages and uses different units. Table 1.5 gives the different ways of describing the amount of radiation present.

TABLE 1.3
Range of Alpha Particles

Energy (MeV)	Mean Range in Air (cm)	Range in Water (μm)
0.5	0.25	—
1.0	0.5	7.2
2.0	1.0	—
3.0	1.5	—
4.0	2.5	—
5.0	3.5	45
6.0	4.6	—
7.0	6.0	60
8.0	7.4	80

Note: An alpha particle requires at least 7.5 MeV to penetrate the protective layer of skin (0.7 mm or 70 μm).

TABLE 1.4
Characteristics of Different Ionizing Radiations

Radiation	Mass (AMU)	Charge	LET (keV/μm)
X rays	0	0	0.1
Gamma rays	0	0	0.1
Beta particle	1/2000	+ or 1	10
Alpha particle	4	+2	100
Neutron	1	0	10

TABLE 1.5
Units of Radiation Exposure

Measured	Quantity	Unit	Symbol
How many	Exposure	C/kg	C/kg
Energy imparted	Absorbed dose	gray	Gy
Adjust for different radiations	Equivalent dose	sievert	Sv
Adjust for nonuniform exposure	Effective dose	sievert	Sv
Amount of radioactivity	Activity	becquerel	Bq

EXPOSURE

Exposure measures how many X rays or gamma rays are present. It is really a measure of how much ionization is produced in air and is measured in coulombs per kilogram (C/kg) of dry air. An older unit still used in some areas is the roentgen, named after the discoverer of X rays. The symbol for the roentgen is R; 1 R = 2.58×10^{-4} C/kg.

Dose

The energy deposited by ionizing radiation is termed the *dose*. The dose is the critical factor in determining the amount of radiation damage resulting from a radiation accident. The unit of dose is the gray (Gy). An older unit still observed in the literature is the rad; 1 Gy = 100 rad.

Equivalent Dose

Different radiations have different biological effects. As a result of energy deposition differences 1 Gy of alpha radiation produces much more severe reactions than 1 Gy of X or gamma radiation. To account for the differences in energy deposition by different types of radiation, a radiation weighting factor is used. The absorbed dose multiplied by the radiation weighting factor (Table 1.6) results in the equivalent dose. The unit of equivalent dose is the sievert (Sv). The older unit of equivalent dose is the rem; 1 Sv = 100 rem.

TABLE 1.6
ICRP Radiation and Organ Weighting Factors

Radiation Type		Radiation Weighting Factor
Photons (all energies)		1
Electrons (all energies)		1
Neutrons	<10 keV	5
	10–100 keV	10
	>100 keV to 2 MeV	20
	>2–20 MeV	10
	>20 MeV	5
Protons	>2 MeV	5
Alpha particles, fission fragments, heavy nuclei		20

Organ	Tissue Weighting Factor
Gonads	0.20
Red bone marrow, colon, lung, stomach	0.12 each
Bladder, breast, liver, esophagus, thyroid	0.05 each
Skin	0.01
Bone	0.01
Remainder organs	0.05

Effective Dose

Most radiation accidents involve nonuniform exposure of the victims. To account for exposures that do not irradiate the body uniformly, and to account for the fact that some organs are more sensitive than others to radiation, the concept of effective dose (ED) has been introduced. The unit of ED is the sievert, with the older unit, the rem, still in use. An accident that results in a whole-body exposure of 4 Sv is very serious, perhaps life-threatening. An accident resulting in a dose of 4 Sv only to the hand is serious, but not life-threatening.

Effective dose must be calculated. It cannot be measured. It is calculated by estimating the average equivalent dose to an organ, multiplying by the organ-weighting factor (Table 1.6) and summing the values from all the organs. The ED tissue-weighting factors are based on cancer induction and other nonfatal effects of ionizing radiation. The ED is a more inclusive measure of radiation detriment at doses below 1 Sv. When accidents involve high doses to the organs resulting in substantial cell killing, the clinical outcome is best predicted using absorbed dose to specific organs.

RADIOACTIVITY

GENERAL

In the current model, the atom has a dense central core surrounded by electrons moving in specific orbits. The nucleus contains positively charged protons and uncharged neutrons. Nuclei with the same number of protons but different numbers of neutrons are called isotopes. Isotopes have the same chemical properties and hence occupy the same place on the periodic table. Almost all naturally occurring isotopes are stable, but some nuclei have too many or too few protons. These nuclei are unstable and spontaneously transform by emitting an alpha or a beta particle. The rules for nuclear stability are complex, but the number of neutrons in stable nuclei is always slightly larger than the number of protons.

Nuclei with an excess number of neutrons, or an insufficient number of protons, decay by negative electron emission, or beta emission. Although the actual process is much more complicated, beta decay can be thought of as the nucleus changing one of the excess neutrons into a proton by emitting a negative electron. Most beta emitters are produced in nuclear reactors.

Nuclei with excess protons usually decay by positive electron or positron emission. After emissions, the positrons combine with ordinary negative electrons in a process called annihilation which results in two 0.511-MeV X rays. This annihilation radiation is very penetrating. Some nuclei with excess positive charge can decay by alpha emission.

NUCLEAR TRANSFORMATIONS

The amount of radioactive material present at any time is determined by its half-life. The half-life is the time taken for one half the original material to be transformed. In dealing with radiation accidents involving radioactive materials, the half-life has two components, the physical and the biological half-lives.

The physical half-life is the amount of time required to reduce the amount present by physical decay to one half the original value. The biological half-life is the time taken for one half the material to be excreted from the body. The effective half-life, which is the combination of the physical and biological half-lives, is less than either. Equation 1.1 gives the relation between the effective, physical, and biological half-lives.

$$1/T_{1/2\text{eff}} = 1/T_{1/2\text{phys}} + 1/T_{1/2\text{biol}} \qquad (1.1)$$

The effective half-life is used in calculations to determine the dose to victims of radiation accidents involving radioactive materials. If a radioactive material is cleared rapidly from the body, its effects will be reduced. This is the basis for some dose reduction methods following ingestion or inhalation of radioisotopes during a radiation accident.

BIOLOGICAL RESPONSE

When ionizing radiation interacts with a cell, several results are possible. Figure 1.4 presents the major cell responses following irradiation. The cell may be killed resulting in some scarring. The cell may be damaged, resulting in repair and return to normal function, or the cell may experience some type of transformation, which may or may not lead to altered cell behavior. Cellular death rarely occurs at doses less than 50 mGy, although there may be some genetic damage. Damage to the DNA that is incorrectly repaired may lead to radiation carcinogenesis.[4–5]

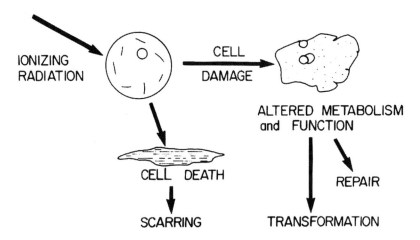

FIGURE 1.4 Possible cell responses following irradiation.

Ionizing radiations interact with tissues and cells in two ways, directly and indirectly. Direct interactions involve the radiation breaking a DNA bond, damaging a cell wall or some other direct interaction between the radiation and the cell. An indirect effect occurs when the radiation produces a free radical, which then damages the cell. Free radicals are uncharged atoms or molecules with an unpaired electron. Radiation interactions with oxygen and water can produce large numbers of free radicals. Free radicals may inactivate cellular mechanisms, or break bonds in the DNA or RNA molecules.

Because oxygen and water are easily involved in the formation of free radicals, they can become modifiers of radiation effects. A reduction in the oxygen or water content of a tissue will render it relatively more radioresistant. The "oxygen effect" describes the ability of oxygen to enhance the effect of radiation. The formation of free radicals in the initial step of radiation damage has implications for development and use of both radioprotective and radio-sensitizing agents. For the most part, radioprotective agents are free-radical scavengers that prevent free radicals from interacting with other cellular compounds and thus avert radiation injury. Radioprotective agents must be in the cells at the time the radiation is absorbed. The introduction of protective agents, even a short time after radiation exposure, has little or no effect.

The sensitivity of cells, tissues, and organs in the body depends on many factors, but one of the most important is the rapidity of cell division. Cells are most sensitive during mitosis, when the DNA is being divided. Table 1.7 presents the radiosensitivity of normal cells. Notice that rapidly dividing cells are more radiosensitive.

Because the body has repair mechanisms in place to repair damage to the cells, the amount of radiation damage depends on the rate at which the radiation is delivered. A dose delivered over several months allows the repair mechanisms to fully function. The same dose delivered in a few minutes may overwhelm the repair mechanisms resulting in more severe damage. The dose rate is an important factor in estimating the effects of any radiation accident exposure.

If the accidental exposure has just occurred and the absorbed dose is high, clinical effects that might be evident include manifestations of cell death in a rapidly dividing system such as skin, bone marrow, and gastrointestinal tract. If the exposure has occurred days or even months ago, clinical findings may include symptoms related to cellular death of the more slowly dividing systems and perhaps cellular death due to narrowing of blood vessels with subsequent ischemia.

Most physicians indicate three clinical phases of human biological response to ionizing radiation: (1) acute, (2) subacute, and (3) late clinical period.[4] In the acute clinical period, there is an initial destructive process with various repair mechanisms in any organ system. Survival of the victim during this period depends on the dose received and the radiosensitivity and volume of the

TABLE 1.7
Radiosensitivity[a] of Normal Cells

Radiosensitivity	Cell Type
Very high	Lymphocytes
	Immature hematopoietic cells
	Intestinal epithelium
	Spermatogonia
	Ovarian follicular cells
High	Urinary bladder epithelium
	Esophageal epithelium
	Gastric mucosa
	Epidermal epithelium
	Epithelium of the optic lens
Intermediate	Endothelium
	Growing bone and cartilage
	Fibroblasts
	Glial cells
	Glandular epithelium of breast
	Epithelium of the lung, liver pancreas, thyroid, adrenal gland, or kidney
Low	Mature hematopoietic cells
	Muscle cells
	Mature connective tissue
	Mature bone and cartilage
	Ganglion cells

[a] Radiosensitivity refers to cell killing and not potential for tumor induction.

tissue irradiated. Later, in the subacute period (6 to 12 months after exposure), underlying damage in parenchymal tissues may become manifest due to vascular deterioration, fibrosis, myointimal proliferation, and sclerosis of small arteries and arterioles. During the late clinical period, 12 months and more after irradiation, an organ system may demonstrate continued deterioration of the vascularity, decreased resistance to stress, and dense fibrosis. Several years after the radiation exposure, the major biological sequela identified is that of radiation carcinogenesis.

TYPES OF RADIATION ACCIDENTS

Radiation accidents can arise from problems with nuclear reactors, industrial sources, and medical sources. Although there are some differences between these three types of accident sources, there are common elements in all of them. Regardless of where the accident occurs, there are two general categories of radiation accidents. The first is external exposure, which is irradiation from a source distant or in close proximity to the body, and the second is contamination; there could also be a combination of the two. Almost all industrial accidents, most reactor accidents, and many medical accidents result in irradiation of the victim. There does not have to be direct contact between the victim and the radiation source, which may be a radiation-producing machine or a radioactive source. Once the person has been removed from the source of radiation, or the machine has been turned off, the irradiation ceases. The victim is not a secondary source of radiation and individuals providing support and treatment are in no danger of receiving radiation from the victim. A person exposed to external irradiation does not become radioactive and poses no hazard to nearby individuals.

External irradiation can be divided into whole-body exposures or local exposures. In either case, the effective dose can be calculated as discussed above, taking into account the attenuation of the body and the steep gradients of absorbed dose throughout the body.

The second category of exposure, contamination, results in an entirely different approach to the care and treatment of victims. Contamination is defined as unwanted radioactive material in or on the body. Figure 1.5 illustrates the different types of exposures that may result from a radiation accident. A simple way to think about contamination is as radioactive dirt. It may be outside or inside the body, but will continue to irradiate the patient until it is removed or decays away. Contamination may be in the form of radioactive gases, liquids, or particles. Care givers and support personnel must be careful not to spread the contamination to uncontaminated parts of the victim's body, themselves, or the surrounding area. Internal contamination can result from inhalation, ingestion, direct absorption through the skin or penetration of radioactive materials through open wounds.

PRINCIPLES OF DOSE REDUCTION

The three factors of radiation dose reduction are time, distance, and shielding. Figure 1.6 illustrates these three principles. Reduction of radiation exposure comes about by reducing the time of exposure and increasing the distance to the radiation source and the amount of shielding between the source and the individual.

TIME

The radiation dose from a source is directly proportional to the time of exposure. Doubling the time of exposure doubles the absorbed dose. If the monitoring instrument reads in mR/h or mGy/h

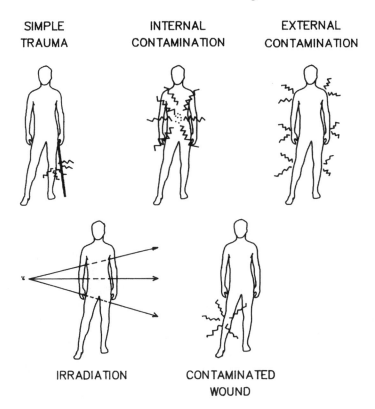

FIGURE 1.5 Different types of exposure that may result from a radiation accident.

Fundamentals of Radiation Accidents

the dose received can be estimated by multiplying the meter reading by the time in hours, or fractions of hours, spent in the radiation area.

DISTANCE

Distance is perhaps the most effective way of reducing radiation exposure. The greater the distance to the radiation source, the lower the radiation dose. Figure 1.7 illustrates the effect of distance on radiation exposure. Doubling the distance to the source will reduce the dose by a factor of four. The relation between dose and distance is called the inverse square law because it is an inverse relation. As the distance increases, the dose decreases as the square of the distance.

SHIELDING

Adding attenuating material between the radiation source and the individual will reduce the absorbed dose to the individual. The amount of attenuation depends on the HVL of the material. Lead and

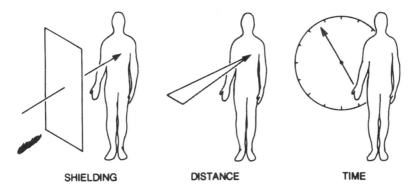

FIGURE 1.6 Three ways of reducing radiation dose.

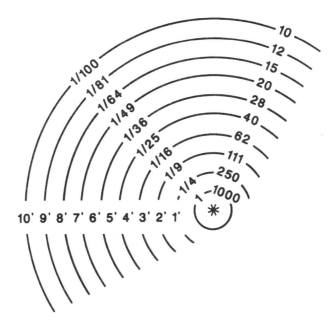

FIGURE 1.7 Effect of distance on radiation dose.

concrete are the most common shielding materials. In many industrial accidents involving cesium-137, cobalt-60, or iridium-192 shielding is not very practical because the energy of the radiation is so high, and the radiation is so penetrating that it becomes impractical to work with even a few HVLs. Table 1.8 gives the HVL in lead, and the thickness required to reduce the dose by a factor of two (HVL) and ten (TVL) for cesium-137, cobalt-60, and iridium-192. Note that this means, for example, that to reduce the radiation from a victim contaminated with cobalt-60 by a factor of 10, an individual would have to wear 80 radiology-type lead aprons that were 0.5 mm thick.

TABLE 1.8
Penetration Capability in Lead (cm) of Several Radionuclides

Isotope	^{137}Cs	^{60}Co	^{192}Ir
Half value layer	0.65	1.2	0.60
Tenth value layer	2.1	4.0	2.0

DOSE LIMITS

To control individual risk during both public and occupational radiation exposure, recommended international and national radiation protection commissions have established dose limits.[5,6] In addition, national and local regulatory authorities also have published limits. Not surprisingly, these are not the same. The current values of some organizations are given in Table 1.9. It should be noted that the values apply to standard operating procedures and practices and are not to be used in accidental situations. Use of numerical values of dose during accidental situations is discussed in Chapters 32 and 38.

TABLE 1.9
Recommended Annual Dose Limits

	International Commission on Radiological Protection (1990)	U.S. National Council on Radiation Protection & Measurements (1993)	U.S. Nuclear Regulatory Commission (1995)
Occupational			
Whole body	20 mSv/year averaged over 5 years	50 mSv in 1 year Cumulative 10 mSv × age	50 mSv in 1 year
Lens of the eye	150 mSv	150 mSv	150 mSv
Skin	500 mSv	500 mSv	500 mSv
Hands and feet	500 mSv	500 mSv	500 mSv
Embryo/fetus	5 mSv		
Public			
Whole body	1 mSv in a year	1 mSv continuous or frequent 5 mSv infrequent	1 mSv from a licensed operation or 5 mSv if operation can be justified
Lens of the eye	15 mSv	15 mSv	
Skin	50 mSv	50 mSv	
Embryo fetus		0.5 mSv	

Note: Whole-body limits are given in effective dose, and organ limits are typically in equivalent dose to that organ.

REFERENCES

1. International Commission on Radiological Protection (ICRP), Protection of the public in the event of major radiation accidents: principles for planning, *Ann. ICRP*, 40, 2, 1984.
2. International Atomic Energy Agency, Diagnosis and Treatment of Radiation Injuries, Safety Rep. Series 2, Vienna, 1998.
3. International Atomic Energy Agency, Planning the Medical Response to Radiological Accidents, Safety Rep. Series 4, Vienna, 1998.
4. Mettler, F.A. and Upton A.C., *Medical Effects of Ionizing Radiation*, 2nd ed., W.B. Saunders, Philadelphia, 1995.
5. Rubin, P. and Casarett, G.W., *Clinical Radiation Pathology*, W.B. Saunders, Philadelphia, 1968.
6. ICRP, 1990 Recommendations of the International Commission on Radiological Protection, Publ. 60, *Ann. ICRP*, 21(1–3), Pergamon Press, Oxford, 1991.
7. National Council on Radiation Protection and Measurements, Limitation of Exposure to Ionizing Radiation, NCRP Rep. 116, NCRP, Bethesda, MD, 1993.

2 Medical Characteristics of Different Types of Radiation Accidents

Angelina K. Guskova

CONTENTS

Introduction 15
Characteristics of Large Accidents 17
Characteristics of Accidents Involving Small Geographic Areas 19
Summary 21

INTRODUCTION

There are certain general principles and characteristics for different types of radiation accidents (Tables 2.1 and 2.2). The existence of national and international registries on accidental radiation injuries not only allows preparation of a useful database, but also allows one to find common general factors. One of the goals of such generalizations is separation of accident types according to the character of the damage, the temporal pattern and magnitude of clinical signs, and the type and results of therapy. Critical examination of the data and the general classification will allow optimization of medical care in the future.

Materials in these registries span over five decades. The material includes short-term effects seen in individual patients who had been exposed under circumstances in which the radiation dose can be ascertained reasonably well. In addition to registries, there are studies of larger populations in which there occasionally are radiation effects as well as nonspecific effects that may be attributable to multiple etiologies. This latter category may show some dependence on dose level, but the nature of the dose–effect relationship has a much more complicated character.

Persons exposed in radiation accidents may demonstrate effects that fall into two general categories. The first is direct deterministic effects, and the second is long-term stochastic effects. Direct deterministic effects include the various types of acute and chronic radiation syndrome; these deterministic effects only develop when a certain dose threshold has been exceeded. The long-term stochastic effects include induction of cancer and potential genetic abnormalities, and they theoretically may develop as a result of any radiation dose, although the probability of development is proportional to the dose.

Stochastic effects are typically identified by the presence of a statistically significant increase in malignant disease or genetic effect, in comparison with an adequate control group. Mathematical methods are used to reveal differences between the study and control groups, including use of correlation coefficients, confidence intervals, etc. It is also important to note whether the sex and age distribution, as well as the type of tumors occurring in the populations, are similar. Monographs

TABLE 2.1
Common Radiation Sources, Facilities, and Exposure Modes

Group	Source and/or Facility	External Exposure	Contamination	Mixed
I	Critical assembly	Yes	Yes	Yes
	Reactor	Yes	Yes	Yes
	Fuel element manufacture	Yes	Yes	Yes
	Radiopharmaceutical manufacture	Yes	Yes	Yes
	Fuel reprocessing plant	Yes	Yes	Yes
II	Radiation device, e.g.,			
	Particle accelerator	Yes	—[a]	—[a]
	X-ray generator	Yes	No	No
III	Sealed source (intact)	Yes	No	No
	Sealed source (leaking)	Yes	Yes	Yes
IV	Nuclear medicine laboratory	Yes	Yes	Yes
	In vitro assay laboratory	Yes	Yes	Yes
V	Source transportation	Yes	Yes	Yes
VI	Radioactive wastes	Yes	Yes	Yes

[a] Neutrons may induce radioactivity within the body.

Source: Diagnosis and Treatment of Radiation Injuries, Safety Series Report 2, International Atomic Energy Agency, Vienna, 1998.

TABLE 2.2
Radiological and Nuclear Accidents Resulting in Radiation Injury

Area of Application	Source, Radionuclide	Part of Body Exposed	Possible No. of Persons Injured
Industry			
Sterilization	^{60}Co, ^{137}Cs	Whole body, hands	1–3
Radiography	^{192}Ir, ^{137}Cs	Hands, other parts	1–10
Gauging	^{192}Ir, ^{137}Cs	Hands, other parts	1–2
Medicine			
Diagnostics	X-ray generators	Hands, face	1–10
Therapy	^{60}Co, ^{137}Cs, and accelerators	Whole body, hands, and other parts	1–10 (more in extremely rare cases)
Research	Broad spectrum of sources, including reactors	Hands, face, other parts	1–3 (more at research reactors)
Spent sources	^{60}Co, ^{137}Cs	Hands, other parts, and others	1–20 (more in extremely rare cases)
Nuclear reactors	^{137}Cs, ^{90}Sr	Whole body	1–500 (usually much less than the number of persons affected)
	^{131}I	Thyroid gland	
	^{210}Pu	Lung	

Source: Diagnosis and Treatment of Radiation Injuries, Safety Series Report 2, International Atomic Energy Agency, Vienna, 1998.

and summaries of these data are available through the periodic reports of the United Nations Scientific Committee on the Effects of Atomic Radiation (UNSCEAR), the International Commission on Radiological Protection (ICRP), and the International Agency for Research on Cancer (IARC). All of these documents have summarized the recent literature relative to stochastic effects and have identified risk coefficients for different tumor types and other effects.

Essential factors in evaluating the medical consequences of radiation accidents include information on the following:

- External radiation (neutron, X-ray, or gamma radiation) and depth of penetration;
- Low-energy surface external radiation (beta radiation);
- Initial surface contamination (important for evaluation of oral or transdermal intake of radionuclides);
- Exposure to gaseous forms of radionuclides (e.g., noble gases).

Radiation exposures or doses need to be carefully quantified. Typically, organ or whole-body doses are expressed in international units of equivalent dose (Gy) or effective dose (Sv). Doses are also often expressed as average, midline, entrance, or exit, and, in addition, collective doses are often used for persons exposed to radiation under similar conditions; the unit used for this is the person-Sv. Even in a single event, there can be significant differences in individual exposure. For example, in the atomic bomb explosions at Hiroshima and Nagasaki, there were different combinations of external radiation, including gamma, neutron, and beta radiation. There was a much smaller contribution from internal contamination with fission products. For persons who were at some distance from the epicenter of the explosions, the exposure consisted of radiation that had a rapidly decreasing dose rate.

CHARACTERISTICS OF LARGE ACCIDENTS

Accidents at atomic test sites exposed numbers of people including in the atolls in the Pacific, in Nevada in the United States, in Kazakhstan, and in Novaya Zemlya. These persons were predominantly exposed to specific types of gamma and beta radioactive fallout, usually as a result of iodine-131 and strontium-90 (see Chapters 35 and 37).

Large-scale nuclear accidents, where there was significant release to the environment, also irradiated large numbers of people. The Windscale accident in the United Kingdom released radioiodine. In contrast, the Chernobyl accident released not only large amounts of radioiodine, but also radioactive cesium; which exposed the public to both external and internal contamination from these particular radionuclides. Personnel remaining near the Chernobyl core during the accident were exposed to additional radionuclides, particularly through inhalation at much higher dose levels of external gamma and beta radiation (see Chapter 12).

This type of accident, involving noncriticality accidents at nuclear reactors, usually is the result of human error. The specific features of such accidents include:

1. The presence of a local neutron exposure, as well as gamma radiation.
2. The possibility of contact (usually of the hands) with exposed elements of the reactor fuel that have escaped from the structural framework. This causes gamma and beta exposure.
3. Environmental release of radioactive gases and aerosols, which can result in beta and gamma exposure; relatively low internal exposure as a result of inhalation compared with external beta and gamma dose.
4. A large percentage of the persons involved have high doses and significant injuries.

This type of accident also differs clinically from other types of accidents, as follows:

1. A large percentage of the persons with even mild forms of the acute radiation syndrome also have significant local radiation injuries.
2. The dose may be fractionated as well as heterogeneous. This adds to the difficulty of patient assessment, particularly with regard to initial symptoms.
3. There are often a large number of people involved, and there is a need for rapid triage of those needing prompt medical assistance.
4. There is limited application of dosimetric techniques (such as electron spin resonance or luminescence signal) since these do not reflect the fractionation or heterogeneity of dose distribution. (They usually reflect average whole-body dose.)

Medical evaluation and prognostication of effects from short-term exposures can be accomplished with reasonable accuracy. Assessing exposure from potential internal contamination of dispersed long-lived radionuclides is more difficult. This is because substantial changes in dose received by the public can occur based on control of the food chain and differing lifestyle habits. Long-lived radionuclides have been particularly important in accidental situations; an example is the discharge of nuclear waste into river systems as a result of a storage explosion in the southern Urals. With large accidents, the health implications clearly relate to the extent of the contaminated area and the population contained within that area. However, since radiation usually decreases rapidly with distance from the accident source, the effects in large populations tend to be long-term effects, rather than acute health effects occurring within days to weeks. This is fortunate as these allow relatively more time for assessment and intervention as compared with the effects on persons immediately adjacent to or directly involved in the accident. For example, in the Chernobyl accident, there were approximately 600 people working at the accident site on the night of the accident, and, of these, about 135 developed acute radiation syndrome. In addition, several hundred thousand persons in the republic received measurable radiation doses, but these were typically below 0.1 Gy, and the risk is predominantly of long-term stochastic effects. Similarly, in the accident in the southern Urals, dose levels to the public were not high enough to cause acute effects, and the total value of dose that could reach the threshold for development of chronic radiation syndrome was registered in only three settlements in the upper part of the Techa River. Overall, chronic radiation syndrome was diagnosed in only 66 cases.

As mentioned earlier, in assessment of medical and biological effects of large radiation accidents, it is important to realize why individual long-term studies may produce contradictory results. First of all, the period of investigation is very important. Obviously, in the 3 days following exposure, if the total dose is high enough, there will be acute radiation syndrome. With more chronic doses, marrow depression and cytopenia may be found; however, as the dose rate decreases, there is a characteristic recovery process. As a result of this, it is clear that studying patients with different exposure conditions may lead to completely different conclusions even though the patients received the same total dose.

Many studies compare incidence rates of diseases in the pre- and the postaccident period. As an example, studies that have examined the incidence rate of malignancies in the decade after Chernobyl showed the rate to be increasing. Many authors have incorrectly indicated that these increases were due to the accident. However, when one examines the data in the decade before the accident, there also was an increasing rate of tumors each year, and the rate of increase was no different before the accident than it was after the accident.

There are additional confounding factors in large epidemiological studies conducted after an accident. Usually, in the aftermath of a large environmental release of radioactivity, people will be more likely to seek medical care for conditions they normally would not have consulted a physician about before an accident. There also may be additional programs instituted, which increase the detection rate of diseases that were present, but undetected, prior to the accident.

The selection process used to determine which persons are included in epidemiological results is also important. Obviously, when laboratory studies are conducted (for example, thyroid function), one would expect to find a higher incidence of abnormalities in those who are older and who are already under medical care for some particular problem. The incidence rate in randomly selected nonhospitalized populations would be expected to be significantly lower. Finally, any long-term program needs to be evaluated for similar social, demographic, and ethnic characteristics, uniform principles regarding complete recording and classification of data. The sample size must be large enough to be able to identify effects with significant statistical power (a number of these issues are presented in Chapter 33).

CHARACTERISTICS OF ACCIDENTS INVOLVING SMALL GEOGRAPHIC AREAS

As a rule, accidents in small areas only affect small numbers of people, although the radiation doses can be extremely high. These accidents typically occur as a result of exposure to industrial radiography sources used in nondestructive testing, in industrial sterilization facilities, in radiotherapy machines, as well as from criticality accidents occurring with experimental assemblies or chemical processing. Usually, there are no health effects in most victims of these types of accidents, and clinically significant effects usually are demonstrated only in 1 to 5% of people involved in these localized accidents. Despite this, there have been in excess of 130 fatal outcomes from such accidents.

Localized accidents have been most common and have increased during the last 25 years. The author's experience indicates that there have been about 200 serious injuries resulting from 120 incidents or accidents. The specific features of these accidents are as follows:

1. Increasing number and type of movable and fixed irradiation sources. Usually, these are gamma and less commonly beta sources.
2. A wide range of doses to persons involved, from negligible to lethal.
3. Predominance of local exposures with the movable sources and more whole-body exposure and severe effects with powerful stationary irradiators.
4. With small sources, very high doses to hands, thighs and buttocks as a result of handling sources or putting them in a pocket.
5. If the dose is very inhomogeneous, difficulty evaluating the results of biological dosimetry.

The clinical aspects that occur most commonly in this type of accident are as follows:

1. Many of the patients do not present immediately. As a result, the initial phase can only be clarified by obtaining a detailed history.
2. Criteria for prognosis are complex and not well defined. This makes decisions regarding the necessity and extent of surgery difficult.
3. Local radiation injuries often result in long-term disability because of scarring and amputation.
4. Late clinical presentation confuses many physicians, and radiation specialists are required.
5. Use of new imaging techniques (such as ultrasound and computed tomography) allows visualization of extent and depth of tissue edema and destruction. This information can be used to optimize therapy.
6. Increasing use of radiation sources in industry, medicine, agriculture increases the importance of training general practitioners in recognizing radiation injuries.

Accidents with industrial radioactive sources can be divided into two main groups: (1) situations in which the radiation source was lost, found, or removed from a unit by persons who did not know that the source was radioactive and what its potential hazard was, and (2) accidental situations with personnel involved in improper use of a device or unaware of a malfunction. A few illustrations of this type of accident are presented in subsequent chapters.

Accidents with substantial overexposure have occurred as a result of operator error or defects in policies and procedures. An example occurs with industrial radiography designed to detect defects in metal. These sources usually contain iridium-192, cobalt-60, and cesium-137. All these are gamma emitters, and dose rates on the surfaces of the sources are usually in excess of 50 Gy/min. More than 90% of accident situations with such sources include severe injuries of the hands or the buttocks, hips, and abdomen. The latter occur because the sources are often put in the pockets of clothing (see Chapters 15 and 17).

Radiation sources with cobalt-60 are also used for sterilization of food products and medical equipment. For sterilization, the objects are exposed to radiation doses exceeding thousands of gray. The need for extremely high doses results in stationary units with much more powerful sources than industrial radiography gamma cameras. With these units, even very short exposures can result in serious and lethal injuries. A number of these are discussed in later chapters, particularly the accidents in San Salvador, Soreq (Israel), and Belarus (see Chapter 13). Fatalities have occurred in all these accidents, and typically the problem was poor maintenance of the equipment and not following operational policies. Many workers involved in these types of accidents began vomiting after a few minutes of exposure and left the room. Severe depression of hematopoietic function of the bone marrow occurs, and local injuries necessitating amputations also are probable.

Radiotherapy equipment in hospitals also has been the cause of a number of accidents. There are two types. The first involves a malfunction of the equipment itself, an error in calculations, or a problem with software programs. These cause patients to receive either higher or lower doses than expected (see Chapters 20 and 21). A number of accidents have occurred in the last decade in the United States and Canada involving errors in the computer program for an accelerator, and, in addition, large accidents involving overexposures have occurred both in Spain and Costa Rica. Often, the errors are not discovered for several weeks until there are a substantial number of patients that have been treated. As a result, it is important to use dosimeters to check radiation therapy treatments. The second type of accidents have occurred when radiotherapy machines have been disposed of improperly. A number of these have been taken to junkyards and either broken open or melted for scrap. Such accidents have occurred in Goiânia (Brazil) (Chapter 26) and in Mexico. These accidents may involve powder-type sources, which when broken open result in substantial internal and external contamination, as well as external irradiation. Other radiotherapy sources are sealed or metallic and cause injuries very similar to the industrial radiography sources.

Criticality accidents occur when there is too much of a fissionable material within a specific geographic location. These accidents occur with experimental critical assemblies as well as in chemical processing of nuclear fuel. Criticality accidents have the following specific features:

1. A complex energy spectrum and geometry that results in a very heterogeneous dose distribution in the body.
2. Usually only a small number (between 1 and 10) persons involved. There is typically little if any exposure of the public.
3. Large differences in the extent of the whole-body damage and local radiation injury found in victims of the same accident.
4. Little internal contamination by radionuclides.
5. Heterogeneous dose distribution that makes dose assessment and interpretation of clinical laboratory tests difficult. In noncriticality accidents these parameters are used to make clinical decisions. Experience with the criticality accidents in Russia in 1957, 1959, 1971, and 1997, in Mol (Belgium), Vinca (Yugoslavia), and the recent accident in Tokaimura (Japan) demonstrates the difficulty in evaluating the bone marrow status and determining when surgery and amputation should be used.

In criticality accidents, high-quality medical expertise is required. The specialists required include hematologists, burn surgeons, and radiation experts (Chapter 11).

The general characteristics of these accidents are of very high, nonuniform radiation doses to individuals within several meters of the critical excursion. In addition, there can be substantial exposure not only to penetrating gamma radiation, but also to very soft gamma radiation and neutrons. These accidents have been summarized in Chapter 11.

SUMMARY

Once the type of radiation accident has been classified, specific algorithms can be designed for the medical management of radiation accidents and injuries (Table 2.3). The following steps can minimize the health sequelae.

1. Determine the source of the irradiation. Although there is often confusion in the initial accident stages, usually it is possible to determine which of the following is involved:
   a. Criticality accident (weapons, nuclear fuel facility, or reactor);
   b. Large stationary radiation source (reactor core or powerful stationary industrial irradiator);
   c. Small but intense irradiation source (usually used for industrial radiography); sources can be in the workplace or lost and in the public domain;
   d. Release of unsealed radioactive materials into the environment.
2. Determine the more-detailed circumstances of exposure related to the specific accident:
   a. External and/or internal contamination (inhalation, ingestion, skin or wound contamination);
   b. Radiation spectrum and degree of homogeneity of dose distribution in time, space, and body surface;
   c. Number of people involved, significantly exposed and other injuries;
   d. Basic clinical manifestations to allow clinical prognostication;
   e. Type of therapeutic actions required, where these will be done, and who is qualified to do them;
   f. Other unfavorable factors of the accident.
3. Determine the information required for the following:
   a. Victims and their relatives;
   b. Administrators and governing bodies;
   c. Mass media and general public of the region and nation; this is particularly important for large accidents with environmental releases of radionuclides;
   d. Registration and documentation forms.
4. Evaluate the consequences of the accident and plan for the future. This requires:
   a. Prospective plan for the return to normal living conditions for the patient, agency, region, and public;
   b. Information for the scientific community and international organizations;
   c. Recommendations for optimization of social, economic, and legislative decisions.

In this chapter, classification of accidents was based on the type of source and the peculiarities of the health effects induced. This approach allows one to understand the possible deterministic or stochastic effects, their frequency, and the likely required diagnostic and therapeutic measures.

Accidents also can be classified according to the spatial and temporal distribution of radiation doses from the different sources. Homogeneous penetrating radiation usually is the result of nuclear explosions, early fallout from weapons tests, accidental releases from nuclear power plants, and powerful stationary irradiators. Short-term heterogenous exposure is characteristic of criticality accidents, reactor accidents that involve beta exposure, and situations involving radiation sources where there is shielding and resultant partial body exposure. Significant internal exposure has been rare except during the early experience with radium and plutonium.

TABLE 2.3
Treatment of Exposed Patients at General Hospitals

Type of Exposure	Possible Consequences	Treatment at a General Hospital
External Exposure		
Localized exposure, most often to hands	Localized erythema with possible development of blisters, ulceration, and necrosis	Clinical observation and treatment Securing of medical advice if necessary
Total or partial body exposure, with minimal and delayed clinical signs	No clinical manifestation for 3 hours or more following exposure Not life-threatening Minimal hematological changes	Clinical observation and symptomatic treatment Sequential hematological investigations
Total or partial body exposure, with early prodromal signs	Acute radiation syndrome of mild or severe degree depending on dose	Treatment as above plus securing of specialized treatment Full blood count and HLA typing before transfer to a specialized center
Total or partial body exposure, with thermal, chemical irradiation burns and/or trauma	Severe combined injuries, life-threatening	Treatment of life-threatening conditions Treatment as above and early transfer to a specialized center
External Contamination		
Low-level contamination, intact skin that can be cleaned promptly	Unlikely, mild radiation burns	Decontamination of skin and monitoring
Low-level contamination, intact skin where cleaning is delayed	Radiation burns Percutaneous intake of radionuclides	Securing of specialist advice
Low-level contamination, with thermal, chemical, or radiation burns and/or trauma	Internal contamination	Securing of specialist advice
Extensive contamination, with associated wounds	Likely internal contamination	Securing of specialist advice
Extensive contamination, with thermal, chemical, or radiation burns and/or trauma	Severe combined injuries and internal contamination	First aid, plus treatment of life-threatening injuries; early transfer to a specialized center
Internal Contamination		
Inhalation and ingestion of radionuclides — insignificant quantity (activity)	No immediate consequences	Securing of specialist advice
Inhalation and ingestion of radionuclides — significant quantity (activity) of radionuclide	No immediate consequences	Nasopharyngeal lavage Early transfer to a specialized center to enhance excretion
Absorption through damaged skin (see under external contamination)	No immediate consequences	Securing of specialist advice
Major incorporation, with or without external total, or partial body, or localized irradiation, serious wounds and/or burns	Severe combined radiation injury	Treatment of life-threatening conditions and transfer to a specialized center

Source: Planning the Medical Response to Radiological Accidents, International Atomic Energy Agency, Safety Series Report No. 4, Vienna, 1998.

3 Radiation Sickness Classification

Angelina K. Guskova

CONTENTS

Introduction 23
Classification Schemes 24
Whole-Body Exposure 27
Local Radiation Injury 30
Summary 30
References 30

INTRODUCTION

Radiation sickness refers to a specific combination of health effects resulting from exposure to ionizing radiation.[1,2] The effects are due to deposition of energy in biological tissues (Figure 3.1).[3] Absorption of energy imparted by ionizing radiation occurs in microseconds, and is accompanied by the occurrence of both ionized and electrically excited atoms and molecules. Subsequently, through the formation of free radicals on various molecules, damage may be manifested as cell injury, cell death, or may transform genetic material resulting in subsequent tumors. The clinical changes identified as a result of cell injury or cell death are manifested over a period of hours to months. Such changes may include the acute radiation syndromes, as well as characteristic erythema, blistering, even necrosis due to local radiation injuries. Changes continue to occur even years later as a result of deterministic effects (vascular narrowing of small blood vessels and other abnormalities, such as atrophy and fibrosis of structural tissues and cataract formation) and stochastic effects (cancer and hereditary).

Information on radiation injuries has been collected over a period of 70 to 100 years.[1–10] There are data on accidental and purposeful exposure of humans as well as modeling of radiation health effects from animal experiments.[11] The first information on local injuries to become available was demonstrated in the late 1800s, with skin damage to the hands of radiologists, X-ray technicians, and experimenters.[12] Changes in mucosa and skin during therapeutic application of radium and X rays also were reported. Subsequently, reports were published on diseases occurring in radium dial painters and researchers working with the first cyclotrons.

Since 1945, the world has known the effects of acute radiation sickness and death from radiation damage as a result of atomic bomb radiation in Hiroshima and Nagasaki. The delayed effects became evident over the following decades in these populations.[13–17] Data have also been accumulated relative to severe radiation injuries of personnel at research facilities and nuclear military installations.[18–24] Over the last 30 years, descriptions of health abnormalities in different occupational groups engaged in long-term work with relatively high radiation doses have been documented.[16,21,25,26] One specific form of this has been referred to as chronic radiation sickness.[4,14,15]

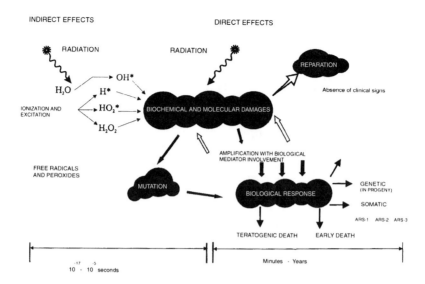

FIGURE 3.1 Schematic diagram of the molecular and cellular basis of radiation injury.

CLASSIFICATION SCHEMES

Initially, radiation sickness was simply classified as local or general, acutely developing or long-term developing changes. This division often was purely descriptive and sometimes poorly substantiated. In addition, the terms *acute* and *chronic radiation sickness* often included clinical syndromes whose occurrence, mechanism, and time of development were different from true radiation effects.[4,23,24–30] As a result of the confusion and classification, there was great difficulty in both diagnosis and development of prognostic criteria following accidental exposure to ionizing radiation. The number of radiation accidents that have occurred and the vast amount of data that have been accumulated have made it clear that it is not easy to develop simple classifications or simple prognostic criteria that would apply to all situations. In spite of this, it is necessary to attempt classification based on scientific principles, which gives one the opportunity to understand the etiology and development of the clinical findings and to be able to develop prognostic criteria. Such work also might allow one to predict clinical events that had not yet been observed in practice, but that would be expected to occur in the future as current barriers are overcome and new treatment modalities are developed.

The majority of manuals devoted to clinical or pathological classification of radiation sickness categorize injuries according to location (local or whole body), the rate at which clinical manifestations develop (acute or chronic), and type of radiation exposure (internal or external). In some cases, classifications are made according to occupation such as those occurring in X-ray technicians, uranium miners, or nuclear industry personnel.

The development of a classification scheme that can be supported by pathophysiological findings is complicated by the fact that the reaction of the organism on a systemic level involves molecular, cellular, and tissue, as well as organ interaction. The typically described syndromes of the acute sickness such as bone marrow, intestinal, toxemic, cardiovascular, or neurovascular have been described as separate syndromes, when often one is predominant but elements of the others are present. Similarly, aplasia and pan myelofibrosis as well as myelodysplastic syndrome have been described as a result of chronic exposure.

Numerous radiation health effects have been described in the literature, including various forms of cancer and sarcoma, leukemia, pneumonitis, aplastic anemia, indurative edema, myelitis, necrosis, etc. These clinical definitions, when accompanied with words like *radiation* or *post-radiation*, indicate a causal relationship of the disease or at the very least suggest an effect of radiation exposure.

Thus, in many cases the literature correctly or incorrectly reflects not only the clinical manifestation, but also the presumptive cause and some assumed information about the underlying injury at the molecular, cellular, and metabolic level.[29-36] In addition, in some literature, the term *radiation stress* has been used when discussing both regulatory and adaptive biological systems. These references are typically in the physiological, neuroendocrine, or immune literature.[5] Finally, the experience of clinicians and experimenters is often viewed subjectively and there can be a tendency to classify various forms of radiation injury according to personal experience. As an example, an experiment may only have used one type of animal or a limited term of observation.

Animal data regarding radiation injuries may have the same underlying basic mechanisms as humans, but there are specific differences in the biological and social aspects relative to humans. These factors are inevitably important and are related to the time of expression as well as the dose threshold in humans. In addition, the spatial dose distribution is often quite different between humans and animals, given the differences in body size.

Assessment of radiation effects in humans is also complicated by prophylactic and corrective measures used to treat patients. Even when only human radiation accident data are examined, the circumstances of exposure and therapies used are often quite different. Despite all these limitations, a classification of radiation sickness was developed in Russia as early as 1962, and has been modified since as experience has accumulated (Figure 3.2).

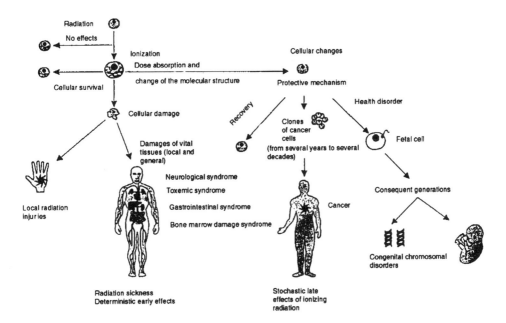

FIGURE 3.2 Schematic diagram of mechanisms involved in the expression of radiation injury.

The basic principle of classification is relating the biological effects observed in tissues and the whole body with the spatial and temporal distribution of the dose. The underlying radiobiologic mechanism allows classification of radiation effects into deterministic and stochastic (probabilistic). Both of these types of effects occur over a wide dose range (Figure 3.3). Deterministic effects are the result of damage to large numbers of cells. If enough cells in a particular organ, for example, are damaged, that organ or system will not be able to function properly. However, damage of a single cell or even a few cells will not be evident. As a result, these effects require a specific threshold of dose and an elevation of dose increases the incidence rate and the severity of the effect (the severity grade of radiation sickness). The development of radiation sickness, therefore, is the final stage in the complex chain of events initiated by ionizing radiation and energy absorption in

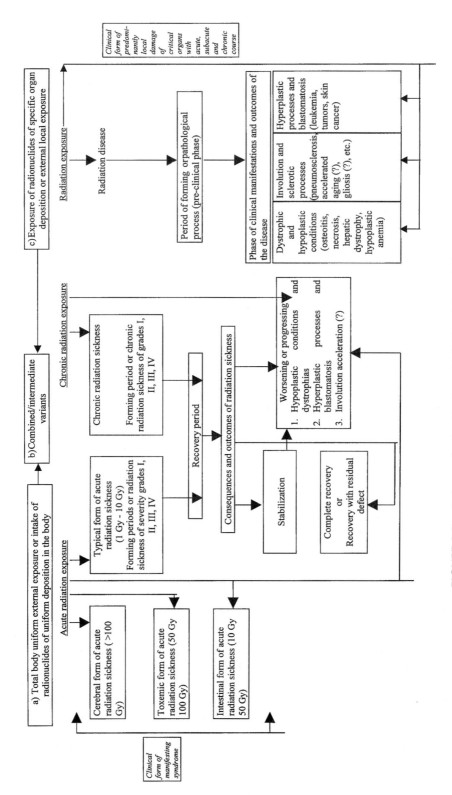

FIGURE 3.3 Pathogenetic classification of radiation sickness in humans.

the tissues. Similar to many other diseases, radiation sickness manifestations are not by themselves specific. However, their combination and temporal sequence is manifest as the typical clinical syndromes.

The primary mechanism for the interaction of radiation with biological tissue is irradiation of the structural elements of DNA. Damage to the genetic material of a single cell can result in cellular death (a deterministic effect that will not be noticed in a single cell), or it may result in transformation of the genetic material and continued viability of the cell. Even if there are damage and death of some cells, there is also a process of reparation and compensation, both in the tissue and organs. For deterministic effects to be evident, the threshold dose that must be reached would require that cell death exceed the ability of cellular reparation and repopulation. Since humans are composed of multiple tissue and organ systems with different radiosensitivities, it is clear that a certain threshold dose would first affect the systems that have the highest sensitivity to radiation, and as one increases the dose to the individual, additional less-radiosensitive tissues will be damaged.

The death of specific lymphocyte fractions, which are immature cells in the bone marrow, and intestinal epithelium happen at the lowest doses (lymphoid exhaustion, bone marrow syndrome, and intestinal syndrome). As the dose is increased, there is damage to the epithelium of the stomach, esophagus, mucosa, skin, and spermatogenesis. The highest resistance to radiation damage occurs in the low proliferative and poorly regenerative cellular elements of adults, including bone, cartilage, muscular, and nerve tissues. The cells of the liver, kidneys, lungs, and thyroid have intermediate resistance to cellular death from radiation.

In addition to identifying absorbed dose as an integral part of the classification scheme, the phases of disease development, recovery, and ultimate outcome also must be considered. Some stages of acute radiation injury take months, or even years, to develop. These include fibrosis, cataracts, and even necrosis. Although these are not evident initially, they are a direct continuation of events that occurred early in the injury. The frequency and severity of these late effects are determined by the magnitude and temporal distribution of the radiation dose. There are other late effects (such as cancer and leukemia), which are stochastic effects, and these are not well substantiated or judged to be a continuation of the initial radiation sickness itself. In a similar fashion, acute radiation sickness does not become chronic radiation sickness, although some researchers have made this connection.[16,19,32,36]

The result of initial, nonfatal radiation-induced changes of the cell can be the initiation or promotion of the development of the pathological cellular clone developing into a malignant neoplasm after some period of latency.[31] The probability of such an event depends on the radiation dose; however, the possibility of cancer development exists for any dose value (the linear nonthreshold concept). These stochastic effects also would include the possibility of inheritable, abnormal genetic information, which may be manifest in the progeny of radiation-exposed individuals. Heritable changes, however, have been difficult or impossible to identify in humans at this time.

In all cases of development of neoplasms, ionizing radiation is only one factor among a set of risk factors that can cause such diseases. The probability that radiation was the factor that caused a certain tumor can only be assessed after one has reviewed the risk factors and sensitivity of the tissue from epidemiological data, and determined the dose and the presence of other endogenous and exogenous risk factors (smoking, chemical carcinogens, genetic predisposition). A number of techniques for such quantitative evaluation have been described in the literature.[21,22,24,26]

WHOLE-BODY EXPOSURE

The classification scheme also presumes the subdivision into clinical syndromes caused by uniform and nonuniform radiation exposure. The extreme example of nonuniform exposure is a local radiation injury of only a single body portion by a radiation beam or high-dose radiation of a particular organ, such as in the case of internal contamination by radionuclides.[30,32] An example of this would be changes in the thyroid after radiotherapy with radioactive iodine. In this case, while there are very high doses within a localized area (the thyroid), the dose is orders of magnitude lower several centimeters away.

In radiation accidents, there is a combination of both local and generalized whole-body damage. This occurs because often there is a complex spectrum of radiation (for example, gamma and neutron plus X rays or beta rays of low energy). Accidental situations also commonly involve partial shielding of organs or a body segment (in the case of external exposure). There are, of course, radionuclides that are relatively uniformly distributed throughout the body (such as tritium and cesium), and these are closer to the first variant of radiation sickness relative to dose distribution.[4,6,7,14,32]

The conditional borderline distinguishing acute from chronic radiation sickness is considered to be the accumulation of the average absorbed body dose of approximately 1 Gy within the time period of several seconds to 3 days.[4,18] A confirmation of this division is obtained empirically from radiation accident data, and comparison with doses in the range of 10 to 12 Gy given over 3 days prior to bone marrow transplantation in patients with leukemia. The classification of acute radiation sickness according to severity for whole-body exposure is presented in more detail in Chapter 4 (Acute Radiation Sickness or ARS). The forms are bone marrow, intestinal, toxemic, cardiovascular, and neurological.

In accidental human overexposure cases, there often is what appears to be an intermediate form between the cerebral and intestinal form of radiation sickness. This is predominantly related to the fact that, in accidental exposure, there is often significantly nonuniform radiation, combined with high total-body exposure. In such circumstances, the disorders of the regulation of the blood circulation can be very important and can be a direct cause of death. As a result, some authors have used the term *cardiovascular form of ARS* with a lethal outcome during the first 3 days. For the bone marrow and intestinal forms of acute radiation sickness, there are usually initial symptoms followed by a latent period and then manifestation of the particular organ damage. With the more severe forms of acute radiation sickness, there has not appeared to be any latent period. Until recently, there have been no survivors beyond the initial phase for the more severe forms of exposure. Typically, death has occurred in 3 to 7 days following clinical manifestation of massive interstitial edema of the brain, lung, pericardium, muscle, and cellular tissue, combined with a hypotensive shocklike or seizure syndrome. The intestinal syndrome without medical treatment causes death within 2 weeks with clinical signs of hypovolemia, abdominal discomfort, and a large loss of liquid, electrolytes, and massive bleeding from intestinal erosions and concurrent ileus and peritonitis.

The bone marrow form has a clear, latent period and shows a typical picture of cytopenia with complications.[33] With medical therapy, or if the dose is not too high, the marrow regenerates, although some cytopenia remains up to several months postexposure. Active reparative and compensatory processes usually continue for 1 to 2 years in the more severe forms of the bone marrow syndrome. Historically, it was considered that, even after the stabilization phase of acute radiation sickness, additional radiation damage might continue to occur. However, with additional experience, this does not appear to be the case as long as radiation exposure has ceased.

Chronic radiation sickness is a clinical syndrome, which develops in the case of long-term radiation exposure to annual doses above 0.1 Gy and to cumulative doses of more than 0.7 to 1.5 Gy. Depending upon the dose rate and the cumulative dose, the time for development of chronic radiation sickness varies from 1 to 2 years up to 5 to 10 years. Data relative to chronic radiation sickness are predominantly in the Russian literature,[1,4] and few, if any, reports exist in Western literature. According to the data of Okladikova, chronic radiation sickness has been identified following relatively uniform whole-body exposure in personnel at atomic facilities where cumulative doses were 2.3 to 10 Gy within 3 to 5 years, and in 1 to 3 years in cases in which the annual whole-body doses were 2 to 2.5 Gy.[14,15] In the author's experience, rapidly progressing cytopenia has been observed in only three patients with chronic radiation sickness with cumulative doses in the range of 4 to 5 Gy. These doses were accumulated in a short time period (less than 2 years). If the radiation exposure was stopped, recovery of the hematological profile to initial levels was observed in the majority of patients within 3 to 5 years. Akleev et al.[21] have indicated that about two thirds of these patients with chronic radiation sickness were diagnosed 6 to 8 years after the beginning of continuous radiation exposure caused by residence in an environment with high external exposure and radionuclide intake (predominantly cesium and strontium). The bone marrow doses in half of the patients at the time of diagnosis were above 0.9 Gy, and the average individual dose was about 1.3 Gy. The majority of these patients were young (approximately 19 years of age) when they received the majority of their radiation dose.[10,27]

Particular features of chronic radiation sickness caused by total-body radiation include:

- A combination of poorly expressed and slowly progressing changes in a number of tissues, but predominantly the hematopoietic tissue. Changes have also been described in neurological, endocrine, and cardiovascular systems; however, these changes are not acceptable as the only criterion for the diagnosis of chronic radiation sickness.
- Severity and persistency of the above-mentioned changes depend on the cumulative dose, as well as the dose rate.
- The duration and wavelike course of the findings over time should reflect variations in dose rate with some expected recovery when the dose rate decreases.

If radiation exposure is prolonged from internal contaminants such as radium, plutonium, or strontium, chronic radiation sickness may not appear for a long time because of the significant abilities of the critical structures to compensate. With very high intakes and doses resulting from internal contamination, and if clinical manifestations do develop, clinical recovery is usually not possible because of the biokinetic and long effective half-life of the radionuclides.[1] Damage to specific organs from prolonged internal exposure is very difficult to detect preclinically, although it can be done if there are informative markers related to the particular organs involved. Such markers may include liver enzymes or changes in chromosomes or even pulmonary function studies in the case of lung damage due to very high intakes of insoluble plutonium.

With chronic radiation sickness, as the dose rate is decreased, the various body systems recover at different rates. Typical persistent changes, however, may include aplasia and hypoplasia of the hematopoietic tissue, signs of demyelinization, and abnormalities of the heart, particularly when the cumulative doses exceed 4 Gy. Chronic radiation sickness is conditionally divided into four grades of severity (I to IV), with IV being extremely severe. If the radiation dose continues, then the severity grade obviously can increase. Once exposure is stopped, as a rule, consequent progression of the disease does not occur.

Similar to acute exposure, chronic radiation exposure outcomes include partial or complete recovery, compensation, or the potential of late health effects such as leukemia and cancer. For nonuniform chronic exposure due to internal contamination, late effects obviously occur in the target organs. For example, with inhalation of large activities of insoluble plutonium compounds, pneumonitis and pulmonary fibrosis are all possible in the late term.[14,15,17,30] In a similar fashion, for radionuclides compounds with liver specificity (soluble compounds of polonium, thorium, and plutonium), increasing hepatic pathology including chronic hepatitis and cirrhosis was identified at high dose levels. Liver tumors also have been observed as a result of such exposures.

For the thyroid, after larger exposures to radioiodine, long-term effects are limited to thyroid aplasia, hypoplasia, and hypofunction. Neoplastic effects also include induction of thyroid nodules and thyroid cancer. Note should be made that radiation-induced thyroid cancer is significantly influenced by multiple factors including age and sex. The adult thyroid appears to be relatively resistant to cancer induction by radioiodine.

LOCAL RADIATION INJURY

The underlying pathological principles related to radiation sickness that were described earlier in the chapter also apply to local radiation injuries caused by external exposure. Local radiation injuries have clearly demonstrated pathophysiological phases of development. As expected, the more severe local radiation injuries caused by very high doses do not have an obvious latent phase. Not all the clinically manifest radiation effects are due to cell killing. For example, in skin, there is an initial erythema and changes due to cell killing typically occur days to weeks later. The chronic forms of local radiation injury include late radiation ulcers and dystrophic and vascular disturbances, which may occur quite some time after tissue (such as skin) has healed from its initial insult.[25,35] In some cases, it is clinically difficult to distinguish the borderline of hyperplastic changes and ulceration or necrosis in skin from the development of cancer. Incorrect terms such as *cancer on scars* or *transformation of a radiation ulcer or hyperkeratosis into cancer* are sometimes used.[36] There is, however, a clear literature that demonstrates both the development of certain types of skin cancer and soft tissue sarcomas following local radiation injuries.[5,6,19,29]

SUMMARY

The subsequent chapters in this book present graphic examples of the phases and progression of radiation injury. The reader should be able to understand these injuries by utilizing the elements of the classification scheme presented here, particularly total dose, type of radiation, dose distribution, and underlying cellular kinetics of both tissue and organ renewal systems.

REFERENCES

1. Guskova, A.K., Diseases caused by the ionizing radiation exposure, in *Occupational Diseases — Manual, Medicina* (Moscow), 2, 186–233, 1996 (in Russian).
2. Doshenko, V.N., Prophylaxis and diagnosis of radiation diseases at the start-up and initial activity period of "Mayak" nuclear industrial facility, *Mag. Med. Radiol. Radiat. Prot.*, Appendices, 71, 1995 (in Russian).
3. Medical consequences of nuclear warfare, in *Textbook of Military Medicine*, Walkner, R.J., Ed., T. Jan Cerveny, TMM Publications, Falls Church, VA, 1997.
4. Guskova, A.K. and Baisogolov, G.D., Radiation sickness of human, *Medicina* (Moscow), 383, 1971 (in Russian).
5. Pobedinsky, M.N., *Radiation Complications of X-ray Therapy*, State Medical Literature Publisher, Moscow, 1954 (in Russian).
6. Mettler, F.A. and Upton, A.C., *Medical Effects of Ionizing Radiation*, W.B. Saunders, Philadelphia, 1995, 125.
7. Radium in Humans: A Review of the U.S. Studies, Argonne National Laboratory, U.S. ANL/ER-3 UC-468, September, 1994.
8. *Effects of A-Bomb Radiation on Human Body*, Bunkodo Conf. Lid, Tokyo, Japan, 1995, 419.
9. Acute radiation effects, *TcniiAtomInform* (Moscow), 79, 1986 (in Russian).
10. Acute early effects in humans induced by high doses of radiation, in *Annex of the UNSCEAR Report to the UN Assembly*, Vienna, 1988, 545–647 (in Russian).
11. Chronic exposure of external gamma radiation in dogs, in *Somatic Effects of Chronic Exposure Abstracts of Symposium*, Moscow, 1972, 190 (in Russian).
12. Rajevsky, B., *Strahlendosis and Strahunwirkung*, George-Thieme-Verlag, Stuttgart, 1956, 206 (in German).
13. Mettler, F.A., Kelsey, C.A., and Ricks, R.C., *Medical Management of Radiation Accidents*, CRC Press, Boca Raton, FL, 1990, 405.
14. Okladnikova, N.D., Pesternikova, V.S., and Sumina, M.N., Consequences of occupational exposure, *Sci. Inf. Methodol. Bull. U.S.S.R. Nucl. Soc.*, 4, 15–16, 1992 (in Russian).

15. Okladnikova, N.D., Early and late effects of occupational exposure, in *Influence of Radiation in Living Nature and Human* (Experience of Cheliabinsk Researchers), Cheliabinsk Emergency Committee–Regional Branch of Russian Nuclear Society, Cheliabinsk–Ozersk, 1995, 56–59 (in Russian).
16. Murhead, K.R., Kendan, G.M., and Little, M.P., Chronic exposure of low doses and mortality recorded by National Registry of Radiation Workers of Great Britain, *Radiat. Risk*, 8, 59, 1996 (in Russian).
17. Koshurnikova, N.A., Okatenko, P.V., and Romanov, S.A., Late effects of occupational exposure, in *Influence of Radiation in Living Nature and Human* (Experience of Cheliabinsk Researchers), Cheliabinsk Emergency Committee–Regional Branch of Russian Nuclear Society, Cheliabinsk–Ozersk, 1995, 66–68 (in Russian).
18. Guskova, A., Acute radiation syndrome in human, in *Internal Conf. on Radiation Effects and Protection*, Japan Atomic Energy Institute, Mito, Japan, 1995, 92–98.
19. Elderle, G.J. and Friedrich, K., East German uranium mines (Wismut); exposure conditions and health consequences, *Stem Cells*, 13, Suppl. 1.
20. Baisogolov, G.D., Guskova, A.K., Lemberg, V.K. et al., *Clinical Anatomy and Pathology of Extremely Severe Forms of Acute Radiation Sickness of Human*, Printhouse No. 5, Moscow, 1955, 155 (in Russian).
21. Akleev, A.V., Goloshapov, P.V., Kosenko, M.M., and Degteva, M.O., Environmental radioactive contamination of south Urals region and its health effects in the population, *Tcniiatominform* (Moscow), 65, 1991 (in Russian).
22. Nikipelov, B.V., Lyzlov, A.F., and Koshurnikova, N.A., Radiation levels and late effects, *Sci. Inf. Bull. Int. Nucl. Soc.*, 27–28, 1992 (in Russian).
23. Barabanova, A.V., Sokolina, L.L., and Novikova, L.V., Clinical dosimetrical relationships in case of local radiation exposure of sources of different energies, *Med. Radiol.*, 10, 46–54, 1974 (in Russian).
24. Guskova, A.K. and Baisogolov, G.D., Peculiarities of diagnosis and therapy of human radiation sickness for different spatial-temporal distribution of dose, in *State Research Center–Institute of Biophysics, Basic Results of 50 Years Activities*, Moscow, 1996, 26-31 (in Russian).
25. Kurshakov, N.A., Radiation sickness, in Manual of Internal Disease, *Meditsina* (Moscow), 10, 213–363, 1962, (in Russian).
26. Methods for Estimating the Probability of Cancer from Occupational Radiation Exposure, IAEA, Tech. Doc. 870, IAEA, Vienna, 1996, 56.
27. Biological Effects of non-uniform radiation exposures, *Atomizdat* (Moscow), 134, 1962 (in Russian).
28. Kurshakov, N.A., *A Case of Acute Radiation Sickness in Human*, State Medical Literature Publisher, Moscow, 1962, 151 (in Russian).
29. Hempelman, L.H., Lisco, M., and Hoffman, J.G., The acute radiation syndrome, *Ann. Intern. Med.*, 36 (279), 102–110, 1952.
30. 1990 Recommendation of International Commission on Radiological Protection, Limits of Annual Intake of Radionuclides Based upon the 1990 Recommendations, *ICRP Recommendations Publ.*, 60(1), 191, 1991.
31. Tokarskaya, Z.B., The input of radiation and non-radiation factors in the lung cancer morbidity of the "Mayak" Nuclear Facility Personnel, in *Influence of Radiation in Living Nature and Human* (Experience of Cheliabinsk Researchers), Cheliabinsk Emergency Committee–Regional Branch of Russian Nuclear Society, Cheliabinsk–Ozersk, 1995, 26–34 (in Russian).
32. Buldakov, L.A., Radioactive substances and humans, *Energoatomizdat* (Moscow), 160, 1990 (in Russian).
33. Baisogolov, G.D., On the pathogenesis of the blood system in case of acute radiation sickness, *Med. Radiol.*, 5, 19–24, 1969 (in Russian).
34. Manual of medical assistance to people exposed to ionizing radiation, *Energoatomizdat* (Moscow), 181, 1986 (in Russian).
35. Barditchev, M.S., *Local Radiation Injuries*, *Meditsina* (Moscow), 240, 1985 (in Russian).
36. Muxinova, K.N. and Mushkatchova, G.S., Cellular and molecular basics of the hemopoiesis changes in case of long-term radiation exposure, *Energoizda* (Moscow), 151, 1990 (in Russian).

4 Acute Radiation Sickness: Underlying Principles and Assessment

Angelina K. Guskova, Alexander E. Baranov, and Igor A. Gusev

CONTENTS

Introduction 33
Criteria for Diagnosis and Prognosis 34
Effect of Local Radiation Injury on Acute Radiation Sickness................................41
Acute Radiation Effects from Internal Contamination 42
Early Identification and Management of ARS Patients 48
References 49

INTRODUCTION

Acute radiation sickness (ARS) is a group of clinical syndromes developing acutely (within several seconds to 3 days) postexposure to penetrating ionizing radiation above average whole-body doses of 1 Gy. Some authors use the term *acute radiation syndrome* or *disease* rather than sickness, but the terms are synonymous. Depending upon the total dose, ARS is manifested as a result of damage to particular systems. Doses in the range of 1 to 10 Gy predominantly cause damage to the hematopoietic system. At doses of 10 to 20 Gy, the initial and lethal manifestations are due to damage to the intestine. At 20 to 80 Gy, there are general disturbances of the cardiovascular system as well as toxemia; above 100 Gy, death appears to be the result of cerebral disorders. If the average whole-body dose or if the dose to a large portion of the body is >10 to 20 Gy, ARS is usually combined with signs of local radiation injuries (LRI) with major tissue damage to the skin, eyes, lungs, intestine, extremities, etc.

The first descriptions of human ARS were made by a number of authors in the 1940s and 1950s.[1-6] The principal description of the underlying pathological mechanisms that result in death from ARS belongs to Rajevsky.[7] The basis of ARS pathogenesis is a disturbance of the physiological recovery of various cellular groups damaged by radiation.[8-14] There is predominant damage of predecessor cell fractions of radiosensitive tissues including hematopoietic cells, skin, epithelium, intestine, and vascular endothelium. These disturbances are accompanied by disorders of regulation and adaptation (nervous, endocrine, and cardiovascular systems). Depending on the dose levels, major manifestations of acute radiation sickness include signs of hematopoietic depression with concurrent infection and hemorrhage. The intestinal, toxemia, and cerebral syndromes occur after large doses with signs of diarrhea, water loss, toxemia, arterial blood pressure drop, and changes of function and structure of the brain. Occasionally, with very high acute doses to the head or trunk, there may be loss of consciousness, which is sometimes referred to as transient incapacitation syndrome.

There are several phases in the development of ARS. These include initial reaction, latent period, disease manifestation, and late outcomes. The severity and time sequence of each of these phases are dependent upon the dose and dose rate. In general, findings of ARS in humans and different mammal species are broadly similar. There are, however, some differences due to spatial distribution of radiation depending on body size, as well as differences in maturation times of different tissues and the interaction of different organ systems. Because the human body is relatively large, in many accidental situations in which patients develop ARS, there is relatively nonuniform distribution of the spatial distribution of dose in the body, and as a result most patients combine variants of ARS.[15–19]

There are a number of national registries that accumulate data on patients with ARS. These exist in Brazil, China, France, Russia, and the United States. In addition, there are international registries maintained by the International Atomic Energy Agency. To date, these registries indicate that there have been about 300 patients with ARS as a result of radiation accidents. Obviously, this number excludes persons who died at Hiroshima and Nagasaki. Historically, approximately 20% of all patients with ARS have fatal outcomes.

There is a large body of information that can be useful in treating patients with ARS. This experience is the result of total-body gamma radiation therapy in preparation for bone marrow transplant in patients with leukemia. Doses typically used are in the range of 10 to 12 Gy. The limitation of such data is the concurrent disease and additional therapy that the patient is undergoing.

Historically, the cases of patients with ARS occurred during development of the early atomic industry. Case observations on single patients or small groups of workers exposed to gamma and neutron irradiation were published. This was the situation until approximately 1970. After this, there were a number of large-scale accidents and even some smaller accidents that have shown important differences in manifestation of ARS, whether the exposure is gamma or a combination of gamma and beta sources (Figure 4.1). Both in the Marshall Islands and at Chernobyl, there was relatively uniform distribution of gamma energy throughout the body, and this would have been expected to produce changes similar to that seen in the A-bomb survivors or patients undergoing radiotherapy. However, the presence of a large amount of beta radiation in these accidents resulted in additional major damage of skin and mucosa. The extensive skin damage often was a major contributing cause of mortality and morbidity. In general, combined injuries such as ARS with other physical trauma (such as open or penetrating wounds) will increase mortality.

The existing clinical experiences have allowed a good description of the basic development, latent period, and manifestation phases related to the bone marrow form of acute radiation syndrome, particularly at doses below 10 Gy. Survival above 10 Gy in accidental situations is very limited, and the pathogenesis and pathological changes that occur remain incompletely understood.

Causes of fatality from the acute radiation syndrome include irreversible damage of hematopoiesis with concurrent infections, hemorrhage, pneumonia, and multiorgan failure. Of those who survive several months postexposure, late effects include dystrophic and sclerotic changes of various tissues including skin, development of cataracts, and subclinical abnormalities in immunity. It also would be expected to have an elevated risk of leukemia 2 to 10 years after exposure and 5 to 10 years or later an increase in the risk of solid cancers. Late changes also include functional insufficiency and difficulties of social and psychological adaptation. Of particular interest is the issue of fertility in such survivors. Most radiation victims exposed to doses below 4 to 6 Gy have revealed rather complete clinical recovery and the ability to parent healthy offspring.

CRITERIA FOR DIAGNOSIS AND PROGNOSIS

There are a number of criteria that have been used for ARS. At this time, the most useful subdivisions of ARS appear to be in three grades of severity with a fourth grade of severity that covers all other forms with an inevitably fatal outcome. With these, it is possible to determine the necessary recommendations, both in terms of diagnosis and for therapy.[20–24] ARS has several forms but all manifest themselves within the first 30 days following exposure and are related to the magnitude of the absorbed dose. The syndromes have hematological, gastrointestinal, cardiovascular, and central nervous system (CNS) forms. Although these are listed in order of increasing absorbed dose, there is considerable clinical overlap of the four forms. The International Atomic Energy Agency (IAEA) has produced useful summary tables on the methods for early diagnosis of radiation injuries as well as the acute, latent, and critical phases of the acute radiation syndrome (Tables 4.1 through 4.4). Even with such classifications, there are essential difficulties in determining the diagnosis and prognosis as well as the outcome, particularly if the situation involves a very uneven distribution of dose or very high doses specifically to the skin, lung, intestine, or hematopoietic tissue.

In accidental situations, dose reconstruction can be difficult.[25] This is because the exposure may involve poorly penetrating and very penetrating gamma and X rays, thermal and intermediate neutrons as well as poorly penetrating beta radiation. Dose reconstruction of each of these will involve different levels of accuracy. At the same time, it is important to note that even when absorbed dose to a particular tissue is known, the relative biological effectiveness of the different radiations is different and even for a similar tissue such as skin (e.g., the relative biological effectiveness of the dose to cause erythema vs. other effects, such as desquamation or necrosis) is different. In any case, a number of prognostic decisions are required for both proper diagnosis and therapy planning, and they must be taken at a relatively early time in the patient course.

Comparatively exact assessment of the severity, grade, and prognosis of damage can be reached for patients who are exposed to relatively uniform radiation (the difference of doses accumulated in body parts is less than threefold). The most confident outcome assessment under these circumstances can be drawn for hematopoietic damage. All other situations of clinical syndromes with predominant damage (or shielding) of separate body segments (head, trunk, extremities, pelvis) or organs (lungs or intestine) have to be analyzed on a case-by-case basis from the viewpoint of the clinical signs and damage identified in these organs and structures.

With relatively uniform exposure, input to the prognosis is provided not only by clinical manifestations, but also by laboratory findings. Early findings include nausea and vomiting but also may involve gastrointestinal distress, fever, arterial hypotension, cutaneous erythema, and acutely developing parotitis. Nausea and vomiting develop in 33 to 50% of patients at 2 to 3 hours after exposure for doses of 1 to 2 Gy. If the doses reach 2 to 4 Gy, these manifestations occur repeatedly in 75 to 80% of victims at 1 to 2 hours. As the dose and dose rate are elevated, nausea and vomiting will occur rapidly in all patients within minutes after exposure. Elevation of body temperature, headache, and hypotension as well as short-term diarrhea suggest that the doses exceed 6 to 8 Gy.

In cases of nonuniform exposure, the patient may have a sensation of heat and there can be rapid erythema and swelling of highly exposed body parts. These initial reactions are most prominent in the region of head, neck, and abdomen. Clinical laboratory studies confirm the importance of identifying persistent lymphopenia as well as depression of young cellular elements (in erythroid stem cells of bone marrow) in the first 3 days postexposure. Data on chromosome aberrations found in peripheral lymphocytes and bone marrow will also provide dose estimates.

The presence of an initial fever, headache, or disorientation is an ominous sign. Duration of fever may also be prolonged, reflecting the influence of toxic components from severe local radiation injuries. For dose levels able to induce cutaneous damage, the time of onset of the secondary erythema is indicative, and in the case of radiation damage to the upper intestine, the time of onset of diarrhea is specific for the diagnosis (4 to 8 days after exposure).

Evaluation of hematopoietic system damage has been investigated over the last two decades.[26–30] The severity of exposure also can be estimated from the timing and severity of effects on blood elements (lymphocytopenia, granulocytopenia, and thrombocytopenia).[31–33] Historically, a number of graphs were developed although the authors rarely indicated what accidents provided the data used. Regardless, such work did form a useful starting point. One such graph is shown in Figure 4.2.

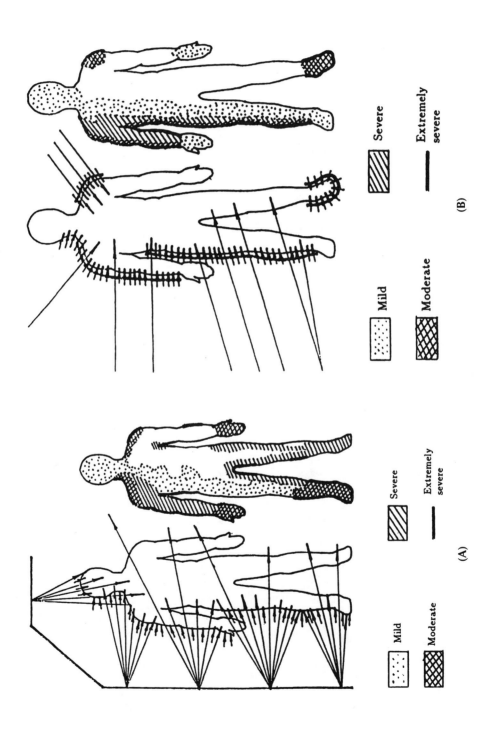

Acute Radiation Sickness: Underlying Principles and Assessment

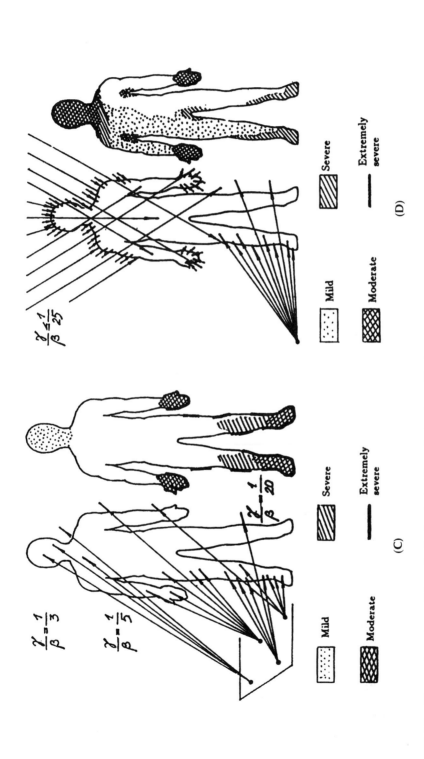

FIGURE 4.1 Four main patterns of dose distribution in the Chernobyl patients. The images on the left show the direction of the exposure and the image on the right shows the effects on the skin. The long arrows are gamma radiation and the short arrows depict beta/gamma contamination on the skin or clothes. (A) Volume source of beta/gamma radiation. (B) Distant gamma sources and thick beta/gamma sources on the skin. (C) Nearby focal sources of radiation on the floor and from nearby objects. (D) Irradiation as in C, but with additional sources on the skin. Note that the gamma/beta ratio changes across the body.

TABLE 4.1
Prodromal Phase of ARS

Symptoms and Medical Response	ARS Degree and the Approximate Dose of Acute WBE (Gy)				
	Mild (1–2 Gy)	Moderate (2–4 Gy)	Severe (4–6 Gy)	Very Severe (6–8 Gy)	Lethal[a] (>8 Gy)
Vomiting					
Onset	2 h after exposure or later	1–2 h after exposure	Earlier than 1 h after exposure	Earlier than 30 min after exposure	Earlier than 10 min after exposure
% of incidence	10–50	70–90	100	100	100
Diarrhea	None	None	Mild	Heavy	Heavy
Onset	—	—	3–8 h	1–3 h	Within minutes or 1 h
% of incidence	—	—	<10	>10	Almost 100
Headache	Slight	Mild	Moderate	Severe	Severe
Onset	—	—	4–24 h	3–4 h	1–2 h
% of incidence	—	—	50	80	80–90
Consciousness	Unaffected	Unaffected	Unaffected	May be altered	Unconsciousness (may last seconds/minutes)
Onset	—	—	—	—	Seconds/minutes
% of incidence	—	—	—	—	100 (at >50 Gy)
Body temperature	Normal	Increased	Fever	High fever	High fever
Onset	—	1–3 h	1–2 h	<1 h	<1 h
% of incidence	—	10–80	80–100	100	100
Medical response	Outpatient observation	Observation in general hospital, treatment in specialized hospital if needed	Treatment in specialized hospital	Treatment in specialized hospital	Palliative treatment (symptomatic only)

[a] With appropriate supportive therapy individuals may survive for 6 to 12 months with whole-body doses as high as 12 Gy.

Source: Adapted from International Atomic Energy Agency, Diagnosis and Treatment of Radiation Injuries, Safety Report Series, No. 2, Vienna, 1998.

Since that time, there has been a large body of data collected from Chernobyl, and this has been particularly valuable in refining previous dose estimation procedures (Figure 4.3). The Chernobyl data have been used to produce better general dose estimation curves than pre-Chernobyl (Figure 4.4) for all three major blood parameters. Subsets of these data also have been used to develop even more detailed graphs (Figure 4.5).

While the peripheral lymphocyte count is the earliest indicator of exposure, the individual error in estimates made from this alone is often in the range of ±1.5 Gy. In an attempt to improve accuracy, Baranov et al.[32] have developed formulas, based on actual patient data, for calculation of the relationships of the magnitude of absorbed dose with uniform exposure to the lymphocyte count at days 4 to 7, minimum counts at days 1 to 8, and a number of other parameters. An example of this work is shown in Figure 4.6.

Similar dose dependence exists for the time period of decreasing granulocyte count, and the measure usually utilized is the day at which the neutrophil count decreases below 500 cells/µl. Since the neutrophil count decreases more slowly than the lymphocyte count, dose estimates of

TABLE 4.2
Change of Lymphocyte Counts (G/L) in the Initial Days of ARS Depending on the Dose of Acute Whole-Body Exposure

Degree of ARS	Dose (Gy)	Lymphocyte Counts (G/L)[a]
Preclinical phase	0.1–1.0	1.5–2.5
Mild	1.0–2.0	0.7–1.5
Moderate	2.0–4.0	0.5–0.8
Severe	4.0–6.0	0.3–0.5
Very Severe	6.0–8.0	0.1–0.3
Lethal	>8.0	0.0–0.05

[a] Expressed as 10^9 cells/L. After 6 days since first exposure.

Source: Adapted from International Atomic Energy Agency, Diagnosis and Treatment of Radiation Injuries, Safety Report Series, No. 2, Vienna, 1998.

TABLE 4.3
Latent Phase of ARS

	Degree of ARS and Approximate Dose of Acute WBE (Gy)				
	Mild (1–2 Gy)	Moderate (2–4 Gy)	Severe (4–6 Gy)	Very Severe (6–8 Gy)	Lethal (>8 Gy)
Lymphocytes (G/L) (days 3–6)	0.8–1.5	0.5–0.8	0.3–0.5	0.1–0.3	0.0–0.1
Granulocytes (G/L)	>2.0	1.5–2.0	1.0–1.5	≤0.5	≤0.1
Diarrhea	None	None	Rare	Appears on days 6–9	Appears on days 4–5
Epilation	None	Moderate, beginning on day 15 or later	Moderate, beginning on day 11–21	Complete earlier than day 11	Complete earlier than day 10
Latency period (days)	21–35	18–28	8–18	7 or less	None
Medical response	Hospitalization not necessary	Hospitalization recommended	Hospitalization necessary	Hospitalization urgently necessary	Symptomatic treatment only

Source: Adapted from International Atomic Energy Agency, Diagnosis and Treatment of Radiation Injuries, Safety Report Series, No. 2, Vienna, 1998.

this sort can only be made after several days to 1 week postexposure. The accuracy of these methods for dose assessment is somewhat better and the individual error is usually ± 1.2 to 1.4 Gy. Dose estimates derived from these sorts of calculations and curves also can be compared with calibration curves for the onset of chromosome aberrations in various portions of the bone marrow at hour 24, and the number of dicentrics in peripheral lymphocyte culture at days 3 to 8.[32] The clinical picture becomes significantly more difficult when a patient is admitted for medical care when bone marrow depression has already occurred, and when previous data on exact circumstances of exposure and early laboratory indices are not available.

TABLE 4.4
Findings of Critical Phase of ARS Following Whole-Body Exposure

	Degree of ARS and Approximate Dose of Acute WBE (Gy)				
	Mild (1–2 Gy)	Moderate (2–4 Gy)	Severe (4–6 Gy)	Very Severe (6–8 Gy)	Lethal (>8 Gy)
Onset of symptoms	>30 d	18–28 d	8–18 d	<7 d	<3 d
Lymphocytes (G/L)	0.8–1.5	0.5–0.8	0.3–0.5	0.1–0.3	0.0–0.1
Platelets (G/L)	60–100 10–25%	30–60 25–40%	25–35 40–80%	15–25 60–80%	<20 80–100%[a]
Clinical manifestations	Fatigue, weakness	Fever, infections, bleeding, weakness, epilation	High fever, infections, bleeding, epilation	High fever, diarrhea, vomiting, dizziness, disorientation, hypotension	High fever, diarrhea, unconsciousness
Lethality (%)	0	0–50, onset 6–8 weeks	20–70, onset 4–8 weeks	50–100, onset 1–2 weeks	100, 1–2 weeks
Medical response	Prophylactic	Special prophylactic treatment from days 14–20; isolation from days 10–20	Special prophylactic treatment from days 7–10; isolation from the beginning	Special treatment from the first day; isolation from the beginning	Symptomatic only

[a] In very severe cases, with a dose >50 Gy, death precedes cytopenia.

Source: Adapted from International Atomic Energy Agency, Diagnosis and Treatment of Radiation Injuries, Safety Report Series, No. 2, Vienna, 1998

It should be pointed out that in cases of nonuniform exposure, evaluation of cytopenia may be somewhat misleading because the cumulative curve of the granulocytes "generalizes" the actual production by different portions of the marrow that had received different doses. Baranov et al.[32] also have examined this issue in detail by examining chromosome aberrations in multiple bone marrow aspirates taken from different body locations and then comparing actual hematological profiles in patients with nonuniform exposure to predicted curves following uniform whole-body exposure (Figure 4.7). Temporal parameters in such cases are more relevant to the magnitude of the dose, and quantitative counts are more correlated to the volume of damaged bone marrow. In addition, in cases of nonuniform exposure, lymphopenia is more prolonged than with uniform exposure.

Most fatalities of patients with the acute radiation syndrome and who have not received medical treatment will occur between days 9 and 60. This is during the period when there are complications of bone marrow (infection and bleeding) or intestinal damage (electrolyte loss and nutrition). If the patient survives the manifest illness portion of the acute radiation syndrome, the majority of patients then show a clear recovery process, which may be complete or incomplete. In most descriptions, the dynamics of the various periods of the radiation sickness is typically limited to about 3 months, although the recovery process may, in fact, take up to 2 years.

The late effects of acute radiation sickness include cataracts, local fibrosis, and atrophy of the skin and other damaged tissues. Ultimately, there would be an increased risk of both leukemia and

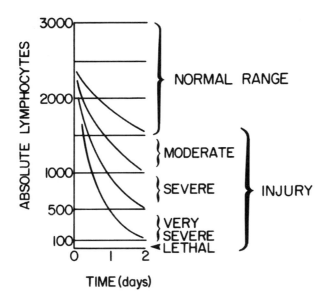

FIGURE 4.2 Historical schematic for patient prognosis based upon initial lymphocyte counts. Lymphocyte count expressed as cells/mm^3.

other malignant neoplasms. Heritable effects on the progeny of radiation-exposed patients appear to be quite low.

Although dose estimates can be obtained from information on the dynamics of neutrophil, thrombocyte, and lymphocyte counts in the peripheral blood as well as aberrations in chromosomes, the most accurate assessment of dose can be obtained using electron spin resonance (ESR). This luminescent signal can be measured from a number of materials including tooth enamel, cloth, and other articles that were exposed at the same time as the patient (see Chapter 40 on biomarkers). The technique consists in the measurement of the ESR spectrum of tooth enamel with consequent calibration done utilizing tooth enamel and a standardized gamma radiation source.[34] Tooth enamel is difficult to use in the evaluation of both the alpha radiation dose and neutron dose of most fission spectra. Usually, the ESR responses in these cases are about 18% and less than 3%, respectively, when comparison is made to the response to gamma radiation. The technique of utilizing ESR tooth enamel can be done with enamel samples without having to extract the whole tooth. Good correlation is found with other dose estimates, particularly in the ranges of 0.2 to 14 Gy. In cases where there was poor coincidence of the ESR dose estimate with other measures, a detailed analysis indicated that there were marked inhomogeneous exposures of the body or secondary exposures of the patient.

EFFECT OF LOCAL RADIATION INJURY ON ACUTE RADIATION SICKNESS

In many accidental situations, there is markedly nonuniform body exposure, causing both ARS and LRI.[35] The reader is referred to Chapter 14 for a more-detailed discussion of local injuries. As a result, some comments relative to the influence of LRI on the course of radiation sickness are important. If more than 25% of the body surface is exposed to gamma radiation doses above 30 Gy, or 10 to 15% of the body surface is exposed to gamma doses in excess of 50 Gy, the patient's status becomes critical. This is particularly true if the dose areas include the chest, head, and abdomen. Sometimes this is called the cutaneous syndrome.

In accidental situations, often the head and neck are highly exposed. This is important because just before the development of agranulocytosis, changes of the mucosa in the mouth and throat

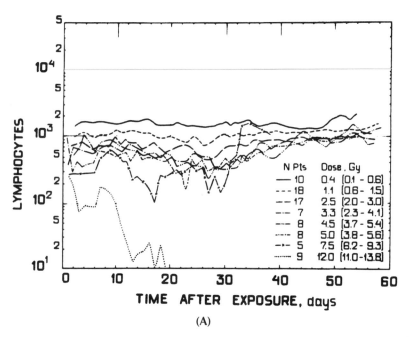

FIGURE 4.3 Composite hematological data from over 82 ARS Chernobyl patients during the first 60 days postexposure. Data include lymphocytes (A), granulocytes (B), and platelets (C).

significantly aggravate the clinical situation. A typical clinical course is that the hyperemia occurring at day 1 with doses of 5 to 10 Gy will gradually disseminate from the mucosa of the cheeks, soft palate, and hypoglossal region to the mucosa of the gum, solid palate, nose, tongue, and larynx. Edema and desquamation of epithelium ensue with painful bleeding erosions and local infection. The recovery process in such cases often is longer than the mucositis seen with more uniform whole-body exposure, and it can continue for several weeks to 2 months.

At doses more than 6 to 10 Gy, the hyperemia and cutaneous edema of the face can be complicated by the occurrence of erosive, necrotic changes, which may occur in the skin of the face, eyelids, and cornea, and even reaction of the iris. If doses are in the range of 15 to 20 Gy, keratitis and conjunctivitis will be present for a long time. Doses in this same range can cause vascular changes in the retina and, often, secondary hemorrhage. When doses are in the range of 50 to 100 Gy, not only is there early damage to the retina, but usually there are also signs of the cerebral syndrome of ARS.

Accidental situations often result in high doses to the anterior chest and abdomen. Acute lethal outcomes have been described for cases when the heart was exposed to doses in excess of 200 Gy, and pericarditis has been observed when the dose to the heart is in the range of 40 to 50 Gy. Doses of 15 to 20 Gy to the intestine can result in early fatality from perforation and hemorrhage, as well as peritonitis, and late changes including stricture and bowel obstruction.

ACUTE RADIATION EFFECTS FROM INTERNAL CONTAMINATION

Although rare, there can be acute deterministic effects from incorporation of radionuclides internally (see Chapters 23 and 27). The particular peculiarities are related to the spatial and temporal accumulation of dose. Usually, there is relatively slow exposure of critical organs that result in slowly developing clinical signs. This is usually seen with long-lived radionuclides, such as strontium, radium, plutonium, and thorium.

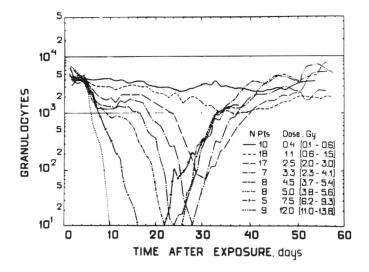

(B)

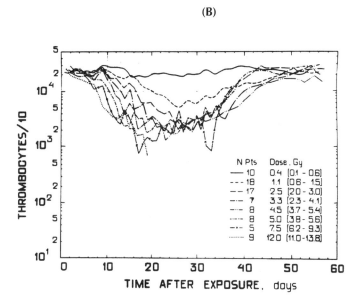

(C)

FIGURE 4.3 (CONTINUED)

Early deterministic effects can occur under the following conditions:

- Relatively uniform or multiorgan deposition of radionuclides in the body (tritium, polonium, cesium).
- Rapid accumulation of radiation doses (some isotopes of iodine).
- Very high dose accumulated during the initial moments of the radionuclide intake or radioactive contamination of the skin and mucosa.
- Presence of radionuclides emitting significant gamma radiation (phosphorus, strontium, yttrium, radium, uranium fission products).

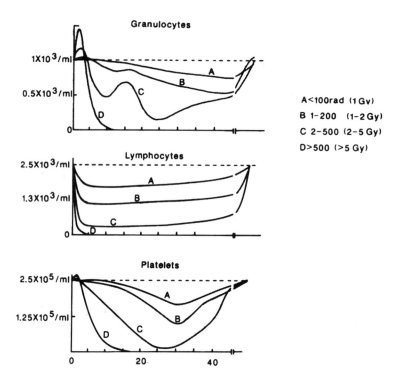

FIGURE 4.4 General schematic data derived from pre-Chernobyl data for dose evaluation at four dose ranges.

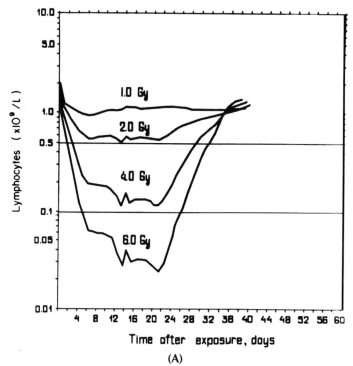

FIGURE 4.5 Specific Chernobyl schematic data at different dose levels and times postexposure for lymphocytes (A), granulocytes (B), and platelets (C).

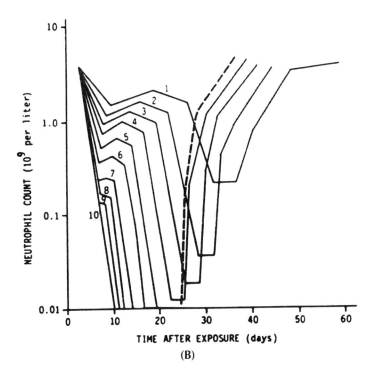

(B)

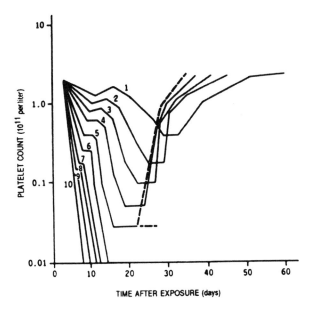

(C)

FIGURE 4.5 (CONTINUED)

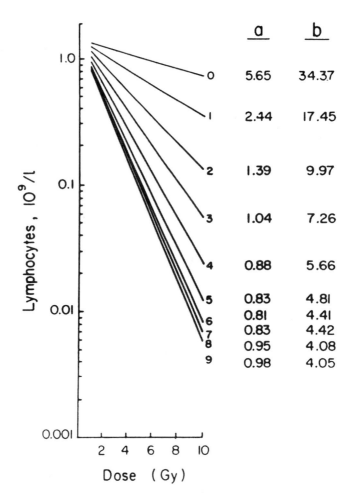

FIGURE 4.6 Mathematical relationship between whole-body gamma dose and peripheral lymphocyte count. Numbers at the end of the lines refer to days postexposure. The formula for the relationship is $D = a - b$ (log y), where D is dose, Gy; a and b are coefficients; and y is lymphocytes expressed $\times 10^9/l$.

The sources of internal exposure that cause acute deterministic effects include explosions of nuclear installations or bombs, damage of a reactor core (when victims are exposed indoors near the core), and with rule violations and mistakes in administration of radionuclides for either medical or research purposes. When doses from such radionuclides occur and result in 1 to 2 Gy to the whole body or bone marrow within a period of 1 to 3 days, certain signs of bone marrow depression and ARS are possible. Such cases have been reported with internal contamination with tritium and cumulative body doses of 10 to 12 Gy, with phosphorus resulting in cumulative body doses of 3 to 6 Gy, with radioactive gold resulting in doses of greater than 4 Gy, and with americium-241 resulting in cumulative body doses of 5.5 Gy.

The exact expression of the bone marrow damage depends upon the radionuclide metabolism as well as the dose rate and distribution. Peculiarities may include lack of initial reactions seen with ARS such as nausea and vomiting and relatively increased involvement when the radionuclides localize in specific organs (such as damage of erythroid hemopoiesis in the case of phosphorus intake and damage of lymphopoiesis in cases of intakes of americium and gold or even damage to the reticular endothelial system following intakes of polonium and colloidal gold). If the dose rate decreases significantly with time, there can be clear signs of recovery even when some radionuclide is still present in the body (tritium, phosphorus). As the dose rate is protracted, the occurrence of

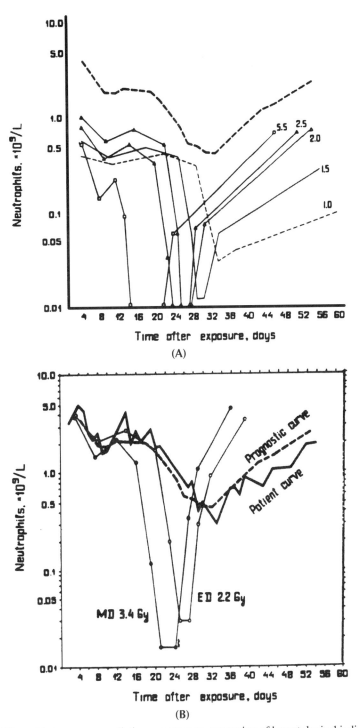

FIGURE 4.7 Effect of heterogenous radiation exposure on expression of hematological indices as an example of prediction of blood neutrophil kinetics using partial curves method. (A) Partial curves of neutrophil count at different dose distributions to the bone marrow in the following dose ranges: 1.0 to 0.1 Gy, 1.5 to 0.15 Gy, 2.0 to 0.25 Gy, 2.5 to 0.20 Gy, and 5.5 to 0.15 Gy. The dashed line represents the summed predictive shape of the curve. (B) Actual patient data on a patient with nonuniform exposure compared with a summed predictive curve (dashed line) and two other prognostic curves for calculated mean physical dose (MD) of 3.4 Gy and equivalent stem cell dose (ED) of 2.2 Gy.

recovery is not as obvious and occurs more slowly. Accumulation of radionuclides in specific organs also has implications for long-term damage to that organ. This may be bone damage in the case of radium intake or damage to the lungs and liver in the case of radium-mesothorium intake. Obviously, iodine radioisotopes can cause a wide range of effects in the thyroid including acute hypoplasia, obvious or biochemical hypothyroidism, occurrence of adenomas, and thyroid cancer. Interpretation of any of these rare cases is complicated, and sophisticated dosimetry and an understanding of the radiobiology are essential.

EARLY IDENTIFICATION AND MANAGEMENT OF ARS PATIENTS

Initial sorting and prevention of additional exposure must be done at the accident site using as many simple techniques as possible. Limitation of access to the radiation area will prevent spread of potential radioactive contamination to other areas. Countermeasures for protection of skin and lungs should be evaluated. If possible, changing the clothing (with individual labeling and consequent storage) should be done. Showering or washing of separate body parts with water is recommended. Urgent medical care for conditions such as loss of consciousness, wounds, fractures, etc. should be provided.

Persons at or near the accident scene who develop nausea, vomiting, or other signs that would lead to a suspicion of radiation doses and who are able to induce ARS of moderate or higher grade should be transported to well-equipped medical facilities. An example of a preliminary accident investigation form (Table 4.5) and information (Table 4.6) that should be obtained is shown below.

TABLE 4.5
Example of a Preliminary Accident Investigation Form

1. Name of patient:
2. Address:
3. Age:
4. Occupation:
5. Affiliation and period of work:
6. Employer:
7. Date and time of incident (dd-mm-yyyy); hh:mm):
8. Date of investigation (dd-mm-yyyy; hh:mm):
9. Circumstances of incident:
    - Characteristics of the technological process and operations done by patient; source term; type of radiation; radiation energy; intensity of radiation (yield); radionuclide half-life; activity and gamma-constant (for radionuclide sources); electrical tension; current; filtering (for X-ray machines and accelerators):
    - Time of the contact with radiation and relative poisoning of the body and radiation source (graphic scheme with scale should be attached together with plans of premises):
    - Radiation situation description at routine and accidental conditions:
    - Positioning of radiation source, plans, and sizes of premises and source compartments:
    - Accountancy and storage of radioactive sources:
    - Presence and reading of individual dosimeter:
    - Systems of source blocking, their maintenance and usage:
    - Date of safety training:
    - Readings of dosimetrical monitoring systems:
    - Measured radioactive contamination of clothes and skin:
10. Preliminary conclusion (external and/or internal exposure), pathway(s) of radionuclide intake (inhalation, ingestion, damaged skin), radionuclide application on skin and mucosa:
11. Approximate maximum doses of local and whole-body exposure:
12. Conclusions on correspondence of elaborated jobs to safety rules and major violation(s):
13. Signatures of specialists and investigators (health physicists, employer, local authorities):

TABLE 4.6
Example of a First Medical Examination Form

Name of patient:
Date of examination: (dd-mm-yyyy; hh:mm):
Characteristics of radiation exposure (whole-body exposures, external, local, combined radiation exposure, radiation exposure combined with nonradiation exposure (thermal burns, trauma):
Date and time of exposure (dd-mm-yyyy; hh:mm):
Individual dose(s) of the exposure (calculation, individual dosimeter):
Early and most significant symptoms of initial reaction:
- Nausea:
- Vomiting:
- Diarrhea:
- Weakness:
- Body temperature elevation:
- Headache:
- Meningeal symptoms:

Initial reaction of skin and mucosa:
- Localization (put on the graphic scheme):
- Time(s) of occurrence:
- Expressiveness:
- Salivary glands:
- Data on palpation of abdominal cavity organs:
- Stool character:
- Heart beat rate:

Mucosa membrane condition:
- Mouth cavity:
- Eyes:

Clinical blood count (dd-mm-yyyy; hh:mm):
Leukocyte counts:
Lymphocyte counts:
Sampling for radiological measurements:
Washing solutions (volume, time of sampling):
Urine (volume, time of sampling):
Feces (mass; time of sampling; way of sampling, independently/stimulated):
Radioactive contamination of skin (yes/no; graphic scheme):
Preliminary diagnosis:
Urgent recommendations and emergency measures:
Signature of physician:

Emergency room management of patients involved in radiation accidents is discussed in more detail in Chapter 31. An example of the information that should be obtained is also provided in a subsequent evaluation form. Various therapies of acute radiation syndrome are discussed in Chapter 5.

REFERENCES

1. De-Cowrsey, E., Human pathological anatomy of ionizing radiation effects of the atomic bomb explosions, *Mil. Surg.*, 102:427, 1948.
2. Leibow, A.A., Warren, S., and De-Cowrsey, E., Pathology of atomic bomb casualties, *Ann. J. Pathol.*, 25(5):853, 1949.

3. Cronkite, E.P., The diagnosis of ionizing radiation injury by physical examination and clinical laboratory procedures, *JAMA*, Vol. 141, 1949.
4. Hempelman, L.H., Lisko, H., and Hoffman, Z.G., The acute radiation syndrome: a study of nine cases and the review of the problem, *Ann. Intern. Med.*, 36(2,1): 290, 1952.
5. Behrens, C.F., Ed., *Atom. Med.* (Moscow), 1951 (in Russian).
6. Guskova, A.K. and Baisogolov, G.D., Two cases of acute radiation syndrome of human, in Action of Radiation in the Organism; Reports of the Soviet Delegation to the 1st International Conference on Peaceful Application of Atomic Energy, Geneva, 1953, U.S.S.R. Academy of Sciences, Moscow, 1953, 23 (in Russian).
7. Rajevsky, B., *Strahlendosis und Strahlenwirkung*, George-Thieme-Verlag, Stuttgart; 1956 (in German).
8. Oughterson, J.M. and Warren, S., *Medical Effects of the Atomic Bomb in Japan*, McGraw-Hill, New York, 1956.
9. Acute Radiation Effects in Man, GosAtomKomitet of the U.S.S.R., 78, 86 (in Russian).
10. Guskova, A.K. and Baisogolov, G.D., Radiation sickness of humans, *MedGIZ* 384, 1973 (in Russian).
11. *Energoatomizdat* (Moscow), 88, 1989 (in Russian).
12. Kurshakov, N.A., Ed., Case of Acute Radiation Sickness in Human, Medical Literature Publisher, Moscow, 1962, 151 (in Russian).
13. Guskova, A.K., Acute radiation syndrome in human: experience of soviet scientists, Japan Mito, International Conference on Radiation Effects and Protection, 1995, 92.
14. Cronkite, E.P., Bond, V.P, and Conard, R.A., Medical effects of exposure of human beings to fallout radiation from a thermonuclear exposure, *Stem Cells*, 3(1), 49, 1995.
15. Radiation Accident in San Salvador, IAEA, Vienna, 1992, 108 (in Russian).
16. Jammet, H., Mathe, G., Pehdic, B. et al., Etude de six cas d'irradiation totale aigue accidentalle, *Rev. Tr. Clin. Biol.*, 4(3), 210–225, 1959 (in French).
17. Soloviev, V.J., Ilyin, L.A., Baranov, A.E. et al., Radiation incidents involving human exposure in the Former USSR before and after Chernobyl, in One Decade after Chernobyl: Summing Up the Consequences of the Accident, IAEA, Vienna, 8–12 April, 1996, 601.
18. The Radiological Accident at the Irradiation Facility in Nesvizh, IAEA, Vienna, 1996, 75.
19. The Radiological Accident in Soreq, IAEA, Vienna, 1993, 78.
20. Planning the Medical Response to Radiological Accidents, Safety Series Rep. 4(32), IAEA, Vienna, 1998.
21. Diagnosis and treatment of radiation injury, in *Abstr. Int. Conf. De Doelen*, Rotterdam, 1998, 30.08–30.09.
22. Diagnosis and Treatment of Radiation Injuries, Safety Series 2(50), IAEA, Vienna, 1998.
23. Proceedings of the 2nd Consensus Development Conference on the Treatment of Radiation Injuries held in Bethesda, MD, April 14–17, 1993. MacVittie, T., Weiss, J.F., Brown, D., Eds., *Adv. Biosci.*, 94, 281, 1994. Pergamon Elsevier Science, London, 1996.
24. Mettler, F.A., Kelsey, C.A., and Ricks, R.C., *Medical Management of Radiation Accidents*, CRC Press, Boca Raton, FL, 1990, 408.
25. Guskova, A.K., Keirim-Markus, I.B., Kleshenko, E.D., Nadejina, N.M., Nugis, V.J., and Baranov, A.E., Comparative assessment of some methods of dose reconstruction and the importance of these data for interpretation of clinical effects, *Health Phys.*, 2000. In press.
26. Baranov, A.E., Selidovkin, G.D., Butturini, G.D., and Gale, R.P., Hematopoietic recovery after 10 Gy acute total body irradiation, *Blood*, 83, 596, 1994.
27. Guskova, A.K., Baranov, A.E., Barabanova, A.V. et al., Acute effects of radiation in victims of Chernobyl NPP accident, *Med. Radiol.*, 12(3), 1987 (in Russian).
28. Baranov, A.E., Guskova, A.K., Nadejina, N.M., and Nugis, V.J., Chernobyl experience: biological indicators of exposure of ionizing radiation, *Stem Cells*, Murphy M.J., Ed., 13(1), 1995.
29. Friesecke, I., Beyer, K., Densow, D., Fliedner, T.M. et al., Acute radiation exposure and early hematopoietic response pattern: an evaluation of the Chernobyl accident victims, *Int. J. Radiat. Med.*, 1, 55, 1999.
30. Guskova, A.K., Nadejina, N.M., Moiseev, A.A. et al., Medical assistance given to personnel of the Chernobyl NPP after 1986 accident, *Sov. Med. Rev. Sect.*, (Moscow), 7(1), 29, 1996 (in Russian).

31. Goans, R.E., Holloway, E.C., Berger, M.E. et al., Early dose assessment following severe radiation accidents, *Health Phys.*, 72(4), 513–518, 1997.
32. Baranov, A.E., Konchalovski, M.V., Yu Soloviev, W., and Guskova, A.K., Use of blood cell count changes after radiation exposure in dose assessment and evaluation of bone marrow function, in *The Medical Basis for Radiation Accident Preparedness,* Ricks, R.C. and Fry, S.A., Eds., Elsevier Science, New York, 1990.
33. Friesecke, I., Beyrer, K., Densow, D. et al., Acute radiation exposure and early hematolopoietic response patterns: an evaluation of the Chernobyl accident victims, *Int. J. Radiat. Med.*, 1(1), 55–62, 1999.
34. Kleshenko, E.D. and Kushnareva, K.K., The uncertainty of the absorbed dose evaluation using the ESR signal analysis from tooth enamel, *Med. Radiol. Radiat. Prot.*, 4(2), 51, 1997 (in Russian).
35. Andrews, G.A., Radiation accidents and their management, *Radiat. Res.*, Suppl. 7, 390–397, 1967.

5 Treatment of Acute Radiation Sickness

Fred A. Mettler, Jr. and Angelina K. Guskova

CONTENTS

Introduction 53
The Lethal Dose 54
Prognostic Categories 55
Early Treatment 57
    Initial Management 57
    Treatment of Early Neurological or Severe Hypotensive Effects 57
Treatment of Gastrointestinal Complications 58
    Nausea, Vomiting, and Diarrhea 58
        Fluid and Electrolyte Imbalance 59
        Enhancing Regeneration 60
    Prevention and Treatment of Infections 60
Treatment of Bone Marrow Depression 61
    Transfusions 61
    Bone Marrow Transplantation 61
    Use of Cytokines 62
Research 64
References 65

INTRODUCTION

There are many circumstances in which humans have been exposed to total-body radiation. These, of course, include the survivors of Hiroshima and Nagasaki, as well as of a multitude of accidental exposures.[1] Worldwide, from 1946 to 2000, there have been over 120 documented fatalities due to radiation accidents. Most acute exposures to the whole body come from external irradiation, although at least one fatality was due to internal contamination following a misadministration of gold-198 (see Chapter 27) and several others as a result of internal and external exposure from cesium in the Goiânia (Brazil) accident (see Chapter 26). The acute radiation syndrome has been described in Chapter 4. This chapter deals with the medical management of acute radiation sickness caused by accidental exposure.

    Although the terms *total-body radiation* and *whole-body radiation* carry the connotation of a homogeneous, uniform dose, this is rarely the circumstance. In almost all situations, the dose is delivered in a fashion that irradiates one part of the body substantially more than another part (Figure 5.1). Perhaps the closest approach to uniform exposure results from those circumstances in which total-body irradiation is utilized for therapeutic purposes prior to bone marrow transplantation. In these cases, the patient is irradiated from front and back.

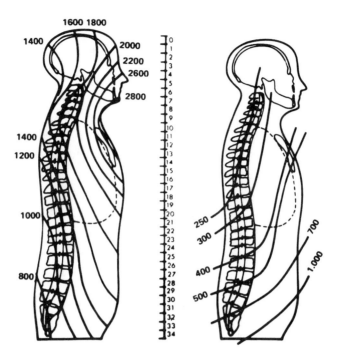

FIGURE 5.1 Isodose curves (in rad) from two different accidents involving whole-body exposure. The patient on the left has most of the maximal dose to the face and chest, while the patient on the right has the highest dose to the pelvis and lower abdomen. Obviously, the clinical presentation, nature of the injuries, and their evolution will be quite different.

The acute radiation syndrome may occur even when the dose is not homogeneous, because some tissues of the body are much more radiosensitive than others or have received the largest dose. This syndrome has several forms but all manifest themselves within the first 30 days following exposure and are related to the magnitude of the absorbed dose. The syndromes have hematological, gastrointestinal, cardiovascular, and central nervous system (CNS) forms. Although these are listed in order of increasing absorbed dose, there is considerable clinical overlap of the four forms.

THE LETHAL DOSE

In medical management it is important to know what dose is survivable. The total-body absorbed dose required to cause death is generally characterized by a median lethal dose (LD_{50}). This abbreviation refers to a dose that is lethal to 50% of the persons irradiated, and it assumes no medical intervention. It is usually necessary to establish a temporal relationship with regard to the mortality, which is usually referred to as the $LD_{50/30}$ or the $LD_{50/60}$. These are highly penetrating doses that, if given, might be expected to result in death in one half of the individuals within 30 and 60 days, respectively, without medical care. The $LD_{50/60}$ in humans is estimated to be 3.5 to 4 Gy (350 to 400 rad) air or surface dose, but this value is usually modified by medical treatment.

A number of estimations of the lethal dose from whole-body radiation (without much medical care) have been reported, and most of these have been derived from analyses of the atomic bomb survivor data. Contributing to uncertainties in atomic bomb data is not only the dosimetry but also other nonradiation factors, such as trauma, nutritional status, and a devastating typhoon on September 17, 1945.[2] The reported doses usually refer to bone marrow dose and $LD_{50/60}$. Estimates by Rotblat[3] using older dosimetry suggested that the $LD_{50/60}$ distance was 892 m from hypocenter and a dose of 1.5 Gy, but more recent computations (using DS 86) of dose at the same distance by Fujita et al.[4,5] estimate a dose of 2.44 Gy. Work done by Young and the U.S. Defense Nuclear Agency[6] reviewing this and other data conclude that if the deaths of the persons who were seriously injured on the first day are excluded, the dose is 3.2 Gy, and, if they are not excluded, the dose would be 2.64 Gy. In a study of 7593 persons (1095 of whom died in the first 60 days), Kamada et al.[7] have made estimates based on a small sample of girls, and with DS 86 dosimetry found a relatively high dose of about 4 Gy. The authors suggest that a young female may be more resistant to whole-body exposure. Fujita et al.[4] using DS 86 dosimetry for each individual have estimated the $LD_{50/60}$ to be in the range of 2.7 to 3.1 Gy when first-day deaths are excluded. Dose estimates of median lethal bone marrow were 2.9 Gy using a logarithmic dose scale and 3.4 Gy using a linear dose scale. Thus, most of the data from Japan yield $LD_{50/60}$ bone marrow dose estimates of about 3 Gy. The Japanese data are a little difficult to use because of the uncertainties in dosimetry. Unfortunately, some authors report the absorbed dose as the skin dose, some do not specify the site, and still others use the midline tissue dose (MTD). In general, for penetrating gamma rays to derive MTD, if one knows the value in air, tissue attenuation in the average person may be corrected for by using a factor of 0.66.[7] Thus, a dose in air of 10 Gy is equivalent to an MTD of about 6.6 Gy for the average adult.

Obviously, the lethal dose of radiation depends upon the dose rate, uniformity, and penetration of the radiation, as well as the pre-exposure status of the irradiated individual. A review of the literature concerning the LD50 has been presented in the 1988 UNSCEAR Report.[8] From the data derived from the Chernobyl accident, it appears that for healthy males who receive medical treatment the $LD_{50/60}$ is at least 5 Gy. Of 21 Chernobyl patients with average whole-body doses in the range of 4.2 to 6.4 Gy, 32% (7) died. Of another 21 Chernobyl patients who were in the 6.5 to 16 Gy range only 5% (1) survived.[9] Half of the Chernobyl patients had severe skin burns and those accounted for 2/3 of the deaths. For ill patients with cancer who are treated with conservative support medications and blood cell infusions, the $LD_{50/60}$ appears to be about 3.0 to 3.5 Gy marrow dose. But a dose of 2 Gy could kill 30 to 40% of very ill patients. With pretreatment, an appropriate bone marrow match, and successful transplantation, a large number of children have survived whole-body acute doses in the range of 9 to 14 Gy.

In accidental exposures where there is good medical care, the $LD_{50/60}$ is probably between 4.5 and 6 Gy. The maximum survivable "whole-body" dose in accidents with good medical care is about 10 Gy. The reason for lack of survival above this dose level is the result of several factors. The maximum acute tolerable dose for the lungs is about 10 Gy and, even with excellent medical care, the respiratory system is a limiting factor in survival after about 9 months postexposure. The other problem is the inhomogeneous dose distribution with the gastrointestinal tract receiving relatively higher doses than the average whole-body dose. Finally, survival is compromised by massive skin, subcutaneous, pulmonary damage, and multiorgan failure.

PROGNOSTIC CATEGORIES

As described in Chapter 4, a number of clinical and laboratory indices can help with patient prognosis.[10,11] Several prognostic categories have been used in evaluating radiation overexposure and to help with medical planning. As with most categorizations, the groupings are somewhat arbitrary, but they are useful from a clinical viewpoint.

For medical management, Fliedner at the University of Ulm and his colleagues have proposed "response categories" based upon early clinical and laboratory findings of a large number of patients involved in accidents.[12]

The categories overlap to a large extent with the grades of acute radiation sickness outlined in Chapter 4, but the response category approach combines specific clinical, laboratory, and therapeutic information. They are as follows:

Response Category 1

Estimated acute whole-body dose 0.4 to 1.4 Sv
Survival almost certain without medical treatment
Clinical signs: Usually none or minimal
Laboratory findings: Granulocytes remain above $2 \times 10^9/l$
Thrombocytes remain above $100 \times 10^9/l$
Lymphocytes between 0.5 and $2 \times 10^9/l$

Response Category 2

Estimated acute whole-body dose 1.3 to 5.5 Sv
Survival usually >60 days with medical treatment
Clinical signs: Few episodes of nausea, vomiting, or diarrhea as well as fatigue
Laboratory findings: Abortive rise in granulocytes day 10 to 20 and nadir at day 25 to 35; spontaneous slow recovery
Treatment includes:
    Antibiotics
    Thrombocyte transfusions if needed
    Follow-up to assure infection-free complete recovery
    Growth factors are not needed

Response Category 3

Estimated acute whole-body dose 4.4 to 8.0 Sv
Survival to be anticipated with therapeutic measures to bridge bone marrow and gastrointestinal problems at 6 days
Clinical signs include nausea, vomiting, fatigue, erythema, temporal disorientation, and epilation beginning at 14 days
Laboratory findings: Initial granulocytosis within 3 days followed by a decline with a nadir during days 16 to 25; thrombocyte count has a shoulder for about 5 days followed by a decline and a nadir during days 15 to 25 with subsequent recovery; lymphopenia of about $0.5 \times 10^9/l$
Treatment includes:
    Reverse isolation
    Replacement therapy (such as thrombocyte transfusions)
    Growth factors to enhance remaining stem cell recovery
    Fluid replacement
    Gut bacterial decontamination

Response Category 4

Estimated acute whole-body dose 9 to 11 Sv
Survival time 10 to 15 days. 100% mortality without stem cell transplant and other advanced medical treatment
Clinical signs include nausea, vomiting, diarrhea, early erythema and edema, and CNS pertubations
Laboratory findings: Initial early granulocytosis and progressive decline within 6 days; thrombocyte count has a shoulder for 4 to 5 days, with a progressive decline and a nadir within 10 to 15 days; lymphocytes decline to minimal levels within 3 days

Treatment includes:
- Reverse isolation and gnotobiotic treatment
- Maintaining fluid and electrolyte balance
- Stem cell transplantation
- Systemic antibiotics and platelet transfusions
- Use of cytokines to enhance regeneration
- Prevention of fungal or viral infections

Response Category 5

Estimated acute whole-body dose above 11 Sv
Survival very unlikely (usually less than 7–12 days)
Clinical signs include disorientation, shocklike syndrome, edema, nausea, vomiting, and disturbances in coordination
Laboratory findings: Initial early granulocytosis but nadir within 5 days
Linear decrease in thrombocytes within 6 to 8 days
Severe lymphopenia within hours
Treatment is palliative only

EARLY TREATMENT

INITIAL MANAGEMENT

Medical management of patients with an acute case of high-dose whole-body radiation exposure begins with triage and necessary immediate lifesaving care. There should be recording and timing of the initial clinical symptoms, evaluation and treatment of hypotension, evaluation of fever and presence as well as location of erythema. Laboratory evaluation for patients suspected of having doses over 0.5 to 1.0 Gy should include a complete blood count, collection of blood for cytogenetic analysis, serum amylase determination, and urine analysis. If neutron exposure is a possibility measurement should be made over the trunk with a Geiger counter, blood should be obtained for sodium-24 analysis, and hair and clothing samples should also be obtained (see Chapter 39). If there is radionuclide contamination present on the skin, it should be removed and the possibility of internal contamination considered. Emergency room management is discussed further in Chapter 31.

During the first day, treatment of whole body irradiation is directed at symptoms and an attempt is made to estimate the dose and dose distribution. A major purpose is to make a prognosis of the supportive treatment that will be required and the likely patient outcome. The "dose" data obtained from most laboratory evaluations (e.g., lymphocyte, granulocyte, and thrombocyte counts or induced sodium-24) give an "average" of the whole-body dose. Even though there are marked inhomogeneities in dose distribution in most accidents, these doses provide general guidance.

Principal measures for treatment have been outlined by the International Atomic Energy Agency[13] and are shown in Table 5.1. A 1993 consensus development conference[14] also has a number of relevant papers and a useful schematic diagram of potential therapy (Figure 5.2).[14]

TREATMENT OF EARLY NEUROLOGICAL OR SEVERE HYPOTENSIVE EFFECTS

When the acute whole-body irradiation dose exceeds 50 Gy, the survival time is usually less than 48 hours. In general, symptoms are identified almost immediately and consist of disorientation, apathy, ataxia, prostration, and often tremor and convulsions. The seizures may result from minimal external stimuli. The cause of death is believed to be a function of several causes, including vascular damage, meningitis, myelitis, and encephalitis. Fluid infiltrates into the

TABLE 5.1
Principal Therapeutic Measures for Acute Radiation Syndrome According to Degree of Severity

	Whole-Body Dose (Gy)				
	1–2	2–4	4–6	6–8	>8
Degree of severity of ARS	Mild	Moderate	Severe	Very severe	Lethal
Medical management	Outpatient observation for maximum of 1 month	Hospitalization and treatment; isolation as early as possible			
		G-CSF or GM-CSF as early as possible (or within the first week)		IL-3 and GM-CSF	
		Antibiotics of broad spectrum activity (from the end of the latent period); antifungal and antiviral preparations (when necessary)			
		Blood components transfusion: platelets, erythrocytes (when necessary)			
			Complete parenteral nutrition (first week)		
			Metabolism correction, detoxication (when necessary)		
				HLA-identical allogene BMT[a] (first week)	Symptomatic therapy only

Note: BMT: bone marrow transplantation; G-CSF: granulocyte–colony stimulating factor; GM-CSF: granulocyte/macrophage–colonystimulating factor; IL-3: interleukin.

[a] See further discussion of bone marrow transplant in text.

Source: Adapted from International Atomic Energy Agency, Diagnosis and Treatment of Radiation Injuries, Safety Rep. Series 2, IAEA, Vienna, 1998.

meninges, brain, and choroid plexus, causing marked edema. The resulting pressure may cause pressure on critical structures. Although these changes can be identified in animals, they have rarely been seen in humans, and some of the deaths in this category may actually result from cardiovascular shock.[15] There has been little pathological examination of human tissue in these circumstances; however, in animals, the brain is grossly congested, with infiltration of granulocytes into the brain tissue. Perivascular hemorrhage and edema, as well as increased vascular permeability, has been identified. Some investigators suggest that in the same dose range there is a syndrome of cardiovascular shock. In humans, a rapid drop in blood pressure has been identified in some accidental situations (usually in which there has been nonuniform exposure, with the greater part being to the upper torso).[16]

TREATMENT OF GASTROINTESTINAL COMPLICATIONS

Nausea, Vomiting, and Diarrhea

A number of articles have examined the effectiveness of various drugs in preventing or treating radiation-induced nausea and vomiting after high-dose whole-body, lower hemibody, or abdominal radiotherapy.[17-22] It appears that much of the nausea and vomiting results from damage to the gastrointestinal mucosa that then release 5-hydroxytryptamine (5-HT3) with subsequent activation of 5-HT3 receptors. Treatment with 5-HT3 receptor antagonists appears to be quite effective at

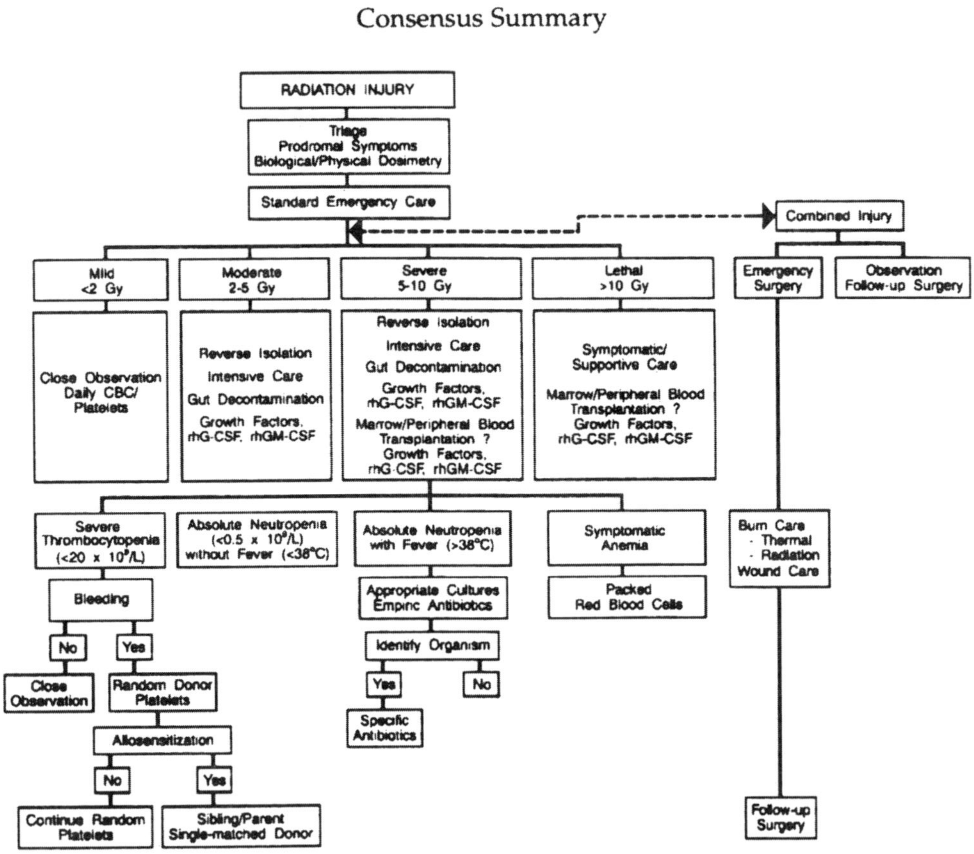

Consensus Summary

FIGURE 5.2 Schematic protocol for treatment of radiation injuries with particular emphasis on whole-body exposure. (From Reference 25. With permission.)

hemibody single doses up to 8 Gy. The drugs that have been used are granisetron, tropisetron, and ondansetron. Whether the 5-HT3 receptors are responsible for postradiation antegrade and retrograde giant migrating contractions of the small bowel and colon is not known. Initial diarrhea probably is the result of altered gastrointestinal motility and transport. Loperamide (an opiate receptor agonist) is effective in treating radiation-induced diarrhea. Other agents that have been suggested are cyclooxygenase inhibitors such as aspirin and indomethacin.[23]

Fluid and Electrolyte Imbalance

When acute absorbed skin doses in the range of 7 to 50 Gy are received, the gastrointestinal syndrome (group IV) may occur. In most circumstances, after the prodromal period, a latent period of approximately 1 to 4 days, during which the patient is asymptomatic, occurs. The clinical progress of the syndrome is a manifestation of the radiosensitivity and failure of both the gastrointestinal syndrome and the bone marrow. The symptoms include lethargy, diarrhea, dehydration, and sepsis. The earliest pathological changes can be identified as degenerative abnormalities in the small bowel epithelium. If the absorbed skin dose does not exceed approximately 12 Gy, regeneration of the bowel epithelium is possible. With higher doses, initial loss of the intestinal stem cells at the base of the mucosal crypts occurs, with subsequent denudation of the mucosa. As the intestinal vascular barrier is broken, there is marked fluid and electrolyte loss into the intestinal lumen and bacteria in the intestine that now have access to the bloodstream cause sepsis. Sepsis, of course, is aggravated by the decrease in granulocytes that normally would be available to combat it. Fluid loss is exacerbated by a failure of reabsorption of fluid in the colon. Many researchers have indicated that the presence of bile in the intestine is one of the main factors causing radiation-induced diarrhea. In animal systems, cannulation or ligation of the bile duct will prevent the diarrhea. Normally, bile salts are reabsorbed in the distal ileum; when reabsorption does not take place, an inordinately large amount of bile salts gains access to the colon.

The abnormalities in secretion of fluid into the bowel and reabsorption may cause a large loss of electrolytes, particularly sodium and, to a lesser extent, potassium. Infection occurs as early as 24 hours. Not only is the white blood cell count reduced, but other mechanisms normally operable to combat infection such as lymphoid elements (Peyer's patches) are depleted. Antibiotics have been demonstrated to reduce the bacteremia, although their effect on the ultimate mortality rate is questionable. Other investigators indicate that treatment with antibiotics may increase the mean survival time. In general, there are very limited human data on the gastrointestinal syndrome, and almost all available findings are derived from animal data. Death resulting from these changes usually occurs in 3 to 14 days postexposure.

Enhancing Regeneration

Treatment at the stage of manifest illness is directed at preservation of the cells in the villi and enhancing regeneration.[23] In this regard, various authors have suggested the use of intestinal growth factors, elemental diets, or gut-specific substrates (such as oral glutamine).[24]

An elemental diet may consist of amino acids, sucrose, and a small amount of fat. There are a wide variety of such products on the market at the present time, but the idea is to give the patient nutrients in their simplest form. This has been shown to decrease pancreatic enzymes and bile that exacerbate lesions, and it eliminates materials that would abrade the damaged epithelium. Total parenteral nutrition is often used in patients who were exposed in severe radiation accidents.

Mucositis is a common problem after radiation exposure. It is the result of direct radiation damage to the mucosal cells and neutrophil dysfunction. A number of authors have noted that mucositis can be reduced by use of mouth-rinse techniques with granulocyte colony–stimulating factor (G-CSF) but not with granulocyte/macrophage colony–stimulating factor (GM-CSF). Good oral hygiene is essential, including brushing, flossing, and rinsing with 3% hydrogen peroxide solution.

Prevention and Treatment of Infections

Radiation damage of the neutrophils and precursor elements in the bone marrow, immune depression, as well as loss of gastrointestinal epithelium leave the patient subject to a variety of infections. Clearly, the best approach is to prevent infection rather than to treat it after it has occurred. Prevention measures in immunocompromised patients have been well established over the last several decades.[25-27] To the extent possible, invasive procedures and placement of intravenous lines, nasogastric tubes, etc. should be kept to a minimum and if they are used, there should be appropriate and regular hygiene of these devices. Since the patient will need a lot of intravenous access, it may be best to place a tunneled central venous access line.

There are a number of methods to reduce the environmental level of pathogens including reverse isolation rooms, laminar airflow with microbial filters, low microbial diet, and hand washing. In recent radiation accidents, hospitalized patients have acquired methicillin-resistant *staphylococcus aureus* (MRSA). Epidemiological studies in hospitals have revealed that the single most common cause of transmission of MRSA is lack of hand washing by the medical staff.

The next step is to suppress or eliminate microorganisms that normally exist on and in the patient. Total microbial suppression is not recommended because it eliminates necessary anaerobes. These methods include use of antibacterial shampoo and use of povidone-iodine or chlorhexidine for skin cleansing. Administration of nystatin or other oral, nonabsorbable antibacterials will preserve anaerobic bacteria. Use of antiviral agents (acyclovir) is often used prophylactically. Physiological methods to reduce microorganisms should also be considered, including maintenance of gastric acidity, avoidance of antacids, and use of sucralfate or prostaglandin analogues for stress ulcer prophylaxis.

Routine culturing of skin, body orifices, urine, and wounds will allow rapid treatment with appropriate antibiotics, should a fever develop. At the time a fever develops, blood cultures should be obtained before treatment is instituted. When therapy is instituted, broad-spectrum antibiotics (particularly directed against gram-negative organisms) are usually used and continued at least until the patient is afebrile for 24 hours and the absolute neutrophil count is above 500/µl. Even if the fever resolves quickly, the treatment regimen should be continued for at least 7 days. If the fever persists, antifungal therapy with amphotericin B is often empirically added. Use of cytokines to prevent infections is discussed below in the section on bone marrow depression.

TREATMENT OF BONE MARROW DEPRESSION

TRANSFUSIONS

In the absorbed average body dose range of 2 to 7 Gy, the hematopoietic syndrome may be encountered. After the prodromal period, the duration of the asymptomatic latent period is 1 to 3 weeks. The signs and symptoms result from radiation damage to the bone marrow, lymphatic organs, and immune response. In this syndrome, rapid reduction in the lymphocytes and a somewhat more delayed reduction of granulocytes, platelets, and red cells occur. The granulocytopenia leads to infection, and the thrombocytopenia leads to hemorrhage. Fliedner[28] has estimated the percent of intact, injured, and destroyed stem cells at various levels of acute whole-body irradiation. His calculations demonstrate (Table 5.2) how few remaining stem cells there are after doses exceeding 5 Gy and also indicate that even a small amount of marrow shielding during an accident can be lifesaving. Shielding portions of the active marrow will have a major effect upon survival in acute exposure situations. In men, it appears that shielding of 10% of the active marrow will enable nearly all to survive when the body receives a dose close to the $LD_{50/60}$. Active marrow in adults is found in approximate percentages at various sites as follows: skull, 7%; upper limbs, 4%; ribs, 19%; sternum, 3%; cervical vertebrae, 4%; thoracic, 10%; lumbar, 11%; pelvis, 30%; lower limbs, 11%. This may explain why some patients (such as patient "S" in the Tokaimura criticality accident) were able to have native marrow recovery following an average whole-body dose in the range of 8 Gy.

Platelet and erythrocyte transfusions are often used prophylactically when the platelet count is less than 20×10^9 cells/l and the hemoglobin is less than 80 to 100 g/L. Actually, in the absence of obvious bleeding a platelet count of 10×10^9 cells/l is probably adequate, but if surgery is to be performed, the platelet count should be at least 75×10^9 cells/l. If possible, platelet and red cell transfusions should have the leukocytes removed and all blood products should be treated with 15 to 20 Gy to eliminate mononuclear cells and risks of cytomegalovirus and alloimmunization. If a stem cell or other transplant is contemplated, transfusions from the donor should be avoided. Granulocyte transfusions also have been considered to deal with neutropenia. One problem was getting enough granulocytes from a donor. Normal persons have been given G-CSF to raise their neutrophil counts prior to neutrophil harvesting, but whether or not this is safe and the efficacy of such transfusions are not clear.

BONE MARROW TRANSPLANTATION

Bone marrow transplantation (BMT) seems to be a logical treatment for victims of accidental whole-body irradiation when the dose is sufficiently high to make spontaneous bone marrow recovery impossible. Nevertheless, BMT has many limitations. These include identification of

TABLE 5.2
Calculation of Stem Cell Pool Sizes after Acute Total-Body Irradiation

Dose (Gy)	Intact Stem Cells, % (number)	Injured Stem Cells, % (number)	Destroyed Stem Cells, %
1.3–2.4	0.008 (1×10^5)	24 (3×10^8)	76
3.4–3.7	0.0024 (3×10^4)	4.8 (6×10^7)	95
3.3–4.3	0.0008 (1×10^4)	2.4 (3×10^7)	97.6
11.1–12.0	0 (0)	0.0006 (7.7×10^3)	99.9994

Source: Adapted from Fliedner, T.M., in *The Medical Basis for Radiation Accident Preparedness*, Ricks, R.C. and Fry, S.A., Eds., Elsevier Science, New York, 1990.

---

histocompatible donors, age constraints, HLA typing in lymphogenic patients, the need for additional immunosuppression, and the risk of graft-vs.-host disease.

Information gained from the accidents at Chernobyl and the Soreq irradiation facility in Israel strongly suggests that nonidentical BMT has a limited role for the treatment of victims of radiation accidents and only a small number of exposed individuals would benefit (Table 5.3).[29] Given these experiences, transplants should rarely be considered for victims receiving doses in the range of 8 to 12 Gy, uniformly distributed, without serious skin injuries, and in the absence of severe internal contamination and conventional injuries.

The timing of grafting is important and all arguments favor early marrow transplantation, even within the first week after exposure. Grafting in the peak period of immunosuppression may reduce the chance of graft rejection. This circumstance underscores the importance of reliable clinical, biological, and dosimetric findings to assess the dose level and dose distribution within the body. In the absence of reliable physical dosimetry and hematological parameters, the use of allogenic bone marrow transplantation is unjustified.

Stem cell transplants and fetal cord transplants have provided an interesting alternative to bone marrow transplantation. Human umbilical cord blood has been used as a viable source of both stem and progenitor cells. A single fetal blood cord collection should provide enough cells for the transplantation of an adult. Specific cord blood banks are being developed, which is especially helpful for rare HLA types. In addition, there appears to be little or no graft-vs.-host disease associated with these. The first umbilical cord transplant in a radiation accident was performed on patient "S" from the Tokaimura accident in Japan, who had received an estimated whole-body dose of 8 Gy. The graft (chromosome XX) was rejected, as the patient's own marrow (chromosome XY) regenerated.

USE OF CYTOKINES

During the past decade, cytokines have been suggested as having the potential to accelerate bone marrow recovery after radiation exposure in the lethal range.[25] G-CSF and GM-CSF increase the rate of hematopoietic recovery in patients after radiation exposure and may obviate the need for BMT when stem cells are still viable. G-CSF increases the functional activity of mature granulocytes and is usually used to decrease the incidence of infection in patients with neutropenia and fever. The typical dose of G-CSF is about 2.5 to 5.0 μg/kg/day (100 to 200 μg/m^2/day), administered subcutaneously or intravenously. The common form of G-CSF used is filagrastim (Neupogen®). Side effects include bone pain, splenomegaly, and, rarely, thrombocytopenia. GM-CSF is used to hasten

TABLE 5.3
Use of Transplants in Recent Radiation Accidents

Accident	Year	Dose (Gy)	Fatal	Final Engraftment	Type of Transplant
Tokaimura (O)	1999	17	Yes d83		BM id
Soreq, Israel	1990	10–20	Yes d36		BM
C-Pra 1023	1986	13.7	Yes d15		FLC
C-Orl 1020	1986	12.4	Yes d17		FLC
Shanghai-S	1990	12	Yes d25		BM
C-Tish 1015	1986	?	Yes d13		FLC
C-Ign 1003	1986	?	Yes d17		BM id
C-Top 1004	1986	11.8	Yes d18		BM
C-Kib 1010	1986	11.1	Yes d14		FLC
Shanghai-W	1990	11	Yes d90		BM
C-Bra 1014	1986	10.9	Yes d18		FLC
C-Nov 1016	1986	10.1	Yes d91		BM
C-Sha 1009	1986	9.5	Yes d23		BM id
C-Vats 1017	1986	9.4	Yes d18		BM
C-Aki 1002	1986	8.9	Yes d15		BM id
C-Iva 1008	1986	8.3	Yes d30		FLC
C-Per 1027	1986	8.2	Yes d24		BM id
C-Tor 1029	1986	8.7	No	No	BM
Tokaimura (S)	1999	8–9	Yes d211	No	CBCT
Egor 3075	?	7.0	Yes d33		BM
C-Sav 1001	1986	6.6	Yes d25		BM
C-Pop 1028	1986	6.4	Yes d48		BM id
Pittsburgh	1967	6.0		?	BM
C-Vers 1006	1986	5.4	Yes d86		BM id
C-Pal 1001	1986	5.4	No	No	
Shanghai-L	1990	5.2	No	No	FLC
C-Sit 1005	1986	4.4	Yes d34		BM
Vinca (V)	1958	4.4	Yes d32		FLC, BM unmatched
Shanghai-J	1990	4.1	No	No	FLC
Shanghai-W	1990	2.5	No	No	FLC
Shanghai-G	1990	2.4	No	No	FLC
Shanghai-J	1990	2.0	No	No	FLC

Note: BM: bone marrow, id: identical, FLC: fetal liver cells, CBCT: umbilical cord blood cell transplant.

neutrophil recovery. Typical dosage of GM-CSF is 5.0 to 10.0 µg/kg/day (200 to 400 µg/m^2/day) subcutaneously or intravenously. The form usually used is sargramostim (Leukine®). Side effects of GM-CSF include mild flulike symptoms, myalgia, fatigue, bone pain, and eosinophilia.

Both G-CSF and GM-CSF are glycoprotein products and both have effects that overlap somewhat but not completely. Both agents have been used in cancer patients undergoing therapy and have reduced the incidence of febrile episodes in patients with neutropenia. In patients with marrow depression, both agents appear to be about equally efficacious. If CSFs have not been used before a patient develops a fever, there is some evidence in patients with cancer that G-CSF therapy still may be beneficial. It is important to note that either agent needs to be continued for an adequate time after the nadir of the granulocytes. There is no clear evidence in the literature of patients with bone marrow suppression that the use of these cytokines actually reduces mortality, even though it can prevent fevers.

Interleukin 3 (IL-3) appears to act in synergy with GM-CSF. IL-3 also affects the lymphoid system by increasing both T-helper and T-suppressor lymphocytes and possibly the B-lymphocyte lineage as well. Doses of IL-3 usually range from 30 to 500 µg/m²/day. Side effects of IL-3 include fever, headache, neck stiffness, chills, bone pain, and local erythema at the subcutaneous injection sites. At high doses, there can be a decrease in the thrombocyte count. CFCs are probably most useful after hematopoietic recovery has begun.

Cytokines have been used in radiation accidents — Goiânia, San Salvador, Soreq, Nesvizh, Peru, Tokaimura — and the results are not clear cut (Table 5.4). A number of authors have indicated that use of cytokines reduces the period of neutropenia and may prolong survival, but to date, no authors have claimed that it affects ultimate mortality. In the Nesvizh accident, both GM-CSF (slow intravenous infusion 11.4 µg/kg/day) and IL3 (slow intravenous infusion 10 µg/kg/day) were used. In the Goiânia accident, after GM-CSF was used, increased neutrophils and bone marrow cellularity were reported; however, those particular patients were probably recovering spontaneously. One reason for the lack of much benefit from CSFs in radiation accidents may be delayed initiation of therapy. Although the data are contradictory, there are some reports that delayed administration results in loss of therapeutic efficacy. In many accidents the growth factors were not administered until 3 to 5 weeks postexposure, and in a number of other accidents it was given even though the total-body radiation dose was in a range that bone marrow depression was mild and significant infections would not have been expected. One note of caution is that in cases of bone marrow depression resulting from internal deposition of long-lived radionuclides, the use of CSFs is potentially detrimental.

TABLE 5.4
Use of G-CSF or GM-CSF without Bone Marrow Transplantation in the Dose Range 4 to 20 Gy

Accident	Date	Dose (Gy)	Used CSF	Fatal
Nesvizh	1991	11–18	Yes	Yes (d113)
San Salvador	1989	8.1	Yes	Yes (d197)
Goiânia	1987	7.1	No	No
Goiânia	1987	6.2	No	No
Mol	1965	5.5	No	No
Goiânia	1987	4–6	Yes	Yes
	1987	4–6	Yes	Yes
	1987	4–6	Yes	Yes
Vinca	1958	4.1	No	No
	1958	4.2	No	No
	1958	4.3	No	No
Iran*	1996	4–5	Yes	No
Peru*	1999	19	Yes	No

* Predominantly local exposure.

RESEARCH

There are a number of areas in which research continues. Due to the relatively small number and different types of radiation accidents, it is not likely that there will be much research on these patients. Most research regarding potential treatments of acute radiation sickness will be conducted on patients who are immunosuppressed as a result of other etiologies and from radiotherapy patients. Other hematopoietic growth factors have also been used in patients with bone marrow depression.

These include interleukin-6 (IL-6), interleukin-11 (IL-11), macrophage colony–stimulating factor (M-CSF), and stem cell factor. IL-3 stimulates the proliferation and differentiation of both early and late progenitor cells in the formation of erythroid, myeloid, and megakaryocyte production.

IL-6 historically has had a number of names including interferon beta, T-cell replacement factor, B-cell-stimulating factor, hybridoma growth factor, and granulocyte differentiating–inducing factor. While IL-6 acts with other cytokines, its main effects are that it increases megakaryocyte size and maturation (increasing circulating platelets) and accelerates multilineage hematopoietic recovery. Use of IL-6 appears to be more effective in irradiated mice than is IL-3 for hematopoietic regeneration. A recombinant cytokine, PIX321, is a fusion protein consisting of GM-CSF and IL-3 and has greater specific activity than either cytokine alone.

M-CSF stimulates proliferation, maturation, and differentiation of macrophage/monocyte cells in the bone marrow and stimulates those to produce prostaglandins, IL-3, tumor necrosis factor (TNF), and C-CSF. Erythropoietin (EPO) regulates the late stages of erythropoiesis and, as such, does not appear to be very useful in radiation accident patients with anemia.

The use of various cytokines has also been proposed to help gastrointestinal recovery. These include epidermal growth factor, growth hormone, and insulin-like growth factor 1, fibroblast growth factors, EPO, and IL-3.

Septic shock is produced by a number of toxins (such as lipopolysaccharides, LPS) released into the bloodstream by Gram-negative bacteria. LPS appears to interact with macrophages to produce TNF as a principal cause of effects from Gram-negative septicemia. IL-1 also may play a role in the development of septic shock. Experimental approaches have included use of LPS-neutralizing proteins, antibodies to LPS, antibodies against TNF, administration of xanthine derivatives (such as pentoxiphylline or HWA 138), IL-1.

Radioprotective agents have been of interest for both military and cancer therapy applications. Thousands of drugs have been tested, and amifostine (WR-2721, ethiofos) has been considered promising. These agents must be given prior to the radiation exposure to be effective. WR-2721 is an aminothil, which is a prodrug and must be metabolized to an active form (WR-1065) to be effective. The drug also may reduce the stochastic long-term consequences of radiation since in mice it reduced the mutagenicity and carcinogenicity of platinum and radiation. Whether this effect applies to humans, or to what extent, is unknown. During infusion, the drug has side effects including somnolence, sneezing, chills, hiccups, vomiting, and, most importantly, hypotension. There is some experimental evidence that the effects of WR-2721 can be enhanced when glucan (an immunomodulator and hematopoietic stimulant) is administered after radiation exposure.[30]

REFERENCES

1. Fry, S. and Hubner, K., *The Medical Basis of Radiation Accident Preparedness*, Elsiever/North Holland, New York, 1980.
2. Fujita, S., Kato, H., and Schull, W., The LD_{50} associated with exposure to the atomic bombing of Hiroshima and Nagasaki, *J. Radiat. Res.* (Suppl):154–161, 1991.
3. Rotblat, J., Acute radiation mortality in a nuclear war, in *The Medical Implications of Nuclear War*, National Academy Press, Washington, D.C., 1986.
4. Fujita, S., Kato, H., and Schull, W., The LD_{50} associated with exposure to the atomic bombing of Hiroshima and Nagasaki: a review and reassessment. RERF Technical Report 17-87, Radiation Effects Research Foundation, Hiroshima, 1987.
5. Fujita, S., Kato, H., and Schull, W., The LD_{50} associated with exposure to the atomic bombing of Hiroshima, *J. Radiat. Res.,* 30:359–381, 1989.
6. Young, R., Human mortality from uniform low-LET radiation. A report presented at the NATO RSG V meeting on LD_{50} held at Gosport, U.K., on May 11, 1987.
7. Kamada, N., Shigeta, C., Kuramoto, A. et al., Acute and late effects of A-bomb radiation studied in a group of young girls with a defined condition at the time of bombing, *J. Radiat. Res.,* 30:218–225, 1989.

8. United Nations Scientific Committee on the Effects of Atomic Radiation, Sources and Effects of Atomic Radiation. Report to the General Assembly with annexes. Acute Effects of Radiation on Man, New York, 1988.
9. United Nations Scientific Committee on the Effects of Atomic Radiation, Sources and Effects of Atomic Radiation. Report to the General Assembly with annexes. Annex G, Exposures and effects of the Chernobyl accident, New York, 2000.
10. Baranov, A.E., Konchalovski, M.V., Yu Soloviev, W., and Guskova, A.K., Use of blood cell count changes after radiation exposure in dose assessment and evaluation bone marrow function, in *The Medical Basis for Radiation Accident Preparedness*, Ricks, R.C. and Fry, S.A., Eds., Elsevier Science, New York, 1990.
11. Friesecke, I., Beyre, K., Densow, D. et al., Acute radiation exposure and early hematolopoietic response patterns: an evaluation of the Chernobyl accident victims, *Int. J. Radiat. Med.*, 1 (1):55–62, 1999.
12. Fliedner, T.M., Presentation at Tokaimura Conference held in Chiba Japan, October, International Atomic Energy Agency, Diagnosis and Treatment of Radiation Injuries, 1999.
13. Safety Report Series, No. 2, Vienna, 1998.
14. Advances in the Treatment of Radiation Injuries: Proceedings of the 2nd Consensus Development Conference on the Treatment of Radiation Injuries, Bethesda, MD, April 14–17, 1993, MacVitte, T.J., Weiss, J.F., and Browne, D., Eds., *Advances in the Biosciences*, Vol. 94, Pergamon/Elsevier Science, Oxford, U.K., 1996.
15. Fanger, H. and Lushbaugh, C.C., Radiation death from cardiovascular shock following a criticality accident, *Arch. Pathol.*, 83:446–460, 1967.
16. Fajardo, L.F. and Stewart, J.R., Cardiovascular radiation syndrome (letter), *N. Engl. J. Med.*, 238:374, 1970.
17. Priestman, S., Priestman, T., Canney, P., A double blind randomised cross-over comparison of nabilone and metoclopramide in the control of radiation-induced nausea, *Clin. Radiol.*, 38:543–544, 1987.
18. Priestman, T., Roberts, J., Lucraft, H. et al., Results of a randomized double-blind comparative study of ondansetron and metoclopramide in the prevention of nausea and vomiting following high-dose upper abdominal irradiation, *Clin. Orthop. Rel. Res.*, 2:71–75, 1990.
19. Scarantimo, C., Ornitz, R., Hoffman, L. et al., Radiation-induced emesis: effects of ondansetron, *Semin. Oncol.*, 19(6 Suppl. 15):38–43, 1992.
20. Sorbbe, B., Berglind, A., and De Bruijn, K., Tropisetron, a new 5-HT3 receptor antagonist, in the prevention of irradiation-induced nausea, vomiting and diarrhea, *Eur. J. Gynecol. Oncol.*, 13:382–389, 1992.
21. Henriksson, R., Lomberg, H., Israelsson, G. et al., The effect of ondansetron on radiation-induced emesis and diarrhea, *Acta Oncol.*, 31:767–769, 1992.
22. Logue, J., Magee, B., Hunter, R. et al., The use of the antiemetic granisetron in lower hemibody radiotherapy, *Clin. Oncol.*, 3:247–249, 1991.
23. Gunther-Smith, P.J. and Dubois, A., Treatment strategies for radiation induced gastrointestinal injuries, in Advances in the Treatment of Radiation Injuries: Proceedings of the 2nd Consensus Development Conference on the Treatment of Radiation Injuries, Bethesda, MD, April 14–17, 1993, MacVitte, T.J., Weiss, J.F., and Browne, D., Eds., *Advances in the Biosciences*, Vol. 94, Pergamon/Elsevier Science, Oxford, U.K., 1996.
24. Klimberg, V.S., Salloum, R.M., Kasper, M. et al., Oral glutamine accelerates healing of the small intestine and improves outcome after whole abdominal irradiation, *Arch. Surg.*, 125:1040-1045, 1990.
25. Consensus summary on the treatment of radiation injuries, in Advances in the Treatment of Radiation Injuries: Proceedings of the 2nd Consensus Development Conference on the Treatment of Radiation Injuries, Bethesda, MD, April 14–17, 1993, MacVitte, T.J., Weiss, J.F., and Browne, D., Eds., *Advances in the Biosciences*, Vol. 94, Pergamon/Elsevier Science, Oxford, U.K., 1996, 325–346.
26. Garilov, O.K., Radiation disease, *Hematol. Rev.*, 7:1–26, 1996.
27. Guskova, A.K., Nadezhina, N.M., Moiseev A.A. et al., Medical assistance given to personnel of the Chernobyl Nuclear Power Plant after the 1986 accident, *Hematol. Rev.*, 7:27–100, 1996.
28. Fliedner, T.M., Hematological indicators to predict patient recovery after whole body irradiation as a basis for clinical management, in *The Medical Basis for Radiation Accident Preparedness*, Ricks, R.C. and Fry, S.A., Eds., Elsevier Science Publishing, New York, 1990.

29. Baranov, A.E., Allogenic bone marrow transplantation after severe, uniform total-body irradiation: experience from recent and previous radiation accidents, in Advances in the Treatment of Radiation Injuries: Proceedings of the 2nd Consensus Development Conference on the Treatment of Radiation Injuries, Bethesda, MD, April 14–17, 1993, MacVitte, T.J., Weiss, J.F., and Browne, D., Eds., *Advances in the Biosciences*, Vol. 94, Pergamon/Elsevier Science, Oxford, U.K., 1996, 281–293.
30. Capezzi, R.L. and Schein, P.S., Chemo and radiation protection with Amifostine, in Advances in the Treatment of Radiation Injuries: Proceedings of the 2nd Consensus Development Conference on the Treatment of Radiation Injuries, Bethesda, MD, April 14–17, 1993, MacVitte, T.J., Weiss, J.F., and Browne, D., Eds., *Advances in the Biosciences*, Vol. 94, Pergamon/Elsevier Science, Oxford, U.K., 1996, 91–102.

6 Direct Effects of Radiation on Specific Tissues

Fred A. Mettler, Jr.

CONTENTS

Introduction 70
Skin and Mucosa 72
    Low-LET (Linear Energy Transfer) Radiation 74
    Neutron Irradiation 77
    Radiation of the Skin by Radionuclides 77
Thyroid 78
    Low-LET Radiation 79
    High-LET Radiation 80
    Internal Radiation 80
Nervous System 81
    Brain 82
        Low-LET Radiation 82
        High-LET Radiation 85
    Spinal Cord 86
        Low-LET Radiation 86
    Peripheral Nerves 87
        Low-LET Radiation 87
        High-LET Radiation 87
Eye 87
    Low-LET Radiation 88
    High-LET Radiation 90
    Radionuclide Irradiation 91
Salivary Glands 91
    General 91
    Low-LET Radiation 91
Respiratory Tract 92
    Trachea 92
    Lung 92
        Low-LET Radiation 93
        High-LET Radiation 95
        Radionuclide Irradiation 96
Heart and Vessels 96
    General 96
    Low-LET Radiation 96
Gastrointestinal Tract 99
    Oral Cavity and Pharynx 99

		Low-LET Radiation 99
		Neutron Radiation 100
	Esophagus...100
		Low-LET Radiation 100
	Stomach..101
		Low-LET Radiation 101
	Small Intestine..101
		Low-LET Radiation 101
	Colon, Sigmoid, and Rectum...102
		General 102
		Low-LET Radiation 102
		Neutron Radiation 103
Liver 103
	Low-LET Radiation 103
	Radionuclide Irradiation 105
Urinary System 106
	Low-LET Radiation 106
	High-LET Radiation 108
	Radionuclide Irradiation 108
Reproductive Organs...108
	Testes..109
		Low-LET Radiation 109
		High-LET Radiation 110
		Radionuclide Irradiation 110
Bone, Cartilage, and Muscle 110
	Low-LET Radiation 110
	Neutron or High-LET Radiation 112
	Radionuclide Irradiation 112
Hematopoietic and Lymphatic Systems 112
	Low-LET Radiation 114
	High-LET Radiation 115
	Internal Irradiation 115
References 116

INTRODUCTION

Direct radiation effects are the most important effects in terms of the medical management of radiation accidents. They represent the major causes of injury and death. This chapter is a detailed review of radiation effects on those tissues that have been shown to be clinically important in radiation accidents. It includes effects on those tissues that are extremely radiosensitive (such as the gastrointestinal tract and bone marrow), as well as tissues that are more resistant but which have typically been included in radiotherapy accidents (such as the central nervous system) and tissues involved in local radiation injury (such as skin, peripheral blood vessels, and bone). The major experience on radiation injury to localized tissues arises from the practice of radiotherapy and therefore the majority of material in this chapter refers to fractionated exposures. Treatment of localized injury is covered in Chapter 14. Where applicable in this chapter, accident data have either been included or other chapters have been referenced. Chapters 3 to 5 review the effects of whole-body radiation exposure.

Direct Effects of Radiation on Specific Tissues

Direct effects of radiation are called *nonstochastic* or deterministic. These effects, whose occurrences are not a function of probability, are determined by dose. The severity of nonstochastic effects varies directly with the absorbed dose. An example of such a nonstochastic, or deterministic, radiation effect is bone marrow depression. Almost all individuals who receive a whole-body, single dose of radiation in excess of 5 Gy will experience bone marrow depression. Additionally, although there is some individual variation, virtually no one who receives less than 0.5 Gy in a single, whole-body exposure will demonstrate clinical bone marrow depression. Thus, for practical purposes, direct, or nonstochastic, effects have a threshold dose.

The direct effects observed in an individual depend on the dose received, volume of tissue irradiated, quality or type of radiation, and time over which the dose is received. Direct effects observed also depend upon the time of observation after irradiation. A given organ is composed of (1) parenchymal cells that have some specific functions for that organ, (2) structural cells that give the organ its form, and (3) vascular tissue that supplies blood to the organ. Each of these three components usually has a different sensitivity to radiation and a different time course of presentation of direct radiation effects. Initial effects that are evident clinically may result from dysfunction of the parenchymal cells; however, if the organ survives, late effects may be due to obliterative vascular changes within the organ (Figure 6.1).

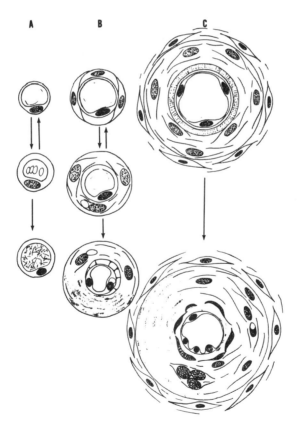

FIGURE 6.1 Diagram of radiation injury involving capillary (A), arteriole (B), and small artery (C). Initially the capillary dilates and has increased permeability; later, with narrowing of the lumen and sclerosis of the wall, a thrombus may form causing occlusion of the lumen. Changes in the arteriole are quite similar to those seen in the capillary. With the small artery, less dilatation of the lumen occurs initially, since the wall is more rigid; later progressive damage to the endothelium with narrowing of the lumen occurs. (From Anderson, W.A.D. and Kissane, J.M., Eds., *Pathology*, C. V. Mosby, St. Louis, 1977. With permission.)

Radiation effects do not produce pathognomonic, histological, or morphological changes that allow a given tissue to be examined and described as having been exposed to ionizing radiation. The tissue can be analyzed for changes that are similar to changes seen following known radiation exposure. If such changes are identified, then radiation can be included in the list of possible etiologies of these changes.

Direct radiation effects on tissues have been classified into a somewhat arbitrary temporal scheme by Rubin and Casarett.[1] In their scheme, *acute effects* are those occurring within the first 6 months; *subacute,* second 6 months; *chronic clinical period,* second through fifth years; and *late clinical period,* after the fifth year. Other authors divide pathological effects into *immediate, acute* (days to weeks), and *delayed* (months to years).[2] The content of this chapter has been largely abstracted from Mettler and Upton[3] and additional material has been added. The reason for inclusion of this material in this book is the belief that in the event of an accident it would be useful to have this material immediately available and contained in one text.

SKIN AND MUCOSA

The skin is injured in most significant radiation accidents. In some cases, there is exposure from a localized source that results in erythema, blistering, ulceration, or necrosis (sometimes called the cutaneous syndrome). Even in cases where there is significant whole-body exposure (such as Chernobyl), accompanying extensive skin injuries resulted in more fatalities than would have been expected on the basis of the whole-body exposure alone. Patients receiving acute doses in the range above 15 Gy often report an immediate sensation of heat and those receiving acute local doses in excess of 25 Gy may report immediate pain or tingling. This is discussed more in the later section on the nervous system.

The skin has a series of layers that must be considered to understand potential radiation effects. The outer group of layers is derived from the embryonic ectoderm and forms the epidermis. The inner layers, which are formed from embryonic mesenchyme, collectively form the dermis. The epidermis is composed of an outer layer of dead cells (stratum corneum). The thickness of this layer, about 20 cells thick, varies markedly in different portions of the body, for example, it is thicker on the palms and soles. A middle epidermal layer (stratum granulosum) is about 4 to 5 cells thick and provides a transition between the dead cells and the underlying viable layers (stratum germinativum and stratum spinosum). These two layers determine the majority of radiation response.

There is an underlying, undulating, and proliferating basal cell layer. Cells derived from the basal layer travel toward the surface and eventually die and are sloughed. This process takes about 14 days (Figure 6.2). The average epidermal layer thickness is 20 to 40 μm on the face and trunk, 40 to 60 μm on the arms and legs, about 85 μm on the backs of the hands, and the greatest thickness on the fingertips is about 150 to 300 μm. Immune functions appear to be a result of Langerhans cells that have migrated from the bone marrow to the skin.

The epidermis is separated from the dermis by a basement membrane. The dermis has two distinct layers: the superficial papillary dermis and the thicker reticular dermis. The dermis is about 1.3 mm thick. The superficial layer is composed of collagen bundles and elastic fibers and is the primary layer for thermoregulation and nourishment of the lower layers of the epidermis. The reticular dermis is densely fibrous and is the primary structural layer of the skin.

In simplistic terms, the clinical radiation response can be visualized after the skin structure is understood. Alpha particles are not able to penetrate even the top two or three layers of dead cells in the stratum corneum. Beta radiation can penetrate farther and often affects the proliferating cells at the basal layer. More-penetrating radiations, such as cobalt-60 X rays, may actually be skin sparing because the dose initially increases with depth, sparing the skin and delivering higher doses to deeper tissues. For appropriate clinical evaluation, it is extremely important to know at least the penetrating ability of the incident radiation, the amount of skin exposed, and the time over which the radiation is delivered. Without this information, inappropriate judgments may be made.

Direct Effects of Radiation on Specific Tissues

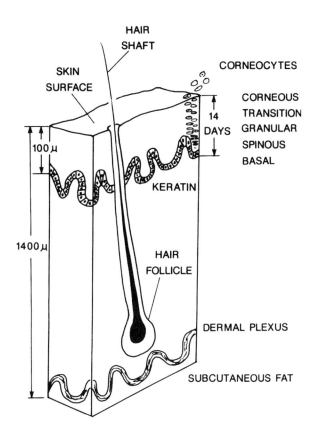

FIGURE 6.2 Structure of the skin.

As early as 1898, Gassmann described histological changes of chronic roentgen ulcers.[4] The "radium burn" and the early radiation pioneers, including Henri Becquerel and Marie Curie, described radiation dermatitis. Comprehensive reports on radiation effects on the skin and a book chapter are recommended to the reader for further reading.[5–7] Basic acute skin changes are summarized in Table 6.1.

TABLE 6.1
Time of Onset of Clinical Signs of Skin Injury Depending on the Dose Received

Stage/Symptoms	Dose range (Gy)	Time of Onset (Days)
Erythema	3–10	14–21
Epilation	>3	14–18
Dry desquamation	8–12	25–30
Moist desquamation	15–20	20–28
Blister formation	15–25	15–25
Ulceration (within skin)	>20	14–21
Necrosis (deeper penetration)	>25	>21

Source: Adapted from International Atomic Energy Agency, Diagnosis and Treatment of Radiation Injuries, Safety Rep. Series, No. 2, IAEA, Vienna, 1998.

Low-LET (Linear Energy Transfer) Radiation

Skin erythema, or reddening, occurs if a single dose of 6 to 8 Gy is given, and it is not identified until 1 to 2 days after irradiation. The higher the radiation dose, the more quickly the erythema may be identified. The early erythema is presumably due to release of vasoactive amines and capillary dilatation.

Erythema increases during the first week and usually fades during the second week. It then may return 2 to 3 weeks after the initial insult and last for 20 to 30 days. The second phase of erythema is due to vessel damage; thermographic studies demonstrate increased blood flow during the first 2 to 3 months. This cyclic behavior of the erythema may continue several times. In general, no erythema is expected if radiation doses are below 5 to 6 Gy, but if the radiation fields are large and there is an acute dose in excess of 2 to 3 Gy, there can be an early erythematous reaction within a few hours. As the dose is fractionated, the threshold for skin erythema rises. If there are 12 daily fractions the dose for erythema of skin rises from about 6 or 8 Gy to about 12 Gy. Acute doses in excess of 8 Gy will produce exudative and erosive changes of the skin. When there are penetrating acute doses in excess of 20 Gy, there is usually nonhealing ulceration.

The late phase of erythema is probably due to blood vessel damage and is characterized by a blue or mauve discoloration of the skin. This was seen in the patients exposed at Chernobyl who received a beta dose at a depth of 1500 μm in the skin of greater than 20 Gy. This was approximately 30% of the dose that was received at a depth of 70 μm.

In addition to erythema, edema may be associated with acute exposures. It can appear in a few hours or a few weeks. The higher the dose, the shorter is the period for appearance; there is enough individual variation that dosimetry is imprecise, at best. If there is an exudative dermatitis in general, the margins correspond to an acute dose to the basal layer of the epidermis of about 18 Gy. For quite large doses of radiation, there may be additional changes of moist desquamation, formation of bullae, or even a sloughing of the skin due to killing of cells in the basal layer.

Changes of the skin that have been described in radiation therapy usually involve a course totaling 40 to 50 Gy from an orthovoltage source in 20 to 25 equal fractions over a 4- to 5-week time period. In such circumstances, patients may demonstrate a faint erythema due to capillary dilatation during the first week of treatment. Some epilation is noted at 10 to 14 days. The true erythema usually occurs in the third week of treatment, with the skin becoming red, warm, and edematous. Moist desquamation begins at the fourth week with oozing of serum and is equivalent to a second-degree thermal burn. The doses required to cause moist desquamation from chronic exposure are shown in Figure 6.3.

In radiotherapeutic situations, desquamation is usually healed by the time treatment is ended because there is compensatory regeneration in the basal layer of the skin. This regenerative capacity usually exceeds the destructive capacity during conventional radiotherapy. Dry desquamation occurs if irradiation is halted during the third week at the 30-Gy level. In these circumstances, the skin may itch, and scaling and increased pigmentation occur. The erythematous changes and desquamation are almost always confined to the treatment field, although occasionally they may extend beyond it. In addition, a generalized skin reaction may occur, perhaps due to indirect effect of a circulating product resulting from breakdown of tissue as a result of radiation. If doses exceed those discussed, necrosis of the structures underlying the epidermis may occur.

Skin ulceration may occur very early with high absorbed doses. These ulcers may heal but ultimately will recur. With more conventional doses such as those used in radiotherapy, painful, slowly healing ulcers may occur and persist for years. The probable cause of these late ulcers is ischemia due to the arteriolar and small-artery changes mentioned earlier.

With relatively large doses of radiation such as a single dose of 20 Gy to 40 Gy or more, a bullous-type, moist desquamation may occur in 4 weeks. In this situation, small blisters tend to coalesce and rupture. If the dose is high enough, blisters may be formed from beneath the basal cell layer. At this stage, the clinical lesion may appear very similar to a second- or third-degree

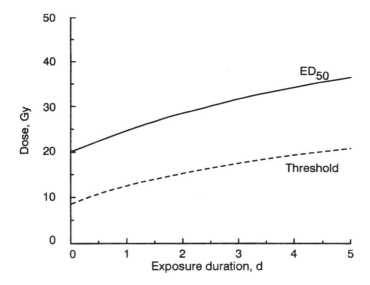

FIGURE 6.3 Variation of dose and duration of low-LET radiation that will cause moist desquamation in 50% of those exposed (ED_{50}). Also shown is the threshold dose that will cause the effect in 1% of those exposed. (From Risk from Deterministic Effects of Ionising Radiation, Documents of the National Protection Radiation Board, Vol. 7, No. 3, Didcot, Oxon, U.K., 1996.)

thermal burn, but an important differential diagnostic point is that the patient will not remember having been burned. In such circumstances, the bullae may become infected, and there also may be sloughing of the epidermis. A week or two after sloughing of the epidermis, the affected areas may become covered with epidermis, although ulcers tend to recur with later arteriolar obliterative changes. In patients who have developed late radiation ulcers following fractionated radiotherapy with doses of 40 to 120 Gy, there is a reduction in circulation.

Some authors have classified skin damage by clinical type.[8] Type I injury is damage limited to the epidermis and dermis without much damage to the subcutaneous tissues. There is an initial erythema, a 3-week latent period, a secondary erythema immediately followed by an exudative epidermatitis, and recovery in 3 to 6 months with or without atrophic changes.

Type II injury is a vascular endothelitis, and at 6 to 8 months postexposure the acute reactions are renewed with necrosis and ulceration usually requiring surgery. This is the result of damage below the basal layer of the epidermis. In type III injury there is necrosis within a few weeks of the acute exposure.

With radiotherapy, temporary loss of hair (epilation) occurs in about 3 weeks with 3 to 5 Gy; hair begins to return during the second month and continues for up to 1 year. Single doses of 7 Gy may cause permanent epilation, with the latent period being less than 3 weeks (Figure 6.4). Not all body areas have the same radiation epilation sensitivity. The scalp and beard are most sensitive, with chest wall, axillary, abdominal, eyebrow, eyelash, and pubic hair less sensitive, respectively. Hair follicles of children are more sensitive than those of adults. Hair that has regrown is always finer and slower-growing than the original hair. It may also be of a different color.

Delayed effects in therapeutic situations or chronic exposure may be apparent at 6 months and may progress slowly. The sequence of pigmentation effects is variable from patient to patient. In some patients, the skin demonstrates gradual hyperpigmentation; however, in blacks, there may be depigmentation of the skin. Increased pigmentation is caused by a radiation-induced increase in enzymatic activity of melanocytes. Depigmentation may occur if the radiation dose has been high enough to destroy the melanocytes. By 1 year, the skin usually demonstrates its final appearance. Diffuse telangiectasia, suppression of sebaceous gland activity, regrowth of hair, and thin, dry, and

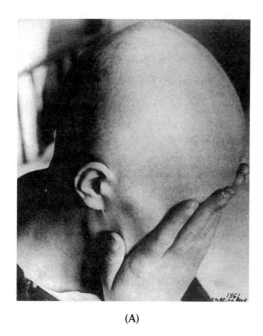 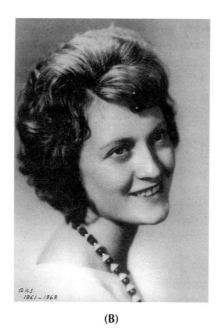

(A)   (B)

FIGURE 6.4 (A) Epilation due to radiation following whole-body exposure in a Russian radiation accident in 1961. (B) Regrowth of hair. Patient seen here 7 years postexposure.

semitranslucent skin may result from atrophy. There have been a number of authors that have reported on the individuality and latent period of late skin telangiectasia. Skin telangiectasia often shows progression up to 10 years but is individually variable.[9,10] If moist desquamation occurs during radiotherapy, there is a higher incidence of telangiectasia.[11] With increasing fibrosis, there may be induration of the skin, as well as limitation of motion.[1] The amount of severe fibrosis is greatly influenced by both dose and fractionation. For example, at 2 fractions/week, severe fibrosis will occur in 20% of persons receiving 36 Gy and 80% of those receiving 43 Gy. For 5 fractions/week, the corresponding values are 46 Gy and 52 Gy. Chronic radiation dermatitis from radioactive gold jewelry has been reported in several patients. Such jewelry has either been contaminated with radon or radioactive gold-198.

Skin reaction varies over the body and is influenced by patient factors, including age. In radiation therapy, moist desquamation rarely occurs in children, probably because of the ability of the epithelium's to recover more rapidly in children than in adults. Hyperthyroidism apparently makes the erythema and skin reaction more brisk than usual. Fairer-skinned people demonstrate more skin reaction than do darker-skinned individuals.

Those portions of the skin that are moist and subject to friction, such as the axilla, groin, and skin folds, are the most radiosensitive. Sensitive areas appear to be the inner aspect of the neck and antecubital and popliteal spaces, followed in decreasing order by the flexor surface of the extremities, chest, abdomen, face, and back. The extensor surfaces of extremities are somewhat less sensitive. The least-sensitive areas appear to be the nape of the neck, scalp, and the palms and soles. Areas of skin grafting in which the graft is less than 3 months old generally demonstrate greater radiosensitivity than does the normal skin. Interestingly enough, skin grafts older than 1 year normally do not demonstrate much reaction to radiation.

Skin tolerance to radiation depends significantly on the volume of tissue irradiated. As the volume of skin irradiated becomes smaller, the dose required to produce necrosis increases. For example, the skin tolerance dose (TD) for a circular field of 150 cm^2 is approximately 15 Gy in a single dose, whereas for a circular field of 50 cm^2 the TD is almost 20 Gy.[12,13] For radiotherapy

Direct Effects of Radiation on Specific Tissues

situations the skin tolerance dose is about 50 Gy for a skin area of 100 cm^2, 58 Gy for 16 cm^2, 84 Gy for 4 cm^2, and 392 Gy for 1 cm^2. Occasionally, there are rare atypical skin reactions after radiotherapy that resemble erythema multiforme, pemphigus, and other entities. Such reactions can begin in the irradiated area but then become more generalized.

Neutron Irradiation

The relative biological effectiveness (RBE) for single doses of neutrons depends upon the neutron energy. The range appears to be between 1.5 and 2.0, and the TD for skin erythema of fast neutrons is approximately 2 Gy. Criticality accident patients who survive the first 2 months may develop severe dermal and soft tissue fibrosis as a result of neutron exposure.

Radiation of the Skin by Radionuclides

The effects on the skin of various radionuclides depend significantly on the half-life and energy spectrum emitted by the radionuclide. In most instances, skin contamination occurs on an accidental basis, with the clinical significance of an accident rarely being a function of the skin dose. Pure alpha-emitting radionuclides pose no skin hazard and predominantly pose an internal contamination hazard. The hazard level of an alpha emitter depends upon the chemical nature and solubility of the contaminant, as well as the integrity of the skin as a natural barrier.

Gamma-emitting radionuclides (such as cesium-137, cobalt-60, and iridium-192) are often accompanied either by beta emissions or possibly soft X rays as a result of interaction with a metallic capsule or covering. Industrial radiography sources are the most common cause of problems and can result in a wide spectrum of skin changes. A number of reports and books on the occurrence and treatment of such lesions are available.[14–17]

Energetic beta particle emitters, if left undetected on the skin surface, may ultimately cause erythema, particularly if they are present in high-specific-activity amounts. Such accidental situations may be possible in a fission product accident at a commercial nuclear facility. Some beta-emitting radionuclides have been carefully studied (particularly phosphorus-32 and strontium-90), and the following values[18] for beta radiation have been derived: threshold erythema, 5 to 15 Gy; dry desquamation, 17 Gy; and bullous epidermitis, 72 Gy.

Skin changes from atomic weapons and discussions of "beta burns" usually arise in many public forums. Beta burns are possible after a nuclear weapon detonation. In early fallout, there are approximately two beta particles for every gamma photon. The maximum range of the beta particles in air (about 6 ft) is much lower than that of the gamma photons. At a planar surface, the beta dose from early-fallout beta particles may be about 140 times that of the gamma dose, falling off very quickly with distance. Practical considerations indicate that under actual field conditions, the beta dose is much lower than one would anticipate because (1) clothing is usually worn (particularly shoes), and the human skin has an outer cornified layer composed of dead cells that stop all beta particles with energies of less than 70 keV; (2) most particles of fallout on the skin are expected to have retention times ranging from 2 h (1000 µm diameter) to 7 h (50 µm diameter); and (3) most fallout on the ground is not deposited on a perfect planar surface but rather on a very irregular surface. Several reports indicate that at 1 m from a fission product fallout-contaminated surface, the beta/gamma ratio is approximately 2 to 3.

In a follow-up study of the Japanese fishermen exposed to accidental radioactive fallout in 1954,[19] skin doses were estimated to have been from 1.7 to 6.0 Gy. The equivalent single acute dose is reported to be approximately half: 0.8 to 3 Gy. The external gamma dose from the fallout particles was accompanied by beta radiation fallout, which produced significant skin lesions, including erythema, erosion, occasional necrosis, and skin atrophy.

In the same fallout accident in the Marshall Islands (see Chapter 35), 23 U.S. radar servicemen were also exposed to fallout in the early 1950s. Many experienced discrete 1- to 4-mm round skin lesions that quickly healed. They also experienced ridging of fingernails several months later.

It should be noted that discussions of fallout experience in the Marshall Islands and the South Pacific might be unique. In the tropical environment, the fission products were attached to calcium oxide from the coral, with the fallout particles sticking to the exposed individuals and clothes. In the continental United States, the situation may be slightly different. In at least one modeling study of fallout,[20] particle size and distribution on the skin significantly affected the calculations. It was concluded that for single particles of less than 500-μm diameter, no particles could cause skin ulceration as long as they were deposited more than 17 min after weapon detonation. Regardless of the particle size distribution, in the multiparticle model, skin damage became virtually impossible after a delay time of 10^7 s following weapon detonation.

The reactor accident at Chernobyl resulted in a large number of workers having skin contamination with high activities of fresh fission products (see Chapter 12). These had a beta/gamma ratio of between 10 and 30. Estimated skin doses to a number of patients were in excess of 40 Gy. The energy of the beta particles was sufficient to damage the basal layer of the skin and cause desquamation and a large portal of entry for infection. More than one half of the acute deaths from Chernobyl were the result of the severe skin changes and infection in the face of a depressed bone marrow and immune system. The survivors have skin that is atrophic, telangectatic, and has underlying fibrosis.

For many years there has been concern about the effects of skin irradiation by small beta or beta/gamma-emitting particles. The reader is referred to a comprehensive NCRP report on the subject.[21] "Hot" particles (also referred to as fleas or specks) are occasionally found in nuclear power plants and commonly contain cobalt-60 of fission products. The cobalt-60 is derived from activation of stable cobalt in the metal of items such as valve seats, while the fission products come from fuel that has escaped through defects in the fuel cladding. The activity of most of the particles is in the range of 400 Bq to 200 kBq (1 nCi to 5 μCi). The particles by definition are less than 1 mm in any dimension, yet they can deliver very high doses to small portions of the skin.

It is clear that the direct effects of radiation in the skin depend markedly upon the area irradiated, with much higher doses tolerated as the field size becomes smaller. A large amount of animal work with small beta-emitting particles has been done, but there is only a limited amount of human data.

THYROID

The thyroid is important in radiation accidents primarily as a result of accumulation of radioiodines produced in the fission process. Potential management of this problem by using stable iodine is discussed in Chapter 23 on internal contamination and Chapter 32 on application of radiation protection principles and intervention in radiation accidents. Of course, there are data on induction of thyroid cancer in children at Chernobyl and this is discussed in Chapter 12.

There is a very large clinical experience of thyroid irradiation. Human data are available from fallout studies, radiotherapy for tumors of the thyroid or the adjacent neck, and radionuclide treatment for hyperthyroidism. The thyroid parenchyma consists of follicles lined by simple epithelium. The follicular cells produce a colloid containing the thyroid hormones. Between the follicles is a very rich network of blood vessels and lymphatics. The epithelial cells are relatively radioresistant. The direct changes following large doses of irradiation identified in the thyroid are mediated by the vasculature and may be manifest as inflammatory and edematous changes, followed later by obliteration of the fine vasculature and, ultimately, by radionecrosis or atrophy. The overall relative radiosensitivity of the thyroid is due to the results of vascular damage.

Low-LET Radiation

The atomic bomb survivors were predominantly exposed to external low-LET radiation. In a study of 477 atomic bomb survivors who were in the 1-Gy-plus group and under the age of 20 at exposure, there was no evidence of an increase in clinical or subclinical hypothyroidism[22] when comparison was made with 501 individuals in the 0-rad group. In addition, there was no evidence of an increase in chronic thyroiditis or in nontoxic diffuse goiter. This is in contrast to a study of Nagasaki atomic bomb survivors reported by Nagataki.[23,24] He found the prevalence of hypothyroidism in the 0.01 to 0.49 Gy group to be elevated at 4.5% compared with 2.5% in controls. The frequency of Hashimoto's thyroiditis was also elevated in the same group (3.2% vs. 0.5% in the controls). Both of these findings are of questionable significance because there was no significant elevation of either entity in the 0.5 to 0.99 Gy group. No evidence of an increase in autoimmune thyroiditis was seen in any group.

Atomic bomb survivors who were under 30 years of age at the time of irradiation have shown a dose-dependent excess of thyroid disease, defined to include nontoxic nodular goiter, diffuse goiter, thyrotoxicosis, chronic lymphocytic thyroiditis, and hypothyroidism.[25] The excess, which became evident within 20 years after irradiation and was not detectable in those exposed at older ages, corresponded to a relative risk of 1.24 at a dose of 1 Gy ($P < 0.003$). Although many of those affected had multiple diagnoses, the exclusion of persons with thyroid cancer or thyroid adenomas did not modify the risk.

Limited data concerning thyroid function after diagnostic medical exposure are available. Kaplan et al.[26] followed 91 women who received an average of 112 fluoroscopic examinations of the chest during tuberculosis treatment by repeated pneumothorax. Autoimmune thyroid disease was found in 15% of the exposed group and in 7% of the comparison group (prevalence ratio 2.2 with 95% confidence interval, or CI, 0.8 to 6.2). The thyroid dose was uncertain but was thought to be between 0.11 and 1.12 Gy. These findings are of questionable clinical significance. No increase in hypothyroidism was seen.

After X-ray therapy of the neck, hyperthyroidism has been reported, but it is quite rare. Reports of the doses needed to cause hypothyroidism from external fractionated irradiation range between 26 and 50 Gy.[27–29] The individual responses to external radiation of the thyroid may be quite variable; some authors indicate that a normal gland can tolerate doses as high as 60 Gy over 6 weeks without clinical evidence of damage, whereas hypothyroidism occasionally may be seen at doses as low as 10 Gy and may occur in a moderate percentage of long-term survivors of bone marrow transplants who were treated with six whole-body fractions of 2 Gy. Laboratory hypothyroidism may be present in approximately half of children irradiated for Hodgkin's disease with fractionated doses to the neck of 22 to 44 Gy. Hancock et al.[30] reviewed the records of 1787 patients treated for Hodgkin's disease. The majority of patients received 44 Gy to cervical lymph node areas. Biochemical hypothyroidism was found in 513 patients. Somewhat less than half required medication, and most cases presented 2 to 3 years after therapy, although some still occurred up to 18 years later. The risk for biochemical hypothyroidism was 44% at 20 years after treatment for patients who had received more than 30 Gy and 27% for those in the 7.5 to 30 Gy range. The comparable figures for overt hypothyroidism were 20 and 5%, respectively. Graves' disease occurred in 30 patients, with a mean onset time of 5.3 years (range 3 weeks to 18 years). Of the patients, 17 also had ophthalmopathy. Silent thyroiditis with transient mildly symptomatic thyrotoxicosis developed in 6 patients about 10 to 24 months after therapy.

Loeffler et al.[31] specifically followed 437 Hodgkin's disease patients treated with mantle fields to ascertain the rate of Graves' disease. The latter was found in seven patients. The O/E ratio was 5.9 for females and 5.1 for males. In a study of 28 patients given mantle therapy for malignant lymphoma (with a thyroid dose of 45 Gy), the incidence of subclinical hypothyroidism was 22%, and no patients had clinical hypothyroidism.[32]

A number of studies have examined hypothyroidism in adults after external radiotherapy. Grande[33] reported biochemical hypothyroidism in 41% of patients after radiotherapy for head and neck cancer. Similar results were reported by Liening et al.[34] and Tami et al.[35] Reports of hypothyroidism after irradiation of supraclavicular nodes during the course of radiotherapy for breast cancer vary widely. Joensuu[36] reported an incidence of clinical and subclinical hypothyroidism of 21%, while Bruning et al.[37] found a value closer to 80%. Both indicated that the cumulative thyroid dose was 45 to 50 Gy. Acute effects of external radiation on the thyroid have been identified in autopsies performed on some of the victims at Hiroshima. Liebow examined patients who died 3 to 6 weeks after exposure and identified only a moderate decrease in the follicular size.[38] There have been radiation therapy accidents in which overexposures of the neck have occurred. In the accident in Costa Rica (Chapter 21), there were a number of patients who died within the first several months who had necrosis of the thyroid gland, although this was not directly responsible for their deaths.

In terms of modifying factors, a large load of stable iodine may cause increased thyroid sensitivity. In one report of patients treated for Hodgkin's disease, those who had a lymphangiogram appeared to be more radiosensitive. It was postulated that the increased radiosensitivity was due to the iodinated contrast material.[39]

High-LET Radiation

Animal studies indicate that the thyroid is not particularly sensitive to neutron radiation when compared with other tissues. The RBE of monoenergetic 14-MeV neutrons was estimated to be 3.2 when 1 Gy of neutrons was used and 1.8 when 5 Gy of neutrons was given.[40]

Internal Irradiation

A large experience with radionuclide irradiation of the thyroid gland in humans with iodine-123, iodine-125, and iodine-131 has been documented. This experience derives from both accidental and therapeutic exposures.

The dose distributions of iodine-125 and iodine-131 are different within the cellular structure of the thyroid. The dose delivered to the cells from iodine-125 is very localized, with most occurring at the colloid–cell interface. It is estimated that the distribution of dose from iodine-125 will spare approximately 30% of the proliferating cells. Iodine-131, on the other hand, delivers a much more homogeneous dose to the gland and produces diffuse damage, as has been confirmed with electron microscopic studies.[41] Iodine-131 delivers seven times the initial mean dose rate to the thyroid compared with that for an equal activity of iodine-125.[42] Iodine-125 has occasionally been used for therapy of hyperthyroid glands. The differences in dose and homogeneity at the cellular level have not caused a significant difference in clinical results, and the use of iodine-125 for treatment of hyperthyroidism has been abandoned.[43,44]

In 1954, a thermonuclear explosion accidentally deposited large amounts of radioactive iodines in the Marshall Islands. The highest dose was received on the Rongelap atoll.[45] The iodines deposited were a mixture of iodine-131, iodine-132, iodine-133, and iodine-135, and they resulted not only in significant internal contamination, but external contamination as well (see Chapter 35). The direct effects identified have included hypothyroidism (both clinical and biochemical). In 4 of 43 subjects biochemical hypothyroidism was demonstrated,[45] and 3 of these subjects were thought to have received a thyroid dose of less than 3.5 Gy. In the course of a 15-year follow-up, 67% of individuals below the age of 10 years developed nodules, as did 15% of the remainder of the population. Thyroid doses in the young age group were felt to range between 10 and 42 Gy and in the older age group, 30 to 50 Gy. An additional study[46] demonstrated that five Marshallese children who were exposed to the fallout showed some growth retardation, and two young males developed hypothyroidism. In a somewhat later study, Robbins and Adams[47] indicated that there were 12 cases of subclinical hypothyroidism.

Direct Effects of Radiation on Specific Tissues

The Chernobyl accident also released very large quantities of radioiodine. Unfortunately, iodine distribution and dosimetry are not well known. The International Chernobyl Project[48] examined the thyroid function of hundreds of persons living in nearby heavily contaminated villages and compared the findings with those on persons living in clean settlements. By 5 years after the accident there was no evidence of thyroid hypofunction in the general population as a result of the accident. Follow-up of the Chernobyl firemen who suffered from both the acute radiation syndrome, with whole-body doses from 1 to 6 Gy, and inhalation of fission products had not revealed clinical hypothyroidism as of 1993. The incidence of hypothyroidism from smaller doses of iodine-131 is difficult to evaluate.

The use of iodine-131 for the treatment of Graves' disease and toxic multinodular goiters has been studied extensively. One problem is that the natural course of Graves' disease often terminates in hypothyroidism, whether treated with iodine-131 or not. Typical doses administered for such treatments range between 110 and 600 MBq (3 to 16 mCi). Some nuclear medicine physicians utilize the lower doses and try to titrate a patient down to a euthyroid state. This approach often requires several treatments. Another procedure is to use high-dose therapy designed to render the patient hypothyroid with a single dose of radioiodine. Most patients become hypothyroid with administered activities of iodine-131 in the range of 370 to 550 MBq (10 to 15 mCi). The actual absorbed dose to the gland is often difficult to calculate in these patients because of uncertainties in the exact size and weight of the gland. Another uncertainty is the biologic half-life of the radioiodine in a hyperthyroid and radiation-damaged gland. When radioiodine therapy is done for Grave's disease or toxic multinodular goiter, there is usually a transient acute radiation thyroiditis. Patients often experience a "sore throat" in 1 to 2 days following ingestion of the radioiodine, which lasts for about 3 to 4 days. Pain is usually relieved by aspirin. If there is a large amount of thyroid hormone stored in the gland that is suddenly released, the patient may experience "thyroid storm" or transient marked hyperthyroidism.

Becker[49] has reviewed the probability in 6000 patients of developing hypothyroidism after surgical and radioiodine treatment for hyperthyroidism. In patients who received 201 to 225 μCi of iodine per gram of gland, there was a 20% probability at 1 year and a 50% probability at 7 years. With 101 to 125 mCi/g, the values were 15 and 30%, respectively. The risk of hypothyroidism in these patients also can be expressed in a different way, i.e., 1.7×10^{-3}/Gy and given that external radiation appears to be more effective per unit dose, then the risk of hypothyroidism after external exposure is about 8.5×10^{-3}/Gy.

Factors modifying the response of the thyroid to internal radiation include preexisting disease, particularly hyperthyroidism. Hyperthyroidism results in an increased radiosensitivity, perhaps due to the increased uptake of iodine or to the more active nature of the gland. There also is some evidence that children have more sensitive glands with regard to induction of hypothyroidism than adults.[50] Sex and prior thioamide therapy do not appear to influence the development of subsequent hypothyroidism.[51]

NERVOUS SYSTEM

The nervous system is rather resistant to radiation effects. Even so, radiation-induced changes have occurred and indeed radiation-induced spinal cord injury has been responsible for a number of cases of paraplegia, quadriplegia, and more than ten deaths secondary to myelopathy after radiation therapy accidents. In cases of very high acute radiation dose accidents, victims have reported an almost immediate feeling of pain, heat, or headache (see Chapters 4, 11, and 13). In cases of localized injuries, medical management often must cope with intense and unrelenting pain caused by irradiation of peripheral nerves (see Chapters 11, 17, and 20). Finally, very high acute doses of radiation may cause transient unconsciousness (transient incapacitation), disorientation, or ataxia. This is most likely the result of transient hypotension, and these effects are discussed in Chapter 4.

On a historical basis, the study of radiation-induced changes in the central nervous system (CNS) received rather late attention compared with effects on other organ systems. Most authors treat the brain, spinal cord, and peripheral nerves as separate entities since their responses are different. The reader is also directed to a recent and superb book on radiation injury to the CNS by Gutin et al.[52] Most of the human data come from radiation therapy of neoplasms,[53] but radiation has been used occasionally for nonmalignant disorders. Scholz and Hsii[54] reported on the use of whole-brain irradiation in schizophrenia and found that 43 Gy delivered in 3 days resulted in brain damage within 20 months. Bailey et al.[55] reviewed the transient use of cobalt-60 wires to perform lobotomies.

The cells of the mature nervous system include the neurons, the glial cells (including satellite cells and peripheral ganglia), the ependymal lining, and the neuroglia. Neurons themselves are very resistant to the direct effects of radiation. Glial cells and Schwann cells are relatively resistant to radiation injury. The myelin sheath surrounding nerve fibers in the brain and spinal cord (particularly in the white matter of the brain) is also resistant to irradiation. However, radiation therapy may accelerate demyelination in diseases such as multiple sclerosis.[56]

The preceding discussion has referred primarily to the mature system. The developing system, which is actively proliferating in the embryo and in early childhood, is less resistant. Thus, the level of maturation substantially influences the radioresistance of the nervous system.

Many of the effects on the nervous system that are manifested, both acutely and at later periods, result from vascular injury, including the diffuse edema identified early and the later necrosis resulting from myointimal proliferation and subsequent fibrosis.

BRAIN

Radiation changes in the brain are of several general types: acute reactions, early delayed reactions, and late delayed reactions.

Low-LET Radiation

Patients exposed to acute, high whole-body or upper-torso doses in criticality and industrial irradiation accidents often report a headache in the first several hours. This is not usually seen below doses of 4 Gy. Headache is moderate and occurs 4 to 24 h postexposure in about 50% of persons receiving 4 to 6 Gy, it is severe and occurs in 3 to 4 h in 80% of those receiving 6 to 8 Gy and headache that is severe and occurs in 1 to 2 h postexposure is indicative of doses in excess of 8 Gy.

Subacute brain damage is usually the result of an insult to the vascular system, although occasionally an acute demyelinating process is observed.[57] Excessively large doses or relatively few fractions of large doses (greater than 70 Gy) have caused radiation-induced brain necrosis.[58] A single case of possible radiogenic dementia has been reported.[59] The tolerance dose of the brain with fractionated radiotherapy over 5 to 6 weeks is thought to be 55 Gy, although small areas of the brain may tolerate doses up to 65 Gy. Overall, the white matter of the CNS is more susceptible to radionecrosis than is the gray matter or the brain stem. The paraventricular and supraoptic nuclei of the hypothalamus appear to be more radiosensitive than white matter.

In the acute clinical period, the response of the brain to irradiation depends on whether the brain was normal initially. The sudden onset of headache, vomiting, and papilledema has often been referred to as "radiation edema," but in most therapeutic circumstances, the clinical presentation has been confused by recent surgery, presence of tumor, and other factors. The actual presence of radiation edema in the usual fractionated radiotherapy scheme appears to be dubious. Elevation of cerebrospinal fluid pressure following fractionated radiotherapy is rare, although single doses in the range of 35 Gy can cause an acute inflammatory reaction with increased capillary permeability and interstitial edema. A single dose in the range of 60 Gy is lethal within 2 to 3 days. Demyelinating lesions have been reported within 10 weeks after 55 Gy of fractionated cobalt-60 radiotherapy.[57]

Early delayed reactions appear from a few weeks to a few months after radiation therapy. They are usually self-limited and are easily mistaken for effects of residual tumor or chemotherapy. In children treated for leukemia with methotrexate and radiation, about 60 to 80% will exhibit anorexia, irritability, and somnolence. In adults there may be ataxia, nausea, vomiting, dysphagia, dysarthria, and nystagmus. The pathogenesis of this reaction appears to be transient interruption of myelin synthesis, perhaps due to abnormalities in capillary permeability.

The late delayed reaction has a number of forms, ranging from asymptomatic periventricular white matter changes to decreased mental status, endocrine changes, and even focal necrosis. Approximately 70% of cases of focal necrosis present themselves within the first 2 years after radiotherapy.[60] Pathologically, areas of focal necrosis occur preferentially in the white matter and extend to the gray–white matter junction. In late stages there can be clumped chalky calcification. Radiation necrosis occurs with a much higher probability when therapy schemes exceed 40 Gy in 20 fractions or 60 Gy in 30 fractions in 5 weeks or when fractions exceed 3 Gy.[61,62] With the advent of radiosurgery, high doses are delivered to small volumes of brain. Even though the volumes are small, there are still reports of significant radiation reactions.[63] The maximum tolerable dose in children up to the age of 3 is 33% less than that for adults, and Bloom[64] has also estimated that for children 3 to 5 years of age, the adult dose has to be reduced by 20%.

Radiation necrosis of the brain occurs with moderate probability when the dose exceeds 50 Gy in 20 fractions. In the Costa Rican radiotherapy accident there were several patients with severe brain injury. The first received 69 Gy in 28 fractions and developed pituitary necrosis and died. The second was a child who received 58 Gy in 20 fractions. He was confined to a wheelchair, unable to speak, and had central and cortical brain atrophy, as well as mineralizing microangiopathy (see Chapter 21).

Imaging of radiation necrosis with computed tomography (CT) often shows a low-density region with surrounding edema, a variable mass effect, and irregular enhancement after administration of contrast material. Magnetic resonance imaging (MRI) shows areas of decreased signal on T1-weighted images and increased signal on T2 images. Unfortunately, residual tumor has the same imaging characteristics, and it is not possible to differentiate between these entities with either modality.[65] Research using positron emission scanning (PET) has been performed, and it appears that using radiotracers (fluorine-18-labeled 2-fluoro-2-deoxyglucose) metabolism can differentiate between these entities. This is because a tumor would have an area of metabolism equal to or greater than that of surrounding brain tissues, while radiation necrosis would have decreased or absent metabolism.[66] Dual isotope methods have also been described by Schwartz et al.[67] using single-photon emission CT. If the area of concern had a high accumulation of thallium-201, there was recurrent tumor rather than necrosis.

Histologically, the most characteristic abnormality in delayed radiation necrosis is the exudation of an amorphous, eosinophilic, and structureless substance that can be identified as fibrin. If there is a fibrin exudate along a hypocellular region occurring along the gray–white junction, the picture is almost diagnostic. There are rare reports of delayed brain hemorrhage several years after radiotherapy for pediatric brain tumors.[68]

With the advent of MRI it became clear that many patients would develop areas of diffusely increased signal in the white matter seen on T2-weighted images (Figure 6.5). Reports indicate that 50 to 100% of patients will show these findings after radiotherapy. The changes occur preferentially in the periventricular white matter and may extend out to the gray–white junction. In mild forms, the patients appear to have no clinical symptoms, while in patients with extensive MRI changes there is more likely to be more mental impairment such as personality change, confusion, seizure disorders, and learning difficulties.[69–71]

Leukoencephalopathy refers to white–matter injury caused by demyelination following treatment with chemotherapeutic agents with or without associated radiation therapy. It is not seen after radiotherapy alone. The most typical situation is after doses of 20 Gy and with use of methotrexate,[72–74] although it has also been reported after whole-body doses of 10 Gy given prior to bone

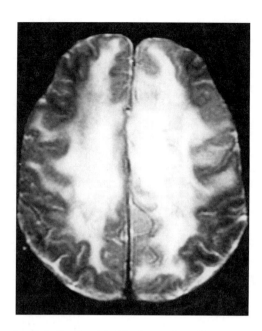

FIGURE 6.5 White matter changes in the brain after radiation therapy. Image from a T2-weighted MRI scan shows symmetrical confluent high signal (white) in a periventricular white matter distribution.

marrow transplantation.[22] On CT and MRI this entity is indistinguishable from the white matter radiation changes. Cortical gray matter and basal ganglia are not affected. Clinical findings are lethargy, poor school performance, ataxia, spasticity, progressive dementia, and even death.

Another change that is sometimes seen in children treated for leukemia with cranial radiation and methotrexate is mineralizing microangiopathy.[75] This is seen as calcification in the gray matter, basal ganglia, putamen, and sometimes in the cortex and even the brain stem.[76] There is calcification in small blood vessels that are surrounded by necrotic mineralized necrotic brain tissue. It is not fatal, and it is unknown if this produces any specific neurological signs, although it is often associated with leukoencephalopathy. The entity is seen in about 25% of patients who received intrathecal methotrexate and cranial radiation of 24 Gy and who survive for more than 9 months.

Another late change that may be seen in about 50% of patients after cranial radiation therapy is cortical atrophy. This is seen either on CT or MRI as enlarged cortical sulci and enlarged ventricles, usually detectable 1 to 4 years after radiotherapy. This is seen in about half of patients who have received more than 30 Gy to the brain with fractionated radiotherapy.

Modifying factors influencing radiation effects appear to be preexisting disease, age, anatomical location, arteriosclerosis, and chemotherapy (including systemically administered vincristine and methotrexate). The increased sensitivity of the nervous system in children requires radiotherapy treatment schedules to be adjusted according to the age of the patient. Arteriosclerosis may lower tolerance of the brain since the occlusive changes due to radiation may be additive with respect to preexisting arteriosclerotic changes. Sheline et al.[77] and others[78] suggest that chemotherapy may add to the radionecrosis and possibly enhance the level of injury.

Both depression and somnolence, probably as a result of a transient encephalopathy, have been reported 6 to 8 weeks after cranial irradiation to dose levels of 24 Gy in 10 to 15 fractions. Such findings have been seen in children and adults treated for acute lymphoblastic leukemia,[79,80] even with normal cerebrospinal fluid. The somnolence is distinct from the more severe neurological abnormalities produced by intrathecal methotrexate.

Follow-up studies have been performed and include both Israeli[81] and U.S.[82] children who received about 1 to 2 Gy during treatment of tinea capitus. In the Israeli study, males with multiple irradiations had a higher rate of admissions to mental hospitals (34.0 vs. 17.4/1000), but this difference was not seen for females. Children irradiated at less than 6 years had an RR of mental hospital admissions of 1.7 (95% CI of 1.1 to 2.8), but for older children there was no increased risk. In the U.S. series, there was a 30% excess of psychiatric disorders among the irradiated children; however, a more recent and detailed study by Omran et al.[83] showed only a borderline difference between the two groups. It should be noted that there does not appear to be a good biologic or pathological basis for effects at these dose levels, and these results are not supported by follow-up studies of children treated for tumors. As with most studies of this type, there is the possibility of recall bias and other potential confounding.

Several interesting reports suggest a decline in intelligence quotient (IQ) scores, as well as cognitive dysfunction in children treated with cranial radiation and intrathecal methotrexate for acute lymphocytic leukemia.[84] Speculation regarding the etiology of such possible effects includes the theory that cranial irradiation may enhance the intracerebral absorption of the methotrexate (which by itself is associated with nervous system dysfunction).

The long-term effects of primary radiation therapy for brain tumors in children have been studied by Danoff et al.[85] Tumor doses were 40 to 65 Gy. Performance status was good to excellent in 89%. Mental retardation was found in 17% of patients, and behavioral disorders were found in 39% of the patients, but also in 59% of mothers and 43% of fathers. Mental retardation was greatest in those younger than 3 years of age and in those who had tumors in the region of the thalamus and hypothalamus.

Neuropsychological abnormalities with behavioral disorders and intellectual impairment are seen in up to 50% of children treated for brain tumors with doses of 40 Gy or more in 1.8 to 2.0 Gy daily fractions. The younger the child, the greater is the IQ loss. The adverse effect may not be evident until 2 to 5 years post-therapy. In general, children who receive 24 Gy of fractionated radiotherapy have a 10 to 15 point loss in IQ. In children treated for leukemia, there does not appear to be neuropsychological impairment if intrathecal methotrexate is used without radiotherapy. When it is used with radiotherapy, the deficit appears to be greater than for radiotherapy alone. A significant reduction in IQ scores occurs when there is 18 Gy of fractionated radiotherapy used with methotrexate. Trautman et al.[86] have noted that social class was a much stronger predictor of ultimate IQ than was age at irradiation or radiation dose, while Bleyer et al.[87] indicate that age at irradiation is the most important factor. This stresses the need for controlling of confounding factors in study design. Some authors have indicated a correlation between calcification and other abnormalities on CT scans and learning disabilities or seizures,[88,89] but these conclusions are not confirmed in other studies.

While the bulk of the literature concerns neuropsychological effects after childhood cranial radiotherapy, there are a few scattered reports concerning mental impairment in adults. Biologically, there seems much less reason for a radiation effect, and there is always the concern about whether the effects seen are the result of the tumor itself, edema, preexisting vascular disease, or other factors. Tucker et al.[90] have indicated that, in adults who received prophylactic CNS radiation for adult leukemia, there were only minimal, subclinical long-term neuropsychological changes.

High-LET Radiation

Neutrons, pi-mesons, and heavy nuclei have been the subject of study in the treatment of brain tumors. In general, neutrons produce more injury to normal tissues than might be expected, and the RBE for the brain appears to be about 4 to 5. Increased brain edema following 13 Gy of neutrons over 4 weeks has been reported. Dementia has occurred in some patients with doses of 15.6 Gy over 4 weeks. It has been speculated that the normal brain tissue may be sensitive as a result of high hydrogen content. The patient series for the other radiation types are generally small, and injury to normal tissues is difficult to ascertain. For further reading in this area, the reader is referred to a chapter on the topic by Laramore.[91]

Spinal Cord

Low-LET Radiation

Direct injury of the spinal cord has been reported many times, particularly in cases of overexposure with radiotherapy of neoplasms that occurred outside the CNS. The radiotherapy accidents in Spain and Costa Rica (Chapters 20 and 21) have had a number of fatalities related to paraplegia and quadriplegia.

In general, radiation-induced lesions of the spine have a shorter latent period to their clinical manifestation than do similar brain lesions. The spinal cord often is unable to tolerate the absorbed dose levels necessary to eradicate malignant tumors. In some cases, the original malignancy may be controlled or cured, with the development of the complication of paralysis associated with the level of the irradiation. The so-called radiation myelitis may be either transient or permanent.

Myelitis was a clearly identified radiation hazard as early as the 1940s. Acute transient myelitis often appears 2 to 4 months after the termination of radiation therapy. The patient may experience electrical shocklike sensations, tingling, and paresthesias. Often the symptoms are exaggerated by either flexion or extension of the spine (Lhermitte's sign). The pathogenesis appears to be transient demyelination of the ascending sensory neurons. This syndrome usually resolves spontaneously without treatment. Reversal of the transient myelopathy may occur at 2 to 40 weeks.

There is a 25 to 50% incidence of thoracic cord myelopathy at dose levels of 60 Gy with 2 Gy fractions, 40 Gy with 3 Gy fractions, and 35 Gy with 4 Gy fractions. In the Costa Rican radiotherapy accident, there were three patients who developed spinal cord complications. Two became quadriplegic (one died of complications) and one became paraplegic. They had received 50 to 57 Gy in 15 to 17 fractions. Myelopathy also was the major cause of fatality in the radiotherapy accident in Zaragoza, Spain.

In many instances, there is a delayed myelitis. The most radiosensitive portion of the CNS appears to be the upper thoracic segments and the lower lumbar and sacral segments. The latent period for delayed myelopathy of the thoracic and cervical spinal cord is about 20 months after radiation therapy, and 75% of cases occur within 30 months. Lumbar myelopathy usually occurs earlier, and the majority of cases appear within 17 months. The signs of radiation myelopathy depend upon the level of the lesion in the spinal cord; however, it is irreversible, and there is a high fatality rate. The incidence of delayed myelopathy rises quickly as the radiation therapy scheme exceeds 30 Gy in 10 fractions, 40 Gy in 20 fractions, or 60 Gy in 30 fractions. The patients may experience paralysis, decreased vibration and position sense, spastic quadriplegia, incontinence, and diaphragmatic breathing. Neurologically, the patient may exhibit the Brown–Sequard syndrome due to involvement of the lateral columns of the spinal cord. During this period, the cerebrospinal fluid and pressure are usually normal. If the lower motor neurons are involved, a flaccid paralysis may result. Fajardo[2] points out that the prognosis for delayed radiation myelitis is usually poor, with rarely any evidence of recovery. Survival in cases of cervical and high thoracic myelitis is about 10 months. Death usually results from either pneumonia or urinary tract infection. Clinically, the neurological level is manifested in anatomical segments lower than the level at which the radiation was given.

The acute reversible form of the myelitis may be due to an abnormality in the synthesis of myelin by the oligodendrogliocytes. Pathologically, the lesions are quite similar to those described in the white matter of the brain with demyelinization and areas of radionecrosis. The delayed form of myelitis has been thought to be due to progressive vascular obliteration and thrombosis, but Withers et al.[92] suggested that the death of slowly dividing cells might be the more likely cause.

The physical factors of the radiation are very important in assessing the risk of myelopathy. If a radiation field is very long, the risk of myelopathy is greater, particularly when adjacent field radiotherapy is performed with overlap in the treatment field. The spinal cord is generally more sensitive than the brain. There is a relationship between the volume of cord irradiated and the tolerance dose. Kramer et al.[58] have indicated the maximum acceptable dose to the cervical and lumbar spinal cord to be 50 Gy in 25 fractions over 5 weeks and, to the thoracic cord, 45 Gy delivered over 4½ to 5 weeks. Other reported tolerance doses range between 35 Gy in 4 weeks and 50 Gy in 5 weeks.[93,94] If these doses are exceeded, transient radiation myelopathy and, perhaps, paralysis may result. Fitzgerald et al.[95] indicated that 13% of patients who received 40 Gy in an accelerated fractionation scheme and survived 11 months developed progressive myelitis.

Dische et al.[96] have examined 754 cases of radiation myelitis that occurred after radiotherapy for lung cancer. They report that the threshold dose for thoracic radiation myelitis in fractionated radiotherapy was 33.5 Gy. Georgiou et al.[97] have reviewed 2410 patients treated with external and internal radiotherapy for carcinomas of the cervix and endometrium. The calculated dose to the lumbosacral plexus was 73 Gy, and only 4 patients developed lumbosacral plexopathy.

Peripheral Nerves

Low-LET Radiation

Peripheral nerves are among the structures most resistant to radiation damage. Although several researchers have reported peripheral neuropathy, including brachial plexus injury, most of the findings are complicated by other forms of therapy that are in themselves neurotoxic (such as misonidazole).[98] Occasionally, it is also difficult to separate changes due to radiation from those due to surgery, such as scarring around the nerves as the cause of the neuropathy. Damage to the brachial plexus has been described in individuals who have received doses in the range of 50 Gy in a fractionated course of therapy to the high axillary nodes. A number of articles concern brachial plexus injuries after radiotherapy for breast cancer. Olsen et al.[99] have indicated that 5% of patients in a Danish series had disabling plexopathy, and 9% had milder symptoms after 50 Gy in 25 fractions over 5 weeks. Clinical manifestations were paresthesia in 100% of cases, hypesthesia in 74%, weakness in 58%, pain 47%, and decreased muscle stretch reflexes in 47%. A higher incidence was found in patients also receiving cytotoxic therapy and if fraction sizes were over 2 Gy. A much lower incidence (1.3%) was reported by Pierce el al.[100] with an axillary dose of less than 50 Gy but 5.6% when the dose exceeded 50 Gy. The median time to occurrence was 10.5 months (range 1.5 to 77 months) and 80% of cases completely resolved. The incidence was 0.6% in patients without chemotherapy and 4.5% in patients receiving chemotherapy. There is controversy as to whether electrophysiological studies are useful in differentiating radiation-induced cases from neoplastic plexopathy. Optic nerve changes are discussed in the section on the eye.

With acute absorbed doses above 25 Gy, patients report the almost immediate sensation of pain or heat. Accidents involving very high acute radiation doses (such as with industrial radiography sources) not only cause necrosis of the skin and underlying soft tissues but also result in severe, disabling, and unrelenting pain. Typically, narcotics do not relieve this pain and often surgery is necessary. The pain can begin days after exposure and continue for many months. The acute threshold dose to cause this effect is about 15 Gy.

High-LET Radiation

The RBE of neutrons for the spinal cord and brain may be equal to or higher than that for skin. Few published data concern the RBE of neutrons for the human spinal cord.

EYE

Effects of radiation on the eye are not usually of immediate concern in accidents although acute conjunctivitis was reported in the 1997 Sarov criticality accident. There are, however, many patients who survived the initial effects of an accident and have gone on to develop cataracts. This has occurred in Chernobyl patients with estimated acute whole exposures in the range of 4 to 8 Gy. Ocular sequelae can also be of importance in radiation therapy accidents.

Direct effects of radiation on the eye were noted as early as 1897, and by 1908, corneal changes were clearly recognized as direct effects. In the 1950s, there was extensive investigation of radiogenic eye damage, particularly concerning cataract formation.[101,102] Most of the tissues around the eye have the same sensitivity as skin; however, the lens is particularly radiosensitive, with subsequent production of opacities within the lens and cataract formation.

Low-LET Radiation

Because a large portion of the eye, particularly the conjunctiva, is composed of epithelial cells, it reacts as the skin does during the acute clinical period. There may be erythema and, if the dose is high enough, dry or moist desquamation. The eyebrows are quite resistant to epilation, even when it occurs at other sites. Permanent epilation of the eyebrows occurs after a fractionated dose of 30 Gy over 3 weeks. Fractionated doses of 20 Gy cause reddening with vascular prominence, and as the orthovoltage dose approaches 40 to 50 Gy, a confluent mucositis appears. At this stage, the lacrimal gland has thick secretions, and the eye easily becomes infected. During this period, the patient may experience photophobia. Lacrimal glands are relatively resistant to radiation and most patients tolerate fractionated therapy schemes to total doses of 30 to 40 Gy without severe symptoms of a dry eye. Atrophy of the glands occurs at cumulative fractionated doses in the range of 50 to 60 Gy. The sclera is quite resistant to radiation effects, although damage has been reported in cases of application of beta-emitting plaques where the doses exceeded 20 Gy in a single exposure. The iris of the eye can be affected, and fractionated doses in excess of 70 Gy can produce an acute iritis.

The cornea demonstrates very few effects until fractionated doses are in the range of 50 Gy. At that point, a superficial punctate keratitis may develop. Deep keratitis and ulceration of the cornea are quite rare unless very high doses are given over a short time period. Changes in the choroid, lens, retina, and optic nerve are almost never seen in the acute period. The changes seen during the acute clinical period are not pathognomonic of radiation, and an effort must be made to ensure that they are not due to infection. At very high dose levels (which may sometimes result from combining several radiotherapy schemes), if the dose level reaches 100 Gy over the course of a year, a panophthalmitis, which may require enucleation, can develop. At least one report of spontaneous corneal rupture after strontium irradiation for a conjunctival carcinoma has been published. This may have been a complication of the tumor rather than a radiation effect alone.[103]

In the period from 6 months to 2 years (subacute clinical period), telangiectasia may develop in the skin and the conjunctiva. During that time, scarring of the cornea may progress if deep keratitis was present during the acute period. Hemorrhage into the vitreous and retina may occur from telangiectatic changes in the retina. Areas of fluffy exudate may be seen in the retina and the choroid, with associated atrophy.[1]

Radiation retinopathy, as a complication of radiotherapy, was described as early as 1930. It can be produced by external beam radiotherapy at doses as low as 15 Gy, but is more common at fractionated doses of 30 to 35 Gy. At total fractionated doses of 70 to 80 Gy, retinopathy will occur in 85% of eyes. Exudates, hemorrhages, microaneurysms, cotton wool spots, telangiectasia, and retinal capillary nonperfusion occur at 4 to 36 months (mean 18 months) after radiotherapy. The earliest changes identified by fluorescein angiography are capillary dilatation, closure, and microaneurysm formation (predominantly on the arterial side). Telangiectatic vessels are a feature of established retinopathy.[104,105] Up to 60% of patients surviving bone marrow transplant therapy after chemotherapy and total-body radiation may develop occlusive microvascular retinopathy.[106]

Several authors have reported on the MRI appearance of radiation-induced optic neuropathy.[107–109] In general, there was gadolinium enhancement of the optic nerve with slight swelling even 6 to 36 months postradiotherapy with dose levels in the range of 55 to 62 Gy.

Cataracts are the most frequent delayed reaction in the eye. Cataracts have been identified as a late effect in atomic bomb survivors and in multiple accidental exposures. The term *cataract* often connotes blindness or at least impaired vision; the vast majority of radiation "cataracts" identified in the atomic bomb survivors were nonprogressive and did not impair vision. There appeared to be a threshold dose below which lenticular opacities were not found.[110,111] A study of the atomic bomb survivors has indicated that the lenses of children may be more sensitive to the induction of cataracts by ionizing radiation than those of adults.[112] The study was based on examination of over 2300 individuals. In Hiroshima, the relative risk for axial opacities and posterior subcapsular changes was 4.8 for individuals exposed to more than 3 Sv while under the age of 15 years. In the age group 15 to 24 years at the time of the bombing, the relative risk was 2.3 as compared with 1.4 in the age group over 25 years. With regard to posterior subcapsular changes alone, the relative risk was 2.8 in the 1 to 1.99 Sv group under the age of 15 years and 4.3 in the 2 to 2.99 Sv group.

Subsequent reports to elucidate the potential effect of neutron exposure (which was higher at Hiroshima than at Nagasaki) have been published. Unfortunately, the answer is not clear because revisions in the dosimetry (DS 86) reduced the estimated neutron component at Hiroshima.[113,114] Another problem is that the posterior lenticular opacities are only present in 76 of the 1983 persons in whom DS 86 dosimetry was available. It should be noted that the posterior lenticular opacities referred to in the atomic bomb survivors are quite subtle and can easily be confused with sequelae of trauma or normal variants in lens structure. Thus, only an ophthalmologist who is very experienced in radiation effects may be able to provide an accurate assessment.

Radiation cataracts are among the few lesions that pathologically are quite characteristic for radiation injury. Most senile cataracts begin in the anterior pole of the lens, whereas radiation cataracts begin as a small dot in the posterior pole. Perhaps the best description of radiogenic cataracts in the literature is that of Cogan et al.[115] As the opacity develops in the posterior pole and enlarges to 3 to 4 mm, a central clear area may be identified. Ultimately, the cataract may progress to the anterior pole of the lens, with development of a nonspecific cataract. Even though the cataract initially appears clinically in the posterior pole, the pathogenesis of the radiation cataract is usually damage to the epithelial cells of the anterior lens. With the inhibition of mitosis and actively proliferating cells, there is interference with differentiation. The damaged cells migrate toward the posterior pole, where they undergo degeneration. While posterior cataracts are characteristic of radiation exposure, they are not pathognomonic; in other words, there are other causes that can result in posterior cataracts.

Lens opacities do not always interfere with vision, and thus a clinical cataract requires higher doses. The latent period for production of cataracts from the time of exposure may range from 0.5 to 35 years, although, on the average, it is 2 to 3 years. The higher the absorbed dose, the shorter is the latent period. The incidence of radiation cataracts is dose, time, and age dependent[116] (Figure 6.6). Single doses of 2 Gy or fractionated doses of 4 Gy can result in the formation of lens opacities.[117] A single dose of 7.5 Gy causes cataract formation in all those exposed. A similar incidence occurs with 14 Gy given over a period of 3 to 12 weeks. In situations in which occupational exposure occurs over a period of years, the threshold for cataract formation appears to be between 6 and 14 Gy.[118,119] Studies of adults who indicate radiation cataracts as a potential complication of radiotherapy as adults have been performed. Sakai et al.[120] report that of 171 patients treated for maxillary carcinoma who survived for 10 years all developed a cataract on the treated side. Studies of children treated for neoplasm relative to the risk of cataracts is hampered, somewhat, by the use of corticosteroids. Many of these patients have received long-term steroids. Posterior subcapsular cataracts have been observed by Ogelsby et al.[121] in 42% of patients with rheumatic disease who were treated with long-term steroids. A corticosteroid-induced cataract is similar to that produced by ionizing radiation. Cataract formation has been reported by Heyn et al.[122] in 90% of children who were treated for orbital rhabdomyosarcoma. Doses to the lens were calculated from less than

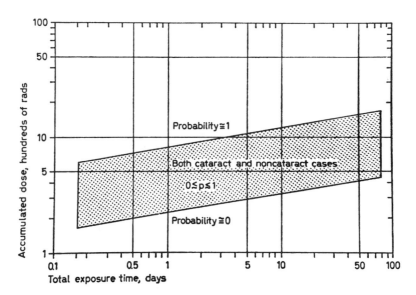

FIGURE 6.6 Probability of cataract formation as a function of dose and exposure time. (From Merriam, G.R., Jr., Szechter, A., and Focht, E.F., in *Frontiers of Radiation Therapy and Oncology*, Vol. 6, Karger, Basel, 1972. With permission.)

10 Gy to greater than 50 Gy, and the appearance of the cataract ranged from 1 to 4 years after radiotherapy.

The incidence of cataracts in children treated for acute leukemia varies widely depending on what literature is examined. Nesbit et al.[123] reported that 2% of survivors of acute leukemia develop posterior subcapsular cataracts, whereas Inati et al.[124] observed a 50% increase in cataract formation in children who were given 24 Gy of fractionated therapy over 2½ weeks; however, these children also received methotrexate and steroids. The incidence of cataracts following bone marrow transplantation in almost 300 patients has indicated that after 10 Gy of single-dose, whole-body radiation, 80% of children will develop cataracts by 6 years compared with 19% given fractionated whole-body radiation of 12 to 15 Gy in 2 to 5 fractions.[125–127] Fractionation for this type of radiation therapy significantly reduces the incidence of cataracts. If a dose of 12 to 15 Gy is given over 6 to 7 days, the cataract incidence is reduced from 50 to 18%. These studies also indicated that about 20% of children treated for aplastic anemia with steroids and given no radiation also developed cataracts. Similar data have been reported by other authors.[128,129] In these cases, the development of cataracts is thought to be of secondary importance since, if and when they occur, they may be surgically corrected.

HIGH-LET RADIATION

Neutrons are known to be especially effective in the formation of cataracts. The literature predominantly concerns animals and indicates that the RBE ranges between 4.5 for 1.8 MeV neutrons and 9 for 0.43 MeV neutrons.[130] Cyclotron workers exposed to neutrons were originally thought to have some changes in the lens, although the doses of neutrons were extremely difficult to calculate and the study was a retrospective analysis of only affected persons.[131] In patients undergoing radiotherapy with fast neutrons, no changes were observed with doses of less than 0.8 Gy given as 12 fractions, but there was a minimal permanent loss of vision at doses totaling more than 2.2 Gy.[132]

Direct Effects of Radiation on Specific Tissues

RADIONUCLIDE IRRADIATION

Beta radiation induction of cataracts following the application of strontium-90 plaques has been examined.[133,134] In the past, strontium-90 applicators were used for orbital radiotherapy in the hope that the beta radiation would not cause damage to structures such as the lens. In fact, unique radiation cataracts occur, with the opacities occurring anteriorly in the lens. The average latent period is 2½ years, and doses causing these changes were similar to those identified for radium applicators. The incidence of lenticular changes ranged from approximately 20% at a dose level of 1.8 to 7.2 Gy, to 42% at 7.2 to 12 Gy, and 73% at doses in excess of 12 Gy to the lens.

SALIVARY GLANDS

GENERAL

Radiation effects on the salivary glands are important following accidents involving whole-body exposure or irradiation of the head and neck. Many patients in criticality accidents and industrial irradiation accidents (Chapters 11 and 13) present with swollen and tender parotid and submandibular glands in the first several hours. This is a reliable clinical indicator of penetrating radiation doses in excess of 2 Gy.

The salivary glands include the parotid, submaxillary, and sublingual glands. They each have secretions that enter the oral cavity through a duct. Both the parenchymal cells of the gland and the duct cells behave as reverting postmitotic cells and, therefore, are relatively resistant to direct effects of radiation. The major exceptions are the relatively large excretory ducts of the parotid, which contain stratified epithelium near the main outlet (similar to that of the oral mucosa, which has vegetative intermitotic cells in the basal layer), and are, therefore, relatively radiosensitive. The pathological effects of radiation on these glands have been well described by Rubin and Casarett,[1] Fajardo,[2] and Ang et al.[135] Most of the data concerning these structures are derived from radiotherapy experience; however, some human data concerning large single absorbed doses are available.

LOW-LET RADIATION

During the acute clinical period, marked swelling of the salivary glands may follow a large dose of irradiation. These changes are predominantly due to increased permeability of the capillaries and may be seen as early as 4 h. This has been described in accidental situations with estimated acute whole-body doses above about 4 Gy. The effects of single acute doses have been studied by Kashima et al.[136] These authors reported results for 33 patients who had received single high doses in the range of 9 to 20 Gy for malignancies in the pharynx. Surgery was performed 24 h after the single dose, and pathological study revealed both neutrophilic and eosinophilic infiltration of the interstitial tissues in the serous acinar tissue. Necrotic cell debris was seen in the ducts. The mucous glands showed little change. Such acute changes usually subside within a few days, even if there are to be later changes of xerostomia. The rise in serum amylase elevation may be a reasonably useful biochemical and biologic dosimeter in cases of accidental radiation exposure. Kashima et al.[136] indicate that a single dose in the region of 1 to 4 Gy will result in hyperamylasemia of 1000 Somogyi units in 24 to 72 h. Those patients who receive less than 10 Gy rarely had elevations in excess of 600 Somogyi units. The peak activity may be identified in 9 to 48 h; these reported enzyme elevations followed treatment of all of the salivary glands.

During a fractionated course of radiotherapy, however, there is rarely any swelling seen early, and dryness of the mouth may occur in 3 to 4 weeks. At that time, there is a rise in the serum amylase level, which can be as much as 10 to 20 times preirradiation levels. Other enzymes, including serum glutamic-oxaloacetic transaminase (SGOT), serum glutamic-pyruvic transaminase

(SGPT), lactate dehydrogenase (LDH), and alkaline phosphatase, remain normal. As one might expect, urinary excretion of amylase also increases.

RESPIRATORY TRACT

The respiratory tract is relatively radiosensitive and radiation effects on this system have been the cause of many deaths in radiation accidents. Pulmonary radiation effects were a common cause of fatality in the radiotherapy accident in Zaragoza (Spain), the industrial irradiator accident in Nesvizh, and the 1999 criticality accident in Tokaimura Japan. Even with advanced medical techniques, at doses in excess of 10 Gy respiratory tract injury is one of the major impediments to survival.

TRACHEA

Radiation effects on the trachea have rarely been of clinical importance. In the radiotherapy accident in Costa Rica, high doses to the mediastinum resulted in six fatalities (see Chapter 21). At autopsy, these patients were reported to have tracheal, laryngeal, and bronchial necrosis. Five of these six patients had doses ranging from 62 to 92 Gy in about 20 fractions of about 3 to 4 Gy.

LUNG

The lung is a relatively radiosensitive organ. An extensive review of the literature on pulmonary responses has been published by Van den Brenk.[137] More recent reviews have been written by Davis et al.[138] and Molls and van Beuningen.[139] The radiosensitivity of the lung is a limiting factor in total-body radiotherapy for treatment of diffuse metastases and prior to bone marrow transplantation.[140] In single-dose treatment, 8 Gy is the accepted maximum since single doses of 7 to 8 Gy may produce radiation pneumonitis. Massive doses to the thorax have occasionally occurred in accidental criticality situations, as well as in industrial irradiator accidents.

Until the last decade, accidental acute whole-body exposures in the range above 4 Gy resulted in death from bone marrow failure and at doses above 6 Gy gastrointestinal damage and fluid and electrolyte loss were causes of death. With advances in critical care and current supportive and prophylactic care, these are no longer the major limiting factor. In recent accidents in Nesvizh (Belarus) and Tokaimura (Japan), the patients were kept alive for several months. They ultimately died of multiorgan failure, but radiation pneumonitis and superimposed pulmonary infection were predominant factors. It appears that at the present time, the radiosensitivity of the lung is a limiting factor for survival at dose levels above 9 to 10 Gy.

The major changes following fractionated pulmonary radiation therapy are radiation pneumonitis (sometimes referred to as *acute radiation pneumonitis*, or ARP) and subsequent pulmonary fibrosis. The exact mechanism of radiation pneumonitis is unclear, but it involves loss of some of the epithelial cells, presence of exudative fluid in the alveolar space, and subsequent thickening of the alveolar walls. In addition to these findings, there have been reported associations with adult respiratory distress syndrome[141] and bronchiolitis obliterans.[142] Recently, some authors have suggested that radiation pneumonitis is the result of a lymphocyte-mediated hypersensitivity reaction, because after unilateral thoracic radiation there was an increase in both lymphocyte lavage and gallium concentration in both lungs.[143] It should be pointed out that many heavily irradiated patients are also immune compromised, and show a higher incidence of infectious pneumonias such as cytomegalovirus and pneumocystis carinii. Whether radiation pneumonitis can be reduced in severity by concurrent treatment with corticosteroids is a subject of debate.[144] Because many patients undergoing radiotherapy are also relatively immunosuppressed, some radiation oncologists also administer broad-spectrum antibiotics when a "pneumonitis" is identified.

Low-LET Radiation

Classic radiation pneumonitis, first described by Grover in 1929, characteristically occurs 3 to 16 weeks after the cessation of radiotherapy. It is characterized by dry cough, rales, dyspnea, and fever. If both lungs are involved, severe respiratory distress, cyanosis, cor pulmonale, and even death from cardiorespiratory failure may occur. The diagnosis is usually made on the basis of radiographic findings of pneumonitis limited to the field of X-ray therapy. Pleural effusions may occur, but they are uncommon.[145] Time, dose, and volume aspects are of particular importance in the development of clinical radiation pneumonitis.

On the basis of several studies, a clinical threshold of 6 to 7 Gy for single doses has been suggested for the development of acute pneumonitis. A single dose of 10 Gy to both lungs will cause pneumonitis in 84% of patients. This percentage is reduced to about 30% if the single dose is 8 Gy. With a dose of 26.5 Gy in 20 fractions over 4 weeks to both lungs, 5% of patients develop pneumonitis. Similarly, 5% of patients receiving a total dose of 20 Gy in 10 fractions over 2 weeks to 1 month develop pneumonitis. As the dose is increased to 30.5 Gy in 20 fractions over 4 weeks to both lungs, 50% of patients will develop pneumonitis, and all patients receiving 30 Gy over 2 weeks in 10 fractions to one lung will develop pneumonitis. Scott and Hahn[146] have shown a clear relationship between dose protraction and mortality as a result of pulmonary injury (Figure 6.7).

There is a delay between radiation exposure and expression of injury (Figure 6.8). Abrupt withdrawal of corticosteroids can unmask subclinical pneumonitis. Clinical radiation pneumonitis is represented pathologically by atypical epithelial cells with congested capillaries and hyaline membrane formation lining the alveolar spaces. In addition, there are mononuclear infiltrates in the alveolar septa.

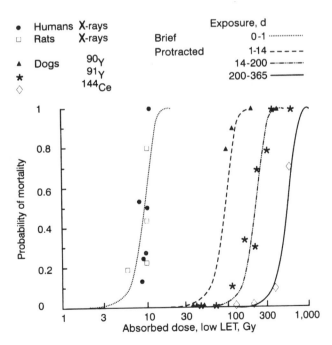

FIGURE 6.7 Relationship between protraction of lung dose and mortality. (From Scott and Hahn.[146])

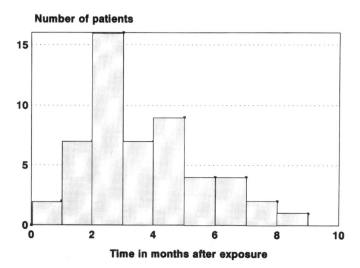

FIGURE 6.8 Radiation pneumonitis.. The time course of radiation pneumonitis in 38 patients is shown graphically in (D). (Adapted from van Dyk, J., Keane, T., Kan, S. et al., *Int. J. Radiat. Oncol. Biol. Phys.*, 7:461–467, 1981.)

At Chernobyl in 1986, there were eight patients who developed ARP and all of them had acute whole-body doses of 6.7 to 11 Gy. Those with doses in the range above 8.8 Gy died in 14 to 24 days with ARP as a major contributing cause.

Radiation pneumonitis was also reported as a cause of death in a patient involved in the commercial irradiator accident in Soreq (Israel) accident in 1990. The estimated dose was 10 to 20 Gy and death occurred on day 36. Another similar radiation accident experience in Nesvizh (Belarus) involved an individual who was exposed in a facility used for sterilization of medical supplies. There was a nonuniform acute whole-body exposure in the range of 16 Gy. Normally, the patient would have succumbed to a bone marrow syndrome; however, Russian physicians, using their experience from Chernobyl, were able to keep the individual alive until there was marrow regeneration. This was probably the first such individual ever to survive this level of acute exposure. Unfortunately, radiation pneumonitis occurred, and the individual died from pulmonary insufficiency about 90 days postexposure (Chapter 12). A similar experience occurred to two patients in the Tokaimura accident (Chapter 11).

The imaging findings associated with radiation pneumonitis have been discussed by many authors.[147–149] The radiological manifestation of radiation pneumonitis is a hazy alveolar infiltrate corresponding to the shape of the radiation port field. As the fibrotic stage progresses, atelectasis, pleural reaction, volume loss, and even calcified plaques may be identified. Radiographic changes of pneumonitis are rare for a dose less than 30 Gy in 3 weeks, but are common when the dose exceeds 40 Gy in 4 weeks. Fibrotic changes appear if the dose exceeds 60 Gy delivered over 6 weeks.

In general, more changes are seen on CT than on standard chest radiographs. Homogeneous or patchy areas of lung opacification and volume loss are the principal findings. The abnormalities are usually, but not always, confined to the radiation fields and are seen in about 80 to 90% of patients within 16 weeks of ending fractionated radiotherapy to the lung, but they may be seen as early as 2 to 4 weeks. At later times, fibrosis may be seen.

The main permanent change that may occur is pulmonary fibrosis or sclerosis, which may occur in patients who have never clinically manifested ARP. If the fibrotic changes are widespread enough, reduction in the pulmonary function of the patient may result. As with most other tissues, the volume irradiated is particularly important in the ability of the patient to tolerate the changes. Irradiation of the total lung may cause reduction in volume and diffusing capacity.[150-152] When smaller volumes of lung are irradiated, diffusing capacity may still be reduced, although patients with previously existing chronic obstructive pulmonary disease (COPD) appear to tolerate the radiation as well as patients without COPD.[153]

The pathology of the chronic or late effects includes replacement of the septa by collagen, reduction in the number of functional capillaries, and decreased volume of aerated alveolar space. This may be a function of ischemia because there is myointimal proliferation of the arterioles, and foamy cells in the intima may be seen. The clinical manifestations include reduction in pulmonary function in the irradiated area, with consolidation, volume loss, and susceptibility to infection (particularly fungal infection).

A large amount of literature is available concerning radiation pneumonitis and late pulmonary function after radiotherapy of adults. The largest literature probably concerns women who received chest wall irradiation for breast cancer. With tangential fields, lung changes should be in the range of 1 to 2% and with a much lower incidence than was seen with earlier radiotherapy methods, and small and reversible changes in pulmonary function may occur.[154,155] In general, the reliability of radiographic, CT, or nuclear medicine findings for prediction of clinical symptoms or amount of ultimate fibrosis has been poor.[156,157]

There is also a great deal of experience and literature relative to pulmonary reactions after radiotherapy in children. Wohl et al.[158] studied children who are survivors of Wilms' tumors irradiated with a median fractionated lung dose of 20 Gy and at age 2 to 4 years. A number of these patients subsequently had dyspnea and interstitial and pleural thickening. A similar study was performed by Littman et al.[159] and, in the study, vital capacity and functional residual capacity were lower in the irradiated group. Both Green et al.[160] and Shaw et al.[161] have reported on the follow-up of patients treated for Wilms' tumor. In these patients sometimes the pneumonitis was traced to an infectious etiology, and in those patients receiving whole-lung irradiation there was reduced pulmonary function.

A number of studies report on patients who have been followed for Hodgkin's disease. In general, those patients who received mantle field therapy with a dose in the range of 20 to 55 Gy demonstrated restricted lung volume and reduced total lung capacity.[162,163] Tarbell et al.[164] have reported on patients treated for Hodgkin's disease with mantle therapy (usually 23 to 43 Gy in 26 fractions); there was about a 3% incidence of radiation pneumonitis, but this rose to about 15% when there was whole-lung radiotherapy. In a group of patients followed by Gustavsson et al.[165] for 10 to 20 years there was right ventricular hypertrophy in half the patients, defects on lung perfusion scintigraphy in 80%, and slight to moderate pulmonary fibrosis in 70%. The abnormalities were generally clinically insignificant. Springmeyer et al.[166] examined patients after bone marrow transplantation for assorted conditions. This generally involved whole-body radiation, and analysis of 79 patients demonstrated restrictive ventilatory changes, with a loss of total lung capacity of almost 1 l.

Whether prednisone and steroid administration affect the development of the fibrosis remains uncertain; however, the effect, if any, is not significant. Inflammatory changes in the bronchi are seen but are generally expressions of superimposed bacterial infections rather than true radiation changes.

High-LET Radiation

Significant human data have not been reported for the RBE of neutrons in humans. Pi-meson treatment of pulmonary metastases in doses of 3980 pion rad in 23 fractions over 4 weeks can produce pneumonitis. There are some data on the normal tissue reactions following high-energy neutron beam therapy, and Cohen et al.[167] indicate that 20 Gy in 12 fractions over 4 weeks represents a practical tolerance limit for most sites.

Radionuclide Irradiation

Although extensive research has focused on inhalation of radionuclides by animals, there is very limited and confusing information with regard to humans. Predicting results of significant internal contamination via inhalation is difficult because the distribution of radionuclide deposition depends initially upon size of the particles inhaled and ultimately upon the solubility of the compound both in the lungs and in the lymph nodes.

The major human database concerning radionuclide inhalation comes from uranium miners who inhale dust, radon, and radon daughter products. Well-documented studies have indicated a higher incidence of lung carcinoma, although the exact relationship to smoking is unknown. Pulmonary fibrosis is difficult to evaluate in uranium miners because they usually have accompanying silicosis and emphysema. A fivefold excess mortality from nonmalignant respiratory diseases (other than tuberculosis) has been found in the Colorado plateau miners.[168] Excess deaths were from silicosis, emphysema, and fibrosis. There was a suggestion in these miners that radon daughter exposure reduced ventilatory function and contributed to the development of emphysema. Even though exposure of animals to high levels of radon daughters leads to interstitial changes and emphysema,[169] most researchers feel that the human epidemiological studies have been unable to separate the possible effects of radon exposure from those of the other occupational exposures.[170] There is some experience with inhalation of plutonium in 26 Manhattan Project workers at Los Alamos Laboratories. An extensive medical follow-up of these workers over 42 years has been performed; no clinically significant deterministic pulmonary changes have been reported.

A report of one patient who ostensibly developed pulmonary fibrosis as a result of thorotrast administration is reported by De Vuyst et al.[171] Whether this case was due to thorotrast or to idiopathic pulmonary fibrosis is unknown. The proportion of thorotrast that is deposited in the lungs is typically only 0.7%, and there would be an estimated average dose to the main pulmonary bronchi of about 0.13 Gy/year.[172] There has been discussion whether pulmonary fibrosis can be the result of occupational inhalation of lanthanides. A pulmonary syndrome is induced by stable rare earths that is not the result of radioactivity.[173]

HEART AND VESSELS

GENERAL

Radiation effects on the heart itself have only been important in massive radiation exposure (Los Alamos criticality, 1958) and are probably a secondary contributing cause to death. Radiation therapy accidents with mediastinal fields have resulted in pericardial effusions and constrictive pericarditis (Costa Rica, 1996). Radiation effects on large peripheral blood vessels are important in accidental high-dose localized exposures since high doses can cause rupture or stenosis. Such effects have occurred in accidents where intensely radioactive industrial radiography sources were placed in pockets or in accidental overdoses in radiotherapy of the neck, shoulder, or groin.

Low-LET RADIATION

Throughout the literature, particularly the early literature, the heart and great vessels were considered to be radioresistant organs. One of the major reasons for this belief was that it was not technically possible to limit radiation therapy to the mediastinal structures without irradiating large portions of the lung that were much more radiosensitive. With appropriate technical advances, it has been possible to localize the radiation more accurately, and direct effects of radiation have now been recognized in the cardiac structures themselves.[174,175] Late effects of radiotherapy on the cardiovascular system include cardiomyopathy, coronary artery disease, pericardial effusions, and constrictive pericarditis.[176]

The myocardium is composed of striated muscle fibers with essentially no regenerative ability. They are classified as fixed postmitotic cells and are thus very resistant to direct effects of radiation. The myocardium itself appears capable of withstanding fractionated radiotherapy doses as high as 100 Gy without obvious clinical or microscopic changes being identified. In one case of exposure to iridium-192 radiography source, there was localized myocardial damage. In that case, the absorbed dose to the myocardium was not calculated; however, the dose was high enough that there was necrosis of the overlying skin, soft tissue, and rib.[177]

There appears to be a great deal of confusion concerning whether radiation can produce myocarditis. The diagnosis of myocarditis prior to 1987 was not well defined; however, after this time, criteria have been proposed.[178] By definition, the diagnosis of myocarditis can be made only if myocyte necrosis or degeneration or both are associated with an inflammatory infiltrate adjacent to the myocytes. Most authors who discuss myocarditis indicate that ionizing radiation is not a cause.[179] With extremely acute doses of radiation (in excess of 30 Gy), edema may be present in the myocardium and cellular infiltrates due to the leakage from the vasculature. This has been reported only in one or two accidental situations where the individual died from other causes within a few days,[180] and the case occurred long before there was an agreed pathological definition of myocarditis.

Radiation changes in the myocardium are probably more correctly called radiation cardiomyopathy. The interval between radiation and development of these changes usually exceeds 10 years. The specific pathological changes seen are similar to idiopathic cardiomyopathy, with a variable amount of interstitial fibrosis and myocardial cell hypertrophy. Overall, data suggests that 40 Gy of fractionated dose is considered a threshold for clinical cardiomyopathy in both adults and children.

"Radiation-induced heart disease" (RIHD) has been described by Stewart et al.[181,182] The majority of these changes have been demonstrated in patients who have received mediastinal irradiation for Hodgkin's disease. The changes most commonly involve the pericardium rather than the heart muscle (myocardium). The changes seen in the pericardium include pericardial effusion, fibrosis, and possibly subsequent constrictive pericarditis. Expressed somewhat differently, pericardial or myocardial disease has been observed in 6 to 7% of patients who have received a mean fractionated total dose of 42.8 Gy in a radiation therapeutic scheme to a large volume of the heart. Administration of 40 Gy in 16 fractions over 4 weeks has been reported to result in pericarditis in about 5% of patients.[183,184] Patients being treated for Hodgkin's disease demonstrate a high incidence of complications when the total dose exceeds 60 Gy.

Carmel and Kaplan[185] reported that pericarditis occurred in 7% of patients who were treated for Hodgkin's disease who had total doses of less than 6 Gy and that this rose to 12% at 6 to 15 Gy, 19% at 15 to 30 Gy, and in 50% of those who received more than 30 Gy.

The fine blood vessels and the connective tissue cells of the heart are only moderately resistant. Following irradiation, both the epicardium and pericardium may demonstrate dense fibrosis, but this always appears to be most prominent in the pericardium. The epicardium may be covered by a thick film of fibrin indistinguishable grossly from fibrinous pericarditis. In the late stages, the myocardium can show diffuse fibrosis, with bands of dense collagen. The exact mechanism of the pericardial fibrosis is uncertain, although ischemia undoubtedly plays a large role.

Brosius et al.[186] performed both clinical and autopsy studies on 16 patients who had received more than 35 Gy in fractionated radiotherapy to the heart 5 to 144 months before death. The patients were between 15 and 33 years old. Essentially all of the patients had thickened pericardium, and eight had some interstitial myocardial fibrosis. There was epicardial coronary artery narrowing seen in almost half the patients who were studied, compared with only 10% of the control subjects. Damage to individual myocardial cells was not detected in any patient by histological study. The authors themselves point out that the high incidence of changes here may be due to the fact that a number of study patients were irradiated with techniques now considered unacceptable by most modern radiotherapists.

Damage to large blood vessels has been reported, although it is much less common than capillary and arteriolar damage. Many case reports of damage to large blood vessels concern patients who have atherosclerotic degenerative changes.[2,187,188] Thus, the causal relationship with radiation has been impossible to prove. Fajardo[2] indicates that spontaneous rupture of large vessels is often blamed on radiation. He has reviewed more than 90 such cases (most of which were fatal) and concluded that in no more than 5 of the 90 cases did radiation appear to be the cause. One case that did appear to be radiation related was adult unilateral occlusion of a pulmonary artery.[189] Many studies in animals have concerned the relationship of radiation with the induction or acceleration of atherosclerosis. These studies confirm that in animals, at least, coronary and proximal atherosclerosis have not been produced by radiation alone.[2] In spite of the animal data, there are a number of articles in the literature indicating narrowed or occluded coronary arteries years after radiotherapy.[190–196]

There are a large number of recent reports regarding higher-than-expected incidence of atherosclerosis and/or stenosis in major arteries.[197] These include the carotid artery,[198–201] brachial artery,[202,203] as well as the aorta[204] and pelvic vessels.[205] Most patients received fractionated radiotherapy in the range of 40 to 70 Gy. In at least one study of carotid disease by Moritz et al.,[206] 30% of patients who received fractionated radiotherapy of 50 Gy had moderate or severe carotid lesions compared with 6% of control patients. In another study by Goodman et al.[207] patients treated for seminoma with unilateral pelvic irradiation with 25 to 26 Gy were followed for an average of 9 years. Only 3 of 19 developed vascular abnormalities, and in 2 patients this was bilateral, indicating that radiation was not likely to be the cause. In the third patient the abnormalities were subclinical.

In these reports arterial lesions tended to develop about 3 to 10 years after radiotherapy. Lesions have been reported as occurring as early as 1 month; however, this does not make sense on a radiobiological basis and almost certainly represents a preexisting lesion. Many patients being treated for tumors with radiotherapy are older and have preexisting cardiovascular disease, and this represents a major bias factor in the case reports. Very few controlled studies are available. In most papers, smoking, as well as the radiation, was thought to play a significant role in the development of atheromatous lesions.

Examination of small arteries, arterioles, and capillaries is most important since changes in these structures are undoubtedly responsible for most delayed radiation injury.[2,208–210] Most veins are relatively resistant to radiation, although phlebosclerosis is occasionally seen and rarely there can be thrombosis of the main hepatic vein.[211] Injury to capillaries has been demonstrated after a single dose to the skin as low as 4 Gy. Smooth-muscle cells and elastic tissues present in large arteries are quite radioresistant. Endothelial cells appear to be the most radiosensitive portions of the entire vascular system. Because capillaries consist only of endothelial cells and are of small diameter, the degenerative changes become apparent earlier in small vessels than in larger vessels. Initially, radiation, even at low doses, causes an increase in capillary permeability, separation of the cell junctions, necrosis or loss of endothelial cells, and damage to the basement membrane. Endothelial renewal and the myointimal proliferation that occur can be concentric but more often are eccentric, causing narrowing or occlusion of the lumen. It should be noted that all capillaries are not equally radiosensitive, e.g., pulmonary capillaries are more sensitive than myocardial capillaries.[212] Overall, it appears that radiation injury to the microvasculature is the most important factor in delayed nonstochastic effects of radiation, particularly in those tissues that have parenchymal cells that are of the slow or nonrenewal type. There are some reports of increased mortality from circulatory diseases in atomic bomb survivors. This is discussed in the section on radiation-induced life shortening near the end of this chapter.

GASTROINTESTINAL TRACT

Radiation effects on the gastrointestinal tract are a major concern and cause of death in radiation accidents. Many patients with whole-body exposure above several gray will acutely develop nausea, vomiting, and diarrhea. Unless a radiation source is known and the effects appreciated, these finding are often misdiagnosed as infectious gastroenteritis or food poisoning. Mucositis is common in patients who have been exposed in industrial irradiator accidents and at Chernobyl.

In many accidental situations, the exposed person(s) are usually facing the radiation source and, as a result, the anterior abdomen usually receives a higher dose than other parts of the body. This inhomogeneous dose distribution and the relative sensitivity of the intestine are causes of death in many accidents. Various portions of the gastrointestinal tract are involved. As an example, in the commercial irradiator accident in Soreq (Israel) in 1990, the patient received an estimated dose of 10 to 20 Gy. He died on day 36 postexposure and the autopsy indicated severe erosive esophagitis and gastritis, complete loss of crypt anatomy, denudation of the epithelium of the small bowel, and edema, thrombosis and pseudomembrane formation in the colon. In a similar accident in Belarus in 1991, the operator received 11 to 20 Gy and he died on day 113. At autopsy there was almost complete denudation of the small bowel with some punctate hemorrhages, but the rest of the gastrointestinal tract was almost normal and it was concluded that partial recovery had taken place (Chapter 14). The patients in the Tokaimura (Japan) criticality accident in 1999 had doses estimated to be 17 Gy and 8 Gy. Both had serious problems with diarrhea, gastrointestinal erosions, and bleeding that were contributory causes of death (Chapter 11). The lethal dose in humans as a result of intestinal irradiation is not clear; however, data from animals indicate an LD_{10} of 10 Gy, an LD_{50} of 15 Gy, and an LD_{90} of 20 Gy.

Effects of a given absorbed dose of radiation on the gastrointestinal tract depend significantly on which portion of the tract is irradiated. Radiation sensitivity varies markedly between the midportion and the ends: the esophagus and rectum are relatively radiation resistant, and the midportions, including the stomach and small intestine, are more sensitive. The reader is referred to a book chapter on the subject by Trott and Herrmann.[213]

With single acute doses to the abdominal region of 10 to 15 Gy, there is rather rapid development of a *gastrointestinal syndrome*. This is manifest initially by diarrhea. At acute doses of 4 to 6 Gy there is the onset of mild diarrhea in <10% of persons at 3 to 8 h postexposure. At doses over 6 Gy the situation changes dramatically. At 6 to 8 Gy over 10% will experience heavy diarrhea in 1 to 3 h and above 8 Gy almost all exposed persons will have heave diarrhea within 1 h.

With fractionation of the radiation dose, the gastrointestinal tract can tolerate much higher absorbed doses. In conventional radiotherapy, doses of up to 40 Gy are tolerated; however, patients receiving 45 to 54 Gy have about a 25% risk of stomach ulcer formation, with occasional perforation of the ulcers.[214,215]

ORAL CAVITY AND PHARYNX

Low-LET Radiation

The epithelial lining of the mouth and pharynx are somewhat more sensitive than the skin because the renewal rate of their cells is higher. Mucositis has been reported in a large number of radiation accidents. At Chernobyl it occurred at a relatively low gamma dose (1 to 2 Gy) and on day 4 to 6 postexposure, but this probably was due to a combined beta/gamma exposure where the beta dose was 10 to 20 times higher than the gamma dose (see Chapter 12). In other accidents, mucositis has been described in almost all patients receiving acute doses in excess of 6 Gy.

The standard descriptions of adverse effects from radiation therapy assume either orthovoltage radiation with 2 Gy five times a week for a total of 50 Gy in 5 weeks or irradiation with cobalt-60 with a daily dose of 2 Gy and a weekly dose of 12 Gy to a total level of 60 Gy in 5 weeks. Because there is increased sensitivity of the mucosa compared with skin, changes of radiomucositis will be noted before radiation dermatitis. In the acute period, the mechanisms of injury are quite similar but vary in time of expression.

At the end of the second week of radiotherapy and dose levels of 20 to 24 Gy, dysphasia, soreness, and pain, as well as dryness of the mouth occur, and taste is deteriorated further. There is definite erythema, and patchy mucositis of the palate may be noted. At 30 to 36 Gy, the saliva is thick, and mucositis is identified in the region of the tonsils and the posterior pharynx. At levels of 50 to 60 Gy, mucositis develops into a pseudomembrane involving all tissues, including the tongue. Clearing of these changes begins in approximately 2 weeks and is completed within 2 months. The volume of the mucosa irradiated influences the reaction. Higher doses are much better tolerated in small areas than in large areas.

In the chronic period, delayed effects include progressive fibrosis of the submucosa, telangiectasia, and interstitial fibrosis of the mucous glands. Areas adjacent to the mucosa, such as Waldeyer's tonsillar ring, demonstrate marked radiosensitivity of the lymphocytes; however, repopulation occurs quite promptly. There has been a lot of recent interest in use of dental enamel as a biologic dosimeter. Through the use of electron spin resonance, a measure of dose can be determined.[216-218]

Neutron Radiation

Hussey et al.[219] have attempted to obtain an RBE for 50-MeV neutrons by utilizing mucosal reactions in patients. Their best estimate is that in relation to cobalt-60 therapy, the neutron RBE is 2.8.

ESOPHAGUS

Low-LET Radiation

The squamous epithelium of the esophagus has approximately the same turnover rate as oral mucosa and, thus, has about the same radiosensitivity. In spite of this, the esophagus is extremely resistant to radiation when compared with the remainder of the gastrointestinal tract. Esophagitis, dysphasia, and later stricture following radiotherapy and accidental exposures have been reported. The appearance of mucositis in the esophagus is very similar to its appearance in the oropharynx. Symptoms include mild to moderate substernal burning and difficulty in swallowing, beginning at the third week after the initiation of radiotherapy, that are sometimes accompanied by sharp chest pain and can be noted at absorbed dose levels as low as 20 Gy. Doses of 20 to 30 Gy over 2 weeks lead to clinical symptoms of esophagitis; however, they are transient. The esophagus can tolerate fractionated doses up to 60 Gy. At higher doses, stricture, perforation, and obstruction may occur. Lepke and Lubshitz[220] identified 40 patients with functional or morphological abnormalities after radiotherapy. These changes included abnormal motility, mucosal edema, strictures, ulcerations, pseudodiverticula, and fistulae.[221-225] Esophageal motility could be impaired as early as 1 week after radiotherapy, but more generally this finding occurred at 4 to 12 weeks. Strictures were reported to develop 4 to 8 months after completion of radiotherapy. Radiation doses in these patients ranged from 30 Gy in 2 weeks to 65 Gy in $6\frac{1}{2}$ weeks. Strictures occurred after 6 to 8 months in some patients who had received 45 Gy over a period of 4 weeks. Higher doses shortened the interval to occurrence, with strictures developing as early as 3 to 4 months.

At 3 months after the usual course of radiation therapy, epithelial regeneration appears to be complete. The epithelium often is thicker than normal but may show occasional areas of atrophy. As with the skin, small-vessel telangiectasia, fibrosis of the muscularis and submucosa, and intimal fibrosis of the arterioles occur.

Stomach

Low-LET Radiation

The earliest changes due to radiation identified in the stomach were reported in 1912 by Regaud, who noted atrophy of the glands of the fundic portion of the stomach. In the 1940s, following high-dose gastric irradiation, other direct effects of radiation on the stomach became apparent. In a series of 256 patients treated for testicular tumors with retroperitoneal node irradiation, 35 proved to have gastric ulceration.[226] Not only can radiation cause ulcers, but historically radiation therapy was also used for treatment of peptic ulcers.[227] Radiation of 15 Gy given over 10 days has been reported to decrease gastric acidity to 30% of pretreatment levels at 11 months and to 58% of pretreatment levels at 30 months.[228] Doses of 16 Gy given in 10 daily fractions to the stomach cause necrosis of glandular epithelium and loss of chief and parietal cell granules within 6 days after the completion of treatment. By 16 weeks after such a course of therapy, the mucosa histologically returns to normal.[2] Fractionated treatments of the upper abdomen of up to 50 Gy produce nausea and vomiting. In this regard it should be noted that whole-body doses as low as 1 Gy may produce the same symptoms. Radiation ulcers in the stomach are usually single, from 0.5 to 2 cm in diameter and antral in location.[215] They have been reported after fractionated doses to the stomach ranging from 48 to 64 Gy. Patients who develop radiation ulcers usually experience epigastric pain 5 to 6 months after the beginning of therapy.

Small Intestine

Low-LET Radiation

The reader is referred to a comprehensive study of small bowel and large intestine published by Becciolini.[229] The small bowel demonstrates mucosal reactions in radiotherapy schemes in which 30 to 40 Gy are given over 4 weeks. Higher doses may cause obstruction and other complications. Prior surgery, with formation of adhesions, reduces the tolerance of the bowel to radiotherapy. The small intestine is quite sensitive to radiation injury because of the rapidly proliferating cells of the mucosal epithelium in the crypts of Lieberkühn. These columnar cells, which divide approximately once every 24 h, push the more mature cells up the villi to the intestinal lumen, where they mature to their final state when they reach the tips of the villi. The epithelium of the crypt is replaced in fewer than 7 days, making this the most rapidly proliferating tissue and one of the most radiosensitive tissues in the body. The relatively high sensitivity of the mucosal lining compared with underlying vascular and stromal components means that acute changes are of the most clinical significance and that late changes due to arteriolar narrowing rarely occur.

Because the small intestine was relatively inaccessible until the advent of endoscopy, there exists little in the way of human observations. A single case of accidental exposure has been reported.[230] Within 7 days after single doses in excess of 15 Gy, superficial erosion, pyknosis, and sloughing of the epithelium into the lumen occur. At somewhat lower doses, mucosal regeneration begins by 7 days. In therapeutic situations, within 12 to 24 h after daily doses of 1.5 to 3 Gy, cell necrosis in the walls of the crypts can be identified. There is progressive loss of cells, as well as atrophy of the villi. During the period of mucosal sloughing, patients experience nausea, vomiting, cramping, pain, diarrhea, fluid and electrolyte imbalance, and sepsis. Hypoproteinemia due to protein leakage through the damaged mucosal cells may occur.

The pathophysiology of radiation enteritis is poorly understood, and increased prostaglandin levels have been implicated; however, Lifshitz et al.[231] have examined patients receiving radiotherapy and have found no increase in prostaglandin levels. Other investigators have concluded that lactose malabsorption is a factor in the nausea, diarrhea, and vomiting experienced by patients undergoing pelvic radiotherapy.[232] Henriksson et al.[233] have pointed out that sucralfate (an aluminum hydroxide complex of sulfated sucrose) can protect against radiation-induced diarrhea and bowel discomfort in patients receiving bowel radiotherapy. The gastrointestinal syndrome that may occur after a large, single, acute absorbed dose usually results in death. It has historically been described to be a combination of fluid–electrolyte derangement and sepsis. With current medical treatment, acute doses of over 10–15 Gy usually result in mucosal loss and massive small bowel bleeding at 5–20 weeks postexposure. A gastrointestinal radiographic contrast examination of the patient during the acute clinical period generally demonstrates rapid transit time of barium from the stomach to the colon. Hypermotility is demonstrated in just under half of patients receiving radiation therapy to the small bowel. Treatment of acute gastrointestinal injury is discussed in Chapter 5.

During the chronic period, delayed effects are generally manifested as intermittent abdominal pain or obstruction. The diagnosis is difficult to make without the history of radiation exposure. Additional symptoms include occasional bleeding, diarrhea, cramping, abdominal bloating, nausea, vomiting, and laboratory findings of hypoproteinemia and malabsorption. Perkins and Spjut[234] have published a radiological–pathological correlative study of nine patients with radiation injury of the small bowel. In general, barium studies demonstrate a lack of distensibility of a bowel segment without sharp margins and the persistence of edematous-appearing mucosa with a "saw-toothed" appearance.

Complications in patients treated with large-field infradiaphragmatic radiation therapy for Hodgkin's disease and seminoma had complications of gastrointestinal injury, such as peptic ulceration, hemorrhage, chronic diarrhea, and intestinal obstruction. The bowel complications occur in about 1% of patients at doses of less than 35 Gy and 3% for doses equal to or greater than 35 Gy. Histologically, during the subacute and chronic period, the villae of the mucosa are often blunt and thickened, and the mucosal cells are often flattened. The lamina propria may be normal or may demonstrate severe fibrosis. Telangiectasia may occasionally occur, as well. Overall, collagen deposition throughout the submucosa is demonstrated most consistently. The arterioles, as in other tissues, show endothelial proliferation and intimal fibrosis.

COLON, SIGMOID, AND RECTUM

General

The mucosal cells of the colon have a somewhat longer turnover time (4 to 8 days) than those of the small intestine. There are also fewer epithelial cells at risk for a given surface area, and some of the cells remain in prolonged interphase. Thus, the epithelial portions of most of the colon have somewhat less radiosensitivity than the small intestine and about the same radiosensitivity as the esophagus. The blood vessels and underlying muscle have radiosensitivity similar to that of the remainder of the gastrointestinal tract. In spite of this, injury of the large intestine has been important in the medical management of radiation accidents (Figure 6.9). These are usually radiotherapy accidents or acute high-exposure situations with very nonuniform exposure (such as criticality accidents).

Low-LET Radiation

In the large bowel the incidence of severe complications is 40% at a dose of 60 Gy given in 2-Gy fractions. In the Costa Rican radiotherapy accident, there were six patients who died with radiation-related bowel complications and many others with increased morbidity. The specifics of these patients are given in Chapter 21.

The pathological basis of radiation-induced changes in the colon and rectum is similar to that already discussed for the small intestine. Acute changes are easily demonstrated during a course of radiation therapy in which the total dose exceeds 30 to 40 Gy. These changes include hyperemic mucosa and abnormalities in mucus production. Pathologically, the peritoneal surfaces are roughened, with variable amounts of fibrin or fibrous plaques, and shallow mucosal ulcers may be present.

When superficial ulcers appear, the changes are usually relatively well healed within a month. Treatment usually consists of low-residue diets and symptomatic management of diarrhea.[235]

By 6 to 12 months after radiation therapy, the patient may exhibit painless rectal bleeding. In mild stages, the rectal changes consist of mucosal thickening and exudate; however, there may ultimately be progression to ulceration, rectal strictures, or fistulas. The mucous membrane is usually granular, and the ulcers may be either solitary or multiple, usually 1 to 4 cm in diameter, and are located in a transverse direction. The appearance on barium enema in these circumstances may be confused with that of a recurrent tumor.

The best method for determining radiation proctitis is by endoscopy. Gehrig et al.[236] have indicated that after fractionated radiotherapy, the incidence of proctitis 1 to 6 years later is 0% at 40 Gy, 20% at 60 Gy, and 50% at 90 Gy. The most characteristic findings described by other authors[237,238] are arteriolar narrowing, telangiectasia, and diminished distensibility. Some relief of radiation proctosigmoiditis can be achieved through the use of rectal steroids or sucralfate.[239] Occurrence of fistulas, perforation, and small-bowel injury can lead to mortalities in the range of 25%.[240,241]

Chronic changes consist of shortening and fibrosis of the colon, with occasional areas of tapered stenosis. At this stage, the mucosa may be normal or atrophic. Occasionally, mucosal glands are present deep in the muscle, probably as a result of healing ulcers.[242] Treatment of these stenotic areas usually is symptomatic. Dilation is sometimes utilized, although occasionally surgical intervention is necessary. The pathology of the late changes is a result of progressive endarteritis and subsequent fibrosis.

The rectum is relatively resistant to radiation, although loss of the epithelium occurs on a transient basis with doses of 30 to 40 Gy. Chau[243] has reported the incidence of bowel complications in supervoltage pelvic irradiation to a total dose of 60 Gy to be between 1 and 3%. As can be expected, the incidence of acute changes increases dramatically with an increase in the volume of tissue irradiated. Daily doses to the entire abdomen in excess of 1 Gy are usually poorly tolerated.

Neutron Radiation

Few available data concern the RBE of neutrons for the gastrointestinal tract of humans. Data from mice would indicate that the RBE of neutrons with regard to the gastrointestinal tract are higher than for other organ systems.[244,245] Issues related to criticality accidents are discussed in Chapter 11.

LIVER

The liver is affected in most high-dose accidents in criticality and industrial irradiator accidents. Liver abnormalities were also noted in Chernobyl patients. In a number of circumstances, the patients received multiple transfusions and it is often not clear whether the changes are due to radiation or hepatitis from transfusions.

Low-LET Radiation

The hepatic changes generally seen following radiation exposure develop over the first month and persist for many months. Single acute doses above 15 to 20 Gy produced hepatic enlargement with necrosis of hepatocytes, central lobular necrosis, and veno-occlusive liver disease. This has been noted in a number of accidents including the 1990 Soreq (Israel) and the 1991 Nesvizh (Belarus) commercial irradiator accidents (Chapter 13).

Radiation-induced changes in hepatic cells were described as early as 1924 by Case and Warthin.[246] Although the liver was considered to be generally radioresistant compared with other upper abdominal viscera, it was clear by the mid-1950s that fractionated doses in excess of 40 to

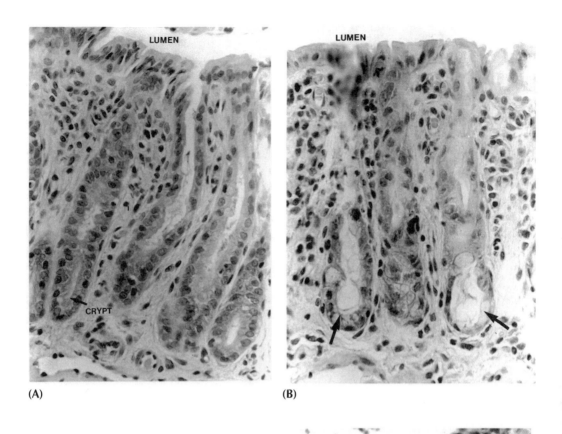
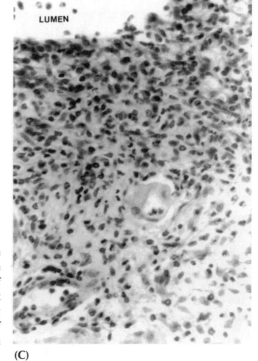

FIGURE 6.9 (A) Normal large intestine mucosa before irradiation. (B) At 7 day postirradiation after a single acute dose of 50 Gy there is loss of cells in the neck of the crypt and abnormally large and pleomorphic cells at the base of the crypts result. Villi are also shortened. By day 13 (C), there is total sloughing of villi and loss of integrity of epithelial barrier. (Case courtesy of William Black, M.D.)

50 Gy resulted in hepatic necrosis. In the mid-1960s, more attention was directed to irradiation of the liver, particularly in terms of radiotherapy schemes.

Clinical signs of hepatic injury induced by radiation include an increase in abdominal girth, hepatomegaly, ascites, jaundice, elevated serum alkaline phosphatase, and, occasionally, a clinical picture resembling the Budd–Chiari syndrome.[247–249] Profound thrombocytopenia, particularly in children, has also been reported.[250] Radiation changes in the liver are primarily due to damage to the fine vasculature and connective tissue. The hepatic cells are relatively resistant to the direct effects of radiation. Both the hepatic cells and ductal epithelial cells are long-lived and behave as reverting postmitotic cells. They do not divide regularly; however, following removal or destruction of a large portion of the liver, there is a marked capacity for regeneration. This induced division of hepatic cells and ductal epithelial cells probably causes regenerating areas to be more radiosensitive than normal liver. The most critical portion of the liver appears to be the small central vein in each lobule, and the few pathological studies that have been done appear to indicate that the most characteristic change following irradiation of the liver is nonspecific venous occlusive damage.

The liver is able to tolerate fractionated doses of 40 to 50 Gy in 4 weeks to a small portion of the organ.[248,251–253] In children there are liver abnormalities noted after radiotherapy to the liver of 12 to 30 Gy. Thomas et al.[254,255] have reported hepatic fibrosis in 3 of 26 long-term survivors of Wilms' tumors who had received at least 30 Gy in 1.5 to 2 Gy fractions. A number of other complications after radiotherapy ranging from thrombocytopenia to death have also been reported. Fajardo and Colby[256] indicate that two total abdominal doses of 5 Gy each is sufficient to cause severe hepatic injury.

In the acute clinical period, symptoms may occur 2 to 6 weeks after completion of a radiation therapy course in which the liver was included in the radiation port. The clinical manifestations are those described earlier and occasionally are termed *radiation hepatitis*. Pathological changes typically identified may include severe sinusoidal congestion, hyperemia, hemorrhage, atrophy of the central hepatic cells with dilation of the central vein, and progressive atrophy of the liver cell plates. Treatment consists of bed rest, high-protein/high-calorie diet, and symptomatic treatment of ascites. Spironolactone and steroids have been used in some cases. During this period, the radionuclide sulfur colloid liver/spleen scan often demonstrates depressed or absent activity of the reticuloendothelial cells. This function may return in a few months after fractionated doses up to 23 Gy.

Hepatic veno-occlusive lesions may occur early, but are more characteristic at 3 to 6 months. Many of the small central lobular or sublobular veins develop a fibrous net that ultimately becomes dense and coalesces. Ultimately, narrowing of the lumen, sinusoidal congestion, and liver cell atrophy occur. If enough liver is included in the radiotherapy treatment field, there may be gradual reduction in liver size due to atrophy with recurrent ascites, jaundice, and liver failure. A 20 to 25% incidence of veno-occlusive disease has been seen after a single acute dose of 10 Gy followed by bone marrow transplantation.[257,258]

Beyond 6 months, pathological examination of the liver reveals markedly less congestion, but there is atrophy due to loss of hepatic cells, with a decreased distance between the central veins and the portal spaces. The veno-occlusive disease identified in the liver after radiation therapy is unique and has been compared to similar conditions caused by various alkaloids,[259] urethane, arsphenamine, and long-term oral contraceptives.

Radionuclide Irradiation

There is a moderate amount of information available concerning effects of internal radionuclide irradiation of the liver in humans. Data stem from four sources: (1) hepatic irradiation for radiotherapeutic purposes, (2) therapeutic intravenous injection of radium, (3) thorotrast given for radiographic contrast studies, and (4) an accidental exposure with gold-198 colloid.

The patients given thorotrast administration for angiography are historically the most interesting. These patients have a high incidence of unusual malignancies; however, they also have a high incidence of nonmalignant liver disease.[260,261] The changes are predominantly those of cirrhosis or fibrosis. Estimates of the exact radiation dose are difficult, but those that have been made are in the range of 5 to 15 Gy. Some of these changes occurred after periods of 20 to 40 years after administration of the thorotrast (thorium-232 oxide).

Injection of radium-224 for ankylosing spondylitis and tuberculosis has resulted in changes in the bone and cartilage. Cirrhosis has been reported in some of these patients, particularly males, but it is not known whether they were secondary to radiation or to alcohol. Therapeutic radionuclide irradiation of the liver has been performed in at least two different circumstances. The first utilized phosphorus-32 phosphate colloid for patients with metastatic colon cancer. Injection of 550 MBq in the hepatic arterial system resulted in doses estimated at 50 Gy. Temporary radiation hepatitis occurred in at least one patient. Arterial injection of yttrium-90 resin microspheres and 5-fluorouracil has also been used for treatment of hepatic metastases. Injection of 3700 MBq (100 mCi) gives an estimated dose of 100 Gy of beta radiation to the liver.[262] In 25 such patients followed for approximately 2 years, no significant abnormalities have been reported.[263] There was an accidental exposure in which a patient was given an overexposure of gold-198 colloid (see Chapter 27), which concentrated in the liver, spleen, and bone marrow. The patient ultimately died from bone marrow failure.

URINARY SYSTEM

The kidney is a relatively radiosensitive organ when compared with the other intra-abdominal organs and tissues. Its radiosensitivity was demonstrated by both experimental and clinical data in the late 1920s. For a review the reader is referred to a chapter by Stewart and Williams.[264] The importance of the urinary system has been illustrated by two recent accidents, one involving whole-body exposure and the other localized exposure. In the 1997 Tokaimura (Japan) criticality accident, there was whole-body exposure of one patient to 17 Gy. The patient's blood urea nitrogen (BUN) was elevated by the end of the first week postexposure and renal insufficiency became a problem 2 to 4 weeks after exposure (perhaps as a result of massive tissue necrosis). The patient ultimately died on day 83 of multiorgan failure. A second patient in this accident received 8 Gy. He had bone marrow recovery but ultimately about 200 days postexposure he developed pneumonia, adult respiratory distress syndrome, and renal failure requiring dialysis. He died on day 211 postexposure. With high-dose whole-body irradiation, many early renal abnormalities are likely the result of massive tissue necrosis at other sites rather than an early direct effect of radiation on the kidneys.

In the 1999 accident in Peru (Chapter 17) an intensely radioactive iridium-192 industrial source was found and placed in a pants pocket. This produced local necrosis of the thigh or buttock, requiring amputation, but it also delivered a substantial dose to the bladder and rectum causing late complications.

Low-LET Radiation

From the time of completion of a standard course of radiation therapy up to about 6 months, renal function is usually relatively normal. Occasionally, at dose levels about 4.5 Gy, there may be a diminution of renal plasma levels; when fractionated doses exceed 20 to 24 Gy, a fall in the glomerular filtration rate (GFR) may occur. Measurements of tubular function (such as those that might be obtained with Hippuran) are highly variable in humans, and most other tests, such as BUN, are usually normal during radiotherapy. There are no human data regarding acute changes after single large doses, but animal studies do not follow the same time course as fractionated doses, and increased diuresis may be noted in dogs.[265] Pathologically, the acute changes that may be identified are hyperemia, increased capillary permeability with interstitial edema, and degenerative changes in the endothelial cells of the fine vasculature. The occlusive changes that follow are usually in the interlobular arteries and afferent arterioles.

In the period 6 to 12 months after radiation (the subacute clinical period) the clinical manifestations of acute radiation nephritis become apparent. The term *acute radiation nephritis* is a poor choice since the condition is neither acute nor a nephritis; pathologically, it is actually a nephrosclerosis.[2] The patients demonstrate anemia, edema, hypertension, proteinuria, uremia, oliguria, and, in some cases, anuria. The hypertension, which may be malignant, is responsible for most deaths occurring before 12 months. Other clinical complaints include the development of peritoneal and pleural effusions, headaches, nausea and vomiting, and, occasionally, photophobia. Following radiotherapy, the development of these signs is often confused with recurrent tumor or the development of distant metastases.

Laboratory studies in patients with acute radiation nephritis occurring after radiotherapy demonstrate albuminuria and a low specific gravity. A normochromic, normocytic anemia with a normal platelet count often occurs. The BUN is elevated (usually to about 80 mg/dl). Hematuria is rarely seen and is usually microscopic. The tolerance dose for the adult kidney appears to be approximately 23 Gy in 5 weeks to the parenchyma of both kidneys. Doses of 28 Gy to both kidneys in 5 weeks carry a high risk of severe radiation nephritis.[266] In children, serious lesions can develop at lower doses, usually when 20 Gy is exceeded.

Reduced creatinine clearance has been reported by Mitus et al.[267] in 18% of 108 children who had nephrectomy for malignant disease and received less than 12 Gy to the remaining kidney and in 33% of those who received 12 to 24 Gy. Radiation nephropathy has also been reported in children receiving bone marrow transplantation therapy.[268,269] After 12 to 14 Gy in 6 to 8 fractions over 3 to 4 days, there was hematuria and elevated creatinine. This is probably the result of both radiation and chemotherapy. Treatment of acute radiation nephritis usually involves transfusions, bed rest, low-protein diet, and restriction of fluid and salt intake. Steroids have occasionally been tried; however, some researchers think that they may actually be harmful rather than helpful. Development of generalized edema, a BUN in excess of 100 mg/dl, or increasing hypertension is a grave prognostic indicator.[1,2]

Chronic radiation "nephritis" develops during the chronic clinical period (usually 1 to 5 years after radiation), with a mean time of 2 to 3 years. The clinical course involves the slow evolution of anemia, hypertension, and impairment of renal function. In general, the kidneys are small, as measured either by ultrasound or on intravenous pyelograms. Nuclear medicine studies utilizing any number of radiopharmaceuticals demonstrate a decrease in renal blood flow. The changes are irreversible and progressive; the treatment is usually symptomatic.

The bladder is relatively more radioresistant than the kidneys; the most resistant portion of the genitourinary system being the ureters. Changes in the ureters and bladder were identified as early as 1930 by Schmitz,[270] who reported the first case of ureteral stricture. Bladder injury, as well as distal ureteral problems, became apparent with the wide clinical experience gained through treatment of cervical carcinoma and other pelvic malignancies, particularly with radium therapy. The effects described for skin and mucosa are generally applicable to the mucosa of the urinary bladder.

Acute cystitis may occur 4 to 6 weeks after a course of radiotherapy. Symptoms include dysuria, nocturia, and frequency. Hyperemia and edema of the mucosa may be seen. At high doses, partial desquamation occurs. In severe cystitis with accompanying infection, ureteritis and transient hydroureter may be identified. The treatment of radiation cystitis is similar to that of cystitis due to other causes. In a series of 527 patients studied after therapy for cervical cancer, Montana and Fowler[271] indicated that the risk of cystitis was 3% for those with a bladder dose of less than 50 Gy and 12% for those receiving fractionated doses in the range of 80 Gy or more to the bladder.

In the subacute clinical period (6 months to 2 years after therapy), painless hematuria may be a sign of trigonal ulcer. Cystoscopically, there is telangiectasia of the vessels in the region of the trigone. If obliteration of the smaller arterioles occurs as well, ulceration and fistula formation may result. The bladder can usually tolerate 55 to 60 Gy in 20 fractions over 4 weeks.[272] A very large study by Lawton et al.[273] reported on 1020 patients followed for at least 7 years after external beam radiotherapy for prostate cancer. Only a total dose greater than 70 Gy was found to have a significant impact on the incidence of urinary complications. The total incidence of complications was cystitis 2.6%, hematuria 3.1%, urethral stricture 4.6%, and bladder contracture 0.7%.

HIGH-LET RADIATION

Only a limited amount of human experience with high-LET radiation exists; however, reports of the use of fast neutrons to control tumors of the bladder suggest an RBE not significantly different from the RBE of photons.[274]

RADIONUCLIDE IRRADIATION

Renal insufficiency has been reported in patients who have received radium-224,[133] occurring in up to 13% of 222 patients who were given radium injections for treatment of ankylosing spondylitis or tuberculosis. It is uncertain how much renal damage was due to the radium. The complicating factors of renal tuberculosis and drug therapy are unknown. Uranium can cause renal damage as a result of its chemical toxicity.

REPRODUCTIVE ORGANS

Most severe radiation accidents to date have involved males, although there have been radiotherapy overexposures of females being treated for pelvic malignancies. In these latter circumstances the effects on the uterus and ovaries have not been a major clinical factor. Accidental exposures in males occur commonly as a result of reactor, commercial irradiator, and radioactive industrial radiography sources. In many of these accidents, if the patient survives, there is a question about testicular function and, particularly, possible sterility. Doses to the testes in these situations have been up to 20 Gy. Sperm counts are rarely done in accidental situations and often the only data are about fathering subsequent offspring. For example, as of 1996, 14 normal children were born to Chernobyl acute radiation sickness survivors and it is stated that as of that time fertility had recovered in all persons who planned to have children.

A vast amount of information on the male and female genital tracts has been accumulated as a result of radiotherapy for pelvic malignancies. Few pelvic malignancies are not treated with radiation; the radiation used is not only external but often interstitial or intercavitary as well. That high doses of radiation can be given to the pelvis indicates that most reproductive organs themselves are not particularly sensitive to radiation necrosis, even though they may demonstrate other changes. One very interesting difference between irradiation of the male and female is that, in the female, radiation may not only cause reduction or obliteration of gamete production but also a decrease in the production of hormones. This, of course, may result in artificial menopause with secondary effects. In the male, there are few, if any, changes in hormone production. Most of the human data were derived from localized radiation, although whole-body radiation has been reported to cause temporary sterility. A review of some of the effects on reproductive organs has been published by Lushbaugh and Ricks,[275] as well as by Ladner.[276]

It should be pointed out that alterations in gonadal function as a result of radiotherapy could occur by a number of mechanisms. In children, cranial irradiation can cause gonadotrophin deficiency or premature puberty,[277] and the reader is referred to the earlier section on brain radiation in this chapter for more details. Direct or scattered radiation to the ovary or testes can cause effects, and finally chemotherapeutic agents, such as alkylating agents, can be toxic to the ovaries but more so to the testes.[278,279]

Testes

Low-LET Radiation

The radiosensitivity of the testes was identified as early as 1906. In fact, the Bérgoni–Tribondeau law was based on work concerning the differential sensitivity of spermatogonia compared with the skin of the scrotum.[280] In general, the human data related to testicular effects come from accidental exposure because the testes are not often irradiated for therapeutic reasons.

The testis itself is a very complicated structure containing seminiferous tubules with a complex epithelium composed of Sertoli's cells (supporting and nutrient cells) and spermatogenic cells. There are numerous interstitial cells, including the Leydig' cells, which produce testosterone. Sperm production begins with type A spermatogonia, which reproduce and give rise to type B spermatogonia. Following several divisions, the type B spermatogonia form primary spermatocytes. As the primary spermatocyte reaches the lumen, it undergoes division and meiosis so that by that time it becomes a secondary spermatocyte. Each secondary spermatocyte then divides to form a spermatid and, finally, mature sperm. The time from stem cell to mature sperm has been estimated to be approximately 60 days. Type A spermatogonia are highly radiosensitive, whereas type B spermatogonia, which are differentiating intermitotic cells, are somewhat less radiosensitive. The Sertoli and Leydig cells are reasonably radioresistant.

Following doses as small as 80 mGy, a reduction in the number of spermatogonia occurs. At these low doses, the more resistant and more differentiated cells in the line may continue normal maturation. A reduction in the sperm count may not be evident until 30 to 60 days have passed. The ultimate degree and duration of depletion of the sperm depend upon the magnitude of the dose received. Sterility following radiation is often a loosely applied term; it may represent complete sterility, temporary subfertility, or, in fact, fertility with a reduced number of sperm produced. A number of discussions concern testicular irradiation from accidental exposures.[38,275,281] The range of effects reported and the doses are distressingly variable. Heller[282] indicates that doses as low as 0.15 Gy may cause oligospermia and temporary sterility. There are suggestions that a single dose in humans in the range of 5 to 6 Gy may cause permanent sterility. Investigation of human volunteers indicates that 25 fractions of 0.15 to 0.20 Gy daily may cause a decrease in the sperm count.[1] It is of interest that in the few patients treated with radiotherapy to one testicle or to the inguinal nodes to dose levels of 0.6 to 2.5 Gy, a significant percentage (34 of 74 patients) were subsequently able to father children.[283–285] Lushbaugh and Casarett[286] have reviewed the literature, finding no case reports of malformed infants from parents who had received prior radiotherapy. Some of these effects may be due to the fact that radiation-damaged spermatogonia are self-destructive. Glucksmann indicated that 5 to 6 Gy in a single dose causes permanent sterility, whereas a single dose of 2.5 Gy causes temporary sterility for 12 months.[280] Hasterlik[287] reported three patients with accidental exposures and average whole-body doses between 0.12 and 1.9 Sv. Results of a sperm count were normal at 10 days, greatly reduced at 7 to 12 months, and normal at 20 months.

A single dose of 5 to 6 Gy will cause permanent sterility in most men; however, in some cases, that dose has been exceeded without causing sterility and a dose of 2.5 Gy certainly may cause sterility for about 12 months. UNSCEAR 1982[285] has reviewed the available literature and indicated the following results: (1) temporary sterility of the testes is reported to occur with single doses ranging from 1.5 to 4 Gy and with fractionated doses of 0.1 to 2 Gy, and (2) permanent sterility occurs with single doses ranging from 5 to 9.5 Gy and with fractionated doses of 2 to 6 Gy.

Sterility may be temporary for a matter of years before returning fertility. Five individuals who received doses of 2.3 to 3.7 Gy in the Oak Ridge criticality accident were aspermic for 4 months and hypospermic for 21 months; at least one demonstrated "sterility" for several years and subsequently had a normal offspring.[288]

Ortin et al.[281] have reviewed data on 148 boys treated for Hodgkin's disease and followed for a median time of 9 years. Sexual maturation was achieved in all boys without the need for androgen replacement. Of eight boys who were treated with radiation alone, three who received 40 to 45 Gy pelvic dose were able to father children. Three others who received 30 to 44 Gy of pelvic radiation were oligospermic. This was contrasted with an 83% incidence of absolute azospermia in boys treated with chemotherapy and no pelvic radiation. Shatford et al.[289] found that long-term follow-up of 13 male children treated for Hodgkin's disease with chemotherapy or abdominal radiotherapy showed normal testosterone levels and secondary sexual characteristics, but 11 of the 13 remarried azoospermic. Patients who have received bone marrow transplantation have been studied by Sanders et al.[28] and Deeg et al.,[27] who report that gonadal failure occurred in almost all boys who were postpubertal at the time of irradiation.

High-LET Radiation

RBE data on the reproductive organs have been derived essentially from animals. These results indicate that, with high-energy neutrons, the RBE ranges from 2.5 to 3.2; at lower energies (1 MeV), values for the RBE range from 4.1 to 5.5.[290–293]

Radionuclide Irradiation

Irradiation of the testes by radionuclides may result from internal or external exposure. In the case of energetic beta radiation, the sperm cells may be irradiated by external radionuclides.[294,295] Although there may be internal deposition of radionuclides such as cesium, few human data are available.

BONE, CARTILAGE, AND MUSCLE

Effects on these tissues have been an issue in a few survivors of criticality accidents, after radiotherapy accidents involving extremities or major joints, but they are most commonly an issue after accidents with industrial radiography sources. The body parts usually involved are hands, thighs, and buttocks.

Low-LET Radiation

Most information about radiation effects on bone and cartilage are derived from experience utilizing radiotherapy for childhood tumors. In young children, age 0 to 6 years, 10 Gy produces mild osseous changes, whereas 10 to 20 Gy in fractionated radiotherapy doses produces severe changes (asymmetrical bone growth).[296–302] In general, the higher the dose and the younger the child, the more deformity results.

Adult bone is much more resistant to the effects of radiation, with effects generally attributable to decreased blood flow. Actual necrosis of the bone is quite rare, and fractionated therapeutic doses up to 65 Gy given in 6 to 8 weeks normally do not cause it. Because bone is extremely dense, the absorbed radiation dose in bone varies markedly, depending upon the energy of the incident radiation. Thus, it is extremely difficult to identify the precise bone dose necessary to produce necrosis since dose levels reported in the literature may be inaccurate.[303]

The changes demonstrated in adult bone usually include decreased ability to resist infection and increased susceptibility to fractures, with poor subsequent healing. One of the bones that most commonly experiences postradiation complications is the mandible, where it is often extremely difficult to differentiate between actual bone necrosis due to radiation and osteomyelitis[304,305] (Figure 6.10).

The incidence or spontaneous rib fractures after postmastectomy irradiation has been reported by Overgaard.[306] High doses per fraction resulted in a 19% incidence of late bone damage compared with 6% in the standard dose fraction. Radiation-induced fractures of the pelvis were identified using radionuclide bone scans in about 30% of women treated for uterine cancer with an average

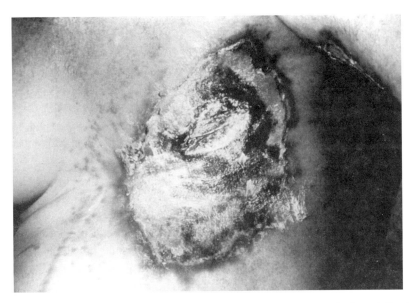

FIGURE 6.10 Necrosis of the left chest wall with visualization of the ribs over the heart following exposure from an intense industrial radiography source.

dose of 46 Gy fractionated radiotherapy. Fractures were often symmetric and 84% of patients had pain.[307]

In growing cartilage and bone, a single dose of 6 Gy has been demonstrated to cause a reduction in mitotic activity of proliferating chondroblasts. The most radiosensitive cells of the skeleton appear to be the intermitotic chondroblasts. After radiation, distortion of the chondroblast columns and interference with normal growth mechanisms occur.[2] At high absorbed doses, osteoblasts may also be killed. If the bone marrow and underlying blood vessels are unable to recover, both bone and cartilage resorption is impaired. In animals, maximal damage is seen with single doses in the region of 30 Gy, causing complete cessation of growth. At lower absorbed doses, the changes identified on a radiograph may appear similar to early epiphyseal closure; however, if the blood supply decreases, the bones become sclerotic.

With mature bone, the direct effects of radiation are not apparent for some time. Some of the earliest changes following radiotherapy are areas of decreased radioactivity on radionuclide bone scans. Such areas do not appear with a total fractionated dose of less than 20 Gy but do appear in 60% of regions receiving more than 45 Gy. These changes appear 4 to 6 months after radiotherapy and may persist for up to 19 months.[308] With high doses, pathologically there is an absence of osteoblasts and osteocytes, with subsequent arteriolar intimal thickening. The bone is then subject to necrosis and fracture with minimal trauma. The skeletal changes evident radiographically have been best described by Bragg et al.,[309] but the doses required to cause such changes are rarely reported. The bone becomes demineralized and has an abnormal coarse trabecular pattern. The process often resembles Paget's disease; however, the appearance of fractures, lack of bone expansion, localized nature, and clinical history generally exclude this diagnosis. It is sometimes difficult to exclude metastases and infection as causes of the radiographic changes identified.

Cartilage, like adult bone, is fairly radioresistant. Doses of 60 to 70 Gy in a prolonged radiotherapy treatment scheme can be tolerated by cartilage.[310,311] Unless there is stress to the cartilage, clinical manifestations of direct radiation effects are rare. There is a case report of localized chondrocalcinosis following radiotherapy.[312]

Direct effects of radiation on muscle are distinctly unusual. Acute radionecrosis of skeletal muscle requires absorbed doses in excess of 500 Gy.[313] At lower fractionated doses, from 22 to 54 Gy, atrophy of fibers can be identified. Finally, ischemia due to arterial narrowing may result in fibrosis.[314] The ultimate clinical result of muscle irradiation probably depends not only on the absorbed dose but also on the length of the muscle segment irradiated. If the muscle is short and is entirely included in the irradiated field, the resultant detriment may be substantially greater than if only a portion of a long muscle is irradiated.

NEUTRON OR HIGH-LET RADIATION

At the present time, there is little, if any, information on the effects of neutron or high-LET radiation on bone and cartilage. There is some animal evidence, but extrapolation to humans is, at best, difficult.[315–318]

RADIONUCLIDE IRRADIATION

Human data concerning effects of radionuclides on bone are derived predominantly from three sources: (1) persons occupationally exposed to radium with subsequent internal contamination, (2) patients receiving therapeutic administration of radium, and (3) individuals having intra-articular administration of radionuclides for treatment of arthritis. Radionuclides that concentrate in bone are referred to as volume seekers or surface seekers. The *volume seekers* ultimately are included in the matrix of the bone, although originally they may deposit on the surface. Examples of such volume-seeking radionuclides include isotopes of calcium, strontium, radium, and the alkaline earth elements. Plutonium and thorium accumulate on the periosteum and endosteal surfaces and are, therefore, considered *surface seekers*.

In the early 1900s, watch dial figures were painted with luminous compounds containing radium. It was a relatively common practice to place the brush between the lips to make the point finer, causing ingestion and internal contamination with large amounts of radium salts. Records for this group have been kept at the Human Radiobiology Section of the Argonne National Laboratory in Chicago.[319] The radioisotopes of radium predominantly involved were radium-226 and radium-228.[320–322] Actual radiographic bone changes include small destructive areas in flat bones, particularly the skull,[321] fractures of long bones, coarsening of the trabecular pattern, bone infarcts, and aseptic necrosis.[321,323–325] These changes were only seen when systemic intake exceeded 148 kBq (4 μCi) or resulted in estimated bone doses in excess of 7 to 8 Sv.[326] The radium dial painters have had a very high incidence of primary bone tumors (osteosarcoma) and tumors of the cranial sinuses.

Radium-224 has been and is still used in Germany for treatment of ankylosing spondylitis. It decays rapidly, and, therefore, its dose is predominantly to the endosteal and periosteal surface of the bone. The longer half-life of radium-226 causes the major dose to be to the bone volume. In children injected with radium-224, growth retardation has been demonstrated in 12 to 70% of the cases. The percentage of children demonstrating growth retardation is a function of the age at injection, with younger children demonstrating more-pronounced changes.[327]

Radionuclides used in intra-articular radiotherapy have included gold-198 colloid, yttrium-90 silicate citrate, phosphorus-32 chromic phosphate, rhenium-186 sulfide, and erbium-169 citrate.[328–332] The main purpose of these injections has been to irradiate the synovial tissue and to sterilize it without causing necrosis of the cartilage. Estimated doses to the synovium of the knee joint utilizing yttrium-90 have been estimated to be approximately 60 to 80 Gy.[333,334] Two cases of joint rupture have been reported, presumably secondary to radiation necrosis of the adjacent cartilage.[335]

HEMATOPOIETIC AND LYMPHATIC SYSTEMS

Effects on the hematopoietic system are of critical importance in radiation accidents that expose significant portions of the thorax, abdomen, or pelvis to doses in excess of 2 to 4 Gy. The crucial role of this tissue in development of the acute radiation syndrome has been pointed out in Chapter 4.

Changes in the hematopoietic system were identified as early as 1904, and by 1906 it was known that myelopoiesis was more radiosensitive than erythropoiesis. In 1913, Shouse et al.[336] demonstrated that aplasia of the bone marrow in animals was a cause of death following total-body irradiation. Lethal accidental exposures in humans and the subsequent blood and bone marrow changes were described in the 1950s by Hempelmann et al.,[337] Guskova and Baisogolov,[338] and Rajevsky.[339] The hematopoietic system is one of the most radiosensitive tissues in the body, and the response to radiation is a classic study in the disturbance of the kinetics of various cellular lines.[339,340] Doses of radiation as small as 0.5 to 1 Gy in a single exposure produce obvious responses.

The reader is referred to a chapter by Nothdurft[341] and to Annex G of the 1988 UNSCEAR Report.[285] The clinical responses of an individual depend markedly upon the amount of tissue irradiated. Radiation of a large portion of the bone marrow results in the hematopoietic form of the acute radiation. The changes discussed in the immediately following text are applicable to either localized radiation or generalized radiation exposure. A major difference in marrow response between localized and generalized radiation is that, in cases in which the bone marrow is irradiated locally, subsequent regeneration may occur more quickly.

The kinetics of human hematopoiesis that form the basis of the responses of the cell lines have been well discussed by Cronkite.[342] Erythrocytes, reticulocytes, granulocytes, mature megakaryocytes, and platelets are fixed postmitotic cells. The reticular cells, macrophages, monocytes, plasma cells, and fibroblasts are reverting postmitotic cells. Both categories are relatively resistant to the direct effects of radiation. Somewhat more sensitive are the differentiating intermitotic cells, including erythroblasts, myeloblasts, and megakaryoblasts. These cells both divide and differentiate and are moderately radiosensitive. Cells that are relatively sensitive to radiation are vegetative intermitotic cells, such as large- and medium-sized lymphocytes and hemocytoblasts.

More recent and detailed descriptions of the hierarchy of the cells in the hematopoietic system by other authors indicate that most cell lines begin with a pluripotent stem cell. From this, there are two distinct pathways, one to lymphopoiesis and another to monocytes, neutrophils, erythrocytes, platelets, and eosinophils. A number of growth factors or cytokines control cell development along different lineages. For example, in the production of neutrophils, cytokines, especially interleukins (IL-1, IL-3, and IL-6) are effective in the development of multipotent progenitor cells from the stem cells. IL-3 and granulocyte/macrophage colony–stimulating factor (GM-CSF) are used to develop granulocyte/macrophage progenitor cells, and finally GM-CSF and granulocyte colony–stimulating factor (G-CSF) are used in the final development of neutrophils.

The kinetic pattern of postradiation events in hematopoietic tissue has been described by a large number of authors but most completely by Fliedner et al.[343] The time-related pattern of changes identified is a function of the time required for each cell type to complete its development from the stem cell. Due to the short life span of neutrophils (7 to 17 h) and of platelets (about 10 days), there is rather rapid development of granulocytopenia and thrombocytopenia after radiation-induced injury of a major proportion of the hemopoietic tissue.

An important exception to this scheme of radiosensitivity is the small lymphocyte. Although it appears to be a nondividing cell and should be relatively resistant to radiation, it is actually very sensitive. It undergoes intermitotic cell death with a D_0 of 0.2 to 0.3 Gy.[344] It is possible that not all the small lymphocytes are radiosensitive and that there may be some very sensitive subpopulations. Lymphocytic depletion may be seen within hours of irradiation, whereas platelets and granulocytes are depleted over days, and depletion of red cells (erythrocytes) occurs over weeks. Late changes of aplastic anemia that are reported in the literature can occur as a result of vascular compromise and fibrosis. Under these circumstances, all cell lines are equally affected. Such changes are not seen with acute marrow doses of less than 10 to 20 Gy in a relatively acute regimen.[2] Marrow depression usually does not occur with chronic exposure unless doses exceed 0.4 Sv per year.

Low-LET Radiation

The acute changes in bone marrow have been studied in patients receiving fractionated radiotherapy. In a typical fractionated radiotherapy treatment regimen (in which the treatment scheme is normally 2 Gy, daily with 5 fractions weekly), the following changes have been identified. At levels of 4 Gy, there is a moderate decrease in nucleated cells with a marked decrease in the precursors of the red cells and granulocytes. When absorbed doses of 10 Gy are reached, there is a total absence of the undifferentiated and differentiating cellular forms, including all "blast" cells. The marrow often is hemorrhagic. By the end of the 5-week course of 50 Gy, extreme hypoplasia of the marrow and difficulty finding anything but a few plasma cells and lymphocytes result.

The typical change identified in the peripheral blood is a fall in the lymphocyte count, with a maximal depression at 10 to 15 days. The count tends to stay depressed until the end of the therapeutic treatment, and recovery occurs 3 to 6 months later.

If either the pelvis or thoracic bone marrow is irradiated in a radiotherapy treatment scheme, it is not unusual for the lymphocyte count to fall to approximately 40% of its original value. The neutrophil count is maximally depressed after 15 to 20 days, again usually to approximately 40% of the pretreatment values. The eosinophil count may change, depending upon the site of irradiation. Pelvic irradiation tends to elevate the eosinophil count, whereas treatment of the upper abdomen and thorax may cause a decrease in the eosinophil count.

There has been some experience in radiotherapy with half-body irradiation. This was usually given to either the upper or lower half of the body, and initially bone marrow tolerance was expected to be the limiting factor. About 60% of the active marrow is located in the upper half of the body. It was found that single doses of 8 to 10 Gy delivered at a rate of 2 Gy/min to the upper half of the body were well tolerated. There was moderate depression in blood cell counts, but these returned to normal in about 3 to 8 weeks.[345,346] Recovery is faster after lower-body irradiation than upper body because there is less active marrow irradiated.

In a patient who is not anemic or treated with chemotherapy prior to localized radiotherapy, the red cell count and platelet (thrombocyte) count are usually not depressed significantly. Major changes may be identified if there is some abnormality in the marrow reserve in other portions of the body. For example, if a patient has extensive marrow infiltration by tumor in portions of the body outside the radiotherapy field, the additional radiation changes on the bone marrow within the field may have effects greater than expected. Regeneration of marrow occurs in many patients after localized radiotherapy. There have been many studies of this subject, and it appears that when the fractionated radiotherapy scheme does not exceed 30 Gy, there is a good chance of marrow regeneration. Some authors report that once dose levels of 40 Gy of localized radiotherapy are exceeded, regeneration in that area is much less likely.[347–349]

When large portions of the bone marrow or the total body are irradiated, the findings are quite different. For acute whole-body irradiation of humans in the dose range of 1 to 6 Gy, clinically important effects result from damage to the bone marrow. This is often referred to as the *hematopoietic syndrome,* and without medical treatment, the following results usually occur:

Absorbed Dose	Survival
<1 Gy	Virtually certain
1–2 Gy	Probable
2–4.5 Gy	Possible
5–6 Gy	Virtually impossible

With current medical measures, whole-body doses as high as 12 Gy in 6 fractions of 2 Gy have been used for bone marrow ablation prior to bone marrow transplantation. The effect of fractionation and total absorbed dose is shown in Figure 6.11. The effects of acute whole-body irradiation on the bone marrow and hematopoietic function has already been discussed in Chapter 4.

Direct Effects of Radiation on Specific Tissues

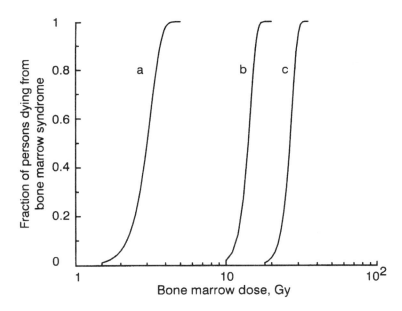

FIGURE 6.11 Dose–response curves for mortality due to the bone marrow syndrome when the dose is given continuously in (a) 1 day or less, (b) 3 months, or (c) 1 year.

HIGH-LET RADIATION

The RBE for neutrons and their effect on the hematopoietic system have been studied by several researchers.[292,350,351] The RBE appears to be low and is probably between 1.0 and 2.0.

INTERNAL IRRADIATION

There is information on the effects of internal irradiation on the hematopoietic system from several sources. The most important from a historical viewpoint is the group of radium dial painters. These female painters were employed between 1915 and 1930 in the United States and became internally contaminated via the oral route with radium-226 and radium-228. In those patients who received very high skeletal doses, an asymptomatic but statistically significant reduction in the hematocrit has been identified, and most received doses in excess of 10 Gy.[352] Sharpe[322] has reported no clinically significant reductions of any peripheral cellular elements in long-term follow-up of the New Jersey radium dial painters. Dose rates to the marrow from radium-226 have been calculated to be 16 mGy annually for a burden of 37 kBq (1 µCi).[352]

The other sources of data in humans predominantly are patients receiving therapeutic administrations of radionuclides. Very large amounts of radioiodine are administered to treat patients with metastatic thyroid carcinoma. Often the limiting consideration is the dose to the bone marrow.[358,359] This effect is usually not severe until there have been four or more treatments, and total activity administered is in excess of 18 GBq (500 mCi). The effect on the bone marrow usually can be assessed with peripheral blood counts. There has been a recent resurgence of interest in treatment of widespread bone metastases with unsealed radionuclides, particularly strontium-89. An unwarranted side effect is marrow depression. For this radiopharmaceutical, the estimated marrow dose is 0.01 Gy per MBq (27 µCi).[356] Lain et al.[357] have examined the depression of platelets at different levels of administered activity and found the following percentage depression, at 0.7 MBq/kg 19%, at 1.5 MBq/kg 24%, and at 3.0 MBq/kg 45%. In general, there is no major bone marrow toxicity in terms of either platelets or leukocytes at administered activity levels of less than 3.0 MBq (81 µCi)/kg unless there has been prior radiotherapy or chemotherapy.

Phosphorus-32 has been used to treat patients with primary polycythemia; generally, multiple administrations are given until the polycythemia is reduced to acceptable levels. The absorbed dose to the bone marrow in such treatment has been calculated by Spiers et al.[358] to be in the range of 0.24 Gy for a 37-MBq (mCi) injected dose. Typically, this is administered with the specific aim of myelosuppression. The typical intravenously administered activity is 85 MBq (2.3 mCi)/m² (not to exceed 185 MBq, or 5 mCi), and this delivers a marrow dose of about 1 Gy.[359] Some authors have reported on the use of sulfur-35 in treatment of chondrosarcomas or chordomas. This treatment is usually limited by marrow damage. When administered activities are in the range of 370 to 1780 MBq/kg of body weight, significant marrow depression can occur.[360]

In one accident, a patient in Wisconsin received a lethal amount of colloidal gold-198 while being treated for serosal metastatic carcinoma of the ovary by instillation of the colloidal radioactive gold into the peritoneal cavity. Through an error, the activity administered was in millicuries rather than microcuries. The patient subsequently died from hematological complications. Had the patient survived, hepatic failure undoubtedly would have also occurred. Other reports of bone marrow depression resulting from radiogold and radiosulfur are presented in the literature.[361,362]

In an accident in Goiânia (Brazil), ingestion of cesium-137 caused radiation doses in 14 persons who were large enough to result in severe bone marrow depression. Of the 14, 4 died as a result of infection and hemorrhage.[363] Eight of these persons received GM-CSF in an uncontrolled manner.[364] Whether there was any benefit remains a matter of speculation.

REFERENCES

GENERAL

1. Rubin, P. and Casarett, G.W., *Clinical Radiation Pathology*, W.B. Saunders, Philadelphia, 1968.
2. Fajardo, L.F., *Pathology of Radiation Injury*, Masson Publishing, New York, 1982.
3. Mettler, F.A. and Upton, A.C., *Medical Effects of Ionizing Radiation*, W.B. Saunders, Philadelphia, 1995.

SKIN AND MUCOSA

4. Gassmann, A., Zur histologie der Röntgenulcera, *Fortschr. Geb. Röntgenstr.*, 2:199–207, 1898.
5. Jammet, H., Daburon, F., Gerber, G. et al., Eds., Radiation damage to the skin, fundamental and practical aspects, in Proceedings of a Workshop, Sacaly, France, October 1985. *Br. J. Radiol.* (Suppl. 19): 1–134, 1986.
6. Trott, K. and Kummermehr, J., Radiation effects in skin, in *Radiopathology of Organs and Tissues*, Scherer, E., Streffer, C., and Trott, K., Eds., Springer-Verlag, Berlin, 1991.
7. International Commission on Radiological Protection (ICRP), The biological basis for dose limitation in the skin, Publ. 59, *Ann. ICRP*, 22, Pergamon Press, Oxford, U.K., 1991.
8. Gongora, R. and Magdelenat, H., Accidental acute local irradiations in France and their pathology, in *Radiation Damage to the Skin: Fundamental and Practical Aspects*, *Proceedings of a Workshop*, Jammet, H., Daburon, F., Gerber, G. et al., Eds., Sacaly, France, October 1985. *Br. J. Radiol.* (Suppl. 19): 12–15, 1986.
9. Turesson, I. and Thames, H., Repair capacity and kinetics of human skin during fractionated radiotherapy: erythema, desquamation and telangiectasia after 3 and 5 years follow-up, *Radiother. Oncol.*, 15:169–188, 1989.
10. Turesson, I., Individual variation and dose-dependency in the progression rate of skin telangiectasia, *Int. J. Radiat. Oncol. Biol. Phys.*, 19:1569–1574, 1990.
11. Bentzen, S. and Overgaard, M., Relationship between early and late normal-tissue injury after postmastectomy radiotherapy, *Radiother. Oncol.*, 20:159–165, 1991.
12. Patterson, R., *The Treatment of Malignant Disease by Radium and X-Rays*, Edward Arnold Press, London, 1956.

13. von Essen, C.F., Roentgen therapy of skin and lip carcinoma: factors influencing success and failure, *AJR*, 83:556–570, 1960.
14. Mettler, F., Ricks, R., and Kelsey, C., *Medical Management of Radiation Accidents*, CRC Press, Boca Raton, FL, 1990.
15. International Atomic Energy Agency, The Radiological Accident in Goiânia, Vienna, 1988.
16. International Atomic Energy Agency, The Radiological Accident in San Salvador, Vienna, 1990.
17. Localized lesions induced by cesium 137 during the Goiânia accident, *Health Phys.*, 60:25–29, 1991.
18. Low-Beer, B.U., External use of radioactive phosphorus: erythema studies, *Radiology*, 47:213–222, 1946.
19. Hubner, K. and Fry, S., Eds., *The Medical Basis for Radiation Accident Preparedness*, Elsevier/North Holland, New York, 1980.
20. Mikhail, S.Z., Beta radiation doses from fallout particles deposited on the skin. Report ESA-TR-71-01 to the Army, Environmental Science Associates, Burlingame, CA, 1971.
21. National Council on Radiation Protection and Measurements, Limit for exposure to "Hot Particles" on the skin, NCRP Rep. 106, Bethesda, MD, 1989.

Endocrine Glands

22. Morimoto, I., Yoshimoto, Y., Sato, K. et al., Serum TSH, thyroglobulin and thyroid disorders in atomic bomb survivors exposed in youth: a study 30 years after exposure, *Technical Report* 20-85, Radiation Effects Research Foundation, Hiroshima, 1985.
23. Nagataki, S., Delayed effects of atomic bomb radiation on the thyroid, in *Radiation and the Thyroid: Proceedings of the 27th Annual Meeting of the Japanese Nuclear Medicine Society*, Nagataki, S., Ed., Nagasaki, Japan, 1987, Excerpta Medica, Amsterdam, 1989.
24. Nagataki, S., Shibata, Y., Inoue S. et al., Thyroid diseases among atomic bomb survivors in Nagasaki, *JAMA*, 272:364–370, 1994.
25. Wong, F.L., Yamada, M., Sasaki, H. et al., Noncancer disease incidence in the atomic bomb survivors: 1958–1986. *Radiat. Res.*, 135:418–430, 1993.
26. Kaplan, M., Boice, J.D., Jr., Ames, D. et al., Thyroid, parathyroid and salivary gland evaluations in patients exposed to multiple fluoroscopic examinations during tuberculosis therapy, *J. Clin. Endocrinol. Metab.*, 66:376–382, 1988.
27. Deeg, H., Storb, R., and Thomas, E., Bone marrow transplantation: a review of delayed complications, *Br. J. Haematol.*, 57:185–208, 1984.
28. Sanders, J., Pritchard, S., Mahoney, P. et al., Growth and development following marrow transplantation for leukemia, *Blood*, 68:1129–1135, 1986.
29. Markson, J.L. and Flatman, G.I., Myxedema after deep x-ray therapy to the neck, *Br. Med. J.*, 1:1228–1230, 1965.
30. Hancock, S., Cox, R., and McDougall, I., Thyroid diseases after treatment of Hodgkin's disease, *N. Engl. J. Med.*, 325:599–605, 1991.
31. Loeffler, J., Tarbell, N., Garber, J. et al., The development of Graves' disease following radiation therapy in Hodgkin's disease, *Int. J. Radiat. Oncol. Biol. Phys.*, 14:175–178, 1988.
32. Feyerabend, T., Kapp, B., Richter, E. et al., Incidence of hypothyroidism after irradiation of the neck with special reference to lymphoma patients, *Acta Oncol.*, 29:597–602, 1990.
33. Grande, C., Hypothyroidism following radiotherapy for head and neck cancer; multivariate analysis of risk factors, *Radiother. Oncol.*, 25:31–36, 1992.
34. Liening, D., Duncan, N., Blakeslee, D. et al., Hypothyroidism following radiotherapy for head and neck cancer, *Otolaryngol. Head Neck Surg.*, 103:10–13, 1990.
35. Tami, T., Gomez, P., Parker, G. et al., Thyroid dysfunction after radiation therapy in head and neck cancer patients, *Am. J. Otolaryngol.*, 13:357–362, 1992.
36. Joensuu, H. and Viikari, J., Thyroid function after postoperative radiation therapy in patients with breast cancer, *Acta Radiol. Oncol.*, 25:167–170, 1986.
37. Bruning, P., Bonfrer, J., DeJong-Bakker, M. et al., Primary hypothyroidism in breast cancer patients with irradiated supraclavicular lymph nodes, *Br. J. Cancer*, 51:659–663, 1985.
38. Liebow, A.A., Warran, S., and DeCoursey, E., Pathology of atomic bomb casualties, *Am. J. Pathol.*, 25:853–1028, 1947.

39. Rogoway, W.M., Finkelstein, S., Rosenberg, S.A. et al., Myxedema developing after lymphangiography and neck irradiation, *Clin. Res.*, 14:133, 1966.
40. Malone, J.F., Hendry, J.H., Porter, D. et al., The response of the thyroid, a highly differentiated tissue, to single and multiple doses of gamma or fast neutron irradiation, *Br. J. Radiol.*, 47:608-615, 1974.
41. Lewitus, Z. and Rechnic, J., Electron-microscopic and isotopic evidence for a difference between the radiobiological effects of iodine 131 and iodine 125, in *Radioaktive Isotope in Klinik und Forschung*, B and II, Hofer, R., Ed., Urban and Schwarzenberg, Vienna, 1975.
42. Snyder, W.S., Ford, M.R., Warner, G.G. et al., Absorbed dose per unit cumulated activity for selected radionuclides and organs, Medical Internal Radiation Dose Committee, Pamphlet No. 11, Society of Nuclear Medicine, New York, 1975.
43. Berger, M.J., Distribution of absorbed dose around point sources of electrons and beta particles in water and other media, *J. Nucl. Med.*, 12(Suppl.):5–23, 1971.
44. Siemsen, J., Wallack, M.S., Martin, R.B. et al., Early results of ^{125}I therapy of thyrotoxic Graves' disease, *J. Nucl. Med.*, 15:257–260, 1974.
45. Larsen, P.R. and Conard, R.A., Thyroid hypofunction appearing as a delayed manifestation of accidental exposure to radioactive fallout in a Marshallese population, Brookhaven National Laboratory BNL-24104, Brookhaven, NY, 1978.
46. Sutow, W.W. and Conard, R.A., The effects of fallout radiation on Marshallese children, in *Radiation Biology of the Fetal and Juvenile Mammal*, Sikov, R. and Mahlum, D.D., Eds., CONF-690501, U.S. Atomic Energy Commission Report, Washington, DC, 1969.
47. Robbins, J. and Adams, W., Radiation effects in the Marshall Islands, in *Radiation and the Thyroid: Proceedings of the 27th Annual Meeting of the Japanese Nuclear Medicine Society*, Nagataki, S., Ed., Nagasaki, Japan, 1987, Excerpta Medica, Amsterdam, 1989.
48. International Atomic Energy Agency, The International Chernobyl Project, Report of an International Committee, Vienna, 1991.
49. Becker, D., Comparison of treatments for hyperthyroidism, in *Radiation and the Thyroid: Proceedings of the 27th Annual Meeting of the Japanese Nuclear Medicine Society*, Nagataki, S., Ed., Nagasaki, Japan, 1987. Excerpta Medica, Amsterdam, 1989.
50. Werner, S.C., Hamilton, H., and Nemeth, M.R., Therapeutic effects from repeated diagnostic doses of iodine 131 in adults and juvenile hypothyroidism, *J. Clin. Endocrinol. Metab.*, 12:1349, 1952.
51. Cunnien, A.J., Hay, I.D., Gorman, C.A. et al., Radioiodine-induced hypothyroidism in Graves' disease: factors associated with increasing incidence, *J. Nucl. Med.*, 23:978–983, 1982.

NERVOUS SYSTEM

52. Gutin, P., Leibel, S., and Sheline, G., Eds., *Radiation Injury to the Nervous System*, Raven Press, New York, 1991.
53. Gilbert, H.A. and Kagan, A.R., *Radiation Damage to the Nervous System*, Raven Press, New York, 1980.
54. Scholz, W. and Hsii, Y., Late damage from roentgen irradiation of the human brain, *Arch. Neurol. Psychiat.*, 40:928, 1938.
55. Bailey, O.T., Woodward, J.S., and Putnam, T.J., Tissue reactions of the human frontal white matter to gamma Cobalt 60 radiation, in *Response of the Central Nervous System to Ionizing Radiation*, Haley, T.J. and Snider, R.S., Eds., Little, Brown, Boston, 1964.
56. Peterson, K., Rosenblum, M., Powers, J. et al., Effect of brain irradiation on demyelinating lesions, *Neurology*, 43:2105–2112, 1993.
57. Rider, W.D., Radiation damage to the brain, a new syndrome, *J. Can. Assoc. Radiol.*, 14:67–69, 1963.
58. Kramer, S., Southard, M.E., and Mansfield, C.M., Radiation effects and tolerance of the central nervous system, *Front. Radiat. Ther. Oncol.*, 6:332–345, 1972.
59. Wachowski, T.J. and Chenault, H., Degenerative effects of large doses of roentgen rays on the human brain, *Radiology*, 45:227–246, 1945.
60. Safdari, H., Fuentes, J., Dubois, J. et al., Radiation necrosis of the brain: time of onset and incidence related to total dose and fractionation of radiation, *Neuroradiology*, 27:44–47, 1985.
61. Lee, A., Ng, S., Ho, J. et al., Clinical diagnosis of late temporal lobe necrosis following radiation therapy for nasopharyngeal carcinoma, *Cancer*, 61:1535–1542, 1988.

62. Marks, L.B. and Spencer, D., The influence of volume on the tolerance of the brain to radiosurgery, *J. Neurosurg.*, 75:177–180, 1991.
63. Tolly, T., Bruckman, J., Czarnecki, D. et al., Early CT findings after interstitial radiation therapy for primary malignant brain tumors, *AJNR*, 9:1177–1180, 1988.
64. Bloom, H., Intracranial tumors, response and resistance to therapeutic endeavors, 1970–1980, *Int. J. Radiat. Oncol. Biol. Phys.*, 8:1083–1113, 1982.
65. Valk, P., Budinger, T., Levin, V. et al., PET of malignant cerebral tumors after interstitial brachytherapy, demonstration of metabolic activity and correlation with clinical outcome, *J. Neurosurg.*, 69:830–838, 1988.
66. Di Chiro, G., Oldfield, E., Wright, D. et al., Cerebral necrosis after radiotherapy and/or intracranial chemotherapy for brain tumors: PET and neuropathologic studies, *Am. J. Roentgenol.*, 150:189–197, 1988.
67. Schwartz, R., Carvalho, P., Alexander, E. et al., Radiation necrosis versus high grade recurrent glioma: differentiation by using dual-isotope SPECT with thallium 201 and technetium 99m HMPAO, *AJNR*, 12:1187–1192, 1991.
68. Allen, J., Miller, D., Budzilovich, G. et al., Brain and spinal cord hemorrhage in long term survivors of malignant pediatric brain tumors: a possible late effect of therapy, *Neurology*, 41:148–150, 1991.
69. Constine, L., Konski, A., Ekholm, S. et al., Adverse effects of brain irradiation correlated with MR and CT imaging, *Int. J. Radiat. Oncol. Biol. Phys.*, 15:319–330, 1988.
70. Curran, W., Hecht-Leavit, C., Schut L. et al., Magnetic resonance imaging of cranial radiation lesions, *Int. J. Radiat. Oncol. Biol. Phys.*, 13:1093–1098, 1987.
71. Tsuruda, J., Kortman, K., Bradley, W. et al., Radiation effects on cerebral white matter, *Am. J. Roentgenol.*, 149:165–171, 1987.
72. Kay, H., Knapton, P., O'Sullivan, J. et al., Encephalopathy in acute leukemia associated with methotrexate therapy, *Arch. Dis. Child*, 47:344–354, 1972.
73. Rubenstein, L., Herman, M., Long, T. et al., Disseminated necrotizing leukoencephalopathy: A complication of treated central nervous system leukemia and lymphoma, *Cancer*, 35:291–305, 1975.
74. Peylan-Ramu, N., Poplak, D., Blei, C. et al., CT in methotrexate encephalopathy, *J. Comput. Assist. Tomogr.*, 1:216–221, 1977.
75. Bleyer, W. and Griffin, T., White matter necrosis, mineralizing microangiopathy, and intellectual abilities in survivors of childhood leukemia, in *Radiation Damage to the Central Nervous System: A Delayed Therapeutic Hazard*, Gilbert, H. and Kagan, A., Eds., Raven Press, New York, 1980.
76. Price, D., Hotson, G., and Loh, J., Pontine calcification following radiotherapy: CT demonstration, *J. Comput. Assist. Tomogr.*, 12:45–46, 1988.
77. Sheline, D.E., Wara, W.M., and Smith, B., Therapeutic irradiation and brain injury, *Int. J. Radiat. Oncol. Biol. Phys.*, 6:1215–1228, 1980.
78. Rubenstein, L.J., Herman, M.M., Long, T.F. et al., Disseminated necrotizing leukoencephalopathy: a complication of treated central nervous system leukemia and lymphoma, *Cancer*, 35:291–305, 1975.
79. Freeman, J.E., Johnston, P.G.B., and Voke, J.M., Somnolence after prophylactic cranial irradiation in children with ALL, *Br. Med. J.*, 4:523–525, 1973.
80. Proctor, S.J., Kernahan, J., and Taylor, P., Depression as component of post-cranial irradiation somnolence syndrome, *Lancet*, 1215–1216, May, 1981.
81. Ron, E., Modan, B., Floro, S. et al., Mental function following scalp irradiation during childhood, *Am. J. Epidemiol.*, 116:149–160, 1982.
82. Shore, R., Albert, R., and Pasternack, B., Follow-up study of patients treated by x-ray epilation for tinea capitis. Resurvey of post-treatment illness and mortality experience, *Arch. Environ. Health*, 31:21–28, 1976.
83. Omran, A., Shore, R., Markoff, R. et al., Follow-up study of patients treated by x-ray epilation for tinea capitis: psychiatric and psychometric evaluation, *Am. J. Public Health*, 68:561–567, 1978.
84. Meadows, A.T., Massari, D.J., Fergusson, J. et al., Declines in IQ scores and cognitive dysfunctions in children with acute lymphocytic leukemia treated with cranial irradiation, *Lancet*, 1015–1018, November 1981.
85. Danoff, B.F., Cawchock, F.S., Marquette, C. et al., Assessment of the long-term effects of primary radiation therapy for brain tumors in children, *Cancer*, 49:1580–1586, 1982.

86. Trautman, P., Erickson, C., Shaffer, D. et al., Prediction of intellectual deficits in children with acute lymphoblastic leukemia, *J. Dev. Behav. Pediatr.*, 9:122–128, 1988.
87. Bleyer, W., Fallavollita, J., Robison, L. et al., Influence of age, sex, and concurrent intrathecal methotrexate therapy on intellectual function after cranial irradiation during childhood: a report from the Children's Cancer Study Group, *Pediatr. Hematol. Oncol.*, 7:329–338, 1990.
88. Brouwers, P. and Poplack, D., Memory and learning sequelae in long term survivors of acute lymphoblastic leukemia: association with attention deficits, *Am. J. Pediatr. Hematol. Oncol.*, 12:174–181, 1990.
89. Chessells, J., Cox, T., Kendall, B. et al., Neurotoxicity in lymphoblastic leukemia: comparison of oral and intramuscular methotrexate and two doses of radiation, *Arch. Dis. Child*, 65:416–422, 1990.
90. Tucker, J., Prior, P., Green, C. et al., Minimal neuropsychological sequelae following prophylactic treatment of the central nervous system in adult leukemia and lymphoma, *Br. J. Cancer*, 60:775–780, 1989.
91. Laramore, G., Injury to the central nervous system after high-LET radiation, in *Radiation Injury to the Nervous System*, Gutin, P., Leibel, S., and Sheline, G., Eds., Raven Press, New York, 1991.
92. Withers, H.R., Thames, H.D., Peters, L.J. et al., Normal tissue radioresistance in clinical radiotherapy, in *Biological Basis and Clinical Implications of Tumor Radioresistance, Proceedings of the Second Rome International Symposium*, Fletcher, G.H., Nervi, C., and Withers, H.R., Eds., Masson et Cie, Paris, 1980.
93. Pallis, C.A., Lowis, S., and Morgan, R.L., Radiation myelopathy, *Brain*, 84:460–478, 1961.
94. Phillips, T.L. and Bushke, F., Radiation tolerance of the spinal cord, *Am. J. Roentgenol.*, 105:659–664, 1969.
95. Fitzgerald, R.H., Jr., Marks, R.D., and Wallace, K.M., Chronic radiation myelitis, *Radiology*, 144:609–612, 1982.
96. Dische, S., Warburton, M., and Saunders, M., Radiation myelitis and survival in the radiotherapy of lung cancer, *Int. J. Radiat. Oncol. Biol. Phys.*, 15:75–81, 1988.
97. Georgiou, A., Grigsby, P., and Perez, C., Radiation-induced lumbo-sacral plexopathy in gynecologic tumors: clinical findings and dosimetric analysis, *Int. J. Radiat. Oncol. Biol. Phys.*, 26:479–482, 1993.
98. Kinsella, T.J., Weichselbaum, R.R., and Sheline, G.E., Radiation injury of cranial and peripheral nerves, in *Radiation Damage to the Nervous System*, Gilbert, H.A. and Kagan, A.A., Eds., Raven Press, New York, 1980.
99. Olsen, N., Pfeiffer, P., Johannsen, L. et al., Radiation-induced brachial plexopathy: neurological follow-up in 161 recurrence free breast cancer patients, *Int. J. Radiat. Oncol. Biol. Phys.*, 26:43–49, 1993.
100. Pierce, S., Recht, A., Lingos, T. et al., Long-term complications following conservative surgery and radiation therapy in patients with early stage breast cancer, *Int. J. Radiat. Oncol. Biol.*, 23:915–923, 1992.
101. Brady, L., Shields, J., Augusburger, J. et al., Eye and ear complications from radiation therapy to the eye, *Front. Radiat. Ther. Oncol.*, 23:238–250, 1989.
102. Alberti, W., Effects of radiation on the eye and ocular adnexa, in *Radiopathology of Organs and Tissues*, Scherer, E., Streffer, C., and Trott, K., Eds., Springer-Verlag, Berlin, 1991.
103. Phillip, W., Daxecker, F., Langmayear, J. et al., Spontaneous corneal rupture after strontium irradiation of a conjunctival squamous cell carcinoma, *Ophthalmologica*, 195:113–118, 1987.
104. Amoaku, W. and Archer, D., Fluorescein angiographic features: natural course and treatment of radiation retinopathy, *Eye*, 4:657–667, 1990.
105. Archer, D., Amoaku, W., and Gardiner, T., Radiation retinopathy—clinical, histopathological, ultrastructural and experimental correlations, *Eye*, 5:239–251, 1991.
106. Lopez, P., Sternberg, P., Dabbs, C. et al., Bone marrow transplant retinopathy, *Am. J. Ophthalmol.*, 112:635–646, 1991.
107. Young, W., Thornton, A., Gebarski, S. et al., Radiation-induced optic neuropathy: correlation of MR imaging and radiation dosimetry, *Radiology*, 185:904–907, 1992.
108. Hudgins, P., Newman, N., Dillon, W. et al., Radiation-induced optic neuropathy: characteristic appearances on gadolinium enhanced MR, *Am. J. Neuroradiol.*, 13:235–238, 1992.
109. Guy, J., Mancuso, A., Beck, R. et al., Radiation-induced optic neuropathy: a magnetic resonance imaging study, *J. Neurosurg.*, 74:426–432, 1991.

110. Schull, W.J., Late radiation responses in man, *Adv. Space. Res.*, 3:231–239, 1983.
111. Otake, M. and Schull, W.J., The relationship of gamma and neutron radiation to posterior lenticular opacities among atomic bomb survivors in Hiroshima and Nagasaki, *Radiat. Res.*, 92:574–595, 1982.
112. Choshi, K., Takaku, I., Mishima, H. et al., Ophthalmologic changes related to radiation exposure and age in the adult health study sample, Hiroshima and Nagasaki, *Radiat. Res.*, 96:560–579, 1983.
113. Otake, M. and Schull, W., Radiation related posterior lenticular opacities in Hiroshima and Nagasaki atomic bomb survivors based on the DS 86 dosimetry system, *Radiat. Res.*, 121:3–13, 1990.
114. Otake, M. and Schull, W., A review of forty-five years study of Hiroshima and Nagasaki atomic bomb survivors. Radiation cataract, *J. Radiat. Res.*, 32(Suppl.):283–293, 1991.
115. Cogan, C.J., Donaldson, D.D., and Reese, A.B., Clinical and pathological characteristics of radiation cataract, *Arch. Ophthalmol.*, 47:55, 1952.
116. Merriam, G.R., Jr. and Focht, F., A clinical study of radiation cataracts and the relationship to dose, *AJR*, 77:759–785, 1957.
117. Merriam, G.R., Jr., Szechter, A., and Focht, E.F., The effects of ionizing radiations on the eye, *Front. Radiat. Ther. Oncol.*, 6:346–385, 1972.
118. Charles, M.W. and Lindop, P.J., Skin and eye irradiation: examples of some limitations of international recommendations in radiological protection, in Application of the Dose Limitation System for Radiation Protection, International Atomic Energy Agency, Vienna, 1979.
119. Bendel, I., Schuttmann, W., and Arndt, D., Cataract of lens as late effect of ionizing radiation in occupationally exposed persons, in *Late Biological Effects of Ionizing Radiation*, Vol. 1, International Atomic Energy Agency, Vienna, 1978.
120. Sakai, S., Kubo, T., Mori, N. et al., A study of the late effects of radiotherapy and operation on patients with maxillary cancer. A survey more than 10 years after initial treatment, *Cancer*, 62:2114–2117, 1988.
121. Oglesby, R.B., Black, R.L., von Sallman, L. et al: Cataracts in patients with rheumatic diseases treated with corticosteroids. Further observations, *Arch. Ophthalmol.*, 66:41–46, 1961.
122. Heyn, R., Ragab, A., Raney, R.B. et al., Late effects of therapy in orbital rhabdomyosarcoma in children. A report from the Intergroup Rhabdomyosarcoma Study, *Cancer*, 57:1738–1743, 1986.
123. Nesbit, M.E., Robison, L.L., Sather, H.N. et al: Evaluation of long-term survivors of childhood acute lymphoblastic leukemia (ALL), *Abstr. Proc. Am. Ass . Cancer Res.*, 23:107, 1982.
124. Inati, A., Sallan, S.E., Cassady, J.R. et al., Efficacy and morbidity of central nervous system "prophylaxis" in childhood acute lymphoblastic leukemia: eight years' experience with cranial irradiation and intrathecal methotrexate, *Blood*, 61:297–303, 1983.
125. Deeg, H.J., Floumoy, N., Sullivan, K.M. et al., Cataracts after total body irradiation and marrow transplantation: a sparing effect of dose fractionation, *Int. J. Radiat. Oncol. Biol. Phys.*, 10:957–964, 1984.
126. Tichelli, A., Gratwhol, A., Egger, T. et al., Cataract formation after bone marrow transplantation, *Ann. Intern. Med.*, 119:1175–1180, 1993.
127. Hamom, M., Gale, R., MacDonald, I. et al., Incidence of cataracts after single fraction total body irradiation: the role of steroids and graft versus host disease, *Bone Marrow Transplant.*, 12:233–236, 1993.
128. Barrett, A., Nicholls, J., and Gibson, B., Late effects of total body irradiation, *Radiother. Oncol.*, 9:131–135, 1987.
129. Applebaum, F.R. and Thomas, E.D., Treatment of acute leukemia in adults with chemoradiotherapy and bone marrow transplantation, *Cancer*, 55:2202–2209, 1985.
130. Merriam, G.R., Jr, Biavati, B.J., Bateman, J.L. et al., The dependence of RBE on the energy of fast neutrons, Part IV: induction of lens opacities in mice, *Radiat. Res.*, 25:123–138, 1965.
131. Abelson, P.H. and Kruger, P.G., Cyclotron-induced radiation cataracts, *Science*, 110:655–657, 1949.
132. Roth, J., Brown, M., Catterall, M. et al., Effects of fast neutrons on the eye, *Br. J. Ophthalmol.*, 60:236–244, 1976.
133. Spiess, H., Gerspach, A., and Mays, C.W., Soft-tissue effects following ^{224}Ra injections into humans, *Health Phys.*, 35:61–81, 1978.
134. Thomas, C.I., Storaasli, J.P., and Gridell, H.L., Lenticular changes associated with beta radiation of the eye and their significance, *Radiology*, 79:588, 1962.

Salivary Glands

135. Ang, K., Stephens, L., and Schultheiss, T., Oral cavity and salivary glands, in *Radiopathology of Organs and Tissues*, Scherer, E., Streffer, C., and Trott, K., Eds., Springer-Verlag, Berlin, 1991.
136. Kashima, H.K., Kirkham, W.R., and Andrews, J.R., Post-irradiation sialadenitis: a study of clinical features, histopathologic changes and serum enzyme variations following irradiation of human salivary glands, *AJR*, 94:271–291, 1965.

Respiratory Tract

137. Van den Brenk, H.A.S., Radiation effects on the pulmonary system, in *Pathology of Irradiation*, Berdjis, C.C., Ed., Williams & Wilkins, Baltimore, 1971.
138. Davis, S., Yankelevitz, D., and Henschke, C., Radiation effects on the lung: clinical features, pathology, and imaging findings, *Am. J. Roentgenol.*, 159:1157–1164, 1992.
139. Molls, M. and van Beuningen, D., Radiation injury of the lung, in *Radiopathology of Organs and Tissues*, Scherer, E., Streffer, C., and Trott, K., Eds., Springer-Verlag, Berlin, 1991.
140. Fowler, J.F. and Travis, E.L., The radiation pneumonitis syndrome in half body radiation therapy, *Int. J. Radiat. Oncol. Biol. Phys.*, 4:1111–1113, 1978.
141. Byhardt, R., Abrams, R., and Almagro, U., The association of ARDS with thoracic radiation, *Int. J. Radiat. Oncol. Biol. Phys.*, 15:1441–1446, 1988.
142. Kaufman, J. and Komorowski, R., Bronchiolitis obliterans. A new clinical-pathologic complication of irradiation pneumonitis, *Chest*, 97:1243–1244, 1990.
143. Roberts, C., Foulcher, E., Zaunders, J. et al: Radiation pneumonitis: a possible lymphocyte mediated hypersensitivity reaction, *Ann. Intern. Med.*, 118:696–700, 1993.
144. Moss, W.T., Haddy, F.J., and Sweany, S.K., Some factors altering the severity of acute radiation pneumonitis: variation with cortisone, heparin, and antibodies, *Radiology*, 75:50, 1960.
145. Jennings, F.L. and Arden, A., Development of radiation pneumonitis: time dose factors, *Arch. Pathol.*, 74:351, 1962.
146. Scott, B.R. and Hahn, F.F., Early occurring and continuing effects, in Health Effects Models for Nuclear Power Plant Accident Consequences Analysis, Evans, J.S., Moeller, D.W., and Cooper, D.W., Eds., U.S. Nuclear Regulatory Commission, NUREG/CR-4214 (SAND85-7185), 1985.
147. Pagani, J. and Lipshitz, H., CT manifestations of radiation-induced change in chest tissue, *J. Comput. Assist. Tomogr.*, 6:243–248, 1982.
148. Ikezoe, J., Takashima, S., Morimoto, S. et al., CT appearance of acute radiation induced injury in the lung, *Am. J. Roentgenol.*, 150:765–770, 1988.
149. Bluemke, D., Fishman, E., Kuhlman, J. et al., Complications of radiation therapy: CT evaluation, *Radiographics*, 11:581–600, 1991.
150. Teates, C.D., Effects of unilateral thoracic irradiation on pulmonary blood flow, *AJR*, 102:875–882, 1968.
151. Miller, R., Fusner, J., Fink, R. et al., Pulmonary function abnormalities in long term survivors of childhood cancer, *Med. Pediatr. Oncol.*, 14:202–207, 1986.
152. Mefferd, J., Donaldson, S., and Link, M., Pediatric Hodgkin's disease: pulmonary, cardiac, and thyroid function following combined modality therapy, *Int. J. Radiat. Oncol. Biol. Phys.*, 16:679–685, 1989.
153. Boushy, S.F., Helgason, A.H., and North, L.B., The effect of radiation on the lung and bronchial tree, *AJR*, 108:284–292, 1970.
154. Lingos, T., Recht, A., Vincini, F. et al., Radiation pneumonitis in breast cancer patients treated with conservative surgery and radiation therapy, *Int. J. Radiat. Oncol. Biol. Phys.*, 21:355–360, 1991.
155. Lund, M., Myhre, K., Melsom, H. et al., The effect on pulmonary function of tangential field technique in radiotherapy for carcinoma of the breast, *Br. J. Radiol.*, 64:520–523, 1991.
156. Rotstein, S., Lax, I., and Svane, G., Influence of radiation therapy on the lung tissue in breast cancer patients: CT assessed density changes and associated symptoms, *Int. J. Radiat. Oncol. Biol. Phys.*, 18:173–180, 1990.
157. Groth, S., Johansen, H., Sorensen, P. et al., The effect of thoracic irradiation for cancer of the breast on ventilation, perfusion, and pulmonary permeability. A one-year follow-up, *Acta Oncol.*, 28:671–678, 1989.

158. Wohl, M.E., Griscom, N.T., Traggis, D.G. et al., Effects of therapeutic irradiation delivered in early childhood upon subsequent lung function, *Pediatrics*, 55:507–516, 1975.
159. Littman, P., Meadows, A.T., Polgar, G. et al., Pulmonary function in survivors of Wilms' tumor. Patterns of impairment, *Cancer*, 37:2773–2776, 1976.
160. Green, D., Finklestein, J., Tefft, M. et al., Diffuse interstitial pneumonitis after pulmonary irradiation for metastatic Wilms' tumor. A report of the National Wilms' Tumor Study, *Cancer*, 63:450–453, 1989.
161. Shaw, N., Eden, O., Jenny, M. et al., Pulmonary function in survivors of Wilms' tumor, *Pediatr. Hematol. Oncol.*, 8:131–137, 1991.
162. Kadota, R.P., Burgert, E.O., Drisscoll, D.J. et al., Cardiopulmonary function in long-term survivors of childhood Hodgkin's lymphoma: a pilot study. Abstr., *Proc. Soc. Clin. Oncol.*, 5:198, 1986.
163. do Pico, G.A., Wiley, A., Rao, P. et al., Pulmonary reaction to upper mantle radiation therapy for Hodgkin's disease, *Chest*, 75:688–692, 1979.
164. Tarbell, N., Thompson, L., and Mauch, P.. Thoracic irradiation in Hodgkin's disease: disease control and long-term complications, *Int. J. Radiat. Oncol. Biol. Phys.*, 18:275–281, 1990.
165. Gustavsson, A., Eskilsson, J., Landberg, T. et al., Long-term effects on pulmonary function of mantle radiotherapy in patients with Hodgkin's disease, *Ann. Oncol.*, 3:455–461, 1991.
166. Springmeyer, S.C., Flournoy, N., Sullivan, K.M. et al., Pulmonary function changes in long-term survivors of allogenic marrow transplantation, in *Recent Advances in Bone Marrow Transplantation*, Gale, R.P., Ed., Alan R. Liss, New York, 1983.
167. Cohen, L., Schultheiss, T., Hendrickson, F. et al., Normal tissue reactions and complications following high-energy neutron beam therapy, *Int. J. Radiat. Oncol. Biol. Phys.*, 16:73–78, 1989.
168. Waxweiler, R.J., Roscoe, R.J., Archer, V.E. et al., Mortality follow-up through 1977 of the white underground uranium miners cohort examined by the United States Public Health Service, in *Radiation Hazards in Mining*, Gomez, M., Ed., American Institute of Mining, Metallurgical, and Petroleum Engineers, New York, 1981.
169. Cross, F.T., Palmer, R.F., Busch, R.H. et al., Development of lesions in Syrian golden hamsters following exposure to radon daughters and uranium ore dust, *Health Phys.*, 41:135–153, 1981.
170. Samet, J.M., Young, R.A., Morgan, M.V. et al., Prevalence survey of respiratory abnormalities in New Mexico uranium miners, *Health Phys.*, 46:361–370, 1984.
171. De Vuyst, P., Dumortier, P., Katelbant, P. et al., Lung fibrosis induced by thorotrast, *Thorax*, 45:899–901, 1990.
172. Health Risks of Radon and Other Internally Deposited Alpha Emitters, BEIR IV Report, National Academy of Sciences, National Academy Press, Washington, DC, 1988.
173. Haley, P., Pulmonary toxicity of stable and radioactive lanthanides, *Health Phys.*, 61:809–820, 1991.

HEART AND VESSELS

174. Cohn, D.E., Stewart, J.R., Fajardo, L.F. et al., Heart disease following radiation, *Medicine*, 46:281–298, 1967.
175. Fajardo, L.F. and Stewart, J.R., Radiation-induced heart disease: human and experimental observations, in *Drug-Induced Heart Disease*, Vol. 5, Bristow, M., Ed., Elsevier/North Holland, Amsterdam, 1980.
176. Schultz-Hector, S., Heart, in *Radiopathology of Organs and Tissues*, Scherer, E., Streffer, C., and Trott, K., Eds., Springer-Verlag, Berlin, 1991.
177. Lister, G.D. and Gibson, T., Destruction of the chest wall and damage to the heart by x-irradiation from an industrial source, *Br. J. Plast. Surg.*, 26:328–335, 1973.
178. Aretz, H.T., Myocarditis: the Dallas criteria, *Hum. Pathol.*, 18:619–624, 1987.
179. Weinstein, C. and Fenoglio, J., Myocarditis, *Hum. Pathol.*, 18:613–618, 1987.
180. Karas, J.S. and Stanbury, J.R., Fatal radiation syndrome from an accidental nuclear excursion, *N. Engl. J. Med.*, 272:756–761, 1963.
181. Stewart, J.R., Cohn, K.E., Fajardo, L.F. et al., Radiation-induced heart disease: a study of twenty-five patients, *Radiology*, 89:302–310, 1967.
182. Stewart, J.R. and Fajardo, L.F., Radiation-induced heart disease, *Front. Radiat. Ther. Oncol.*, 6:274–288, 1972.
183. Fajardo, L.F., Radiation-induced coronary artery disease, *Chest*, 71:563–564, 1977.

184. Stewart, J.R. and Fajardo, L.F., Dose response in human and experimental radiation-induced heart disease: application of the nominal standard dose (NSD) concept, *Radiology*, 99:403–408, 1971.
185. Carmel, R.J. and Kaplan, H.S., Mantle irradiation in Hodgkin's disease. An analysis of technique, tumor eradication and complications, *Cancer*, 37:2813–2825, 1976.
186. Brosius, F.C., Waller, B.F., and Roberts, W.C., Radiation heart disease, *Am. J. Med.*, 70:519–530, 1981.
187. Branch-Zawadzki, M., Anderson, M., DeArmond, S.J. et al., Radiation-induced large intracranial vessel occlusive vasculopathy, *AJR*, 134:51–55, 1980.
188. Painter, M.J., Chutorian, A.M., and Hilal, S.K., Cerebrovasculopathy following irradiation in childhood, *Neurology*, 25:189–194, 1975.
189. Hekali, P., Halttunen, P., Korhola, O. et al., Occlusion of the right pulmonary artery: a rare late complication of radiation therapy, *Ann. Clin. Res.*, 14:7–10, 1982.
190. Maunory, C., Perga, J.Y., Balett, H. et al., Myocardial perfusion damage after mediastinal irradiation for Hodgkin's disease: a thallium 201 single photon emission tomographic study, *Eur. J. Nucl. Med.*, 19:871–873, 1992.
191. Van Son, J.A., Noyez, L., and Van Asten, W.N., Use of internal mammary artery in myocardial revascularization after mediastinal irradiation, *J. Thorac. Cardiovasc. Surg.*, 104:1539–1544, 1992.
192. Sande, L.M., Casariego, J., and Llorian, A.R., Percutaneous transluminal coronary angioplasty for coronary stenosis following radiotherapy, *Int. J. Cardiol.*, 20:129–132, 1988.
193. McEniery, P.C., Dorosti, K., Chiavone, W.A. et al., Clinical and angiographic features of coronary artery disease after chest irradiation, *Am. J. Cardiol.*, 60:1020–1024, 1987.
194. Joensuu, H., Acute myocardial infarction after heart irradiation in young patients with Hodgkin's disease, *Chest*, 95:388–390, 1990.
195. Gustavsson, A., Essikilsson, J., Landberg, T. et al., Late cardiac effects after mantle radiotherapy in patients with Hodgkin's disease, *Ann. Oncol.*, 1:355–363, 1990.
196. Corn, B.W. and Goodman, R.L., Radiation-related ischemic heart disease: review article, *J. Clin. Oncol.*, 8:741–750, 1990.
197. Fajardo, L. and Berthrong, M., Vascular lesions following radiation, *Pathol. Ann.*, 23:297–330, 1988.
198. Atkinson, J.L., Sundt, T.M., Dale, A.J. et al., Radiation-associated atheromatis disease of the cervical carotid artery: report of seven cases and review of the literature, *Neurosurgery*, 24:171–178, 1989.
199. Call, G.K., Bray, P.F., Smoker, W.R. et al., Carotid thrombosis following neck irradiation, *Int. J. Radiat. Oncol. Biol. Phys.*, 18:635–640, 1990.
200. McGuirt, W.F., Feehs, R.S., and Bonds, G., Radiation-induced atherosclerosis: a factor in therapeutic planning, *Ann. Otol. Rhinol. Laryngol.*, 101:222–228, 1992.
201. Phillips, G.R., Peer, R.M., Upson, J.F. et al., Late complications of revascularization for radiation-induced arterial disease, *J. Vasc. Surg.*, 16:921–924, 1992.
202. Atabek, U., Spence, R.K., Alexander, J.B. et al., Upper extremity occlusive arterial disease after radiotherapy for breast cancer, *J. Surg. Oncol.*, 49:205–207, 1992.
203. Hashmonai, M., Elami, A., Kuten, A. et al., Subclavian artery occlusion after radiotherapy for carcinoma of the breast, *Cancer*, 61:2015–2018, 1988.
204. Piedbois, P., Becquemin, J.P., Blanc, I. et al., Arterial occlusive disease after radiotherapy: a report of 14 cases, *Radiother. Oncol.*, 17:113–140, 1990.
205. Pettersson, F. and Swedenborg, J., Atherosclerotic occlusive disease after radiation for pelvic malignancies, *Acta Chir. Scand.*, 156:367–371, 1990.
206. Moritz, M.W., Higgins, R.F., and Jacobs, J.R., Duplex imaging and incidence of carotid radiation injury after high dose radiotherapy for tumors of the head and neck, *Arch. Surg.*, 125:1181–1183, 1990.
207. Goodman, M., Lalka, S., and Reddy, S., Static and dynamic vascular impact of large artery irradiation, *Int. J. Radiat. Oncol. Biol. Phys.*, 26:305–310, 1993.
208. Dunjic, A., The influence of radiation on blood vessels and circulation, Part XI: blood flow and permeability after whole-body irradiation, *Curr. Top. Radiat. Res.*, 10:170–184, 1974.
209. Reinhold, H.S. and Bruisman, G.H., Radiosensitivity of capillary endothelium, *Br. J. Radiol.*, 46:54–57, 1973.
210. Reinhold, H.S. and Bruisman, G.H., Repair of radiation damage to capillary endothelium, *Br. J. Radiol.*, 48:727–731, 1975.

211. Rahmouni, A., Montazel, J.L., Golli, M. et al., Unusual complication of liver irradiation: acute thrombosis of a main hepatic vein, *Radiat. Med.*, 10:163–166, 1992.
212. Fajardo, L.F. and Stewart, J.R., Experimental irradiation-induced heart disease, Part I: Light microscopic studies, *Am. J. Pathol.*, 59:299–316, 1970.

GASTROINTESTINAL TRACT

213. Trott, K. and Herrmann, T., Radiation effects on abdominal organs, in *Radiopathology of Organs and Tissues*, Scherer, E., Streffer, C., and Trott, K., Eds., Springer-Verlag, Berlin, 1991.
214. Amory, N.I. and Brick, I.B., Irradiation damage of the intestines following 1000 kV roentgen therapy. Evaluation of tolerance dose, *Radiology*, 56:49–57, 1951.
215. Hamilton, F.E., Gastric ulcer following irradiation, *Arch. Surg.*, 55:394–399, 1947.
216. Doi, Y., Aoba, T., Okazaki, M. et al., Carbon 13 enriched carbonate apatites studied by ESR: comparison with tooth enamel apatites, *Calcif. Tissue Int.*, 33:81–82, 1981.
217. Pass, B. and Aldrich, J.E., Dental enamel as an in-vivo radiation dosimeter, *Med. Phys.*, 12:305–307, 1985.
218. Aldrich, J. and Pass, B., Determining radiation exposure from nuclear accidents and atomic tests using dental enamel, *Health Phys.*, 54:469–471, 1988.
219. Hussey, D.H., Jardine, J.H., Raulstron, G.L. et al., 50 MeV neutrons: comparison of normal tissue tolerance in animals with clinical observations in patients, *Int. J. Radiat. Oncol. Biol. Phys.*, 8:2083–2088, 1982.
220. Lepke, R.A. and Lubshitz, H.I., Radiation-induced injury of the esophagus, *Radiology*, 148:375–378, 1983.
221. Hishikawa, Y., Taniguchi, M., Kamikonya, N. et al., Esophageal pseudodiverticulum following high dose rate intracavitary irradiation for esophageal cancer, *Radiat. Med.*, 6:267–271, 1988.
222. Yang, Z., Hu Y., and Gu, X., Non-cancerous ulcer in the esophagus after radiotherapy for esophageal carcinoma: a report of 27 patients, *Radiother. Oncol.*, 19:121–129, 1990.
223. Kaplinsky, C., Kornreich, L., Tiomny, E. et al., Esophageal obstruction 14 years after treatment for Hodgkin's disease, *Cancer*, 68:903–905, 1991.
224. Silvain, C, Barrioz, T., Besson, I. et al., Treatment and long-term outcome of chronic radiation esophagitis after radiation therapy for head and neck tumors, *Digest. Dis. Sci.*, 38:927–931, 1993.
225. Ellenhorn, J., Lambroza, A., Lindsley, K. et al., Treatment-related esophageal stricture in pediatric patients with cancer, *Cancer*, 71:4084–4090, 1993.
226. Bowers, R.F. and Brick, I.B., Surgery in radiation injury of the stomach, *Surgery*, 22:20–38, 1947.
227. Doig, R.K., Funder, R.J., and Weiden, S., Serial gastric biopsy studies in a case of duodenal ulcer treated by deep x-ray therapy, *Med. J. Aust.*, 38:828–830, 1951.
228. Findley, J.M., Newaishy, G.A., Sircus, W. et al., Role of gastric irradiation in management of peptic ulceration and esophagitis, *Br. Med. J.*, 3:769–771, 1974.
229. Becciolini, A., Relative radiosensitivities of the small and large intestine, in *Advances in Radiation Biology*, Vol. 12, Academic Press, New York, 1987.
230. Drier, J.S. and Browning, T.H., Morphologic response of the mucosa of human small intestine to x-ray exposure, *J. Clin. Invest.*, 5:194–204, 1966.
231. Lifshitz, S., Savage, J.E., Taylor, KA. et al., Plasma prostaglandin levels in radiation-induced enteritis, *Int. J. Radiat. Oncol. Biol. Phys.*, 8:275–277, 1982.
232. Weiss, R.G. and Stryker, J.A., Carbon 14-lactose breath tests during pelvic radiotherapy: the effect of the amount of small bowel irradiated, *Radiology*, 142:507–510, 1982.
233. Henriksson, R., Franzen, L., and Littbrand, B., Effects of sucralfate on acute and late bowel discomfort following radiotherapy of pelvic cancer, *J. Clin. Oncol.*, 10:969–975, 1992.
234. Perkins, D.E. and Spjut, H.J., Intestinal stenosis following radiation therapy, *AJR*, 88:953, 1962.
235. Geffand, M.D., Tepper, M., Katz, L.A. et al., Acute radiation proctitis in man, *Gastroenterology*, 54:401–411, 1968.
236. Gehrig, J., Hacki, W., Schulthess, H. et al., Strahlenproktitis nach gynaekologischer radiotherapie: eine endoskopische studie, *Schweiz. Med. Wochenschr.*, 117:1326–1332, 1987.

237. den Hartog-Jager, F., van Haastert, M., Battermann, J. et al., The endoscopic spectrum of late radiation damage of the rectosigmoid colon, *Endoscopy*, 17:214–217, 1985.
238. Haboubi, N., Schofield, P., and Rowland, P., The light and electron microscopic features of early and late phase radiation-induced proctitis, *Am. J. Gasteroenterol.*, 83:1140–1144, 1988.
239. Kochhar, R., Patel, F., Dhar, A. et al., Radiation-induced proctosigmoiditis: prospective, randomized, double blind controlled trial of oral sulfasalazine plus rectal steroids versus rectal sucralfate, *Digest. Dis. Sci.*, 36:103–107, 1991.
240. Fischer, L., Kimose, H., Spjeldnaes, N. et al., Late progress of radiation-induced proctitis, *Acta Chir. Scand.*, 256:801–805, 1990.
241. Harling, H. and Balslev, I., Long-term prognosis of patients with severe radiation enteritis, *Am. J. Surg.*, 155:517–519, 1988.
242. Black, W.C., Gomez, L., Yukas, T.S. et al., Quantitation of late effects of x-irradiation of the large intestine, *Cancer*, 45:444–451, 1980.
243. Chau, P.M., Fletcher, G.H., Rutledge, F.N. et al., Complications in high dose pelvis irradiation in female pelvic cancer, *AJR*, 87:22–40, 1962.
244. Hornsey, S. and Field, S.B., The RBE of cyclotron neutrons for effects on normal tissues, *Eur. J. Cancer*, 10:231–234, 1974.
245. Phillips, T.L., Barshall, H.H., Goldberg, E. et al., Comparison of RBE values of 15 MeV neutrons for damage to an experimental tumor and some normal tissues, *Eur. J. Cancer*, 10:287–292, 1974.

LIVER AND BILIARY SYSTEM

246. Case, J.T. and Warthin, A.S., The occurrence of hepatic lesions in patients treated by intensive deep roentgen radiation, *AJR*, 12:27, 1924.
247. Ogata, K., Hizawa, K., Yoshida, M. et al., Hepatic injury following irradiation, a morphologic study, *Terkushime J. Exp. Med.*, 9:240–251, 1963.
248. Ingold, J.A., Reed, G.B., Kaplan, H.S. et al., Radiation hepatitis, *AJR*, 92:200–208, 1965.
249. Reed, G.B. and Cox, A.J., The human liver after radiation injury, a form of veno-occlusive disease, *Am. J. Pathol.*, 48:597–612, 1966.
250. Tefft, M., Mitus, A., Das, L. et al., Irradiation of the liver in children: review of experience in acute and chronic phases in the intact normal and partially resected liver, *AJR*, 108:365–385, 1970.
251. Kurohara, S.S., Swensson, N.L., Usselman, J.A. et al., Response and recovery of liver to radiation as demonstrated by photoscans, *Radiology*, 89:129–135, 1967.
252. Kraut, J.W., Bagshaw, M.A., and Glatstein, E., Hepatic effects of irradiation, in *Frontiers of Radiation Therapy and Oncology*, Vol. 6, Vaeth, J.M., Ed., University Park Press, Baltimore, 1972.
253. Johnson, P.M., Grossman, F.M., and Atkins, H.L., Radiation-induced hepatic injury: its detection by scintillation scanning, *Am. J. Roentgenol.*, 99:453–462, 1967.
254. Thomas, P., Griffith, K., Fineberg, B. et al., Late effects of treatment for Wilms' tumor, *Int. J. Radiat. Oncol. Biol. Phys.*, 9:651–657, 1983.
255. Thomas, P., Tefft, M., D'Angio, G. et al., Radiation associated toxicities in the Second National Wilms' Tumor Study, *Int. J. Radiat. Oncol. Biol. Phys.*, 10(Suppl. 2):88, 1894.
256. Fajardo, L.F. and Colby, T.V., Pathogenesis of veno-occlusive liver disease after radiation, *Arch. Pathol. Lab. Med.*, 104:585–488, 1980.
257. McDonald, G., Sharma, P., Matthews, D. et al., Veno-occlusive disease of the liver after bone marrow transplantation: Incidence and predisposing factors, *Hepatology*, 4:116–122, 1984.
258. Trott, K. and Herrmann, T., Radiation injury of the abdominal organs, *Br. J. Radiol.*, 22(Suppl.):30–32, 1988.
259. Bras, G., Jelliffe, D.B., and Stewart, K.L., Veno-occlusive disease of liver with non-portal type cirrhosis, occurring in Jamaica, *Arch. Pathol.*, 57:285–300, 1954.
260. Da Silva Horta, J., Da Silva Horta, M.E., Da Motta, L.C. et al., Malignancies in Portuguese thorotrast patients, *Health Phys.*, 35:135–137, 1978.
261. Kato, U., Mori, T., and Kumatori, T., Thorotrast dosimetric study in Japan, *Environ. Res.*, 18:32–36, 1979.
262. Grady, E.D., Adjuvant therapy for colon cancer by internal irradiation to the liver, in *Therapy in Nuclear Medicine*, Spencer, R.P., Ed., Grune & Stratton, New York, 1978.

263. Ariel, I.M., Treatment of metastatic cancer to the liver from primary colon and rectal cancer by the intraarterial administration of chemotherapy and radioactive isotopes, in *Therapy in Nuclear Medicine*, Spencer, R.P., Ed., Grune & Stratton, New York, 1978.

URINARY SYSTEM

264. Stewart, F. and Williams, M., The urinary tract, in *Radiopathology of Organs and Tissues*, Scherer, E., Streffer, C., and Trott, K., Eds., Springer-Verlag, Berlin, 1991.
265. Maier, J.G. and Casarett, G.W., Pathophysiologic Aspects of Radiation Nephritis in Dogs, Atomic Energy Commission Report, UR-626, University of Chester, 1963.
266. Luxton, R.W. and Kunkler, P.B., Radiation nephritis, *Acta Radiol.*, 2:169–178, 1964.
267. Mitus, A., Tefft, M., and Fellers, F., Long-term follow-up of renal function in 108 children who underwent nephrectomy for malignant disease, *Pediatrics*, 44:912–921, 1969.
268. Tarbell, T., Guinan, E., Chin, L. et al., Renal insufficiency after total body irradiation for pediatric bone marrow transplantation, *Radiother. Oncol.*, 18(Suppl. 1):139–142, 1990.
269. Van Why, S., Friedman, A., and Wei, L., Renal insufficiency after bone marrow transplantation in children, *Bone Marrow Transplant.*, 7:383–388, 1991.
270. Schmitz, H., Complications of the urinary tract due to carcinoma of the cervix or radiation treatment, *AJR*, 24:47, 1930.
271. Montana, G. and Fowler, W., Carcinoma of the cervix: analysis of bladder and rectal radiation dose and complications, *Int. J. Radiat. Oncol. Biol. Phys.*, 16:95–100, 1989.
272. Morrison, R. and Deeley, T.J., The treatment of carcinoma of the bladder by supervoltage x-rays, *Br. J. Radiol.*, 38:499–458, 1965.
273. Lawton, C., Won, M., Pilepich, M. et al., Long term treatment sequelae following external beam irradiation for adenocarcinoma of the prostate: analysis of RTOG studies 7506 and 7706, *Int. J. Radiat. Oncol. Biol. Phys.*, 21:935–939, 1991.
274. Batterman, J.J., Results of d-T neutron irradiation on advanced tumors of the bladder and rectum, *Int. J. Radiat. Oncol. Biol. Phys.*, 8:2159–2164, 1982.

REPRODUCTIVE ORGANS

275. Lushbaugh, C.C. and Ricks, R.C., Some cytokinetic and histopathologic considerations of male and female irradiated gonadal tissues, *Front. Radiat. Ther. Oncol.*, 6:228–248, 1972.
276. Ladner, H., Reproductive organs, in *Radiopathology of Organs and Tissues*, Scherer, E., Streffer, C., and Trott, K., Eds., Springer-Verlag, Berlin, 1991.
277. Livesey, E. and Brook, C., Gonadal dysfunction after treatment of intracranial tumors, *Arch. Dis. Child.*, 63:495–500, 1988.
278. Clayton, P., Shalet, S., Price, D. et al., Ovarian function following chemotherapy for childhood brain tumors, *Med. Pediatr. Oncol.*, 17:92–96, 1989.
279. Byearne, J., Mulvihill, J., Myers, M. et al., Effects of treatment on fertility in long-term survivors of childhood or adolescent cancer, *N. Engl. J. Med.*, 317:1315–1321, 1987.
280. Glucksman, A., The effects of radiation on reproductive organs, *Br. J. Radiol.*, 1 (Suppl.):101–109, 1947.
281. Oakes, W.R. and Lushbaugh, C.C., Course of testicular injury following accidental exposures to nuclear radiation: report of a case, *Radiology*, 59:737–747, 1952.
282. Heller, C.G., Radiobiological factors in manned space flights, in Report of the Space Radiation Study Panel of the Life Sciences Commitee, Langham, W.R., Ed., National Academy Press, Washington, DC, 1967.
283. Ortin, T., Shostak, C., and Donaldson, S., Gonadal status and reproductive function following treatment for Hodgkin's disease in childhood, *Int. J. Radiat. Oncol. Biol. Phys.*, 19:873–880, 1990.
284. Smithers, D.W., Wallace, D.M., and Austin, D.E., Fertility after unilateral orchidectomy and radiotherapy for patients with malignant tumors of the testes, *Br. Med. J.*, 4:77–79, 1973.
285. United Nations Scientific Committee on the Effects of Atomic Radiation (UNSCEAR): early effects in man of high doses of radiation, Report to the General Assembly, Annex G, United Nations, Vienna, 1988.

286. Lushbaugh, C.C. and Casarett, G.W., The effects of gonadal irradiation in clinical radiation therapy, *Cancer*, 37:1111–1120, 1976.
287. Hasterlik, R.J. and Marinelli, L.P., Physical dosimetry and clinical observations on 4 human beings involved in an accidental assembly excursion, in *Proceedings of International Conference on Peace Uses of Atomic Energy*, Geneva, 1956.
288. Andrews, G.A., Hubner, K.F., Fry, S.A. et al., Report of 21 year medical follow-up of survivors of the Oak Ridge Y-12 accident, in *The Medical Basis of Radiation Accident Preparedness*, Elsevier/North Holland, New York, 1980.
289. Shafford, E., Kingston, J., Malpas, J. et al., Testicular function following treatment of Hodgkin's disease in childhood, *Brit. J. Cancer*, 68:1199–1204, 1993.
290. Silini, G., Hornsey, S., and Bewley, D.K., Effects of x-ray and neutron dose fractionation on the mouse testis, *Radiat. Res.*, 19:50–63, 1963.
291. Hornsey, S., Myers, R., and Warren, P., RBE for the two components of weight loss in the mouse testis for fast neutrons relative to x-rays, *Int. J. Radiat. Biol.*, 32:297–301, 1977.
292. Geraci, J.P., Jackson, K.L., Christensen, G.M. et al., Cyclotron fast neutron RBE for various normal tissues, *Radiology*, 115:459–463, 1975.
293. De Ruiter, J., Bootsma, A.L., Kramer, M.F. et al., Response of stem cells in the mouse testis to fission neutrons of 1 MeV mean energy and 300 kV x-rays: methodology, dose-response studies, relative biological effectiveness, *Radiat. Res.*, 67:56–68, 1976.
294. Casey, R., Jewitt, M.A., and Facey, R.A., Effective depth of spermatogonia in man, measurements of scrotal thickness, *Phys. Med. Biol.*, 27:1349–1356, 1982.
295. Facey, R.A., Effective depth of spermatogonia in man, Part II: calculations for external high energy beta rays, *Phys. Med. Biol.*, 27:1347–1365, 1982.

BONE, CARTILAGE AND MUSCLE

296. Desjardins, A.U., Osteogenic tumor: Growth injury of bone and muscular atrophy following therapeutic irradiation, *Radiology*, 14:296, 1930.
297. Stevens, R.H., Retardation of bone growth following roentgen irradiation of an extensive nevocarcinoma of the skin of an infant four months of age, *Radiology*, 25:538–546, 1935.
298. Spangler, D., The effect of x-ray therapy for closure of the epiphysis: preliminary report, *Radiology*, 37:310–315, 1941.
299. Neuhauser, E.B.D., Wittenborg, M.H., and Berman, C.Z. et al., Irradiation effects of roentgen therapy on the growing spine, *Radiology*, 9:637–650, 1951.
300. Probert, J.C. and Parker, B.R., The effects of radiation therapy on bone growth, *Radiology*, 114:155–162, 1975.
301. Gauwerky, F., Uber die Strahlenschadigung des wachsenden Knochens, *Strahlentherapie*, 113:325–350, 1960.
302. Rausch, L. and Ander, E., Untersuchungen zur Beziehung zwischen ortlicher und allgemeiner Strahlenempfindlichkeit, *Sonderb. zur Strahlenther.*, 62:198–205, 1966.
303. Parker, R.G., Tolerance of mature bone and cartilage in clinical radiation therapy, in *Frontiers of Radiation Therapy and Oncology*, Vol. 6, Vaeth, J.M., Ed., Karger, Basel, 1972.
304. Seldin H.M., Radio-osteomyelitis of the jaw, *J. Oral Surg.*, 13:112–119, 1955.
305. Regen, E.M. and Wilkins, W.E., On rate of healing of fractures and phosphatase activity of callus of adult bone, *J. Bone Joint Surg.*, 18:69–79, 1936.
306. Overgarrd, M., Spontaneous radiation-induced rib fractures in breast cancer patients treated with postmastectomy irradiation. A clinical radiobiological analysis of the influence of fraction size and dose response relationships on late bone damage, *Acta Oncol.*, 27:117–122, 1988.
307. Abe, H., Nakamura, M., Takahashi, S. et al., Radiation-induced insufficiency fractures of the pelvis: evaluation with technetium 99m methylene diphosphonate scintigraphy, *Am. J. Roentgenol.*, 158:599–602, 1992.
308. Hattner, R.S., Hartmeyer, J., and Wara, W.M., Characterization of radiation-induced photopenic abnormalities on bone scans, *Radiology*, 145:161–163, 1982.
309. Bragg, D.G., Shidnia, H., Chu, F.C. et al., The clinical and radiographic effects of radiation osteitis, *Radiology*, 97:103–111, 1970.

310. Baclesse, F., Clinical experience with ultrafractionated roentgen therapy, in *Progress in Radiation Therapy*, Grune & Stratton, New York, 1958.
311. Fletcher, G.H. and Klein, R., Dose-time-volume relationship in squamous cell carcinoma of the larynx, *Radiology*, 82:1032–1041, 1964.
312. Collis, C., Dieepe, P., and Bullimore, J., Radiation-induced chondrocalcinosis of the knee articular cartilage, *Clin. Radiol.*, 39:450–451, 1988.
313. Gerstner, B., Lewis, R.B., and Rickey, E.O., Early effects of high intensity x-irradiation on skeletal muscle, *J. Gen. Physiol.*, 37:445–459, 1954.
314. Zeman, W. and Solomon, M., Effects of radiation on striated muscle, in *Pathology of Irradiation*, Berdjis, C.C., Ed., Williams & Wilkins, Baltimore, 1971.
315. Kember, N.F., Radiobiological investigations with fast neutrons using the cartilage clone system, *Br. J. Radiol.*, 42:595–597, 1969.
316. Dixon, B., The effect of radiation on the growth of vertebrae in the tails of rats, Part II. Split doses of x-rays and the effect of oxygen, *Int. J. Radiat. Biol.*, 15:215–226, 1969.
317. Dixon, B., The effect of radiation on the growth of vertebrae in the tails of rats, Part III: The response to cyclotron neutrons, *Int. J. Radiat. Biol.*, 15:541–548, 1969.
318. Kember, N.F., Cell survival and radiation damage in growth cartilage, *Br. J. Radiol.*, 40:495–505, 1967.
319. Rowland, R.E., Failla, P.M., Keane, A.T. et al., Some dose–response relationships for tumor incidence in radium patients, ANL-7760, Argonne, IL, 1970.
320. Aub, J.C., Evans, R.D., Hempelmann, L.H. et al., The late effects of internally-deposited radioactive materials in man, *Medicine*, 31:221–329, 1952.
321. Looney, W.B., Hasterlik, R.J., Brues, A.M. et al., A clinical investigation of the chronic effects of radium salt administered therapeutically, *Am. J. Roentgenol. Radium Ther. Nucl. Med*., 73:1006–1037, 1955.
322. Sharpe, W.D., Chronic radium intoxication: clinical and autopsy findings in long-term New Jersey survivors, *Environ. Res.*, 8:243–383, 1974.
323. Evans, R.D., The effects of skeletally deposited alpharay emitters in man (Silvanus Thompson Memorial Lecture), *Br. J. Radiol.*, 39:881–895, 1966.
324. Hasterlik, R.J., Finkel, A.J., and Miller, C.E., The cancer hazards of industrial and accidental exposure to radioactive isotopes, *Ann. N.Y. Acad. Sci.*, 114:832–837, 1964.
325. Spiers, F.W,, Whitwell, J.R., and Dorley, P.J., Dose in bone marrow cavities from radium 226, in *The Effects of Radiation on the Skeleton*, Clarendon Press, Oxford, 1973.
326. Keane, A., Kirsch, I,, Lucas, H. et al., Non-stochastic effects of radium 226 and radium 228 in the human skeleton, in Biological Effects of Low-Level Radiation, IAEA-SM 226/24, International Atomic Energy Agency, Vienna, 1983.
327. Spiess, H., ^{224}Ra induced tumours in children and adults, in *Delayed Effects of Bone-Seeking Radionuclides*, Mays, C.W., Jee, W.S., Lloyd, R.D. et al., Eds., University of Utah Press, Salt Lake City, 1969.
328. Ansell, B.M., Crook, A., Mallard, J.R. et al., Evaluation of intra-articular colloidal gold 198 Au in the treatment of persistent knee effusions, *Ann. Rheum. Dis.*, 22:435–439, 1963.
329. Makin, M., Robin, R.C., and Stein, J.A., Radioactive gold in the treatment of persistent synovial effusion, *Isr. J. Med. Sci*., 22:107–111, 1963.
330. Topp, J.R. and Cross, E.G., The treatment of persistent knee effusions with intra-articular radioactive gold, *Can. Med. Assoc. J*., 102:709–714, 1970.
331. Rosenthal, L., Use of Radiocolloids for intra-articular therapy for synovitis, in *Therapy in Nuclear Medicine*, Spencer, R.P., Ed., Grune & Stratton, New York, 1978.
332. Ingrand, J., Characteristics of radioisotopes for intraarticular therapy, *Ann. Rheum. Dis.*, 32(Suppl.):3–9, 1973.
333. Stevenson, A.C., Bedford, J., Dolphin, G.W. et al., Cytogenetic and scanning study of patients receiving intra-articular injections of gold 198 and yttrium 90, *Ann. Rheum. Dis*., 32:112–123, 1973.
334. Bowring, C.S. and Keeling, D.H., Absorbed radiation dose in radiation synovectomy, *Br. J. Radiol.*, 51:836–837, 1978.
335. Davis, P. and Jayson, M.I.V., Acute knee joint rupture after ^{90}Y, *Ann. Rheum. Dis.*, 34:62–63, 1975.

HEMATOPOIETIC SYSTEM

336. Shouse, S.S., Warren, S.L., and Whipple, G.H., Aplasia of marrow and fatal intoxication in dogs produced by roentgen irradiation of all bones, *J. Exp. Med.*, 53:421, 1913.
337. Hempelmann, L.H., Lisco, H., and Hoffman, J.G., The acute radiation syndrome. A study of 9 cases and a review of the problem, *Ann. Intern. Med.*, 36:279, 1952.
338. Guskova, A.K. and Baisogolov, G.D., Two cases of ACS in humans, in Action of Radiation in the Organism, Reports of the Soviet Delegation to the First International Conference on the Peaceful Applications of Atomic Energy, Geneva, U.S.S.R. Academy of Science, Moscow, 1953 (in Russian).
339. Rajevsky, B., *Strahlendosis und Strahlenwirkung*, 2 verbeste und vermehrteauflage, G. Thieme Verlag, Stuttgart, 1956 (in German).
340. Bond, V.P., Fliedner, T.M., and Archambeau, J.O., *Mammalian Radiation Lethality*, Academic Press, New York, 1965.
341. Nothdurft, W., Bone Marrow, in *Radiopathology of Organs and Tissues*, Scherer, E., Streffer, C., and Trott, K., Eds., Springer-Verlag, Berlin, 1991.
342. Cronkite, E.P., Kinetics of human hematopoiesis, in *Effects of Ionizing Radiation on the Hematopoietic Tissue*, International Atomic Energy Agency, Vienna, 1967.
343. Fliedner, T., Nothdurft, W., and Steinbach, K., Blood cell changes after radiation exposure as an indicator for hemopoietic stem cell function, *Bone Marrow Transplant*, 3:77–84, 1988.
344. Tubiana, M., Clinical treatments of leukemia by splenic irradiation, in *Cell Survival after Low Doses of Radiation: Theoretical and Clinical Implications*, Alper, P., Ed., John Wiley & Sons, London, 1975.
345. Fitzpatric, P. and Rider, W., Half body radiotherapy, *Int. J. Radiat. Oncol. Biol. Phys.*, 1:197–207, 1976.
346. Salazar, O., Rubin, P., Keller, B. et al., Single-dose half body irradiation for palliation of multiple bone metastases from solid tumors. Final Radiation Therapy Oncology Group Report, *Cancer*, 58:29–36, 1986.
347. Sykes, M.P., Chu, F.C., Savel, H. et al., The effects of varying dosages of irradiation upon sternal marrow regeneration, *Radiology*, 83:1084–1087, 1964.
348. Sacks, E.L., Goris, M.L., Glatstein, E. et al., Bone marrow regeneration following large field irradiation: Influence of volume, age, dose and time, *Cancer*, 42:1057–1065, 1978.
349. Rubin, P., Landman, S., Meyer, E. et al., Bone marrow regeneration and extension after extended field irradiation in Hodgkin's disease, *Cancer*, 32:699–711, 1973.
350. Field, S.B., The relative biological effectiveness of fast neutrons for mammalian tissues, *Radiology*, 93:915–920, 1969.
351. Broerse, J.J. and Barendsen, G.W., Relative biological effectiveness of fast neutrons for effects on normal tissues, *Curr. Top. Radiat. Res. Q.*, 8:305–350, 1973.
352. Polednak, A.P., Long-term effects of radium exposure in female dial workers: hematocrit and blood pressure, *Environ. Res.*, 13:237–249, 1977.
353. Marshall, J.H. and Hoegerman, S.F., Estimation of alpha particle dose from radium 226 to blood, Argonne National Laboratory Report 75-3, 1974.
354. Benua, R.S., Cicalie, N.R., Sorenberg, M. et al., The relation of radioiodine dosimetry to results and complications in treatment of metastatic thyearoid cancer, *AJR*, 87:171–182, 1962.
355. Keldsen, N., Mortensen, B., and Hansen, H., Haematological effects from radioiodine treatment of thyearoid carcinoma, *Acta Oncol.*, 29:1035–1039, 1990.
356. Breen, S., Powe, J., and Porter, A., Dose estimation in Sr-89 radiotherapy of metastatic prostate cancer, *J. Nucl. Med.*, 33:1316–1323, 1992.
357. Laing, A., Ackery, D., Bayly, R. et al., Strontium 89 chloride for pain palliation in prostatic skeletal malignancy, *Br. J. Radiol.*, 64:816–822, 1991.
358. Spiers, F.W., Beddoe, A.H., King, S.D. et al., The absorbed dose to bone marrow in treatment of polycythemia by phosphorus 32, *Br. J. Radiol.*, 49:133–140, 1976.
359. Chauduri, T., The role of phosphorus 32 in polycythemia vera and leukemia, in *Therapy in Nuclear Medicine*, Spencer, R., Ed., Grune & Stratton, New York, 1978.
360. Mayer, K., Pentlow, K., Marcove, R. et al., Sulphur 35 therapy for chondrosarcoma and chordoma, in *Therapy in Nuclear Medicine*, Spencer, R., Ed., Grune & Stratton, New York, 1978.
361. Rubin, P. and Levitt, F.H., The response of disseminated reticulum cell sarcomas to the intravenous injection of colloidal radioactive gold, *J. Nucl. Med.*, 5:581–594, 1964.

362. Andrews, J.R. et al., The effects of 1 curie of sulfur 35 administered intravenously as sulfate to a man with advanced chondrosarcoma, *AJR*, 83:123–124, 1960.
363. Brandao-Mello, C., Oliveira, A., Valverde, N. et al., Clinical and hematological aspects of cesium 137: the Goiânia radiation accident, *Health Phys.*, 60:31–39, 1991.
364. Butturini, A., DeSouza, P., Gale, R. et al., Use of recombinant granulocyte-macrophage colony stimulating factor in the Brazil radiation accident, *Lancet*, 2:471–475, 1988.

7 The Safety of Radiation Sources and the Security of Radioactive Materials

Abel J. Gonzalez

CONTENTS

Introduction 133
Quantifying the Problem...134
Current Issues...135
A Yardstick for Safety and Security 137
Requirements for Safety 137
The Agency's Current Program 145

INTRODUCTION

Sources of ionizing radiation (or radiation sources, for short) are used throughout the world for a wide variety of beneficial purposes, in industry, medicine, research, defense, and education. There is currently an increase in developing and promoting the application of techniques that use radiation properties, particularly in the developing world. Today additional radiation sources are used for diagnosing or treating illnesses that were before undetectable or incurable, for producing more and better food for a demanding and growing population, and for facilitating the technical processes required by modern industries. These sources can be in the form of radiation generators, such as X-ray apparatuses and particle accelerators, or devices containing radioactive materials. Many applications involve sealed devices with the radioactive materials firmly contained or bound within a suitable capsule or housing. Some also involve radioactive materials in an unsealed form. The risks posed by these sources and materials vary widely, depending on the radionuclides, the forms, the activities, etc. Unless breached or leaking, sealed sources present a risk from external radiation exposure only. However, breached or leaking sealed sources, as well as unsealed radioactive materials, may lead to contamination of the environment and the intake of radioactive materials into the human body. Thus, radiation sources can be detrimental to human health.

The International Atomic Energy Agency (IAEA) is the organization within the United Nations system with statutory functions relative to radiation. These functions are to establish international standards of radiation safety, and to provide for the applications of these standards at the request of any state. The relevant IAEA standards are the International Basic Safety Standards for Protection against Ionizing Radiation and/or the Safety of Radiation Sources, the so-called BSS. Broadly, the BSS are intended to ensure:

- The protection of individuals and the population as a whole against the radiation exposure that they are expected to incur as a result of the normal uses of radiation sources;

- The safety of the radiation sources to prevent the occurrence of accidents and, should they happen, to mitigate their consequences; and
- The security of the radioactive materials to prevent any relinquishing of their control and consequent misuse.

Routine radiation protection is proving to be extremely good. Very small radiation doses are routinely incurred by occupationally exposed workers and by the public at large as a result of the normal operation of radiation sources. The application of the principle of optimization of radiation protection (that is, keep doses as low as reasonably achievable, or ALARA), in conjunction with stringent individual dose limitation, has been successful in achieving large reductions in radiation doses.

There was also the dogma that radiation accidents would be prevented. But this presumption has proved to be wrong. In fact, many accidents have occurred during the last two decades, demonstrating serious problems with the safety of radiation sources and, recently, also with the security of the radioactive materials.

While the meaning of the term *protection* is self-evident, *safety* and *security* are two distinct terms in English and French only; a common word is used for these concepts in all other major languages. Not surprisingly, therefore, many people wonder, "What is the distinction?" If they reached for their dictionaries, they would perhaps be none the wiser, because one of the definitions of security is safety, and vice versa. "Safety of radiation sources" is used to mean the assembly of technical and managerial features that diminish the likelihood of something going wrong with a source, resulting in people being overexposed. "Security of radioactive material" is used to mean the assembly of technical and managerial features that prevent any unauthorized activity with radioactive materials by ensuring that their control is not relinquished or improperly transferred.

The safety issue covers all types of radiation sources, i.e., radiation generators and radioactive materials. The former is relevant when the generated radiation has enough energy and its flux is important enough to be a cause of radiological accidents. The latter are relevant when the activity of the material, and sometimes its activity concentration, is sufficient to create serious radiological situations.

The security issue is usually limited to radioactive materials alone and not to radiation sources (as a whole) because apparatus, which generates ionizing radiation, such as X-ray machines and accelerators, is less likely to be a security threat. Security of radioactive materials is required for two major purposes: (1) to prevent lost or misplaced radioactive materials from causing harm to people, and (2) to prevent the diversion of those radioactive materials that are also special fissionable (nuclear) materials, such as uranium-235 and plutonium-239, from legal to illegal, even criminal, uses. The IAEA has a full program dealing with activities in the security of nuclear materials for safeguard purposes.

This chapter describes the problems caused by breaches in the safety and security of radiation sources and the current international responses to the problem.

QUANTIFYING THE PROBLEM

Breaches in the safety of sources have resulted in accidents and overexposure of people, many with fatal consequences. Sometimes these occurred as a result of equipment failure. Other breaches have been the consequences of human mistakes. Many have been the result of underlying problems in the regulatory oversight that governments presumably have to enforce.

There is no complete database on all the accidents that have occurred worldwide. The IAEA has made a compilation of the more important among those reported in the open literature, and this list is presented in Table 7.1. In addition, after the accident in Goiânia (Brazil), the IAEA has assessed a number of accidents with the support of local authorities, and published specific accident reports with the purpose of fostering information exchange and lesson learning.

Breaches in security result in radioactive materials that are lost, stolen, or simply abandoned. There are no complete data sources of how many of these events are occurring worldwide. But, in the United States alone, where the regulations for controlling radioactive sources are particularly restrictive and where the regulatory authority is particularly efficient, the Nuclear Regulatory Commission (NRC) receives about 200 reports of lost, stolen, or abandoned radioactive sources each year. The NRC recognizes that "the volume of reports received probably represents only the tip of the iceberg."

The world metal recycling industry has been particularly vulnerable to the problem of "orphan" sources. Sources that are no longer under regulatory control may be mixed with metal scrap destined for recycling. Simple economic benefits, or sometimes ignorance, lead the "relinquishing" individual to sell the source for its metallic value to scrap dealers who usually are not aware of the radioactive content. Thus, the source enters into the worldwide scrap metal inventory, which, because of the recent global opening of the markets, has become essentially uncontrollable. More than 60 events of highly radioactive sources appearing in scrap metal have been reported to the U.S. NRC (Table 7.2). Sometimes, these events are discovered only after melting and because some commodity has been detected with contamination of radioactive materials (Table 7.3). No international registry is available of cases of melting of radioactive sources, or contaminated scrap, or of detected radioactively contaminated commodities.

In spite of this situation, it is reassuring that the theft and smuggling of radioactive materials for malevolent purposes have, historically, been a rarity. However, the uses of chemical, biological, and, possibly, radioactive materials by terrorists as weapons may be crimes of the future. Not surprisingly, governments have been anxious about the illicit movement of radioactive and nuclear materials. Custom officers seize some materials, but others may cross the borders of countries undetected, particularly where customs officers are unprepared in knowledge and equipment to deal with this problem. The World Custom Organization has reported 234 confirmed cases of seizures of illicit radioactive material between 1993 and 1998 (Table 7.4). The seizures by element are reported in Table 7.5. The International Criminal Police Organization (INTERPOL) has also been active in the field.

CURRENT ISSUES

The turning point in global interest of radiation safety and security problems was the International Conference on the Safety of Radiation Sources and the Security of Radioactive Materials. The conference was cosponsored by the IAEA together with INTERPOL, the World Customs Organization, and the European Commission. It took place from September 14 to 18, 1998 in Dijon, France.

The major findings of the Dijon Conference, as summarized by the chairman of the Conference Program Committee, were as follows:

> The attention of the radiation protection community was in the past focused on the prevention of accidents involving radiation sources subject to regulatory control, but the rise in the incidence of illicit trafficking in radioactive materials during the early 1990s led to greater awareness of the problem of radiation sources that are — for various reasons — not subject to regulatory control. Bearing this in mind, the Conference concluded that:
>
> (a) Sources of ionizing radiation must have sufficient protection to allow for safe normal operations.
> (b) The possibility of accidental exposures involving radiation sources must be anticipated and there must be appropriate safety devices and procedures. In this connection:
>   (i) weaknesses in the design and construction of radiation sources must be corrected;
>   (ii) a high level of safety culture in the handling of radiation sources must be promoted, so that — inter alia — human errors are minimized through good training; and
>   (iii) regulatory infrastructures for the control of radiation sources must be supported by governments and be able to act independently, and the regulatory authority in each country

must maintain oversight of all radiation sources in that country — including those which have been imported.
(c) Radiation sources should not be allowed to drop out of the regulatory control system. This means that the regulatory authority must keep up-to-date records of the person responsible for each source, monitor transfers of sources and track the fate of each source at the end of its useful life.
(d) Efforts should be made to find radiation sources that are not in the regulatory authority's inventory, because they were in the country before the inventory was established, or were never specifically licensed or were lost, abandoned or stolen (such radiation sources are often referred to as "orphan" sources).
(e) Because there are many "orphan" sources throughout the world, efforts to improve the detection of radioactive materials crossing national borders and moving within countries by carrying out radiation measurements and through intelligence-gathering should be intensified. Optimum detection techniques need to be developed, and confusion would be avoided if international agreement could be achieved on quantitative levels that would trigger investigations at border crossings.

It is clear from these points that the key common element which would have the greatest part to play both in the avoidance of "orphan" sources — with their potential for misuse or accidents — and in the achievement and maintenance of safe and secure operating conditions is effective national regulatory authorities operating within suitable national infrastructures.

Governments are urged to create regulatory authorities for radiation sources if they do not exist. Whether the regulatory authority is newly created or has been in existence for some time, the government must provide it with sufficient backing and with sufficient human and financial resources to enable it to function effectively. Only in this way can the problem of the safety of radiation sources and the security of radioactive materials be tackled at its roots and eventually brought under control.

Further efforts should be made to investigate whether international undertakings concerned with the effective operation of national regulatory control systems and attracting broad adherence could be formulated.

It is surprising that the issue of the safety of radiation sources and security of radioactive materials has become high in the international agenda now, after three quarters of a century of radiation protection, and nearly half of a century of IAEA activity. In its 70 years of existence, the International Commission on Radiological Protection (ICRP) has produced around 100 publications with recommendations for protection against ionizing radiation; national and international organizations have used these recommendations for establishing radiation protection standards. However, only two ICRP publications deal with the problem of the safety of radiation sources, and none has ever dealt with the issue of the security of radioactive materials. For the IAEA, the balance is similar. The IAEA has taken the leading role in the United Nations system in establishing standards of safety and has issued more than 100 documents on the subject. However, again until the appearance of the BSS, the subject of radiation source safety had been loosely addressed in the IAEA standards by the simplistic requirement that "accidental exposures shall be prevented" (a fine "motherhood and apple pie" statement), which offered no guidance on to how to achieve safety. The security issue was also completely ignored by international standards. With the BSS, some progress was achieved and a full set of requirements for safety and security was established. However, they are general in nature and with very little quantification.

It appears that professionals and authorities alike were assumedly convinced that appropriate requirements for safety and security were somehow automatically established and implemented. It seems that it was automatically presumed, for example, that all governments had radiation safety infrastructures in place, which at least included a system of notification, registration, licensing, and inspection of radiation sources. But many of these assumptions and presumptions proved to be wrong.

In the early 1980s, the IAEA launched the Radiation Protection Advisory Teams (RAPAT) program as a diagnostic tool. The IAEA was surprised to learn that among its member states visited by RAPAT, nearly half lacked the minimum radiation safety infrastructure, more than 50 countries. In addition, there are at least 60 countries, which are not members of the IAEA, where we can only guess the situation may be even worse. In summary, more than 110 countries do not have the minimum infrastructure to control radiation sources properly. This is certainly not encouraging.

The IAEA response has been to launch an aggressive, proactive technical cooperation program, which aims to solve the problem. The so-called Model Project in Radiation Protection is one of the largest efforts in the history of the United Nations to enhance radiation safety infrastructure in states that need it most urgently. This IAEA initiative involves a proactive approach rather than the traditional reactive approach to technical cooperation on the part of UN organizations. The initial phase covered just the 53 IAEA member states in most urgent need. The IAEA Board of Governors has recently decided that the IAEA should also provide for the application of the BSS in its nonmember states.

A YARDSTICK FOR SAFETY AND SECURITY

To solve a problem, one first needs a standard yardstick for measuring its extent. In the UN family and for the specific case of the many problems related to the safety of radiation sources and the security of radioactive materials, such a yardstick is provided by the BSS. A main purpose of the BSS is simply to promote coherent and consistent approaches to radiation safety. The BSS include a preamble, entitled Principles and Fundamental Objectives, which presupposes the governmental responsibilities for radiation safety and security. The main standards, entitled Principal Requirements, include some obligations on safety and few on security. Also included is a series of Technical Appendices and Schedules, including a relatively modest appendix devoted to the safety of sources.

REQUIREMENTS FOR SAFETY

The BSS do not (and indeed may not) impose responsibilities on governments. Instead, they presuppose that governments have discharged their responsibilities. The preamble indicates that the BSS are based on the presumption that governments have proper legislation and regulations in place to deal with problems of the safety of radioactive sources and the security of radioactive materials and that they have established independent regulatory authorities who license sources, inspect them, and enforce safety requirements. The BSS have assumed that in every country there is a regulatory authority with the necessary powers and resources and with effective legal independence. But resources, in particular, are something that regulatory authorities in developing countries are usually lacking. The BSS have also assumed that governments can provide, either directly or indirectly, essential support such as personal dosimetry services, calibration services, information exchange mechanisms, and, of course, personnel training. All are idealistic hypotheses for most of the world.

Many of these assumptions, made back in the early 1990s when the BSS were being prepared, have proved to be wrong. It is not true that there is proper legislation in most countries — indeed, many countries have no legislation at all. It is not true that all countries have proper regulations in place. Many have no regulations at all. It is not true that in most countries there are independent regulatory authorities invested with the necessary powers to perform the work required of them. Finally, it is not true that when a regulatory authority exists it always has the necessary resources at its disposal. The existence of governmental infrastructures of radiation safety is a precondition for the actual safety of radiation sources and security of radioactive materials in the years ahead.

In light of what we have learned in recent years, it would now seem that the administrative requirements, which were previously thought to be of secondary importance — simply because

TABLE 7.1
Major Radiation Accidents (1945 to 2000)

Year	Place	Source	Dose (or Activity Intake)	Significant Overexposures[a]	Deaths
1945/46	Los Alamos, USA	Criticality	Up to 13 Gy (mixed[b] radiation)	10	2
1952	Argonne, USA	Criticality	0.1–1.6 Gy (mixed[b] radiation)	3	—
1953	USSR	Experimental reactor	3.0–4.5 Gy (mixed[b] radiation)	2	—
	Melbourne, Australia	^{60}Co	Unknown	1	—
1955	Hanford, USA	^{239}Pu	Unknown	1	—
1958	Oak Ridge, USA	Criticality (Y-12 plant)	0.7–3.7 Gy (mixed[b] radiation)	7	—
	Vinca, Yugoslavia	Experimental reactor	2.1–4.4 Gy (mixed[b] radiation)	8	1
	Los Alamos, USA	Criticality	0.35–45 Gy (mixed[b] radiation)	3	1
1959	Johannessburg, South Africa	^{60}Co	Unknown	1	—
1960	USA	Electron beam	7.5 Gy (local)	1	—
	Madison, USA	^{60}Co	2.5–3 Gy	1	—
	Lockport, USA	X rays	(to 12 Gy, nonuniform)	6	—
	USSR	^{137}Cs (suicide)	~15 Gy	1	1
	USSR	Radium bromide (ingestion)	74 MBq	1	1 (4 yr later)
1961	USSR	Submarine accident	1.0–50.0 Gy	>30	8
	Miamisburg, USA	^{238}Pu	Unknown	2	—
	Miamisburg, USA	^{210}Po	Unknown	2	—
	Switzerland	^{3}H	3 Gy	3	1
	Idaho Falls, USA	Explosion in reactor	Up to 3.5 Gy	7	3
	Plymouth, UK	X rays	Local overdosage	11	—
	Fontenay-aux-Roses, France	^{239}Pu	Unknown	1	—
1962	Richland, USA	Criticality	Unknown	2	—
	Hanford, USA	Criticality	0.2–1.1 Gy (mixed[b] radiation)	3	—
	Mexico City, Mexico	^{60}Co capsule	9.9–52 Sv	5	4
	Moscow, USSR	^{60}Co	3.8 Gy (nonuniform)	1	—
1963	China	^{60}Co	0.2–80 Gy	6	2
	Saclay, France	Electron beam	Unknown (local)	2	—
1964	FRG	^{3}H	10 Gy	4	1
	Rhode Island, USA	Criticality	0.3–46 Gy (mixed[b] radiation)	4	1
	New York, USA	^{241}Am	Unknown	2	—
1965	Rockford, USA	Accelerator	>3 Gy (local)	1	—
	USA	Diffractometer	Unknown (local)	1	—
	USA	Spectrometer	Unknown (local)	1	—
	Mol, Belgium	Experimental reactor	5 Gy (total)	1	—
1966	Portland, USA	^{32}P	Unknown	4	—

TABLE 7.1 (CONTINUED)
Major Radiation Accidents (1945 to 2000)

Year	Place	Source	Dose (or Activity Intake)	Significant Overexposures[a]	Deaths
1966	Leechburg, USA	^{235}Pu	Unknown	1	1
	Pennsylvania, USA	^{198}Au	Unknown	1	—
	China	"Contaminated Zone"	2–3 Gy	2	—
	USSR	Experimental reactor	3.0–7.0 Gy (total)	5	—
1967	USA	^{192}Ir	0.2 Gy 50 Gy (local)	1	—
	Bloomsburg, USA	^{241}Am	Unknown	1	—
	Pittsburgh, USA	Accelerator	1–6 Gy	3	—
	India	^{60}Co	80 Gy (local)	1	—
	USSR	X-ray medical diagnostic facility	50 Gy (head, local)	1	1 (after 7 yr)
1968	Burbank, USA	^{239}Pu	Unknown	2	—
	Wisconsin, USA	^{198}Au	Unknown	1	1
	FRG	^{192}Ir	1 Gy	1	—
	La Plata, Argentina	^{137}Cs	Local 0.5 Gy (WB)	1	—
	Chicago, USA	^{198}Au	4–5 Gy (bone marrow)	1	1
	India	^{192}Ir	130 Gy (local)	1	—
	USSR	Experimental reactor	1.0–1.5 Gy	4	—
	USSR	^{60}Co irradiation facility	1.5 Gy (local, head)	1	—
1969	Wisconsin, USA	^{85}Sr	Unknown	1	—
	USSR	Experimental reactor	5.0 Sv (total) nonuniform	1	—
	Glasgow, UK	^{192}Ir	0.6 Gy	1	—
1970	Australia	X rays	4–45 Gy (local)	2	—
	Des Moines, USA	^{32}P	Unknown	1	—
	USA	Spectrometer	Unknown (local)	1	—
	Erwin, USA	^{235}U	Unknown	1	—
1971	Newport, USA	^{60}Co	30 Gy (local)	1	—
	UK	^{192}Ir	30 Gy (local)	1	—
	Japan	^{192}Ir	0.2–1.5 Gy	4	—
	Oak Ridge, USA	^{60}Co	1.3 Gy	1	—
	USSR	Experimental reactor	7.8; 8.1 Sv	2	—
	USSR	Experimental reactor	3.0 total	3	—
	USSR	Criticality	8–60 Gy	4	2
1972	Chicago, USA	^{192}Ir	100 Gy (local)	1	—
	Peach Bottom, USA	^{192}Ir	300 Gy (local)	1	—
	FRG	^{192}Ir	0.3 Gy	1	—
	China	^{60}Co	0.4–5.0 Gy	20	—
	Bulgaria	^{137}Cs capsules (suicide)	>200 Gy (local, chest)	1	1
1973	USA	^{192}Ir	0.3 Gy	1	—
	UK	^{106}Ru	Unknown	1	—
	Czechoslovakia	^{60}Co	1.6 Gy	1	—
1974	Illinois, USA	Spectrometer	2.4–48 Gy (local)	3	—
	Parsipany, USA	^{60}Co	1.7–4 Gy	1	—
	Middle East	^{192}Ir	0.3 Gy	1	—

TABLE 7.1 (CONTINUED)
Major Radiation Accidents (1945 to 2000)

Year	Place	Source	Dose (or Activity Intake)	Significant Overexposures[a]	Deaths
1975	Brescia, Italy	^{60}Co	10 Gy	1	1
	USA	^{192}Ir	10 Gy (local)	1	—
	Columbus, USA	^{60}Co	11–14 Gy (local)	6	—
	Iraq	^{192}Ir	0.3 Gy	1	—
	USSR	^{137}Cs irradiation facility	3–5 Gy (total) + >30 Gy (hands)	1	—
	GDR	Research reactor	20–30 Gy (local)	1	—
	FRG	X rays	30 Gy (hand)	1	—
	FRG	X rays	1 Gy (total)	1	—
1976	Hanford, USA	^{241}Am intake	>37 MBq	1	—
	USA	^{192}Ir	37.2 Gy (local)	1	—
	Pittsburg, USA	^{60}Co	15 Gy (local)	1	—
1977	Rockaway, USA	^{60}Co	2 Gy	1	—
	Pretoria, South Africa	^{192}Ir	1.2 Gy	1	—
	Denver, USA	^{32}P	Unknown	1	—
	USSR	^{60}Co irradiation facility	4 Gy (total)	1	—
	USSR	Proton accelerator	10.0–30.0 Gy (hands)	1	—
	UK	^{192}Ir	0.1 Gy + local	1	—
	Peru	^{192}Ir	0.9–2.0 (total)	3	—
1978	Argentina	^{192}Ir	12–16 (local)	1	—
	Algeria	^{192}Ir	Up to 13 Gy (for max. exposed person)	7	1
	UK	—	—	1	—
	USSR	Electron accelerator	20 Gy (local)	1	—
1979	California, USA	^{192}Ir	Up to 1 Gy	5	—
1980	USSR	^{60}Co irradiation facility	50.0 Gy (local, legs)	1	—
	GDR	X rays	15–30 Gy (hand)	1	—
	FRG	Radiography unit	23 Gy (hand)	1	—
	China	^{60}Co	5 Gy (local)	1	—
1981	Saintes, France	^{60}Co medical facility	>25 Gy	3	—
	Oklahoma, USA	^{192}Ir	Unknown	1	—
1982	Norway	^{60}Co	22 Gy	1	1
	India	^{192}Ir	35 Gy local	1	—
1983	Constitu, Argentina	Criticality	43 Gy (mixed[b] radiation)	1	1
	Mexico	^{60}Co	0.25–5.0 Sv protracted exp.	10	—
	Iran	^{192}Ir	20 Gy (hand)	1	—
1984	Morocco	^{192}Ir	Unknown	11	8
	Peru	X rays	5–40 Gy (local)	6	—
1985	China	Electron accelerator	Unknown (local)	2	—
	China	^{198}Au (mistake in treatment)	Unknown, internal	2	1
	China	^{137}Cs	8–10 Sv (subacute)	3	—
	Brazil	Radiography source	410 Sv (local)	1	—
	Brazil	Radiography source	160 Sv (local)	2	—

TABLE 7.1 (CONTINUED)
Major Radiation Accidents (1945 to 2000)

Year	Place	Source	Dose (or Activity Intake)	Significant Overexposures[a]	Deaths
1985/86	USA	Accelerator	Unknown	3	2
1986	China	^{60}Co	2–3 Gy	2	—
	Chernobyl, USSR	Nuclear power plant	1–16 Gy (mixed[b] radiation)	134	28 (+2 nonrad. deaths)
1987	Goiânia, Brazil	^{137}Cs	Up to 7 Gy (mixed[b] radiation)	50[c]	4
	China	^{60}Co	1.0 Gy	1	—
1989	El Salvador	^{60}Co irradiation facility	3–8 Gy	3	1
1990	Israel	^{60}Co irradiation facility	>12 Gy	1	1
	Spain	Radiotherapy accelerator	Unknown	27	18[d]
1991	Nesvizh, Belarus	^{60}Co irradiation facility	10 Gy	1	1
	USA	Accelerator	>30 Gy (hands and legs)	1	—
1992	Vietnam	Accelerator	20–50 Gy (hands)	1	—
	China	^{60}Co	>0.25–10 Gy	8	3
	USA	^{192}Ir brachytherapy	>1000 Gy (local)	1	1
1994	Tammiku, Estonia	^{137}Cs source from waste rep.	1830 Gy (thigh) + 4 Gy (WB)	3	1
1996	Costa Rica	^{60}Co radiotherapy	60% overdosage	115	13[d]
	Gilan, Iran	^{192}Ir radiography	2–3 Gy? (WB) + 100 Gy? (chest)	1	—
1997	Kremlev, Russia	Criticality experiment	5–10 Gy (WB) + 200–250 (hands)	1	—
1998	Turkey	^{60}Co	Various doses, up to 3 Gy WB, up to 100 Gy locally; leg amputation	10	—
1999	Japan	Criticality	1–17 Gy	3	2
	Peru	^{192}Ir radiography	Up to 100 Gy locally; leg amputation	1	—
2000	Thailand	^{60}Co	Unknown	3	3
	Egypt	?	?	?	2

Note: WB = whole body.

[a] ≥0.25 Sv to the whole body, blood-forming organs or other critical organs; ≥6 Gy to the skin locally; ≥0.75 Gy to other tissues or organs from an external source, or exceeding half of the annual limit on intake (ALI).
[b] Mixed radiation refers to various types of radiation with different LET values, such as neutrons and gamma rays, or gamma and beta rays.
[c] The number is probably lower (some of the 50 contaminated persons received doses of less than 0.25 Sv).
[d] To June of 2000.

TABLE 7.2
Meltings of Radioactive Materials

No.	Year	Product	Origin	Contaminant	Activity (GBq)
1	—[a]	Gold	NY	^{210}Pb, ^{210}Bi, ^{210}Po	Unknown
2	1983	Steel	Auburn, NY	^{60}Co	930
3	1983	Iron/steel	Mexico[b]	^{60}Co	15,000
4	1983	Gold	Unknown, NY	^{241}Am	Unknown
5	1983	Steel	Taiwan[b]	^{60}Co	>740
6	1984	Steel	US Pipe & Foundry, AL	^{137}Cs	0.37–1.9
7	1985	Steel	Brazil[b]	^{60}Co	Unknown
8	1985	Steel	Tamco, CA	^{137}Cs	56
9	1987	Steel	Florida Steel, FL	^{137}Cs	0.93
10	1987	Aluminum	United Technology, IN	^{226}Ra	0.74
11	1988	Lead	ALCO Pacific, CA	^{137}Cs	0.74–0.93
12	1988	Copper	Warrington, MO	Accelerator	Unknown
13	1988	Steel	Italy[b]	^{60}Co	Unknown
14	1989	Steel	Bayou Steel, LA	^{137}Cs	19
15	1989	Steel	Cytemp, PA	Th	Unknown
16	1989	Steel	Italy	^{137}Cs	1000
17	1989	Aluminum	Russian Federation	Unknown	Unknown
18	1990	Steel	NUCOR Steel, UT	^{137}Cs	Unknown
19	1990	Aluminum	Italy	^{137}Cs	Unknown
20	1990	Steel	Ireland	^{137}Cs	3.7
21	1991	Steel	India[b]	^{60}Co	7.4–20
22	1991	Aluminum	Alcan Recycling, TN	Th	Unknown
23	1991	Aluminum	Italy	^{137}Cs	Unknown
24	1991	Copper	Italy	^{241}Am	Unknown
25	1992	Steel	Newport Steel, KY	^{137}Cs	12
26	1992	Aluminum	Reynolds, VA	^{226}Ra	Unknown
27	1992	Steel	Border Steel, TX	^{137}Cs	4.6–7.4
28	1992	Steel	Keystone Wire, IL	^{137}Cs	Unknown
29	1992	Steel	Poland	^{137}Cs	Unknown
30	1992	Copper	Estonia/Russian Federation	^{60}Co	Unknown
31	1993	Unknown	Russian Federation	^{226}Ra	Unknown
32	1993	Steel (?)	Russian Federation	^{137}Cs	Unknown
33	1993	Steel	Auburn Steel, NY	^{137}Cs	37
34	1993	Steel	Newport Steel, NY	^{137}Cs	7.4
35	1993	Steel	Chaparral Steel, TX	^{137}Cs	Unknown
36	1993	Zinc	Southern Zinc, GA	U (dep.)	Unknown
37	1993	Steel	Kazakhstan[b]	^{60}Co	0.3
38	1993	Steel	Florida Steel, FL	^{137}Cs	Unknown
39	1993	Steel	South Africa[c]	^{137}Cs	<600 Bq/g
40	1993	Steel	Italy	^{137}Cs	Unknown
41	1994	Steel	Austeel Lemont, IN	^{137}Cs	0.074
42	1994	Steel	US Pipe & Foundry, CA	^{137}Cs	Unknown
43	1994	Steel	Bulgaria[b]	^{60}Co	3.7
44	1995	Steel	Canada[d]	^{137}Cs	0.2–0.7
45	1995	Steel	Czech Republic	^{60}Co	Unknown
46	1995	Steel (?)	Italy	^{137}Cs	Unknown
47	1996	Steel	Sweden	^{60}Co	87
48	1996	Steel	Austria	^{60}Co	Unknown

TABLE 7.2 (CONTINUED)
Meltings of Radioactive Materials

No.	Year	Product	Origin	Contaminant	Activity (GBq)
49	1996	Lead	Brazil[b]	^{210}Pb, ^{210}Bi, ^{210}Po	Unknown
50	1996	Aluminum	Bluegrass Recycling, KY	^{232}Th	Unknown
51	1997	Aluminum	White Salvage Co., TN	^{241}Am	Unknown
52	1997	Steel	WCI, OH	^{60}Co	0.9(?)
53	1997	Steel	Kentucky Electric, KY	^{137}Cs	1.3
54	1997	Steel	Italy	$^{137}Cs/^{60}Co$	200/37
55	1997	Steel	Greece	^{137}Cs	11 Bq/g
56	1997	Steel	Birmingham Steel, AL	$^{137}Cs/^{241}Am$	7 Bq/g
57	1997	Steel	Brazil[b]	^{60}Co	<0.2
58	1997	Steel	Bethlehem Steel, IN	^{60}Co	0.2
59	1998	Steel	Spain	^{137}Cs	>37
60	1998	Steel	Sweden	^{192}Ir	<90

[a] Multiple cases reported, earliest circa 1910.
[b] Contaminated product exported to the United States.
[c] Contaminated vanadium slag exported to Austria; detected in Italy.
[d] Contaminated by-product (electric furnace dust) exported to the United States.

TABLE 7.3
Products Contaminated with Radioactive Materials Imported into the United States

Item No.	Product	Contaminant Discovered	Year	Country of Origin
1	Steel, iron	^{60}Co	1984	Mexico
2	Steel	^{60}Co	1984	Taiwan
3	Steel	^{60}Co	1985	Brazil
4	Steel	^{60}Co	1988	Italy
5	Steel	^{60}Co	1991	India
6	Ferrophosphorus	^{60}Co	1993	Kazakhstan
7	Steel	^{60}Co	1994	Bulgaria
8	Furnace dust	^{137}Cs	1995	Canada
9	Lead	^{210}Pb, ^{210}Bi, ^{210}Po	1996	Brazil
10	Steel	^{60}Co	1998	Brazil

they appeared to be so obvious — have become very significant. The administrative requirements of the BSS are extremely simple: the BSS rely on the existence, in every single country, of a system for the notification, registration, and licensing of radiation sources. Indeed, many countries are not even aware of the need to meet this requirement, and consequently the authorities in those countries do not know how many sources exist within their territories or where the sources are, and, it follows logically, there is no registration or control of radiation sources. That is the reason the administrative requirements are so important.

Although the BSS took the existence of the administrative requirements for granted, they placed more emphasis on two technical requirements: "defense in depth" and good engineering practice. With the benefit of hindsight, it was very naive to place so much emphasis on technical requirements when the basis — the administrative requirements — had not been universally established. Defense

TABLE 7.4
Seizures of Radioactive Sources (by country, 1993 to 1998)

Country	No. of Cases	Percentage of Cases
Germany	67	28.6
Russian Federation	52	22.1
Poland	18	7.7
Ukraine	17	7.2
Lithuania	17	7.2
Turkey	14	6.0
Bulgaria	10	4.3
Estonia	8	3.4
Czech Republic	7	3.0
Belarus	6	2.6
Azerbaijan	3	1.3
Italy	3	1.3
New Zealand	1	0.4

TABLE 7.5
Seizures by Element (1993 to 1998)

Element	No. of Cases	Percentage of Cases
Uranium	129	55.1
Cesium	53	22.6
Plutonium	10	4.3
Radium	5	2.1
Americium	3	1.3
Other	34	14.5

in depth refers to a multilayered system of safety provisions for the purpose of preventing accidents, mitigating the consequences of accidents, and restoring sources to safe conditions. Good engineering practice is something that has also been taken for granted at times but which is not always in place. The BSS presume that sources are always reliable and built to approved engineering standards, with sufficient safety margins, and (this is very important) that they take account of research and development results — not being fossilized in time.

The management requirements include, besides quality assurance, attention to human factors, and the use of qualified experts, the so called "safety culture." Safety culture is a very elusive requirement. The expression is not the most felicitous, and when it is translated into other languages there are problems. Basically, what was intended with the concept of safety culture was to make it clear that safety should be the highest priority in organizations handling radiation sources, which should be prepared to identify and correct problems promptly; that clear lines of responsibility should be established, not only for organizations in handling sources but also in the governmental agencies controlling the use of sources. The lines of authority for decision making should be clearly defined, but this is not normally the case — particularly in the medical field, where the highest authorities in hospitals are often unaware of the safety conditions in their radiology and nuclear medicine services. The problem of safety culture — or lack of safety culture — is particularly critical, since the dissolution of eastern European states, and the consequent appearance of "newly independent states," where there is a lack of regulatory instruments and technical tradition for the control of radiation sources. Quality assurance is essential for radiation safety. Its importance was demonstrated at the accident in Costa Rica, where at least 13 people were killed because this requirement was not being met.

Human factors are the final step to manage radiation sources safely. The main issue is that operating personnel should be properly trained and qualified. In many of the accidents reported to the IAEA, lack of training and qualifications was a common cause of failure. Also important are design in accordance with ergonomic principles, the availability of equipment and software for reducing the likelihood of human error, and the provision of means for detecting human error and facilitating intervention when it occurs.

Verifying safety is the ultimate requirement, but it does not exist in many countries. Many are failing to identify potential exposure pathways, to estimate probabilities and magnitudes of potential exposure, and to assess the quality and extent of safety provisions. Last but not least, monitoring for the verification of compliance and record keeping are things that the BSS call for very specifically.

The security requirements in the BSS are minimal. They focus on the prevention of theft, damage, and unauthorized use by ensuring that control is not relinquished, that sources are not transferred to unauthorized users, and that periodic inventories are conducted, particularly of movable sources. This requirement covers all essential security issues. The problem of security cannot be tackled by controlling illicit traffic at borders or by asking the police to find sources. Rather, it will be solved only when there are national systems everywhere that ensure that control is not relinquished, that sources are not transferred to unauthorized users, and that periodic inventories are conducted. But, unfortunately, the world is far from this ideal situation. That is the reason the help of customs, of border controls, and of the police is essential at the moment. That is the reason the IAEA has an active program on illicit movement of radioactive sources.

The BSS requirements are a necessary but not a sufficient condition for ensuring safety and security. First, they are not sufficiently quantitative: new ICRP recommendations on the subject have been recently issued and can close the gap to quantification. Second, the essential issue is not the existence of standards, but their application. Under its statute, the IAEA must provide for the application of the BSS. There are several ways to provide for the application of such standards, a very important one, particularly for those countries where the situation is critical, is the provision of assistance through the IAEA Technical Co-operation Program.

For the purpose of providing for the application of its safety standards, the IAEA renders radiation safety services, fosters information exchange, promotes education and training, coordinates research and development, and, last, but not least, provides technical cooperation and assistance in this subject area. The IAEA has been using these mechanisms from its inception. In the last years, responding to the findings of RAPATs and to the initiatives of the Model Project, its programs in this area were enlarged. After the Dijon Conference, however, it became clear that they had to be reinforced.

THE AGENCY'S CURRENT PROGRAM

The main relevant current agency activities are summarized below:

1. Support in strengthening regulatory infrastructures. The following have been made available to member states:
    - IAEA-TECDOC-1067 on "Organization and Implementation of a National Regulatory Infrastructure Governing Radiation Protection and the Safety of Radiation Sources."
    - The Regulatory Authority Information System (R, 4IS), which provides the management of regulatory programs with information on the location of radiation sources and facilities, on the authorization process, on inspection and enforcement actions, and on the dosimetry of occupationally exposed personnel.

2. The development of guidance on how to undertake peer reviews of regulatory programs. A draft safety report on "Assessment by Peer Review of the Effectiveness of Regulatory Programs for Protection against Ionizing Radiation and the Safety of Radiation Sources" is available. It contains a methodology for preparing, conducting, and reporting on peer reviews and is seen as a prelude to a service for the provision to states, on request, of assistance with the regulatory control of radiation sources.
3. An education and training program. Educational course manuals are available (in several languages), and courses are held in all regions. However, other training materials are needed.
4. Prevention, detection, and response to illicit trafficking:
    - A memorandum of understanding (MOU) between the agency and the World Customs Organization, signed in May 1998. The MOU will serve to promote cooperation between customs and regulatory authorities at the national level and information exchange, cooperation and harmonization at the international level, with the aim at improving the control of radioactive materials.
    - The development of a "Safety Guide on Prevention, Detection and Response to Illicit Trafficking in Radioactive Materials," which is being cosponsored by the World Customs Organization and INTERPOL.
    - A set of technical manuals will contain information on materials typically involved in illicit trafficking, on prevention, detection, and response, and on training for customs and police officers; a database on illicit trafficking incidents involving nuclear and other radioactive materials has been operated by the agency since 1994.
5. Work connected with the installation of radiation monitoring systems at airports, seaports, and border crossings.
    - A report on the agency's Illicit Trafficking Radiation Monitoring Assessment Program (ITRAP) is being prepared.
    - A laboratory/field study sponsored by the Austrian Government and carried out by the Austrian Research Centre Seibersdorf will provide information about radiation measuring and monitoring equipment (handheld, portable, and fixed) available on the international market and suitable for the detection of illicit movements of radioactive materials.
6. An international database on unusual radiation events, referred to as RADEV, is being developed. It will cover accidents resulting in exposures or radioactive contamination and any other event that is relevant to safety. In addition, it will provide information on causes and contributing factors and on lessons to be learned.
7. Work connected with emergencies:
    - The development of documents on the recognition of radiation injuries and how to deal with them. Safety reports on "Diagnosis and Treatment of Radiation Injuries" and "Planning the Medical Response to Radiological Accidents" and an IAEA-TEC-DOC-869 on "Assessment and Treatment of external and Internal Radionuclide Contamination" are available.
    - A recently finalized technical document on "Generic Procedures for Assessment and Response during a Radiological Emergency" provides the tools and data required for the initial response to a radiological emergency. A technical document on "Generic Procedures for Monitoring during a Nuclear or Radiological Emergency " has been published (IAEA-TECDOC-1 092). The secretariat is developing standard training materials on the basis of those two technical documents and plans to use the materials at regional workshops.
    - A technical document on "Method for the Development of Emergency Response Preparedness for Nuclear or Radiological Accidents" (IAEA-TECDOC-953) provides tools and approaches to develop emergency response preparedness. Training material

exists and is used in regional workshops. A technical document "A Model National Emergency Response Plan for Radiological Accidents" (IAEA-TECDOC-718) provides an outline for a national response plan.

8. The Model Project on Upgrading Radiation Protection Infrastructure was developed to assist those member states that have inadequate infrastructures and are already receiving IAEA assistance so that they can comply with the BSS. Currently more than 50 countries are involved in the project.

9. Guidance on the management of disused sources is provided by a number of documents, such as:
   - "Handling Conditioning and Disposal of Spent Sealed Sources" (IAEA-TECDOC-548),
   - "Nature and Magnitude of the Problem of Spent Radiation Sources" (IAEA-TECDOC-620),
   - "Methods to Identify and Locate Spent Radiation Sources" (IAEA-TECDOC-804), and
   - "Reference Design for Centralized Spent Sealed Sources Facility" (IAEA-TECDOC-886)

   (Direct assistance is provided to member states on conditioning their radium inventories and demonstrating methods and procedures for conditioning and storage of spent sealed radiation sources.)

10. The IAEA operates an Emergency Response Centre that can respond to requests for assistance under the terms of the Convention on Assistance in the Case of a Nuclear Accident or Radiological Emergency. Such emergency assistance includes medical response and radiological surveys, technical assessment or advice, or assistance in accident mitigation.

8 Review of Chinese Nuclear Accidents

Pan Ziqiang

CONTENTS

Introduction 149
Status of Radiation Protection and Accidents in the Nuclear Industry 149
Application of Radioisotopes and Nuclear Technology..150
Accidents Leading to Acute Radiological Syndrome and Deaths..............................150
    Sanli'an Accident..150
    Shanghai "6.25" Cobalt-60 Source Accident 152
    Xinzhou Accident..153
Accident Registration and Management..153
References 154

INTRODUCTION

The nuclear industry began in China in 1955 and the initial Chinese nuclear fuel cycle system as an aspect of the nuclear industry was completed in the late 1960s. Research activities relating to nuclear power plants were initiated in the 1970s. Furthermore, at the end of 1991, a 300-MWe prototype reactor nuclear power plant at Qinshan was connected to an electricity network. In 1994, Guangdong Daya Bay Nuclear Power Station with two units, each with installed capacity of 900 MWe, was placed into commercial operation. At present, there are a total of eight units with 6500 MWe under construction. Within the context of development of the nuclear industry, a comparatively comprehensive system of research, development, production, and applications of both radioisotope and irradiation technology has been gradually established.

STATUS OF RADIATION PROTECTION AND ACCIDENTS IN THE NUCLEAR INDUSTRY

With more than 40 years of history, the nuclear industry in China has established a good safety record. The external doses to the workers at a reprocessing plant and production reactor were elevated to some extent in the initial years. The annual average individual dose to the workers at the reprocessing plant from 1968 to 1987 was about 15.3 mSv. From 1983 to 1987, the annual average individual dose decreased to 3.87 mSv and the percent of workers who received doses in excess of 50 mSv was only 0.11%.

    The annual average individual dose to workers at production reactors from 1968 to 1987 was about 14.2 mSv, with the highest value of 32 mSv in 1969. The dose then decreased to around 10 mSv after 1983, with the number of workers having received the doses in excess of 50 mSv accounting for about 1%. Around 1970, higher doses were received by the workers at reprocessing plants and production reactors, which are attributable to accident and overhaul. The maximum dose was up to 0.25 Gy in a short time, but there was no case that received a single dose higher than 1 Gy. Neither acute radiation-induced death nor acute radiological syndrome has occurred.[1]

Cases that resulted in local skin burns and injuries have occurred. In respect to skin burns, beta ray–induced skin injuries are dominant, accounting for about 93%, and mainly found in the hands. The statistics of 67 cases of beta ray–induced skin injuries show that there are 53 cases found in hands and the dose to skin is generally distributed on the palms, especially on the fingers. Skin injury involves small areas, generally less than 2% of the whole-body area, and is usually accompanied by gamma external exposure to either part of or the entire body, or by nuclide contamination. Statistics show that, among 50 cases of beta ray–induced skin injuries, there are only three cases that had significant initial reaction. The incubation period for a patient receiving a 5-Gy radiation dose is about 20 days; for those receiving 7 to 14 Gy, it is about 8 to 25 days (13 days on average). The incubation period for severe skin injury may be less, generally only 3 to 5 days. Second-degree skin injury (blister) may enter the recovery phase after 2 to 3 weeks, while third-degree skin injury (ulcer or necrosis) may enter the recovery phase after 3 to 5 weeks. Usually, injured skin area is minor, so the syndrome is relatively slight. Typical beta radiation injuries are presented in Reference 2.

APPLICATION OF RADIOISOTOPES AND NUCLEAR TECHNOLOGY

With respect to application of radioisotope and nuclear technology application, individual dose-monitoring work was initiated in the mid 1980s and, at present, is being updated. The available monitoring reports indicate that, under normal conditions, the doses to workers are minor. In the time period from 1985 to 1989, the annual average doses to workers were 1.39 mSv for nuclear medicine, 1.25 mSv for radiotherapy, and 2.01 mSv for industrial radiography, respectively. But there are many accidents that have occurred, including three accidents resulting in seven deaths. Table 8.1 presents a summary of the accidents resulting from sealed source-based irradiation installation and Table 8.2 lists accidents due to "spent" sources that were not under regulatory control. In total, 17 accidents have occurred, 12 of which are attributable to fixed irradiation installations, including 3 that have led to deaths. Among the ten accidents listed in Table 8.1, seven are attributable to interlock failure and safety device fault, which led to allowed entry of workers/personnel into the irradiation room. Of the seven accidents resulting in public exposure shown in Table 8.2, five accidents are due to irradiation installations. Thus, it is necessary to strengthen the safety of irradiation installations.

ACCIDENTS LEADING TO ACUTE RADIOLOGICAL SYNDROME AND DEATHS

From 1949 to 1988, there have been 14 severe accidents that resulted in 47 cases of acute radiological diseases (including 3 cases of subacute diseases) and at least 3 accidents that delivered radiation doses of about 1 Gy and led to 4 cases of slight radiological syndrome, totaling 51 cases of disease. These accidents do not include the 1972 Wuhan radiotherapy unit accident, which was caused when a cobalt-60 source fell out of a machine; the accident led to acute radiological syndrome in 15 patients with tumors.

Reference 19 provides a comprehensive summary of the progress in diagnosis and treatment of acute radiological disease in China. The following are descriptions of several accidents leading to deaths.

SANLI'AN ACCIDENT[3]

In 1960, Anhui Agriculture Institute, located in Hefei City in Anhui Province of East China, purchased a cobalt-60 source for the purpose of radiation research. The source was then placed in

TABLE 8.1
Accidents Leading to Radiation Injuries at Irradiation Facilities with Sealed Sources

Date	Location	Brief Account	Consequence	Ref.
02/1972	Sichuan	Workers accidentally entering the irradiation room with a 2.65×10^{14} Bq ^{60}Co source	0.55–1.47 Gy whole-body radiation exposure	3
12/1972	Wuhan	A 5×10^{12} Bq ^{60}Co source for radiotherapy purposes falling on copper filter plate for 16 days; the design did not meet international standards	A total of 20 patients and 8 workers received doses in range of 0.05–2.45 Gy	4
12/1980	Shanghai	Worker entering irradiation room with a 2.2×10^{15} Bq ^{60}Co source after a power failure and interlock out of order	A worker incurred a 5.22-Gy radiation exposure	5
06/1985	Shanghai	Worker entering a 1.5-MeV Van de Graff accelerator hall while main motor running	A worker incurred local radiation exposure in range of 25–210 Gy	6
03/1986	Beijing	Workers entering a 0.2 PBq ^{60}Co source radiation room when it is on irradiation position with failed drive system and door open	Two workers received doses of 0.7 and 0.8 Sv, respectively	7
05/1986	Henan	Workers entering a 0.3-PBq ^{60}Co source room when it is on irradiation position which was manually raised due to power loss	Two workers incurred 3.5 and 2.6 Gy acute radiological syndrome	8
03/1988	Liaoning	Workers taking source in bare hands when removing a radiography source of 1.1×10^{12} Bq in failure	Six workers incurred doses in range of 0.1–12.6 Gy on hands	9
06/1990	Shanghai	Workers entering a 0.85-PBq ^{60}Co source room when one protection door was broken and tand removed and another had failed due to power loss	Seven workers were exposed to 2–12 Gy radiation, resulting in two deaths	10
12/1992	Wuhan	Out of order interlock, and the design did not meet the safety standards	Four workers overexposed to radiation, one of whom incurred acute radiological sickness	11
01/1998	Harbin	Workers entering irradiation room after safety equipment failure	One worker suffered acute radiological sickness	12

a lead cask on open farmland within its affiliated farm, near a water pond, in the suburb of the city. The screws used for fixing the lead can were loose and fell off. At 2 P.M. on January 11, 1963, an 18-year-old farmer went to the pond to fish. He found the lead cask and took the source out of the cask and put it into his fish basket. At 4 P.M. that afternoon, upon returning home, he moved the source from the basket to the left pocket of his upper outer garment. At midday on January 20, the management department involved in this event searched and located the source in a box at the farmer's bedside. Six people who lived in the home were sent to the hospital for medical help. The source, identified at that time as 43 PBq, remained in the farmer's home for 212 h and in his pocket for 52 h. The source was also kept in the left pocket of his 7-year-old brother's trousers for 18 h.

The average whole-body dose to the farmer and his younger brother was estimated to be 806 and 40 Gy. Both died on January 23 and 25, respectively, due to failure to respond to any medical treatment. Four other people, who received doses of 8, 6, 4, 2 Gy, respectively, survived after medical treatment. Two of them have not fully recovered from local injuries; the other two are

TABLE 8.2
Accidents Due to Radiation Sources out of Control

Date	Location	Brief account	Consequence	Ref.
1963	Anhui	A 0.43 TBq ^{60}Co source not in use for irradiation study purpose was taken home as a result of improper storage	2–80 Gy doses to individuals, with two deaths and four acute radiological injuries	13
1969	Beijing	A 3.7×10^{10} Bq ^{60}Co source of unknown origin was poured into the basement of a reinforced concrete statue	A collective dose 1010 Bq ^{137}Cs source was taken home	14
1978	Henan	An unused 5.4×10^{10} Bq ^{137}Cs source was taken home	Red marrow doses to 29 individuals in the range of 0.01–0.53 Gy	15
1982	Hanzhong	A 1.03 TBq ^{60}Co source not in use was stolen	Doses to stem cell ranging from 0.42–3 Gy were received	16
1985	Mudanjiang	A 3.7×10^{11} ^{137}Cs source not in use was removed	Accumulated local doses 8–15 Gy, with three acute radiological injuries	17
1988		A 2.2×10^{11} Bq ^{192}Ir radiography source fell to the ground, and was later picked up by a worker and placed in his home for about 50 hours	The worker received a dose of 0.5–1 Gy	18
1992	Shanxi	A 4×10^{11} Bq Co source was picked up by a worker and taken home	Three deaths	19

doing well. A follow-up study, together with involved medical treatment, has shown that in 17 years after the exposure, they had fully recovered with good physical and mental condition and memory. Local effects are mainly long-term injuries to the skin and skeleton. There have been no significant changes in their lenses.

SHANGHAI "6.25" COBALT-60 SOURCE ACCIDENT[10]

As of June 24, 1990, an irradiation installation containing a 8.5×10^{14} Bq cobalt-60 gamma source at a radiological medicine laboratory in Shanghai was operated to irradiate traditional Chinese medicine. The second protection door installed for shielding purposes had not been in use for a long time period as a result of motor failure. At 9 A.M. on June 25, 1990, someone opened the safety/protection door with a key but without a personal dose monitor. The main power supply control was not switched on, and the interlock of the safety/protection door did not operate. This allowed entry of seven workers into the irradiation room, thus exposing them to a cobalt-60 source. Because the raised or lowered source position of the hoist mechanism was wholly covered with 30-cm-diameter thin-metal shielding, the radiation position could not be observed from outside the room. The seven workers suffered acute external radiation exposure of the whole body at widely varying degrees at different distances from the source in a short time. Within 30 min after the accident, one worker felt nauseated and within 2 h, the others began vomiting. At 11 A.M. that day, the seven workers were sent to the hospital.

Dose reconstruction was made for the measurement and estimation of the radiation doses received by the seven workers, along with biological dose measurements, as summarized in Table 8.3. The table shows that both measurements are in agreement. Chromosome aberration analysis and physical measurements agree within 10%. Two of the seven workers, who received

TABLE 8.3
Physical Measurements and Biological Dose Estimates

		Biological Dose (Gy)			
Patient No.	Reconstruction, Measurement, Estimation	Chromosome Analysis		Micronucleus Analysis	
1	12.0			>10	
2	11.0			>10	
3	5.2	5.1	5.2	6.6	5.1
4	4.1	3.5	3.5	3.9	3.7
5	2.5	2.5	2.7	2.4	3.0
6	2.4	2.9	3.0	4.0	3.6
7	2.0	1.9	2.1	1.9	2.5

12 and 11 Gy radiation exposure, respectively, died after being treated for 25 and 90 days. The other five workers have recovered after treatment.

XINZHOU ACCIDENT

On the morning of November 19, 1992 in Xinzhou, a city of Shanxi Province of North China, a farmer who was working at a site in demolishing a cobalt-60 irradiation installation picked up a cylindrical steel bar and put it into his jacket pocket. That afternoon, he was sent to the hospital feeling nauseated and beginning to vomit; he died on December 2 that year. His father and elder brother who were taking care of him in the hospital following the accident died on December 7 and 10, respectively. On December 19, 1990, his wife went to the Beijing Medical University–affiliated People's Hospital to seek medical help and was suspected to be suffering from radiological disease. The diagnosis was confirmed with peripheral lymphocyte chromosome analysis; she was identified as having acute radiological disease.[20] On December 18, 1990, Shanxi Provincial authorities requested that the radiological source be located. The investigation found that a cylindrical steel bar had fallen out of the farmer's pocket when he was in the hospital and the bar was then thrown into a wastebasket. The radiological source was located on February 1, 1991 and later stored in a temporary radioactive waste repository in the locality on February 2, 1991. Measurement indicated that a 4×10^{11} Bq cobalt-60 source was contained in the cylindrical steel bar. Through reconstruction, measurement, and estimation, the doses to the farmer, his brother, and father were all higher than 8 Gy and that to his wife about 2.3 Gy. Another 14 persons exposed received doses in excess of 0.25 Gy.

ACCIDENT REGISTRATION AND MANAGEMENT

In China, registration of accidents arising from the applications of radioisotopes and nuclear technology is the responsibility of Industry Hygiene Research Institute under the Ministry of Health, whereas the accidents in relation to nuclear fuel cycle are registered by the China Institute for Radiation Protection. Beijing North Taiping Street Hospital has accumulated a lot of experience in diagnosis and treatment of radiological syndromes. Since the late 1980s Beijing Radiological Medicine Institute has developed an extensive registry of 630 cases of acute radiological diseases involving exposures above 0.2 Gy. It also has established a computerized database and consultative system, which primarily includes acute radiological disease.[22]

As indicated above, all accidents relating to radiation exposure have occurred in the field of the application of radioisotopes and nuclear technology. For the purpose of strengthening the management of safety of radiation sources, especially irradiation installation, the relevant authorities have developed Regulations on Management of Health and Protection for Gamma Irradiation Processing Equipment (1991/02/26), Regulations on Radiation Protection for Co-60 Irradiation Installation in Use for Irradiation Processing (GB10252), and Design Criteria for Safety and Protection for Co-60 Irradiation Facility (EJ-377-89). These regulations provide impetus to strengthening the safety of irradiation facilities. However, these regulations are mainly directed to radiation protection, and contain little regarding radiation source safety. More detail of potential exposure and radiation source safety will be included in Basic Safety Standards for Protection against Ionization Radiation and for Safety of Radiation Source to be issued. This will improve the management/administration of radiation source safety.

REFERENCES

1. Pan, Z. et al., *Radiation Level and Effects of China's Nuclear Industry*, Atomic Energy Publishing, Beijing, 1996 (in Chinese).
2. Sun, S. et al., *Clinics of Over-Exposed Individuals*, Atomic Energy Publishing, Beijing, 1989 (in Chinese).
3. Pan, Z. et al., *Environmental Quality Assessment of Nuclear Industry of China over past 30 Years*, Atomic Energy Publishing, Beijing, 1990 (in Chinese).
4. Jin, C. et al., A 10 year follow-up observation of Wuhan individuals exposed to Co source in respect of chromosome abbreviation, *Chin. J. Radiol. Med. Prot.*, 5(1), 14, 1985 (in Chinese).
5. Yang, J. et al., A four year follow-up study of micronucleus rates in peripheral lymphocytes of a patient with acute radiation syndrome, *Chin. J. Radiol. Med. Prot.*, 7(1), 47, 1987 (in Chinese).
6. Zhou, Z. et al., Cause investigation and dose assessment in an accident of a Van de Graff accelerator, *Chin. J. Radiol. Med. Prot.*, 10(2), 116, 1990 (in Chinese).
7. Gou, Y. et al., Dose estimates for two cases accidentally exposed to a Co-60 source, *Chin. J. Radiol. Med. Prot.*, 9(2), 115, 1989 (in Chinese).
8. Wang, G. et al., Clinical report of acute radiation sickness, *Chin. J. Radiol. Med. Prot.*, 8(6), 396, 1988 (in Chinese).
9. Zhang, W. et al., Dose estimation of a case of exposed patient sustaining Ir-192 radiograph source, *Chin. J. Radiol. Med. Prot.*, 10(4), 278, 1990 (in Chinese).
10. Liu, B. et al., *Dose Estimation for Shanghai "6.25" Co-60 Source Radiated Person*, P15, Beijing Science and Technology Press, Beijing, 1994 (in Chinese).
11. Li, M., Zhang, Y., Zhang, D. et al., Clinical report of four cases of acute radiation sickness in a 60 Co radiation accident in Wuhan, *Chin. J. Radiol. Med. Prot.*, 18(4) 230, 1998 (in Chinese).
12. Guo, Z. et al., Clinical report of a case of serious acute radiological sickness, Report Abstracts of National Conference on Radiological Medicine and Protection to meet the Century 21, 101, 1998 (in Chinese).
13. Shi, Y. et al., Dose analysis for Sanli'an radiation accident, in *Proceedings of Clinical Study of 23 Acute Radiological-Disease Patients*, Atomic Energy Publishing, Beijing, 1985 (in Chinese).
14. Yang, X. et al., unpublished, 1994.
15. Yao, S. et al., Chromosome aberrations in persons accidentally exposed to Cs-137 gamma rays, *Chin. J. Radiol. Med. Prot.*, 4(6), 22, 1984 (in Chinese).
16. Task Group Dealing with Hanzhong Co-60 Source Accident, Five year observation on cases accidentally exposed to Co-60 gamma rays, *Chin. J. Radiol. Med. Prot.*, 9(2), 73, 1989 (in Chinese).
17. Huang, S. et al., A clinical report of three cases of acute radiation sickness, *Chin. J. Radiol. Med. Prot.*, 9(2), 82, 1989 (in Chinese).
18. Gan, Y., Dealing with an accident involving loss of a cs-137 source for purpose of field well logging, *Radiol. Hyg.*, 4(2), P82, 1991 (in Chinese).
19. Ye, G. et al., Advances in diagnosis and treatment of acute radiation syndrome in China, *Chin. J. Radiol. Med. Prot.*, 18(5), 316, 1998 (in Chinese).
20. Lou, B. et al., Clinical report of eight chief victims in Co-60 radiation accident in Xinzhou, *Chin. J. Radiol. Med. Prot.*, 18(4), 225, 1998 (in Chinese).

21. Bai, Y. et al., Chromosome aberration analysis and dose estimation for 34 examined persons exposed in Xinzhou accident, *Chin. J. Radiol. Med. Prot.*, 15(2), 84, 1995 (in Chinese).
22. Tang, Z. et al., Data Bank and Consulting System for Medical Management of Paitents with Acute Radiation Sickness, *Chin. J. Radiol. Med. Prot.*, 15(4), 306, 1995 (in Chinese).

9 Radiation Accidents in the Former U.S.S.R.

Vladimir Soloviev, Leonid A. Ilyin, Alexander E. Baranov, Anjelika V. Barabanova, Angelina K. Guskova, Natalia M. Nadejina, and Igor A. Gusev

The Chernobyl accident changed many people's perception of the safety of nuclear power. Hundreds of thousands of people were evacuated, and almost as many were involved in the cleanup efforts. In all, 134 patients suffered from acute radiation syndrome and 28 people died in the acute period as a result of radiation exposure. It is instructive to look at accidents in the former Soviet Union before and since Chernobyl.

The State Research Center of Russia (Institute of Biophysics) has provided medical assistance, observation, and treatment for the majority of patients involved in radiation accidents in the former U.S.S.R. At least 172 radiation accidents with serious human exposure occurred between 1950 and 2000. When compared to previous reports[1] the information presented here has been updated. In previous literature, some incidents were erroneously classified as criticality accidents due to insufficient information. This information has been clarified and some diagnoses also have been revised.[2] More than 900 individuals received significant exposures in these accidents. In addition to the accidents listed, there were accidents in the southern Urals, nuclear submarine accidents, fallout from nuclear explosions, as well as incidents without clinically significant health effects.

There have been at least 435 patients in the territory of the former Soviet Union who have experienced the acute radiation syndrome (ARS), significant local radiation injury (LRI), or a combination. As a result of radiation exposure, 59 deaths occurred in the first 3 months postaccident. There have been one to four radiation accidents per year over the last three decades and about one case every 2 years with a fatal outcome in the acute period. On average, there have been five to six people a year who have had serious clinical effects; although in recent years the number and severity of incidents have declined.

During the 1940–1970 period, most accidents (including criticality accidents) occurred in the atomic industry. Thereafter, radioisotope devices became predominant (more than half of cases: 88 out of 172). In addition there have been gamma and beta incidents which have affected a large number of people including members of the public. Accidents that involve the public require comprehensive organizational measures to distinguish those people actually irradiated. Accidents involving a large number of people have also occurred in other countries (Mexico, 1983; Brazil, 1987).

It is clear from our data that the direct human health impact of nuclear power, radioisotope uses, and X-ray devices used in industry, medicine, and research is significantly lower than that for other industries in Russia. At the same time, lessons of Chernobyl show the great importance of safety discipline in nuclear power and the indirect economical and social harm. The accidents and accompanying facts are listed in Tables 9.1 and 9.2.

TABLE 9.1
Radiation Incidents in the Territory of the Former U.S.S.R. and the Structure of Early Medical Effects

Date[a]	Place		Major Radiation Features			No. of People Involved			
	Current Name of the Country	City, Region, or Medical Facility	Incident Type[b]	Major Radiation Factor	Kind of Exposure	Total	Those with Significant Clinical Symptoms		
							Total ARS + LRI	ARS Only	Died
05.07.50	Russia	Chelyabinsk-40 (Ozersk)	R	γ-β	External	5	5	1	—
19.08.50	Russia	Chelyabinsk-40 (Ozersk)	R	γ-n	External	1	1	1	—
28.09.50	Russia	Chelyabinsk-40 (Ozersk)	R	γ-n	External	1	1	1	—
??.01.51	Russia	Chelyabinsk-40 (Ozersk)	R (FR)	γ-β	External	1	1	—	—
01.10.51	Russia	Chelyabinsk-40 (Ozersk)		γ-β	External	7	4	4	1
02.12.51	Russia	Chelyabinsk-40 (Ozersk)	R (FR)	γ-n	External	2	2	2	—
??.??.52	Russia	Chelyabinsk-40 (Ozersk)		β(HTO)	Internal	2	2	—	2
??.??.52	Russia	Chelyabinsk-40 (Ozersk)		γ	External	1	1	—	—
??.??.52	Russia	Chelyabinsk-40 (Ozersk)		γ-β	External	3	3	—	—
04.07.52	Russia	Chelyabinsk-40 (Ozersk)	R (FR)	γ-n	External	1	1	1	—
??.??.53	Russia	Chelyabinsk-40 (Ozersk)		β(HTO)	Internal	2	2	2	—
15.03.53	Russia	Chelyabinsk-40 (Ozersk)	crit	γ-n	External	2	2	2	—
09.09.53	Russia	Moscow	crit	γ-n	External	7	4	4	—
18.09.53	Russia	Chelyabinsk-40 (Ozersk)	R (FR)	γ-n	External	2	1	1	—
13.10.53	Russia	Chelyabinsk-40 (Ozersk)	R (FR)	γ-n	External	5	5	5	—
28.12.53	Russia	Chelyabinsk-40 (Ozersk)	R (FR)	γ-n	External	9	7	7	—
11.03.54	Russia	Obninsk	crit	γ-n	External	10	1	—	—
28.06.54	Russia	Arzamas-16 (Sarov)	source	$\beta(^{210}Po)$	External	2	2	2	1
24.01.55	Russia	Moscow	source	$\gamma(^{124}Sb)$	External	1	1	1	—
03.06.55	Russia	Chelyabinsk-40 (Ozersk)	R	γ-n	External	2	2	2	—
??.06.57	Russia	Moscow	accel.	e	External	1	1	—	—
21.04.57	Russia	Chelyabinsk-40 (Ozersk)	crit	γ-n	External	9	6	6	1
02.01.58	Russia	Chelyabinsk-40 (Ozersk)	crit	γ-n	External	4	4	4	3
??.??.60	Kazakhstan	?	source	γ	External	>1	1	—	—
08.06.60	Russia	Moscow	suicide	γ	External	1	1	1	1

Radiation Accidents in the Former U.S.S.R.

Date	Country	Location	Type	Radiation	Exposure			
20.03.61	Russia	Moscow	I	γ(^{60}Co)	External	1	—	—
26.06.61	Russia	Moscow	crit	γ-n	External	4	4	—
14.07.61	Russia	Tomsk-7 (Seversk)	crit	γ-n	External	1	1	—
30.09.61	Russia	Moscow	source	γ	External	1	—	—
06.02.62	Russia	Moscow	I	X	External	1	—	—
10.04.62	Russia	Moscow	source	γ	External	1	—	—
02.11.62	Russia	Obninsk	crit	γ-n	External	2	2	—
??.??.63	Russia	Chelyabinsk-40 (Ozersk)		α-β	Ext+Int	1	—	—
??.??.63	Russia	Chelyabinsk-40 (Ozersk)	R (FR)	γ	External	1	2	—
11.03.63	Russia	Arzamas-16 (Sarov)	crit	γ-n	External	6	—	—
28.06.63	Russia	Sverdlovsk (Ekaterinburg)	source	γ	External	3	1	—
26.07.63	Russia	Chelyabinsk-40 (Ozersk)		β(HTO)	Internal	1	—	—
29.05.65	Russia	Moscow	accel.	e	External	1	—	—
11.06.66	Russia	Kaluga	I	X	External	1	—	—
??.??.66	Russia	Chelyabinsk-40 (Ozersk)	source	γ	External	1	—	—
20.05.66	Russia	Moscow		β	External	1	—	—
15.04.67	Kirgizia	Frunze	I	X	External	1	—	—
24.05.67	Russia	Moscow	I	X	External	1	—	—
09.12.67	Russia	Moscow	I	X	External	1	—	—
22.12.67	Russia	Moscow	source	γ-β(^{46}Sc)	External	2	2	2
05.04.68	Russia	Chelyabinsk-70 (Snezhinsk)	crit	γ-n	External	1	—	—
??.05.68	Russia	Moscow	I	X	External	3	—	—
27.06.68	Russia	Arzamas-16 (Sarov)	I	β(^{210}Po)	Internal	2	2	1
10.12.68	Russia	Chelyabinsk-40 (Ozersk)	crit	γ-n (Pu)	External	1	—	—
07.12.68	Russia	Moscow	I(SI)	X	External	1	—	—
??.??.69	?	?	I	γ	External	1	—	—
02.01.69	Russia	Moscow	R(FR)	X	External	2	2	—
20.01.69	Russia	Obninsk	accel.	γ	External	1	1	—
11.02.69	Russia	Moscow	I	e	Beam	1	—	—
11.03.69	Russia	Melekes	R	γ(^{60}Co)	External	4	2	—
22.04.69	Russia	MSF-99?	R (FR)	γ-β	External	2	1	—
07.05.69	Russia	Voronezh NPP		γ	External	2	2	—
24.09.69	Russia	Tomsk-7 (Seversk)	I(IR)	γ-β	External	1	—	—
13.10.69	Russia	Far East		γ(^{192}Ir)	External	1	—	—
??.??.69	Russia	Chelyabinsk-40 (Ozersk)		α, β	Internal	3	—	—
24.11.69	Russia	Novomoskovsk	I	γ(^{137}Cs)	External	3	—	—

TABLE 9.1
Radiation Incidents in the Territory of the Former U.S.S.R. and the Structure of Early Medical Effects

	Place			Major Radiation Features			No. of People Involved		
								Those with Significant Clinical Symptoms	
Date[a]	Current Name of the Country	City, Region, or Medical Facility	Incident Type[b]	Major Radiation Factor	Kind of Exposure	Total	Total ARS + LRI	ARS Only	Died
??.??.69	Russia	Moscow	I	X	External	1	1	—	—
13.09.69	Russia	Moscow	I	X	External	1	1	—	—
20.12.69	Russia	Moscow	I	X	External	1	1	—	—
04.02.70	Ukraine	Kiev	crit?	γ-n	External	2	1	1	—
13.02.70	Russia	?	I	γ(^{60}Co)	External	1	1	1	—
15.04.70	Russia	Moscow	accel.	e	Beam	1	1	—	—
??.09.70	Russia	Chelyabinsk	source	γ(^{137}Cs)	External	1	1	—	—
18.01.70	Russia	Sormovo, Gorky region	R	γ-β	External	7	5	5	3
15.02.71	Russia	Moscow	crit	γ-n	External	4	3	3	—
??.03.71	Russia	Tula	source	γ(^{137}Cs)	External	1	1	—	—
26.05.71	Russia	Moscow	crit	γ-n	External	7	4	4	2
05.12.71	Russia	Arkhangelsk region	source	γ(^{137}Cs)	External	>20	3	—	—
??.??.71	Russia	Ufa	source	γ(^{137}Cs)	External	1	1	—	—
??.09.71	Russia	Voronezh NPP		γ-β	External	1	1	—	—
31.03.72	Russia	Moscow	I	X	External	1	1	—	—
??.06.72	Russia	Moscow	I	X	External	1	1	—	—
09.10.72	Russia	Primorsky Region	crime	γ(^{192}Ir)	External	1	1	—	—
04.10.72	Russia	Moscow	I	X	External	1	1	—	—
22.12.72	Russia	Irkutsk	I	X	External	>1	>1	—	—
11.01.73	Russia	Moscow	source	γ(^{60}Co)	External	>1	>1	—	—
17.03.73	Ukraine	Odessa	crime	γ(^{60}Co)	External	1	1	1	—
??.03.73	Russia	Kaliningrad, Moscow region	I	X	External	1	1	—	—
??.04.73	Russia	Moscow	I	X	External	1	1	1	—
26.07.73	Russia	Elektrogorsk, Moscow region	I	γ(^{60}Co)	External	2	1	—	—
05.09.73	Russia	Khokhol, Vladimir region	source	γ(^{137}Cs)	Ext/Int	>100	4	—	—

Radiation Accidents in the Former U.S.S.R.

Date	Country	Location	Type	Radiation	Exposure	N			
??.12.73	Ukraine	Donetsk	source	$\gamma(^{137}Cs)$	External	>1	1	—	—
09.01.74	Russia	Novosibirsk	I	X	Beam	1	1	—	—
24.05.74	Russia	Tomsk-7 (Seversk)	source	$\beta(^{106}Rh)$	External	1	1	—	—
24.10.74	Russia	Perm'	source	$\gamma(^{60}Co)$	External	1	1	—	—
15.12.74	Russia	Lipetsk	crime	$\gamma(^{137}Cs)$	External	2	2	2	—
??.??.74	Russia	Sverdlovsk (Ekaterinburg)	source	X	External	1	1	—	—
20.06.75	Russia	Kazan'	I	$\gamma(^{60}Co)$	External	2	2	2	—
11.07.75	Russia	Sverdlovsk (Ekaterinburg)	source	$\gamma(^{60}Co)$	External	3	3	3	—
??.03.76	Russia	Moscow	I	X	External	1	1	—	—
12.07.76	Russia	Moscow	I	$\gamma(^{60}Co)$	External	1	1	1	—
22.07.76	Russia	Melekes	I	γ-β	External	1	1	—	—
01.03.77	Russia	Obninsk	I	γ-β	External	1	1	1	—
05.03.77	Ukraine	Kiev	accel.	p+	Beam	1	1	—	—
07.03.78	Russia	Primorsky Region	I(IR)	$\gamma(^{192}Ir)$	External	1	1	—	—
04.04.78	Russia	Primorsky Region	I(IR)	$\gamma(^{192}Ir)$	External	1	1	—	—
03.06.78	Russia	Protvino, Kaluga region	accel.	p+	Beam	1	1	—	—
21.09.78	Russia	Moscow	accel.	e	Beam	1	1	—	—
17.10.78	Russia	Moscow	R	β	External	1	1	—	—
25.11.78	Russia	Udmurtia	I(IR)	$\gamma(^{192}Ir)$	External	1	1	—	—
13.12.78	Russia	Tomsk-7 (Seversk)	crit	γ-n	External	7	3	3	—
08.05.79	Russia	Sverdlovsk (Ekaterinburg)	R (FR)	γ-β	External	1	1	—	—
20.07.79	Russia	Leningrad (S.-Peterburg)	accel.	e	Beam	2	2	2	—
20.09.79	Kirgizia	Frunze	I(IR)	$\gamma(^{192}Ir)$	External	1	1	—	—
01.12.79	Kazakhstan	Semipalatinsk	I	$\gamma(^{60}Co)$	External	1	1	—	—
23.05.80	Russia	Chelyabinsk-40 (Ozersk)	I	X	Beam	1	1	—	—
01.09.80	Russia	Leningrad (S.-Peterburg)	I(SI)	$\gamma(^{60}Co)$	External	1	1	1	—
19.09.80	Russia	Yuzhno-Sakhalinsk	source	$\gamma(^{192}Ir)$	External	2	2	1	—
03.12.80	Russia	Vladivostok	I(IR)	$\gamma(^{192}Ir)$	External	1	1	—	—
15.03.82	Russia	Krasnodar	source	$\gamma(^{192}Ir)$	External	>20	1	—	—
19.05.82	Russia	Smolensk NPP	I(IR)	$\gamma(^{192}Ir)$	External	4	1	—	—
14.06.82	Turkmenia	Ashkhabad	crime	$\gamma(^{60}Co)$	External	13	7	1	1
09.01.82	Ukraine	Kramatorsk	source	$\gamma(^{137}Cs)$	External	5	2	0[c]	2
05.10.82	Azerbaidjan	Baku	source	$\gamma(^{137}Cs)$	External	22	18	5	5
18.12.82	Russia	Urengoy	I(IR)	$\gamma(^{192}Ir)$	External	2	2	—	—
27.01.83	Russia	Moscow	I	X	Beam	1	1	—	—
28.04.83	Ukraine	Kharkov	I(IR)	$\gamma(^{137}Cs)$	External	2	2	1	—

TABLE 9.1
Radiation Incidents in the Territory of the Former U.S.S.R. and the Structure of Early Medical Effects

Date[a]	Current Name of the Country	Place City, Region, or Medical Facility	Incident Type[b]	Major Radiation Factor	Kind of Exposure	Total	Total ARS + LRI	ARS Only	Died
17.05.83	Russia	Volgograd	I(IR)	$\gamma(^{192}Ir)$	External	1	1	—	—
11.06.83	Russia	Ufa	I(IR)	$\gamma(^{137}Cs)$	External	1	1	—	—
07.12.83	Russia	Ufa	I(IR)	$\gamma(^{192}Ir)$	External	1	1	—	—
07.02.84	Russia	Perm'	I(IR)	$\gamma(^{192}Ir)$	External	7	5	—	—
21.04.84	Russia	Chelyabinsk-40 (Ozersk)	I	X	External	1	1	—	—
12.06.84	Russia	Ufa	I(IR)	$\gamma(^{192}Ir)$	External	1	1	—	—
15.06.84	Russia	Gorky (Nijny Novgorod)	source	$\gamma(^{192}Ir)$	External	11	8	4	—
24.10.84	Russia	MSF-13?	I(IR)	$\gamma(^{124}Sb)$	External	1	1	—	—
03.03.85	Russia	Norilsk	source	$\gamma(^{137}Cs)$	External	3	3	—	—
26.09.85	Lithuania	Ignalinskaya NPP	I(IR)	$\gamma(^{192}Ir)$	External	1	1	—	—
16.10.85	Russia	Podolsk, Moscow region		γ	External	1	1	—	—
26.04.86	Ukraine	Chernobyl NPP	R	γ-β	External	>384[d]	134	134	28
11.06.86	Russia	Obninsk	1	$\gamma(^{60}Co)$	External	1	1	—	—
05.08.86	Russia	Kalinin NPP	I(IR)	$\gamma(^{192}Ir)$	External	1	1	—	—
01.02.87	Russia	Moscow	1	X	Beam	1	1	—	—
22.03.88	Russia	Sverdlovsk (Ekaterinburg)	source	$\beta(^{90}Sr+^{90}Y)$	External	3	3	—	—
05.04.88	Uzbekistan	Tashkent	I(IR)	$\gamma(^{192}Ir)$	External	2	2	—	—
18.08.88	Latvia	Riga	crime	n-$\gamma(^{252}Cf)$	Beam	1	1	—	—
20.03.89	Russia	Moscow	1	X	External	1	1	—	—
04.08.89	Russia	???	I(IR)	$\gamma(^{192}Ir)$	External	1	1	—	—
14.08.89	Russia	Zagorsk (Sergiev Posad)	accel.	e	Beam	1	1	—	—
30.10.89	Russia	Moscow	1	X	Beam	1	1	—	—
27.02.90	Russia	Kalinin NPP	source	$\gamma(^{192}Ir)$	External	1	1	—	—
13.03.90	Russia	Moscow	accel.	e	Beam	1	1	—	—
13.09.90	Ukraine	Kharkov	source	$\gamma(^{192}Ir)$	External	1	1	1	—

Radiation Accidents in the Former U.S.S.R.

Date	Country	City	Type	Radiation	Exposure	N1	N2	N3
30.10.90	Russia	Komsomolsk-on-Amur	I(IR)	γ(^{192}Ir)	External	1	—	—
24.08.91	Russia	Bratsk	crime	γ(^{137}Cs)	External	3	1	—
26.10.91	Belarus	Nesvij	I(SI)	γ(^{60}Co)	External	1	1	1
09.01.92	Russia	Riazan'	I(IR)	γ(^{192}Ir)	External	2	1	—
25.05.92	Kazakhstan	Axay	I(IR)	γ(^{192}Ir)	External	4	—	—
14.04.93	Russia	Moscow	crime	γ(^{137}Cs)	External	23	0[c]	1
07.08.93	Russia	Dimitrovograd	R	γ-n	External	1	—	—
11.07.93	Estonia	Tallinn	source	γ(^{137}Cs)	External	9	4	1
12.07.93	Russia	Vologda	source	γ(^{192}Ir)	External	1	—	—
09.11.93	Russia	Tula region	source	γ(^{192}Ir)	External	1	—	—
28.11.94	Russia	Voronezh	I(IR)	γ(^{192}Ir)	External	1	—	—
18.03.95	Russia	Pervouralsk	I(IR)	γ(^{192}Ir)	External	1	—	—
23.05.95	Russia	Smolensk	source	γ(^{192}Ir)	External	1	—	—
07.07.95	Russia	Moscow	crime	γ(^{137}Cs)	External	1	0[c]	—
11.09.95	Russia	Moscow	source	γ(^{137}Cs)	Internal	1	—	—
03.10.95	Russia	Nijny Novgorod/Gorky/	I(IR)	γ(^{192}Ir)	External	1	—	—
23.02.96	Russia	Moscow	accel.	e	Beam	1	—	—
08.06.96	Russia	Nijny Novgorod/Gorky/	I(IR)	γ(^{192}Ir)	External	1	0[c]	—
??.??.97	Georgia	Tbilisi	source	γ(^{137}Cs)	External	35	1	1
17.06.97	Russia	Sarov/Arzamas-16/	crit	γ-n	External	1	—	—
02.12.97	Russia	Volgograd	source	γ(^{192}Ir)	External	1	—	—
29.11.97	Russia	Grozny	source	γ(^{60}Co)	External	4	3	—
18.03.98	Russia	Moscow	source	γ(^{60}Co)	External	1	—	—
16.08.2000	Russia	Samara	I(IR)	γ(^{192}Ir)	External	3	3	—
13.10.2000	Russia	Dubna	accel.	p+	External	1	—	—

[a] "?" Date or other information on incident is unknown correctly.

[b] Following abbreviations are applicable: Accelerator, *accel.*; atomic reactor incidents, *R*; atomic reactor incidents with fuel rod manipulations, *R(FR)*; lost control of criticality of fissile materials, *crit*; X-ray or radioisotope installation, *I*; radiation sterizilation unit, *I(SI)*; industrial radiography unit, *I(IR)*; incidents with radioisotope sources, *source*; criminal cases, *crime*; suicidal cases, *suicide*.

[c] Chronic radiation injuries are not considered.

[d] Excluding recovery operation workers.

Source: Registry of SRC, Institute of Biophysics, November 1, 2000.

TABLE 9.2
Major Types of Radiation Incidents in the Territory of the Former U.S.S.R. and the Structure of Their Early Medical Effects

Incident Classification	Major Radiation Factors	No. of Radiation Incidents			No. of People Involved Including Those with Significant Clinical Symptoms of:			
		Total	Including Those with Two or More Victims	Including Those with Fatal Outcomes	Total	Total	ARS	Died
Incidents with radioisotope units and their sources (total)		88	26	10	>378	163	45	16
^{60}Co	γ	17	4	3	>36	28	15	3
^{137}Cs	γ	19	10	4	>234	59	13	9
^{192}Ir	γ	34	6	1	>81	50	10	1
Other γ emitters	γ	8	1	—	>10	10	2	—
γ-β emitters	γ-β	2	—	—	2	2	—	—
β emitters	β	8	5	2	15	14	5	3
Reactor incidents and the loss of control of critical fissile materials (total without Chernobyl)		34	20	7	118	83	73	13
Criticality	γ-n	16	12	6	70	42	42	10
Reactor incidents (other causes)	γ-β	18	8	1	48	41	31	3
X-ray units and accelerators (total)		38	1	—	39	39	1	—
X-ray units	X	26	—	—	26	26	—	—
Electron accelerators	e	9	1	—	10	10	1	—
Proton accelerators	p+	3	—	—	3	3	—	—
Other incidents (total)		11	2	2	20	16	6	2
Total without Chernobyl		171	49	19	>555	301	125	31
Chernobyl accident	γ-β	1	1	1	>384*	134	134	28
TOTAL		172	51	20	>939	435	259	59

* Excluding recovery workers.

Source: SRC, Institute of Biophysics Registry data, November 1, 2000.

REFERENCES

1. Soloviev, V., Ilyin, L., Baranov, A., Guskova, A., Nadejina, N., and Gusev, I., Radiation accidents in the former U.S.S.R. territory before and after Chernobyl (IAEA-CN-63/6), in *One Decade after Chernobyl: Summing up the Consequences of the Accident*, Poster presentation – Vol. 2, International Conference held in Vienna, April 8–12, 1996, IAEA, September 1997, p. 601–607.
2. McLaughlin, T., Monahan, S., Puvost, N., Frolov, V., Ryazanov, B., and Sviridov, V., A Review of Critical Accidents, 2000 Revision, Los Alamos National Laboratory, LA-1368, May 2000, p. 142.

10 Radiation Accidents in the United States

Robert C. Ricks, Mary Ellen Berger, Elizabeth C. Holloway, and Ronald E. Goans

CONTENTS

Introduction 167
Background 168
The Registries 168
The U.S. Registry (1944 to June 30, 2000) 169
Summary 171
References 172

INTRODUCTION

Serious injury due to ionizing radiation is a rare occurrence. From 1944 to the present, through years of research, development, and use of nuclear materials in industry, energy production, and medicine, only 30 people have lost their lives in 13 separate radiation accidents in the United States (Table 10.1). Information about these and 233 other less serious U.S. accidents is documented in the U.S. Radiation Accident Registry, maintained at the Radiation Emergency Assistance Center/Training Site (REAC/TS) in Oak Ridge, Tennessee.

TABLE 10.1
U.S. Radiation Accidents Resulting in Deaths (1944 to June 2000)

State	No. of Deaths	Accident Circumstances
Idaho	3	Trauma/reactor criticality (non-radiation death)
New Mexico	3	2 — Research with critical assembly
		1 — Chemical operations/criticality
Ohio	10	Radiation therapy
Oklahoma	1	Self-inflicted injury (probable)
Pennsylvania	1	Radiation therapy (brachytherapy)
Rhode Island	1	Chemical operations/criticality
Texas	9	7 — Nuclear medicine therapy
		2 — Radiation therapy/computer programming
Washington	1	Radiation therapy (nonradiation death)
Wisconsin	1	Nuclear medicine therapy

BACKGROUND

REAC/TS was established in 1975 and is operated by the Oak Ridge Institute for Science and Education (ORISE) in Oak Ridge, Tennessee for the U.S. Department of Energy. The REAC/TS program provides 24-h direct or consultative assistance regarding medical and health physics problems associated with radiation accidents in local, national, and international incidents. The REAC/TS facility serves not only as a treatment facility, but also as a central training and demonstration unit where U.S. and foreign medical, nursing, paramedical, and health physics personnel receive intensive training in medical management of radiation accidents.

One of the objectives of the REAC/TS program has been to broaden knowledge of the early and late effects of radiation injury in humans, with the goal of developing better diagnostic, therapeutic, and prognostic modalities. REAC/TS maintains registries to further this aim through preservation of valuable historical and medical records for use in research and medical and health physics training. Medical aspects and subsequent follow-up of many serious accidents are reviewed in a series of conference proceedings on the Medical Basis for Radiation Accident Preparedness (1980, 1990, 1991).[1-3]

The REAC/TS registries include the Worldwide Accident Registry, comprising the U.S. Radiation Accident Registry and the Non-U.S. Accident Registry. Figure 10.1 indicates the registries maintained at REAC/TS and their status on June 30, 2000.

THE REGISTRIES

Information for the REAC/TS accident registries is gathered from many sources. These include reports from the World Health Organization (WHO), the International Atomic Energy Agency (IAEA), the Nuclear Regulatory Commission (NRC), state radiological health departments, medical and health physics literature, personal communications, the Internet, and, most frequently, from physicians, health physicists, and other involved individuals who call REAC/TS for assistance when an incident occurs.

REAC/TS takes an average of 55 calls for assistance each year. Although each of these calls is about a real or perceived event involving ionizing radiation, not all "incidents" involve significant exposures. For purposes of the registry, designation as a "significant exposure" requires the

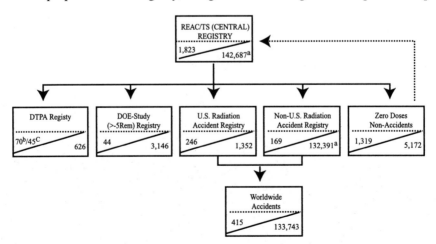

[a] Includes Chernobyl — 116,500; Brazil — 249; Mexico — 4000; Kyothm — 10,180; Spain — 27.
[b] Former and current DTPA sites.
[c] Current coinvestigators.

FIGURE 10.1 Status of REAC/TS registries, June 2000. The numerator indicates the number of registered events or sites. The denominator indicates the number of persons in the events or at the sites. (From Radiation Emergency Assistance Center/Training Site Radiation Accident Registries.)

following conditions and dose criteria: 250 mSv (25,000 mrem) to the bone marrow of the whole body or to the gonads; 6,000 mSv (600,000 mrem) to the skin of the extremities; 750 mSv (75,000 mrem) to organs such as the eye or thyroid; internal contamination levels exceeding one half of the maximum permissible body burden (currently under revision); and medical misadministrations resulting in any one or more of these conditions. Significant "accidental ionizing radiation exposures" are defined as levels at which early biological changes and clinical symptoms might be detected.

Most calls for assistance to REAC/TS are concerned with one or more individuals who, through history, diagnostic testing, and/or dose estimation, are shown to have had little or no exposure. Information about these "incidents" is maintained, but the "incident" is not counted as an "accident" for inclusion in the registry. Examples of such incidents include:

- Discovery of a radium therapy source that had been in a file cabinet in a busy city office environment over a period of many years.
- Low-level contamination in a residence that occurred when a discarded exit sign containing tritium (^{3}H) was brought home and broken.
- Unexplained exposure recorded by dosimeter (film badge, thermoluminescent dosimeter).

Approximately one in five calls for REAC/TS assistance involves significant radiation exposure to one or more persons. Information about these "accidents" is recorded in the registry. Every person who received any radiation exposure in the accident is listed in the registry as "involved." All such information is handled with discretion, under strict considerations for privacy, protection of human subjects, and other legal and ethical concerns.

THE U.S. REGISTRY (1944 TO JUNE 30, 2000)

The U.S. Registry contains records from 246 accidents involving 1352 persons, including 793 whose exposures met the criteria for inclusion in the registry. There is good reason to believe this number does not represent all radiation accidents in the United States. Some accidents are unreported because of legal or financial concerns, lack of knowledge of radiation hazards or radiation effects, or because unsuspecting persons were unaware of an exposure.

Accidents have been reported in 41 states, the District of Columbia, and Puerto Rico, with the greatest number of accidents involving radiation devices. These devices include sealed sources used in industrial radiography, radiotherapy, and industrial processes, X-ray-generating devices used in medicine, research, and industrial processes and quality assurance, and accelerators used in medicine and research. Table 10.2 lists the number of accidents by state, and Table 10.3 lists the major accidents in the United States classified by the type of device involved in the accident.

Of the recorded accidents, 140 took place in industrial settings, with sources used in industrial radiography accounting for 51 accidents. There was a marked decrease in the number of industrial radiography accidents in the early 1990s. Equipment changes, training, and regulations contributed to this drop, along with a reduced need for radiography of high-pressure pipe welds, valves, and vessels (i.e., less construction of nuclear power plants, oil refineries, etc.). Ten accidents occurred in irradiation facilities; 46 accidents happened in industrial research and development. Other industrial uses accounted for 33 accidents.

A total of 11 individuals were injured by neutron and gamma exposures in criticality accidents during activities in nuclear weapons research and development, reactor engineering development, or production of enriched uranium. No one in the United States has received a significant exposure in a criticality accident since 1962.

The greatest number of accidental deaths and significant exposures were associated with diagnostic or therapeutic procedures in medical facilities. The registry (1944 to June 2000) includes information from 80 accidents in U.S. medical facilities. One of these accidents alone accounts for

TABLE 10.2
Number of Accidents in Registry by State (including the District of Columbia and Puerto Rico)

State	No. of Accidents	State	No. of Accidents
Alabama	1	Nebraska	0
Alaska	0	Nevada	4
Arizona	2	New Hampshire	0
Arkansas	0	New Jersey	12
California	16	New Mexico	12
Colorado	2	New York	10
Connecticut	4	North Carolina	1
Delaware	0	North Dakota	0
District of Columbia	3	Ohio	8
Florida	1	Oklahoma	4
Georgia	4	Oregon	2
Hawaii	3	Pennsylvania	16
Idaho	3	Rhode Island	1
Illinois	12	South Carolina	2
Indiana	9	South Dakota	0
Iowa	2	Tennessee	9
Kansas	2	Texas	30
Kentucky	1	Utah	1
Louisiana	6	Vermont	0
Maine	1	Virginia	3
Maryland	6	Washington	9
Massachusetts	7	West Virginia	0
Michigan	7	Wisconsin	6
Minnesota	5	Wyoming	1
Mississippi	2	Puerto Rico	3
Missouri	2	Unknown	11
Montana	0		

403 of the 790 individuals with significant exposures in the United States. Seven accidents involved the use of X-ray devices in medical facilities; these resulted in significant exposures to 12 individuals. Of the 80 accidents, 30 occurred with sealed sources of radioactive materials, with 617 individuals involved, 457 significantly exposed, and 11 deaths. An additional 38 of the recorded accidents occurred with use of radiopharmaceuticals. These involved 112 persons, with 46 having significant exposures and 8 deaths. There were five accidents with accelerators used in radiation therapy in which two persons lost their lives and three were seriously injured. These accidents in hospitals and other medical facilities occurred because of classical errors: wrong patient, wrong dosage (for example, mistaking "milli" for "micro"), wrong medication, or because of irradiation of the wrong area of the body. Other errors resulting in injury or death included failure to determine if a female was pregnant or nursing, incorrect calibration of therapy devices, incorrect computer programming, errors in equipment maintenance or repair, negligence, and malpractice. Registry information about these and other cases is occasionally sketchy, incomplete, or not made available to REAC/TS, usually because of legal considerations.

Valuable information about several medical cases can be found in published works. For example, Flynn et al.[4] describes a case involving a 136.9 GBq) (3.7 Ci) iridium-192 brachytherapy source that was left in a patient for 92.75 h, resulting in death of the patient and involvement of 95 persons.

TABLE 10.3
Major Radiation Accidents in the United States (1944 to June 2000)

Classification	No. of Accidents	No. of Persons Involved	No. of Persons with Significant Exposure
Criticalities	11		
Critical assemblies	4	74	19
Reactors	2	14	5
Chemical operations	5	61	18
Radiation Devices	162		
Sealed sources	110	848	578
X-ray devices	38	58	55
Accelerators	13	15	15
Radon generators	1	9	6
Radioisotopes	73		
Transuranics	24	118	26
Fission products	7	31	19
Diagnosis and therapy	38	117	48
Other	4	7	5
TOTAL	**246**	**1352**	**793**

Newman et al.[5] describes deaths and serious injuries due to errors in the computer programming of a therapy device. Shope[6] describes serious skin injuries caused by prolonged periods of fluoroscopy.

The most common type of radiation injury in the United States has been a local injury to some part of the body. Of all documented local injuries, 77% involved the fingers and hands. Another 6% were extremity injuries involving the arms, legs, or feet. A further 9% of local injuries involved the head or neck, and the remainder was injuries to the thorax and other areas. The radiation sources in these cases of local injury were predominantly sealed sources of iridium-192 and cobalt-60.

Accidents resulting in significant exposures due to internally deposited radioactive materials occurred in research and development activities, in industry, and, most frequently, in hospitals. In medical therapy, 43 individuals given iodine-131 or iodine-125 had significant exposures. Two of these accidents involved pregnant women and another involved a nursing mother. Other radionuclides implicated in injuries and deaths include yttrium-99, plutonium and americium compounds, phosphorus-32, uranium compounds, gold-198, strontium-85, and mixed fission products.

SUMMARY

Serious radiation accidents in the United States have been rare. The safety record, unmatched by other technologies, is due in large part to careful regulation and control provided by regulatory agencies and radiation protection specialists (medical and health physics professionals). Although not all accidents result in injury, a serious radiation injury can be physically, psychologically, and economically debilitating to an individual; treatment is complex and prolonged and the outcome may not be satisfactory. Control, strict safety precautions, and training are absolutely essential elements in prevention of injuries. In these regards, the REAC/TS registry for documentation of accidents serves useful purposes: (1) weaknesses in design, safety practices, training, or control can be identified, and trends noted; (2) information regarding the medical consequences of injuries and the efficacy of treatment protocols is available to the treating physician; and (3) registry case studies serve as valuable teaching tools.

REFERENCES

1. Hubner, K.F. and Fry, S.A., Eds., *The Medical Basis for Radiation Accident Preparedness*, Elsevier/North-Holland, New York, 1980.
2. Ricks, R.C. and Fry, S.A., *The Medical Basis for Radiation Accident Preparedness II, Clinical Experience and Follow-Up since 1979*, Elsevier, New York, 1990.
3. Ricks, R.C., Berger, M.E., O'Hara, and F.M., Eds., *The Medical Basis for Radiation Accident Preparedness III, The Psychological Perspective*, Elsevier, New York, 1991.
4. Flynn, D.F., Mihalakis, I., Mauceri, T., and Pins, M.R., Gastrointestinal Syndrome after Accidental Overexposure during Radiotherapy, Loss of an Iridium-192 Source and Therapy Misadministration at Indiana Regional Cancer Center Indiana, Pennsylvania, on November 16, 1992, NUREG-1480, U.S. Nuclear Regulatory Commission, Washington, DC, February 1993.
5. Newman, F.H., Ricks, R.C., and Fry, S.A., Eds., The malfunction 54 accelerator accidents 1985, 1986, 1987, in *The Medical Basis for Radiation Accident Preparedness II, Clinical Experience and Follow-Up since 1979*, Elsevier, New York, 1990, 165–171.
6. Shope, T.B., Radiation-induced skin injuries from fluoroscopy, presented at the Scientific Assembly and Annual Meeting of the Radiological Society of North America, November 26–December 1, 1995, *Radiology*, 197P(Suppl.), P449 and *Radiographics*, 1996.

11 Criticality Accidents

*Fred A. Mettler, Jr., George L. Voelz,
Jean-Claude Nénot, and Igor A. Gusev*

CONTENTS

Introduction 173
Los Alamos, New Mexico, U.S.A. (August 1945) 174
Los Alamos, New Mexico, U.S.A. (May 1946) 175
Argonne, Illinois, U.S.A. (June 1952)..176
Mayak, Russia (March 1953) 176
Mayak, Russia (April 1957) 181
Mayak, Russia (January 1958) 183
Oak Ridge, Tennessee, U.S.A. (June 1958) 183
Vinca, Yugoslavia (October 1958) 185
Los Alamos, New Mexico, U.S.A. (December 1958) 186
Idaho Chemical Processing Plant, U.S.A. (October 1959) 186
Siberian Chemical Combine, Russia (July 1961) 187
Hanford, Washington, U.S.A. (April 1962) 187
Sarov Vniief, Russia (March 1963) 187
Wood River Junction, Rhode Island, U.S.A. (July 1964) 187
Mol, Belgium (December 1965) 188
Chelyabinsk-70 (April 1968) 188
Mayak Production Facility, Russia (December 1968) 189
Kurchatov Institute, Moscow, Russia (February 1971) 189
Kurchatov Institute, Moscow, Russia (May 1971) 189
Siberian Chemical Combine, Russia (December 1978) 190
Constituyente, Argentina (September 1983) 190
Sarov (Arzimas-16) Vniief, Russia (June 1997) 190
Tokaimura, Japan (September 1999) 191
Summary 192
References 193

INTRODUCTION

Criticality accidents are rare. They usually occur during the assembly/disassembly of nuclear weapons, radiochemical operations with fissionable materials, and unexpected nuclear reactor excursions. The accident at Chernobyl is not included in this chapter since it was the result of a steam explosion in an operating reactor and it is covered in detail in Chapter 12.

Heat and blast are not present in critical excursion accidents although there often is a flash of blue light. The spectrum of radiation energies and types received by the patients is a function of the specific accident. A significant portion of the dose to individuals and the subsequent tissue damage may be from neutrons. Despite their rather high energy, thermal neutrons have limited penetration ability in tissue and are usually absorbed in the first few inches of flesh. The rest of the dose is from gamma rays released in the fission process. The depth dose distribution approximates that of unfiltered 80-kV X rays. Many of the patients have received sufficient penetrating dose to develop the acute radiation syndrome with hematological, gastrointestinal, and central nervous system complications. Most patients close to a critical excursion receive very nonuniform doses.

The unique features of criticality accidents are the relatively increased damage in superficial tissues as compared with accidents involving gamma rays and the induced radioactivity in body tissues, metal objects, and clothing. The latter feature can help with dosimetric analysis. The quality factor for neutrons in producing damage in various tissues is not well known and there is virtually no human data regarding neutron exposures to allow a firm assessment of long-term carcinogenic risk in the survivors. The RBE or radiation-weighting factor for neutrons is different for different tissues, usually between 1 and 2 for acute deterministic effects. It is even different for various effects in the same tissue. As a result, a calculated dose is often at variance with clinically observed effects.

Criticality accidents happen in two different types of settings: processing facilities (22 accidents worldwide) and during criticality experiments or operations with research reactors (39 accidents worldwide). As of July 2000, there have been 23 criticality accidents that resulted in exposures high enough to cause bone marrow depression (Table 11.1), 18 fatalities, and four accidents where amputations were required. There are some characteristics of criticality accidents that have implications for medical management. The exposures are almost all instantaneous and with a very sharp dose decrease with distance. The fission yield in criticality accidents has ranged from 10^{15} to 4×10^{19} fissions, but most accidents are about 1 to 2×10^{17} fissions. Approximate doses with distance from the criticality are shown in Table 11.2. From these data, it is clear that the probability of fatality is high within 3 m, but is unlikely if a person is located more than 5 m away. It also is clear that extremities very near or touching the apparatus may be very highly exposed (necessitating amputation) even though the individual's whole-body dose may be low enough for survival.

Exposure to the public from criticality accidents is usually minimal. The remainder of the chapter is devoted to descriptions of those accidents where there was significant human exposure and of the medical details that are available. An attempt has been made to present the medical data in a uniform fashion for the very seriously overexposed patients. To do this in the accompanying tables (Table 11.3a, b, and c), data have been interpolated if a specific test was not available on that day for a given patient. At the end of the chapter is a summary of lessons learned from these accidents as a group.

LOS ALAMOS, NEW MEXICO, U.S.A. (AUGUST 1945)

In the Los Alamos I accident, the operator (designated case 1) was adding tungsten carbide bricks to a plutonium assembly when the neutron flux began to increase rapidly. He accidentally dropped a brick onto the center of the assembly and a flash occurred that was easily visible to a guard 12 ft away. For such a glow to be visible, the radiation intensity must have been on the order of 7 million R/s. The operator then removed the last brick with his right hand and partially dismantled the assembly. He was seen at the hospital 30 min after the accident and complained of numbness and tingling of his swollen hands (Figure 11.1).

The operator received an estimated dose of 2 Gy (neutrons) and 1.1 Gy (gamma). He died 24 days postexposure from the acute radiation syndrome (see Color Figure 1*) (hematological). The guard (case 2) received 0.08 Gy (neutrons) and 0.001 Gy (gamma). He died at age 62 (32 years postexposure) from acute myeloblastic leukemia. His brother also died of leukemia (and three other siblings are believed to have had cancer), so a familial component may have contributed to the disease.

---

* Color figure follows page 202.

Criticality Accidents

TABLE 11.1
Criticality Accidents with Serious Exposures

Accident	Date	Victims with Doses > 0.25 Gy	Estimated Average Whole-Body Dose to Victims	Fatalities
Los Alamos, New Mexico, U.S.A.	August 1945	1	2 Gy neutron and 0.1 gamma	1 (day 24)
Los Alamos, New Mexico, U.S.A.	May 1946	8	21, 3.6, 2.5, 1.6, 1.1, 0.65, 0.47, 0.37 Sv	1 (day 9)
Argonne, Illinois, U.S.A.	June 1952	3	1.59, 1.26, 0.61 Gy	0
Mayak, Russia	March 1953	2	10, 1 Gy	0
Mayak, Russia	April 1957	6	30 Gy and five workers with 3+ Gy	1 (day 12)
Mayak, Russia	January 1958	4	60 Gy for three workers and 6 Gy for the fourth	3 (days 5–6)
Oak Ridge, Tennessee, U.S.A.	June 1958	7	3.65, 3.39, 3.27, 2.70, 2.36, 0.69, 0.69 Gy	0
Vinca, Yugoslavia	October 1958	6	4.36, 4.26, 4.19, 4.14, 3.23, 2.07 Gy	1 (day 32)
Los Alamos, New Mexico, U.S.A.	December 1958	3	45, 1.35, 0.5 Gy	1 (35 h)
Idaho, U.S.A.	October 1959	2	0.5, 0.3 Sv	0
Siberia, Russia	July 1961	1	2 Gy	0
Hanford, Washington, U.S.A	April 1962	2	1.1, 0.43 Sv	0
Sarov, Russia	March 1963	2	5.5, 3.7	0
Rhode Island, U.S.A.	July 1964	3	100, 1, 0.6 Gy	1 (49 h)
Mol, Belgium	December 1965	1	5 Gy	0
Chelyabinsk	April 1968	2	5–10, 20–60 Gy	2
Mayak, Russia	December 1968	2	24.5, 7 Gy	1 (about day 30)
Kurchatov, Moscow, Russia	February 1971	2		0
Kurchatov, Moscow, Russia	May 1971	4	60, 20, 9, 9 Gy	2 (24 h and 2 weeks)
Siberia, Russia	December 1978	?	2.5 Gy and seven other workers with 0.05–0.5 Gy	0
Constituyentes, Argentina	September 1983	3	23 Gy gamma and 17 neutron and two others with 0.2 Gy gamma and 0.15 neutron	1 (48 h)
Sarov, Russia	June 1997	1	45 Gy neutron and 3.5 Gy gamma	1 (66 h)
Tokaimura, Japan	September 1999	3	17, 8, 1–2 Gy	2 (day 83 and 211)

LOS ALAMOS, NEW MEXICO, U.S.A. (MAY 1946)

The Los Alamos I (August 21, 1945) and II (May 21, 1946) accidents were similar in that an experimental plutonium assembly unexpectedly became critical during a manual procedure. In both instances the operator died.[1] In the Los Alamos II accident, criticality occurred in a plutonium sphere when two beryllium hemispheres accidentally surrounded the plutonium mass (Figure 11.3). The operator (designated case 3) was attempting to teach another individual (designated case 4) how to do experiments even though there were six other people in the area. Even in a sunlit room

TABLE 11.2
Approximate Dose Related to Distance from a Criticality

Distance from Criticality (m)	Total Dose Gy (Neutron and Gamma)[a]
0.3	50–200
0.5	30–100
1	10–30
2	3–8
3	1–3
5	0.6–1.5
10	0.15–0.40
20	0.05–0.10
50	0.007–0.002
100	0.002–0.005

[a] Normalized to 10^{17} fissions.

a blue glow was easily visible as criticality occurred. The yield was about 3×10^{15} fissions. The eight people in the room received 15 to 21, 3.6, 2.5, 1.6, 1.1, 0.65, 0.47, and 0.37 Sv, respectively.

The operator received an estimated 15 to 21 Gy and died 9 days postexposure from the gastrointestinal type of the acute radiation syndrome. Of the seven initial survivors, one refused to participate in long-term follow-up but was alive as of 1978. Of the others, one patient who received 1.66 Gy (neutrons) and 0.26 Gy (gamma) experienced moderate to severe fatigue for 6 months, epilation, and aspermia. He died 20 years later of a myocardial infarction. Another who received 0.51 Gy (neutrons) and 0.11 Gy (gamma) had no acute radiation response but died 29 years later with clinical aplastic anemia and bacterial endocarditis. Another individual who had received 12 rad (neutrons) and 4 rad (gamma) died 18 years later of acute myelocytic leukemia.

ARGONNE, ILLINOIS, U.S.A. (JUNE 1952)

The accident at the U.S. Argonne National Laboratory occurred as a result of reactor criticality on June 2, 1952. A large reactivity change was made manually during testing control rods in the ZPR assembly causing a power excursion. Three workers (A, B, and C) were on a platform surrounding the reactor tank while another worker (D) leaned over the tank and unclamped and withdrew a control rod. A dull "thud" was heard and a blue light emanated from the top of the reactor. The control rod was dropped back in and the workers left the room. The patients were seen within 10 min by a physician. They were asymptomatic and transported to a hospital. The doses were about 1.59, 1.26, 0.61, and 0.11 Gy. Only patient A was symptomatic. No fatalities resulted from this accident.

MAYAK, RUSSIA (MARCH 1953)

The accident occurred on March 15, 1953 in a building where processing was being carried out to recover plutonium from irradiated uranium rods. Transfer of plutonium solution was made between two vessels assuming that one was empty (which was not the case). The vessel became hot, there was a gas release and the solution foamed. The yield was estimated to be about 2×10^{17} fissions. This was not recognized as a criticality accident by the two workers and they continued to carry

TABLE 11.3
Summary of Very Seriously Exposed Patients

Site	Los Alamos	Los Alamos	Los Alamos	Argonne	Oak Ridge	Oak Ridge
Year	1945	1946	1946	1952	1958	1958
Case No.	1	3	4	A	A	B
Whole-body dose	5.5–20 Sv	13–21Sv	3.6 Gy	1.59 Gy	3.65 Gy	2.7 Gy
Incapacitation	NR	No	No	No	No	No
Early hypotension	Mild 100/60	No	No	No	No	No
Nausea	1.5–24h	<1–12h	6h	4h (1×)	2–4h	4–11h
Vomiting	1.5–24h	<1–12h	6h	4h (1×)	2h–2d	4–11h
Diarrhea	No	4–8h	No		No	No
Headache	NR	No	No		No	No
Weakness	Days	1h–9d	1d–70d		Mild	No
Initial fever	1h–26d	6h–9d	No (5–9d)			
Numb/tingling hands	0.5h					
Edema	0.5h	3h	No		No	No
Blistering	36h (finger)	28h	No		No	No
Epilation	17d		17d	No	17d	17d
WBC						
1h	7800	9600	8000	9100	7850 at 2h	8250 at 2h
1d	16000	11000	7000	7000	9500	5300
2d	14000	1600	8000	6000		4400
4d	17000	8000	10000	4900	4500	9100
8d	5500	400	3500	3500	2300	4700
16d	8000		7000	5500	3200	4000
24d	1800		4000	4800	2200	3600
32d					1200	2800
40d				2800	3800	3100
Lymphocytes						
1h	2000	2200	2000	2000	2370 at 2h	1320 at 2h
1d	1800	0	800	2100	1000	1000
2d	800	200	1400	1500	1200	900
4d	500	0	400	1000	450	700
8d	400	0	200	1000	500	800
16d	1200		900	1500	1000	1100
24d	300		1000	1000	500	1200
32d					900	1000
40d				950	1300	1400
Thrombocytes						
1d					300000	200000
16d					130000	200000
24d					15000	50000
32d					70000	70000
40d					400000	100000
Death	24d	9d	No	No	No	No

TABLE 11.3 (CONTINUED)
Summary of Very Seriously Exposed Patients

Site	Oak Ridge	Oak Ridge	Oak Ridge	Vinca	Los Alamos	Sarov
Year	1958	1958	1958	1958	1958	1963
Case No.	C	D	E	V	K	M
Whole-body dose	3.39 Gy	3.27 Gy	2.36 Gy	4.36 Gy	45–120 Gy	300 Gy
Incapacitation	No	No	No	NR	Immediate	No
Early hypotension	No	No	No	NR	Immediate	In minutes
Nausea	No	2h–3d	2–11h	Yes–24h	NR	20m
Vomiting	No	2–11h	No	Yes–24h	NR	1–6h
Diarrhea	No	No	No	Yes on 4d	0.5h	No
Headache	No	2–11h	No	NR		20m
Weakness	Mild	No	No	NR	Disabled	20m–4d
Initial fever						
Numb/tingling hands						
Edema	No	No	No	NR	2h, hands[a]	NR
Blistering	No	No	No	NR	NR	NR
Epilation	17d			NR	No	13d, head
WBC						
1h	17350 at 2h	10450 at 2h	11400 at 2h	5500	5500 at 1.5h	
1d	12300		6500		6100 at 4h	5600 at 6h
2d			7000	3000 at 3d	10000 at 6h	
4d	6000		7000	3000 at 6d	19000 at 11h	4200
8d	4100		3600	500 at 11d	28000 at 14h	
16d	4500		4300		14000 at 33h	4000 at 14d
24d	1800		3900			3000
32d	1500		2800			1200 at 33d
40d	5000		3100			2700 at 50d
Lymphocytes						
1h	1995 at 2h	1358 at 2h	2450 at 2h	1248	1800 at 1.5h	
1d	2000	1700	1000	452 at 14h	1000 at 4h	615 at 6h
2d	2100	1300	1100	200 at 3d	0 at 6h	
4d	1100	1000	1700	100 at 5d	100 at 11h	650
8d	900	1300	1300		0 at 14h	
16d	1200	1300	1500		0 at 33h	600 at 14d
24d	1000	1300	1400			600
32d	800	1200	1450			500 at 33d
40d	1900	1600	1600			750 at 50d
Thrombocytes						
1d	220000		230000	90000		250K at 6h
16d	120000		150000	40000 at 8d		200K at 15d
24d	28000		40000			100K at 23d
32d	18000		60000			17K at 33d
40d	110000		250000			
Death	No	No	No	32d	35 h	No

TABLE 11.3 (CONTINUED)
Summary of Very Seriously Exposed Patients

Site	Sarov	Mol	Sarov	Tokaimura	Tokaimura	Tokaimura
Year	1963	1965	1997	1999	1999	1999
Case No.	KH	1	1	O	S	Y
Whole-body dose	4.5 Gy	5.5 Gy	48.5 Gy	17 Sv	8 Sv	1–4.5 Gy
Incapacitation	No	No		Minutes	No	No
Early hypotension	Minutes	No	Yes, 80/40	Yes, 86/?	No	No
Nausea	Minutes	2h	1h	20 min	<1h	2–4h, slight
Vomiting	Minutes	2h	1h	20 min	1h	No
Diarrhea	NR	No	No	<1h	No	No
Headache	Minutes	No	1h	No	No	No
Weakness	0.1h–4d	Yes	1h	NR	NR	No
Initial fever		No, 21–60d	4h	4h	No	
Numb/tingling hands						
Edema	NR		6h	4h	1d and 22d	No
Blistering	NR		30h	21d	3 weeks	No
Epilation	NR			~20d	3 weeks	No
WBC						
1h	9300		4500	22800	12700	
1d		16500	15000 at 3h	29100	13000	15000
2d		7000	9000 at 5h	22300	18000	5500
4d		4000	12700 at 12h	8100	19000	17000[d]
8d		800	14300 at 1d	200[b]	0[c]	13000
16d		900	11700 at 2d	1000	0	5500
24d	800 at 27d	300		12600	500	3000
32d	1000 at 33d	4500		8200 at 28d	4000 at 28d	7500 at 29d
40d	4000 at 50d	6500				
Lymphocytes						
1h	1100		900	1600	270	
1d		1300	600 at 3h	400	170	800
2d		280	180 at 5h	0	125	950
4d		130	130 at 12h	80	50	800
8d		300	300 at 1d	0	0b	650
16d		380	0 at 2d	210	0	600
24d	250 at 27d	200		1210 at 25d	9	700
32d	300 at 33d	1100			100 at 28d	1000 at 28d
40d	700 at 50d	800				
Thrombocytes						
1d		300000		280K at 1h	205000	175000
16d	20K at 14d	30000		218K at 1d	51000	50000[e]
24d	20K at 27d	14000		180K at 2d	19000	60000
32d	40K at 33d	80000		63K at 4d	30000 at 28d	90000 at 28d
40d	160K at 50d	220000		39K at 16d		
Death	No	No	66h	83d	211d	No

[a] Erythema at 20 min
[b] Peripheral blood stem cell transplant received on day 7.
[c] Cord blood cell transplant received on day 9.
[d] G-CSF received from day 2 to 28.
[e] Three platelet transfusions received from day 17 to 24.

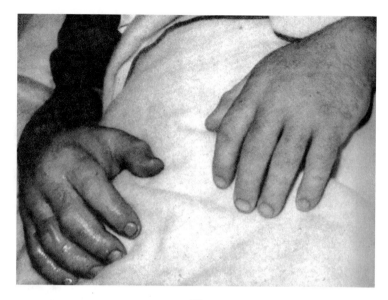

(A)

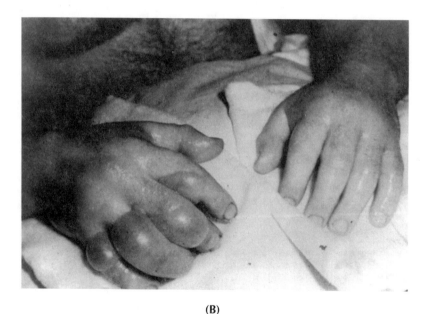

(B)

FIGURE 11.1 View of the hands of case 1 from the Los Alamos I accident. At 42 h postexposure (A), there is swelling of both hands and early blistering of the fingers of the right hand. At 3½ days postexposure (B), the blisters of the right hand have markedly enlarged. At 15 days postexposure (C), the right hand has patches of gangrene with loss to the epidermis over the knuckles. By day 24 (D), there was marked progression of gangrene. This was also the day of death.

out their work plans for the shift. Two days later one of the workers became abruptly ill. He was estimated to have received about 10 Gy and he suffered severe radiation sickness and amputation of both legs. He died 35 years after the accident. The other worker was estimated to have received about 1 Gy.

Criticality Accidents 181

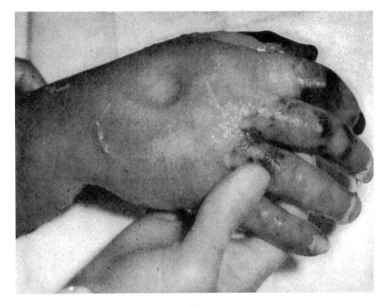

(C)

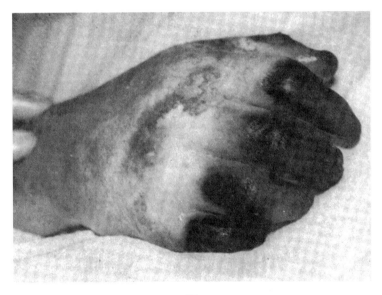

(D)

FIGURE 11.1 (CONTINUED)

MAYAK, RUSSIA (APRIL 1957)

On April 21, 1957, there was an accident in a building that housed various operations concerning highly enriched uranium. The accident occurred in a glove box in which there was an excess accumulation of uranium during filtration of uranyl oxalate precipitate. The operator was looking through the glove box window and saw a bulge in the vessel fabric and there was a release of gas and precipitate. The yield was estimated to be about 1×10^{17} fissions. The operator picked up the

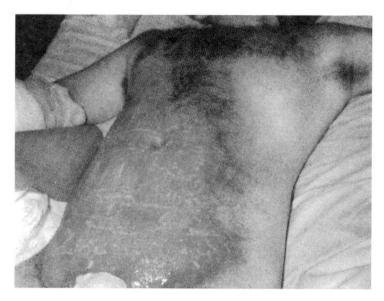

FIGURE 11.2 Los Alamos I case 1. View of the anterior abdomen and chest 24 days postexposure showing effects of inhomogeneous exposure. There is loss of epidermis with fibrin covering the dermis. Also note the loss of hair on the right lower chest. Obviously the intestinal and right lung dose were much higher than the "average" whole-body dose.

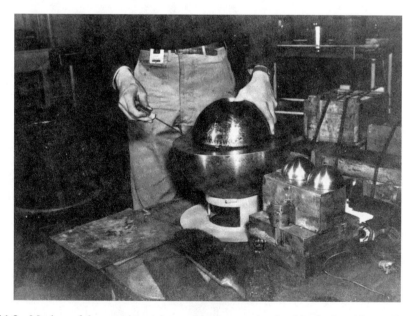

FIGURE 11.3 Mockup of the experimental assembly that was involved in the Los Alamos II accident.

precipitate and put it back into the filter vessel. Within seconds he became ill. Within 17 h after the accident the specific activity of sodium-24 in the operator's blood was 245 Bq/cm^3. This correlated to an estimated dose of about 30 Gy. The operator died 12 days after the accident. There were five other workers in the room, and they received doses upward of 3 Gy and all suffered from radiation sickness but recovered.

MAYAK, RUSSIA (JANUARY 1958)

The accident occurred on January 2, 1958 and involved enriched uranyl nitrate solution that was being transferred from an experimental vessel to bottles with more favorable geometry. Rather than use a drain line as prescribed, the three workers lifted the experimental vessel and began to move it to pour the contents manually into other bottles. There was an immediate blue flash and fissile material was ejected about 5 m above the vessel. Yield was estimated to be about 2×10^{17} fissions. A fourth worker, who was 2.5 m away, was also exposed. They were all decontaminated and transferred to a hospital. The estimated exposures were 60 Gy for the three workers who lifted the tank and 6 Gy for the fourth worker. The three massively exposed workers died in 5 to 6 days. The fourth worker was exposed to a very heterogeneous of gamma and neutron radiation (20 Gy on the left side of the body and 3 Gy on the right) and developed an acute radiation sickness and subsequently suffered a number of health problems, including cataracts. She survived more than 25 years after exposure.

OAK RIDGE, TENNESSEE, U.S.A. (JUNE 1958)

This accident occurred at the Y-12 facility of the U.S. Oak Ridge National Laboratories at 2 P.M. on June 16, 1958.[2] A solution of enriched uranium unexpectedly became critical as it was transferred from a 40- to a 55-gal drum. There were several fission spikes and the total fission yield was estimated to be about 1.3×10^{18} fissions.

Initial dose estimates ranged from 2.98 to 4.61 Sv for five individuals. The patients were admitted to the hospital at 1 A.M. on June 17, 1958. There were eight individuals exposed (five severely), but no fatalities resulted. The final total doses for the eight individuals (designated A though H) were as follows:

Patient	Dose	Location
A	4.61 Sv	6 ft from source
B	3.41	15 ft from source
C	4.28	17 ft from source
D	4.13	16 ft from source
E	2.98	22 ft from source
F	0.86	1 floor above Patient E
G	0.86	1 floor above and 6 ft farther from source than Patient F
H	0.29	50 ft from source

Induced radioactivity was of interest. Initial examinations showed maximal skin surface activity of 0.3 mR/h It was estimated that about 10 µCi of sodium-24 had been induced in the five patients with the highest doses. At 3 days after the accident, activity measured in the patients was almost down to background level and by 4 days only background activity could be detected.

Hematological changes were evident in most patients; however, it was noted that even with the final dose estimates that the order of severity of dose estimates did not correlate very well with the hematological and clinical data. The possibility of using bone marrow transplantation for Patients A and E was considered but rejected because of potential harmful effects. None of the patients received transfusions during the course of their hospital stay. Figure 11.4 shows a composite of the hematological parameters and symptoms in the five most seriously exposed patients. This is a useful picture of what can be expected in patients who receive doses just below the LD_{50}.

The platelet counts remained rather stationary until day 15, and then they fell progressively, reaching the lowest levels between day 25 and 35. Patients A and C developed petechiae on day 25 postexposure when the platelet count was 2500/cc and 12,500/cc, respectively. The other patients' platelet counts remained above 20,000/cc.

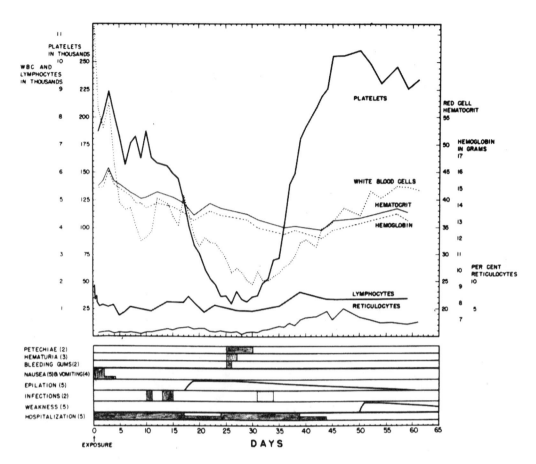

FIGURE 11.4 Composite hematological and clinical findings in the five most seriously exposed patients in the Oak Ridge Y-12 criticality accident.

The patients were admitted approximately 12 h after the accident. Admission absolute lymphocyte values per cubic millimeter for Patients A through E were as follows: 1256, 1316, 1703, 1980, and 1050. These patients had values in the range of 2000 to 4300 from preaccident medical data. By 48 h postexposure the average value was about 1000 although in Patient A the value on one occasion decreased to 500. For the less-exposed patients (F through H), initial values were between 1900 and 2600.

The white blood cell counts of the patients reached their nadir at about 30 days. For Patient A this was 800/mm^3 on day 29 and it increased to 3600 at 44 days. Patient B had his lowest white count of 1650 on day 33 and this was 3250 by day 44. Patient E had his lowest white cell count on day 36 when it was 2050. This increased to 3750 by day 44. The red cell counts, hemoglobin, and hematocrit in the five most exposed patients decreased slowly by about 20% over the 55 days postexposure.

Gastrointestinal symptoms occurred in the patients. Patients A and B experienced nausea and vomiting 2 to 4 h after the accident and Patient E became nauseated about 5 h after the accident but did not vomit. The patients were treated with prochlorperazine dimaleate. Patient C had neither nausea nor vomiting. All patients were free of these symptoms 18 h after exposure, although several had more transient nausea and vomiting about 40 h postexposure. Some of this latter episode was felt to have psychological origins.

Only two patients developed a fever. Patient A developed a fever on day 31 and was noted to have a sore throat and tonsillitis. He was treated with tetracycline and his temperature returned to normal in 72 h. Patient B developed a furuncle in the left gluteal region on day 10, which was incised and drained. He also developed a fever and pharyngitis, which was treated successfully with tetracycline. Epilation began on day 17 in Patients A through E. Soreness of the scalp was reported 2 to 3 days earlier by three of the patients. The greatest hair loss occurred in the occipital region probably related to the mechanical rubbing of the back of the head on the pillow while lying in bed (Figure 11.5). The hair loss had stopped in all patients by day 44. All recovered their hair completely in 6 months.

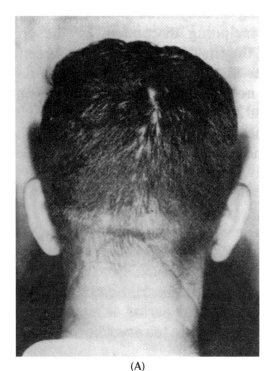
(A)

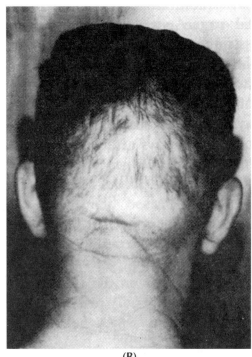
(B)

FIGURE 11.5 Oak Ridge accident Patient D. (A) Posterior view of head at 7 days postexposure. (B) Epilation occurring several weeks later.

Few if any patients experienced weight loss, hematuria, and melena or complained of significant weakness or fatigue. There were quite a number of other studies performed including serum uric acid, plasma alpha-amino acid nitrogen, urinary volume, creatinine, taurine excretion, beta aminoisobutyric acid in urine and other compounds. Overall, although there were some elevations noted, there was little useful information that could be used for either dosimetric evaluation or clinical guidance.

VINCA, YUGOSLAVIA (OCTOBER 1958)

The Vinca reactor criticality accident occurred on October 15, 1958. The facility had a reactor using natural uranium rods moderated by heavy water. An experiment was in progress to activate metal foils. Detectors had reached a maximum saturation value and were reading a constant value even though the power level was rising. The reactor became supercritical. The exposure period was about 5 to 8 min before one of the experimenters smelled ozone and inserted safety rods to stop the reaction.

The accident exposed six individuals and resulted in one fatality. The individuals were designated H, V, G, M, D, and B. The total doses they received were 3.23, 4.36, 4.14, 4.26, 4.19, and 2.07 Gy, respectively. Exposure was relatively uniform over the body. By day 10 postexposure all patients except Patient B had granulocyte levels between 800 and 1500/µl and by day 20 the values had fallen to 20 to 100. For Patient B with a dose of 2.07 Gy (207 rad) the granulocyte level had decreased to 1000/µl by day 20.

LOS ALAMOS, NEW MEXICO, U.S.A. (DECEMBER 1958)

A third criticality accident (LA-III) at Los Alamos occurred at 4:35 P.M. on December 30, 1958 in a plutonium recovery plant.[3-5] Plutonium-rich solids that normally would have been handled separately were washed from two tanks into one large vessel. The operator (designated CK) was standing on a ladder looking through a viewport into the top of the tank and his waist was at the level of the midportion of the tank. His hands were on the tank. The tank was about 110 cm tall and was approximately half-full of solution; when he started a stirrer, a critical reaction took place with a blue flash and what was described as a dull thud. The exposure was from mixed fast neutrons and gamma rays and the number of fissions was calculated to be about 1.5×10^{17}. The operator either fell or was knocked to the floor. He was confused, disoriented, and ataxic. All he could say was "I'm burning up." His co-workers immediately took him to a decontamination shower where he was unable to stand up and became unconscious. The immediate incapacitation was followed by severe hypotension. At 4:46 P.M. a nurse noted CK to be unconscious, in shock, and to have erythema. After about $1^1/_2$ h he became more coherent. His body temperature rose to 103.5°F during the first several hours and decreased to 100°F after about 8 h. After the first several hours, he complained of acute abdominal pain and was anoxic and hypotensive with circulatory failure. His hematocrit remained stable. He was treated with demerol (50 mg), thorazine (25 mg), calcium gluconate (10% in 20 ml of saline), sodium luminal (60 mg), and intravenous administration of 5% dextrose in saline. Vasopressor amines had little effect on his hypotension. Abrupt decreases in systolic blood pressure were noted when rate of flow of saline infusion was decreased. He had intense dermal erythema (anterior surface of the face, thorax, abdomen, genitalia, upper thighs) and conjunctival hyperemia, and there was edema of both hands and forearms. This stage was followed by coma. He died approximately 35 h postexposure.

The average total-body dose from gamma and neutron exposure was estimated to be 45 Gy with the head and upper abdominal area receiving about 104 Gy. Surface gamma ray reading indicated 15 mR/h as a result of sodium activation. The sodium-24-induced activity in the body at the time of the accident was estimated to be 293 µCi. Activity in the various body organs at autopsy was relatively uniform and corrected to the time of the accident ranged from 1.5 to 12 nCi/g with an average of about 4 to 5 nCi/g. Activity in serum was 12 nCi/g and for whole blood the value was 5.3. The average total-body fast neutron dose estimated from sodium-24 activity was 8.35 to 9.68 Gy. Hair was analyzed for induced phosphorus-32. The phosphorus and sulfur mass was 0.063 mg P/g hair and 45 mg S/g. The results indicate a P/S ratio of 0.001. The phosphorus-32 activity was 24 decays/min/mg S for an estimated fast neutron dose of 26 Gy. Metallic buttons on the coveralls were analyzed for the presence of copper-64 and averaged 11,200 counts/m for an estimated fast neutron dose of 19 Gy. The ratio of the gamma/neutron dose was felt to be about 3 for the upper portion of the body and 10/1 at the feet due to neutron absorption in the chemical solution in the tank.

Of the two individuals (RD and JR) who survived, one had a dose of about 1.35 Gy and the other 0.35 to 0.54 Gy of mostly gamma rays. RD was located about 40 ft from the vessel and was shielded by a wall of tanks. Neither had nausea, vomiting, diarrhea, erythema, or epilation. RD's lymphocyte count never went below 1000/mm^3.

IDAHO CHEMICAL PROCESSING PLANT, U.S.A. (OCTOBER 1959)

The accident in a plant dealing with enriched uranium and was caused by an inadvertent siphoning action that resulted in transfer of 200 l of solution to another tank. The critical reaction resulted in a yield of about 4×10^{19} fissions. Thick shielding was present so no significant exposure occurred from prompt gamma rays or neutrons. Airborne fission product gases exposed one person to 0.5 Sv (50 rem); another person received 0.32 Sv and 17 others received smaller amounts. No medical consequences were reported.

SIBERIAN CHEMICAL COMBINE, RUSSIA (JULY 1961)

The accident occurred in a gaseous diffusion facility as a result of enriched uranium accumulation in oil in a vacuum pump. When an operator turned on the pump, the criticality alarm sounded and he saw a flash of light. Fission yield for two excursions was estimated to be 1.2×10^{15}. The operator was sent to the hospital with an estimated dose of about 2 Gy. He experienced mild radiation sickness.

HANFORD, WASHINGTON, U.S.A. (APRIL 1962)

This accident resulted during processing of plutonium solution in a transfer vessel due to improper operation of valves. The fission yield was estimated to be about 8×10^{17}. Three workers received estimated doses of 1.1, 0.43, and 0.19 Sv. There were no fatalities.

SAROV VNIIEF, RUSSIA (MARCH 1963)

The accident involved an experimental reactor and there was an excursion during inadvertent closure of a lithium deuteride reflector around a plutonium core. There was a flash of light and two experimenters left the area. The yield was estimated to be about 5×10^{15} fissions. There were two individuals involved: a facility chief, age 26, and an operator, age 36. The facility chief was close to the reactor and received an estimated gamma and neutron dose of about 3 to 3.7 Gy.

Theoperator was also in close proximity to the reactor and received an estimated gamma and neutron dose of 5.5 Gy. During the maximal period of bone marrow depression, the patient had petechiae, bleeding from the gums, and fevers.

Treatment of both patients was similar. Both patients received penicillin from the first day and streptomycin was added to the regimen at about day 15. Transfusions of whole blood (200 ml) were given every 3 to 5 days. Patients were also given vitamins C and K. Cardiac drugs such as caffeine and cardiasol were also given, as well as a high-protein diet. To stimulate the marrow sodium nucleinate thesan, pentoxyl, and campolon were given.

The facility chief was fully recovered 3 months after exposure and returned to nonradiation work. For the operator there was essentially full bone marrow recovery at the end of the fourth month postexposure and the patient was able to return to work. Both were alive for more than 25 years.

WOOD RIVER JUNCTION, RHODE ISLAND, U.S.A. (JULY 1964)

The facility involved a chemical processing accident at United Nuclear Fuels recovery plant. Scrap material was shipped to the plant from which highly enriched uranium was recovered. A bottle containing a high concentration of uranium was added to a vessel producing a critical reaction. The yield was estimated at 1.1×10^{17} fissions. There was a flash of light and the operator was either knocked to the floor or was transiently incapacitated, but then recovered and left the area. His estimated dose was about 100 Gy. He died 49 h later. Of note is that the local hospital refused to admit this patient because of its own fear of radiation.

An hour and a half after the initial incident, a supervisor and operator entered the area to drain the vessel, but their actions caused a second criticality excursion with an estimated yield of 3×10^{16} fissions. They did not realize that another excursion had occurred, and they drained the tank. They received an estimated dose of 1 and 0.6 Gy, respectively.

MOL, BELGIUM (DECEMBER 1965)

The accident occurred on December 30, 1965 and was a criticality excursion from a small experimental reactor.[6-9] The accident was a result of improper manipulation of control rods; a technician removed one control rod before another was inserted and a critical excursion occurred. The technician was on a grating over the tank. He noticed a glow in the tank and felt an immediate sensation of heat in his left lower leg. Nausea and vomiting occurred within 2 h but only lasted a few hours. The patient was admitted to the hospital within 8 h. Early erythema was observed for the first several days.

The chest dosimeter indicated a gamma dose of 5.5 Gy and evaluation of the activated sodium-24 in the blood indicated a neutron dose of 0.5 Gy. The mean marrow dose was essentially the same. A bone marrow transplant was contemplated, but no suitable donors were located. The patient was felt to be at high risk of lethality, but he ultimately recovered because of inhomogeneous dose distribution and surviving native marrow in his upper spine. The dose reconstruction indicated isodose curves of about 10 Gy (1000 rad at the pelvis) and 2 to 5 Gy in the chest. The percentage of bone marrow that received 2 to 3 Gy was estimated to be 16% and the mean bone marrow dose was estimated to be 5 Gy. Chromosome analysis revealed about 65 dicentrics/100 cells examined.

Initial treatment was directed to resolve hypotension and prevent infection. The patient was placed in a sterile room, fed sterilized food, and had his skin and orifices disinfected daily. The patient experienced a latent period for about 3 weeks. After about 3 weeks, the patient experienced oral *Candida albicans*, fevers, and bacteremia for about another 4 weeks. A radionecrotic lesion developed on his left foot.

The hematological picture indicated a rise in granulocytes to 16,500/µl in the first 24 h followed by a decline to 1000 by 9 days and 20 at 21 days. The lymphocytes decreased to 140 cells/µl by day 4 postexposure and remained near this level for the next 4 weeks. Platelets slowly decreased to 25,000/µl by day 20. Therapy included isolation, antibiotics, fluids and transfusions. Recovery began to occur in most blood elements by 35 days postexposure and was complete by 12 weeks. At 12 weeks, epilation of the head and complete azoospermia were still present.

The left foot was the most heavily irradiated since it was on the top of the reactor at the time of the accident. The estimated dose was 50 Gy with local skeletal doses of 25 to 40 Gy. There was intense erythema for the first 1 to 3 weeks. Pain became severe at 3 weeks postexposure with peeling of the skin. On week 6 the toenails fell off. A sympathectomy was done at 24 weeks postexposure because of unbearable pain. Amputation was carried out at 25 weeks postexposure at the level of the thigh where the dose was estimated to be 15 Gy. The patient was followed at the Curie Institute annually for 15 years and then about every 5 years. He had no long-term sequelae related to either the whole-body exposure or the amputation and he is still alive.

CHELYABINSK-70 (APRIL 1968)

The accident occurred on April 5, 1968 at the Russian Federal Nuclear Center (VNITF) located in the Southern Ural mountains between the cities of Ekaterinburg and Chelyabinsk. Criticality experiments began at VNITF in 1957 using an FKBN vertical lift assembly machine. FKBN is a Russian acronym for "a physics neutron pile." The FKBN assembly consisted of upper and lower reflectors and core. The core of the assembly consists of uranium spherical metal shell with an internal cavity with a polyethylene sphere inside. The upper and lower reflectors were the natural uranium. The accident occurred on a Friday evening after regular working hours. Two specialists decided to continue work to complete the assembly. Using a hand-held controller panel, the senior specialist operated an overhead tackle to lower the upper half of the reflector to make contact with the core (the operation of lowering the upper half of the reflector could not be carried out under remote control). The junior specialist stood next to the FKBN with both hands on the upper reflector to guide it into place. The accident occurred as the upper half of the reflector was being lowered onto the core and was about to make contact with it. The emergency instrument system was operating and responded after the power level of the excursion reached the kilowatt level. The system dropped the lower half of the reflector, which was sufficient to drive the system deeply subcritical and terminate the excursion.

The junior specialist received an accumulated neutron plus gamma dose in the 20–60 Gy range and about 700 Gy local dose in the left hand. The senior specialist received an accumulated neutron plus gamma dose of 5–10 Gy. Following the accident, both specialists were admitted to the local hospital and immediately evacuated to the specialized hospital in Moscow. The junior specialist died 55 hours after the accident. The senior specialist survived for 54 days after the accident.

MAYAK PRODUCTION FACILITY, RUSSIA (DECEMBER 1968)

This accident resulted from unfavorable geometry in a vessel containing plutonium-bearing organic liquids. There were two critical excursions about 1 h apart. A 20-l bottle was emptied into a 60-l vessel when the operator saw a flash of light and felt a pulse of heat. He immediately left the area and informed his supervisor. The excursion was estimated to have resulted in about 3×10^{16} fissions. An hour later a shift supervisor entered the area against instructions and attempted to manipulate the vessel when another excursion occurred. The second excursion yield was estimated at 1×10^{17} fissions.

Both men were flown to Moscow for medical treatment. Blood samples (adjusted to the time of exposure) showed 5000 decays/min/ml (83 Bq/cm^3) for the operator and 15,800 decays/min/ml (263 Bq/cm^3) for the shift supervisor. The total absorbed neutron and gamma doses were estimated to be 7 Sv for the operator and 24.5 for the shift supervisor. The shift supervisor had acute severe radiation sickness and he died about a month after the accident. The operator also had acute severe radiation sickness and survived but had to have amputations of both legs and one hand. He was still alive 31 years later.

KURCHATOV INSTITUTE, MOSCOW, RUSSIA (FEBRUARY 1971)

The accident occurred during an experiment to evaluate iron and beryllium reflectors for power reactors. The error occurred when the operators assumed that iron and beryllium would act similarly and that no additional calculations were needed. When water was added to the dry assembly (an untested change in procedure), there was a blue glow in the tank. Both the supervisor and the scientist received about 15 Sv to their feet.

KURCHATOV INSTITUTE, MOSCOW, RUSSIA (MAY 1971)

This accident occurred on May 26, 1971. Researchers were in the process of shutting down a structurally fragile reactor. This involved draining the assembly of water that was used as a moderator. Instead of a normal drain, the researchers were in a hurry and used a large emergency drain, which caused the bottom fuel rod support to buckle. The rods fell out of the upper support into a configuration, which resulted in a critical mass. There was a blue flash, the rods melted, and the configuration became subcritical.

A technician standing nearby was estimated to have received 60 Gy and he died the next day from a "heart attack." Most likely this was cardiovascular collapse as a result of the exposure. A second researcher was estimated to have received over 20 Gy and he died 2 weeks later. Another two researchers received estimated doses of 8 to 9 Gy and apparently were saved, but had unknown types of long-term health problems.

SIBERIAN CHEMICAL COMBINE, RUSSIA (DECEMBER 1978)

The accident occurred in a facility dealing with plutonium metal ingots. In violation of procedures, multiple metal ingots of about 11 kg (in excess of the administrative limit of 4 kg or less) were put into a glove box. Operator A saw a flash of light and noted an instantaneous rise in the temperature near his hands. As a result of thermal expansion, one ingot was expelled and the operator removed two more. The yield of the excursion was estimated to be 3×10^{15} fissions. The operator received an estimated whole-body dose of 2.5 Gy and more than 20 Gy to the hands and forearms. Ultimately, amputation up to the elbows was necessary. Later he developed cataracts. Seven other workers received doses from 0.05 to 0.50 Gy.

CONSTITUYENTE, ARGENTINA (SEPTEMBER 1983)

A criticality accident occurred on September 23, 1983 at the RA-2 facility of the Nuclear Research Center "Constituyente" in Buenos Aires Argentina. An operator was instructed to modify the configuration of the core of a light water reactor for pulsed neutron experiments. Apparently he was in a hurry and overconfident and violated at least three procedures. One of these was complete removal of the moderator and this was only partially done. A power excursion of approximately 3×10^{17} fissions took place over a few tens of milliseconds.

The operator was estimated to have received 23 Gy of gamma radiation and 17 Gy of neutron radiation. About 25 min after exposure he had nausea, vomiting, headache, and diarrhea. He died about 48 h later, at which time he had edema of the forearms and hands, neurological findings, and pulmonary edema.

Other exposed persons included two persons on the control room who received an estimated 0.20 Gy of gamma radiation and 0.15 Gy of neutron radiation, five persons who received 40 to 200 mGy of total gamma and neutron radiation and two persons who received about 10 mGy total dose.

SAROV (ARZIMAS-16) VNIIEF, RUSSIA (JUNE 1997)

This accident occurred in a copper-reflected 90% enriched uranium core assembly. The operator incorrectly transcribed the thickness of the reflector to be used and dropped the upper copper hemisphere onto the bottom assembly. When this happened, he saw a flash of light. He then left the area and reported the accident to the engineer and health physicist. The fission yield was estimated to be about 2×10^{17} in one burst and a total of 1×10^{19} fissions. The experimenter received an unusually high neutron/gamma ratio (about 15) with estimated doses of 45 Gy from neutrons and 3.5 Gy from gamma rays. Doses to the hands were estimated to be 200 to 300 Gy.

He was transported to Moscow. Initial medical therapy included antiemetic drugs (metoclopramide hydrochloride and atropine) as well as polyvidone 6%, glucose 5%, and prednisolone (90 mg). The initial hypotension was treated with phenylephrine (10 mg), which helped transiently. After that, the hypotension persisted in spite of dopamine (200 mg intravenously). He also received heparin (20,000 IU/day), Acyclovir (6 mg/8 h), ketoconazole (200 mg twice a day), and Ciproflloxin (250 mg twice a day). An antinecrotic drug, Aprotinine (1 M IU/day) was also administered.

Edema on the hands and forearms, as well as pain, was severe and by 24 h there was moist desquamation. Also at 24 h postexposure the chest radiograph indicated interstitial edema. At the end of the second day, there was marked hypotension and oliguria which was treated with furosemide, methylprednisolone (125 mg once), dexamethasone (8 mg/8 h), and increased fluid volume to 2800 ml on the second day compared with a urinary output of 1200 ml. Because of the life-threatening nature of the combined local and whole-body injuries, amputation of both arms at the mid-humeral level was performed on the third day. After this, there was continued hypotension in spite of treatment with dopamine (4 mg/h), albumin 20% (200 ml), sodium 4% (100 ml), and frozen plasma (1000 ml). The patient died 66 h postexposure.

In this case the approximate depth–dose distribution calculated at the anterior chest level was approximately as follows: 100% at 0 cm, 90% at 2 cm, 73% at 4 cm, 46% at 8 cm, 20% at 14 cm, and 12% at 20 cm. The air kerma was 100% at 0 cm, 86% at 2 cm, 65% at 4 cm, 35% at 8 cm, 11% at 14 cm, and 5% at 20 cm.

TOKAIMURA, JAPAN (SEPTEMBER 1999)

This accident is a sentinel event in medical management of radiation accidents. Exposures to two patients were very high. The technology, labor, and medical expertise brought to bear on the problems were extensive and state of the art. The patients ultimately died, but they were kept alive much longer than has been possible before and new problems were confronted. This accident is very similar to the Los Alamos III (1958) accident. In this case the workers were in contact with a tank of enriched uranium solution (rather than plutonium) when a critical excursion occurred.[10]

The accident occurred in Tokaimura, Ibaraki Prefecture on September 30, 1999 during preparation of fuel for the Joyo reactor. Three workers (designated Y, O, and S) dissolved 20% enriched uranium oxide powder in stainless steel buckets and poured the solution into a precipitation tank, which had unsafe geometry dimensions. The volume reached 40 l and criticality occurred. Patient O was standing on a platform beside the tank holding a funnel, while Patient S stood on a platform and poured the solution into the tank through the funnel. Patient Y was about 15 m away in another room.

There was a blue flash and an alarm sounded at 10:35 A.M. Patient S recalls feeling pain in the neck, chest, arms, and hands and had numbness in some fingers. Patients O and S left for a decontamination shower 20 m away. Patient O vomited several times within 5 to 25 min and lost consciousness for about 2 to 3 minutes. When he awoke, his level of consciousness was still low and he had amnesia for about 70 min.

An ambulance arrived at 10:46 A.M. and the patients were taken to a regional hospital at 11:49. During transport, Patient O vomited twice and had two episodes of diarrhea. Patient O was hypotensive and was treated with lactated Ringer's solution. All three patients were then transferred to the National Institute of Radiological Sciences Hospital in Chiba by 15:25 h. Upon arrival, Patient O had erythema of the arms, face, and trunk and complained of pain in the jaw and abdomen. His blood pressure recovered after injection of prednisolone. Diarrhea continued for 4 days. The dose, estimated by various methods, was lymphocyte decrease (16 to 18 Gy), sodium-24 in the blood (18.4 Gy), and cytogenetics (>20 Gy).

Patient S felt nausea within an hour and vomited several times in the ambulance. Upon arrival in Chiba his face was tender and swollen and there was salivary inflammation with elevated amylase levels. His dose was estimated by the same methods with the following results: lymphocyte decrease (6 to 10 Gy), sodium-24 in the blood (10.4 Gy), and cytogenetics (7.8 Gy). This patient never experienced diarrhea. Patient Y had slight nausea on the way to the hospital but never had vomiting or diarrhea. He did have transient hypoxemia. There was never any epilation. Patient Y had a estimated dose of 1 to 4.5 Gy. He had mild bone marrow depression that recovered and he was discharged on day 82 postexposure.

Treatment of Patients O, S, and Y during the first 3 days was directed at several issues. The patients were administered 250 ml of sodium bicarbonate for possible inhalation of radioactive uranium. To control the gastrointestinal syndrome and digestive tract decontamination the patients were given vancomycin, polymyxin B sulfate, and Fungison syrup (amphotericin B). There was stimulation of crypt cells by L-glutamine (50 g/day) and elementary diet. Electrolytes and fluid were balanced by routine intensive care and residual granulocytes were activated by administration of granulocyte colony–stimulating factor (G-CSF). Bone marrow failure was controlled by administration of G-CSF (200 to 500 µg/day) and administration of bone marrow stem cell transplants. Finally, vascular injury was controlled administration of the vasodilator pentoxifylline (900 mg/day orally).

Patient O was transferred to an isolation room at the University of Tokyo Hospital on day 3 postexposure as his urine volume and oxygen saturation both decreased. Cross-reactive protein and BUN levels were increased. During days 3 to 8 chest radiographs revealed edema and atelectasis. He also received Acyclovir (750 mg), gamma globulin (10 g every other day), Ambizome, FK506, and vancomycin. He received a peripheral bone marrow stem cell transplant from an HLA identical sister on day 7 to 8 postexposure. After the transplant he received steroids (predonisolone, 80 mg daily) and platelet transfusions. Beginning on day 23 he received cyclosporin A (140 to 200 mg/day). Renal insufficiency was a problem during weeks 2 to 4. On day 17 skin blisters appeared and both herpes and *Candida* were cultured. Diarrhea resumed on day 26 and liver function values became elevated. Later, there also was massive bleeding from the stomach, colon, and small bowel as a result of absent mucosa and bleeding telangectasias. Intra-arterial vasopressin reduced the bleeding but had to be stopped after a cardiac arrest on day 58. The patient was resuscitated, but he died from multiple organ failure on day 83 postexposure.

Patient S had an estimated average dose in the range of 8 Sv. He was transferred to the Hospital of the Medical Research Institute of the University of Tokyo on day 4 postexposure. There, as a result of having no HLA-identical donor available, he received a female fetal cord blood transplant of approximately 2.1×10^7 cells/kg, or a total of about 10^9 cells. To prevent graft-vs.-host disease he was given premedication with antithymocyte globulin (ATG) (2.5 mg/kg for 2 days) and subsequently received cyclosporin A (3 mg/kg/day) and prednisilone. He was also given rG-CSF (5 to 10 µg/kg) and erythropoeitin (EPO, 100 IU/kg) to stimulate cell lines and differentiation. He was also given thrombopoietin (TPO, 5 µg/kg) to promote platelet recovery during days 10 through 25. Radiation stomatitis appeared at day 10 postexposure and erythema and blistering of the hands and feet began on day 21. Epilation also occurred about the same time.

Bone marrow examination 9 days post-transplant showed a mixed chimerism with 41% XY and 57% XX chromosomes. By day 16 post-transplant the ratio was 66% XY and 34% XX. His own marrow eventually recovered and replaced the transplant. Various skin grafts were required. During the first several weeks post-transplant, it was very difficult to determine whether the clinical abnormalities were due to radiation effects, graft-vs.-host disease, or drug toxicity.

He had started to recover in January and February and was able to move about the hospital in a wheelchair. Through March and early April, he developed chronic, antibiotic-resistant pneumonia and severe radiation fibrosis of the skin/pneumonitis and required a respirator. He also had gastric bleeding. In April, he developed renal failure and required dialysis. As a result he was transferred to the University of Tokyo Hospital on April 10, 2000. He died on April 27, 2000 (211 days postexposure).

Shortly after the accident, radiation levels around the plant site were analyzed; at the plant boundary the level was about 100 mSv. In addition to the three heavily exposed workers there were about 90 people in the plant who received less than 50 mSv.

SUMMARY

There are a number of observations and lessons that can be gleaned from criticality accidents as follows:

- Location within 3 meters of a critical excursion has a high probability of fatality.
- The doses to persons close to an excursion are very inhomogeneous, and if the dose is survivable, there may still be a necessity to amputate limbs.
- Since the operators are usually facing the critical reaction, there are extremely high doses to the anterior abdomen, chest, and face (cutaneous syndrome).

Criticality Accidents

- The transient incapacitation syndrome with neurological findings due to hypotension has been seen in at least three accidents and has always been associated with fatal outcomes.
- Fever in the first few hours post-exposure is an ominous finding and usually is associated with fatality.
- The wide spectrum of radiation that results from a critical excursion makes dosimetry and clinical prognostication very difficult. There are fast and slow neutrons as well as soft and very penetrating gamma rays. Neutrons have differing abilities to cause different effects in the same tissue (Figure 11.6). For example, neutrons are about 2.5 times more effective per gray than gamma rays in causing erythema but are about four times more effective in terms of epidermolysis and late skin effects. Fast neutrons are more damaging to the germinal epithelium than to skin itself. Thus, in assessing dose, the RBE to be used for neutrons varies by tissue, effect, and dose rate. Often a value of 1.5 is used. In criticality accidents, if average doses exceed 10 Gy and the patient survives >2 months, extreme skin and subcutaneous fibrosis should be expected.
- Location more than 5 m from a critical excursion usually results in radiation doses that are survivable.
- At more than 50 m, doses usually do not exceed regulatory limits.

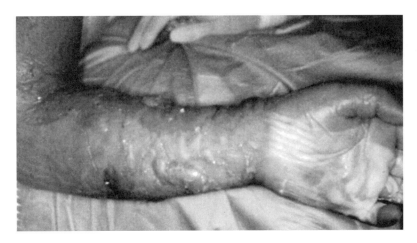

FIGURE 11.6 Blisters on the arm about 20 days postexposure in a patient in a recent accident.

REFERENCES

1. Brucer, M., The Acute Radiation Syndrome: A Medical Report on the Y-12 Accident, ORINS-25 Biology and Medicine, U.S. Atomic Energy Commission, April 1959.
2. Hemplemann, L.H., Lisco, H., and Hoffman, J.G., The acute radiation syndrome. A study of nine cases and a review of the problem, *Ann. Intern. Med.*, 36, 279, 1952.
3. Shipman, T.L., Acute radiation death resulting from an accidental nuclear excursion, *J. Occup. Med.*, 3(3), 146–191, 1961.
4. Bond, V.P., Fliedner, T.M., and Archambeau, J.O., *Mammalian Radiation Lethality*, Academic Press, New York, 1965.
5. Hempelmann, L.H., Lushbaugh, C.C., and Voelz, G.L., What happened to the survivors of the early Los Alamos nuclear accidents, in *The Medical Basis for Radiation Accident Preparedness*, Hubner, K.F. and Fry, S.A., Eds., Elsevier North Holland, New York, 1980, 19–32.
6. Jammet, H.P., Gongora, R., Le Go, R., Marble, G., and Faes, M., Observation clinique et traitment d'un cas d'irradiation globale accidentelle in *Proceedings of the First International Congress of Radiation Protection*, Rome, Italy, September 5–10, 1966, Pergamon Press, Oxford, 1968, 1249–1290.

7. Parmentier, N.C., Nénot, J.C., and Jammet, H.J., A dosimetric study of the Belgian (1965) and Italian (1975) accidents, in *The Medical Basis for Radiation Accident Preparednesss*, Hubner, K.F. and Fry, S.A., Eds., Elsevier North Holland, New York, 1980, 105–112.
8. Jammet, H.J., Gongora, R., Le Go, R., Doloy, M.T., Clinical and biological comparison of two acute accidental irradiations: Mol and Brescia, in *The Medical Basis for Radiation Accident Preparedness*, Hubner, K.F. and Fry, S.A., Eds., Elsevier North Holland, New York, 1980, 92–104.
9. Jammet, H.J., Gongora, R., Le Go, R., Marble, G., and Faes, M., Observation clinique et traitment d'un cas d'irradiation globale accidentalle, in *Proceedings of the First International Congress of Radiation Protection*, Pergamon Press, Oxford, 1968, 1249–1290.
10. Proceedings of the International Symposium on the Criticality Accident in Tokaimura, December 14–15, 2000, Chiba, Japan.

12 Medical Aspects of the Accident at Chernobyl

Angelina K. Guskova and Igor A. Gusev

CONTENTS

Introduction 195
Initial Accident Details 196
Expected Clinical Symptoms as a Function of Dose..198
Initial Medical Response 198
Acute Radiation Sickness 198
Therapy and Outcomes of Patients with ARS..201
Follow-Up of the ARS Survivors 203
Evaluation of People without ARS...205
Cancer after the Chernobyl Accident 206
Principles of Organizational Decisions 206
Chernobyl Accident Lessons 208
References...209

INTRODUCTION

The accident happened on April 26, 1986 in Unit 4 of a functional and active nuclear power plant at Chernobyl. The reactor core, cooling system, and building were destroyed in a steam explosion with a large radiation exposure occurring to plant personnel, recovery staff, and the public. Factors that influence the potential health effects in a nuclear power plant accident include the amount and type of environmental releases, either as an aerosol or as larger fragments of the reactor core. These releases result in external exposure by gamma and beta particles and to a lesser extent internal exposure from inhaled radionuclides. The radioactive materials that are emitted in the form of a cloud can be dispersed through a populated area resulting in short-term exposure of the public to the passing cloud, as well as short- and long-term internal exposure from inhaled and ingested radioactive materials.

The largest potential danger for both plant staff and members of the public results initially from external gamma exposure and radioisotope intake (particularly radioactive iodine and radioactive cesium isotopes). Both distance from the reactor and time since the accident play a role in exposure of the population. As the distance from the reactor increases, the external gamma and beta radiation dose rate usually decreases. Since the radioactive iodines are somewhat short-lived, their importance is usually only in the first days and months after exposure. Other fission products such as cesium, which are long-lived, contribute relatively more to dose as the time since the accident increases. Exposure of Chernobyl plant personnel to strontium and transuranic radionuclides occurred, but the absolute quantities were relatively low compared with other exposures.[1-4]

Population exposure is usually limited by sheltering, evacuation, and control of food substances. All these countermeasures were employed in the days and months after the accident. Control of the food pathways of meat and milk are particularly important and radiation dose to the thyroid is decreased by using stable iodine prophylaxis. This chapter will focus primarily on the victims with acute radiation sickness, but some details on long-term effects are also included.

INITIAL ACCIDENT DETAILS

The Chernobyl Nuclear Power Plant is situated in northwestern Ukraine on the bank of the Pripjat River, which discharges into the Dnieper River, and then flows past Kiev. At the beginning of 1986, the total number of people living within the 30-km radius zone of the nuclear power plant was about 100,000. This included 49,000 people living in the town Pripjat (situated 3 km to the west of the nuclear power plant) and 12,500 people living in the town of Chernobyl (15 km to the southeast of the nuclear power plant). The first two units of the reactor started their operation in 1977 and units three and four began operation in 1983. Two additional units were under construction at the time of the accident.

In 1986, the nuclear power plant was equipped with four boiling water reactors utilizing water as a coolant and graphite as a moderator (Soviet design RBMK-1000). These are heterogeneous channel reactors utilizing thermal neutrons and having uranium dioxide of poor enrichment as the fuel. Graphite is the moderator.

The accident happened as a result of a violation of safety standards when experimental research was being done on the night of April 26 to 27, 1986. The experiment caused a large, sudden fluctuation of power over a period of milliseconds with a marked elevation in temperature and steam explosions, resulting in the destruction of the reactor. Containment was breached, allowing significant environmental release of radionuclides. The release had four phases. During phase I, there was release of reactor fuel with radioactive iodine, tellurium, cesium, and radioactive noble gases. During phase II (April 26 to May 2), the rate of environmental release decreased; however, a fire in the graphite allowed releases similar in radionuclide content to that of reactor fuel. Measures had been taken during this time to extinguish the graphite fire. In phase III (May 2 to May 6) there was an increase in the release rate of uranium fission products similar to that released initially. During phase IV (after May 6), there was a rapid decrease in the release rate. The total environmental release of fission products was about $3^1/_2$% of the total amount of radionuclides present inside the reactor at the time of the accident. The total activity of released radionuclides is estimated to be about 1850 PBq (radioactive noble gases excluded).

On April 27, the altitude of the released cloud exceeded 1200 m with maximum radionuclide concentration observed at about 600 m. Volatile radionuclides of iodine and cesium were measured as high as 6 to 9 km. Fallout beyond the U.S.S.R. occurred and was measured in Sweden on April 27. Over the next 10 days, the meteorological and wind conditions changed altitudes and directions many times. The fallout pattern became very complex and Western European countries registered contamination on April 29 and 30. In the beginning of May, there were reports of elevated radioactivity from Israel, Kuwait, and Turkey, from Japan on May 2, from China on May 4, and from the United Stated and Canada on May 5 and 6.

Based upon radiation monitoring data, inhabitants of the town of Pripjat were evacuated on April 27, and after this there were further evacuations from regions north of Kiev, in Gomel, Bryansk, and Zhitomir. Approximately 115,000 people were evacuated. No acute radiation injuries were found among the evacuated people. The total committed collective effective dose resulting from the Chernobyl accident is estimated to be approximately 600,000 man-Sv, where the percentage of this dose is as follows: 53% European countries, 36% republics of the former U.S.S.R., 8% Asia, 2% Africa, 3% Northern Central and South America.[5,6] The local and regional cesium-137 deposition covered vast areas in a heterogenous pattern (Figures 12.1 and 12.2).

Medical Aspects of the Accident at Chernobyl

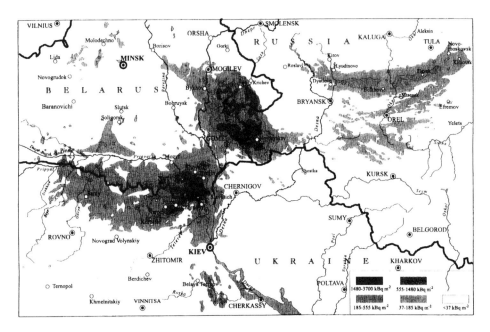

FIGURE 12.1 Map of cesium-137 deposition across the Ukraine, Belarus, and Russia. Note the very heterogeneous fallout pattern over vast distances. The distance from Chernobyl to Kiev is about 120 km, Gomel 150 km, Minsk 350 km, and to the fallout near Tula over 500 km. (From UNSCEAR 2000 report.)

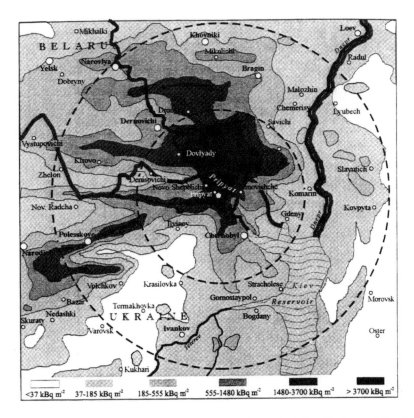

FIGURE 12.2 Ground cesium deposition locally around the Chernobyl site. Circles are 30 and 60 km from the plant. (From UNSCEAR 2000 report.)

EXPECTED CLINICAL SYMPTOMS AS A FUNCTION OF DOSE

Initial evaluation is done based on the clinical manifestations of external gamma exposure. Symptoms begin to occur with whole-body acute doses of around 1 Gy.[7] At doses in excess of 1 Gy to 5 Gy, there is cytopenia, which is particularly manifest in peripheral lymphocytes as well as neutrophils (granulocytes) and platelets (thrombocytes). The higher the dose, the more severe is the cytopenia. High doses also result in thrombocytopenia. Even with advanced medical treatment, fatalities almost always occur at dose levels in excess of 10 to 12 Gy acute whole-body dose, and they are common at doses in excess of 5 to 6 Gy. In addition to gamma exposure, there was large beta exposure and many workers had a significant portion of the body surface irradiated in this manner. There were a number of fatalities as a result of beta exposure from several tens to hundreds of gray.

The threshold for acute effects from such radionuclides as cesium-134 and cesium-137 is also 1 Gy since they are relatively uniformly distributed inside the body and have high-energy gamma rays. Approximately 111 to 148 MBq (3 to 4 mCi) of these radionuclides are sufficient to cause bone marrow aplasia if there is an internal dose rate of 0.1 to 0.2 Gy/day.[8] Effects on the thyroid as a result of radioiodine exposure also should be expected. If the thyroid dose is in the range of 200 to 300 Gy, there is destruction of thyroid parenchyma with transient hyperthyroidism. This usually results from acute single intakes of 370 to 740 MBq (10 to 20 mCi) of iodine-131. At later times and at lower doses, hypothyroidism may become evident, usually occurring at 1 to 5 years. In the case of children, thyroid dose per unit intake of radioiodine can be three times more than in adults, depending on the child's age and diet.

Doses resulting from radionuclide inhalation may cause acute damage of the bronchi and pulmonary system, but the threshold dose to cause these effects has not been satisfactorily evaluated. It is clear, however, that with external low-LET (linear energy transfer) gamma radiation, acute doses in the range of 20 to 30 Gy and higher results in radiation pneumonitis approximately 1 to 3 months postexposure.[8] The threshold of acute damage of the nasal mucosa and nasopharynx mucosa (oropharyngeal syndrome, acute rhinotracheitis) is close to the same value.[9]

INITIAL MEDICAL RESPONSE

During the first several hours after the accident, a number staff members and firemen were admitted to the local hospital with a diagnosis of possible radiation injury. Emergency dosimetry was virtually nonexistent. Based on expected radiation effects, there appeared to be about 150 victims identified within 4.5 h after the explosion who would probably need advanced treatment at the Radiation Medicine Department at the Institute of Biophysics in Moscow (Figure 12.3). The time of evaluation, transportation of victims to Kiev and Moscow, and additional measures taken are presented in Table 12.1.

ACUTE RADIATION SICKNESS

The possible diagnosis of acute radiation sickness was initially entertained for 237 persons. Of this group, 115 patients were transported to the Radiation Medicine Department of the Institute of Biophysics. Within several days, the acute radiation syndrome (ARS) was verified in 104 of these persons. An additional 30 patients were also verified to have ARS when considered retrospectively, for a total of 134.[10–13] The doses and outcomes of these patients are shown in Table 12.2.

Analysis during the first 2 days was also performed to ascertain the degree of radioactive contamination of the skin and potential levels of internal radionuclides, including radioiodine and radiocesium. These evaluations were carried out on 75% of all patients. The majority of patients did not show radionuclide body burdens above 1.5 to 2.0 MBq (40 to 50 mCi); 6% of patients had internal burdens approximately two to four times higher than this. Patients were also analyzed for the presence of sodium-24, to ascertain the potential magnitude of neutron exposure. Ultimately,

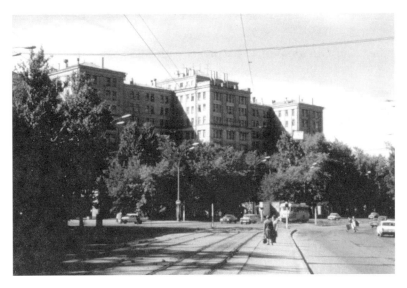

FIGURE 12.3 Hospital 6, of the Institute of Biophysics, where 108 of the 134 patients with ARS were treated.

TABLE 12.1
Dynamics of Information Exchange; Basic Organizational Decisions at Different Times

	Time after the Accident
1. Information is provided to the Radiation Medicine Department from the Ministry of Health and from local medical facilities	$2^1/_2$–$4^1/_2$ h
2. Decision is taken for complete hospitalization of people and the emergency team is called; information is provided to Hospital 6 as support organization	$4^1/_2$–6 h
3. Hospital 6 is ready for patient admission; emergency team is sent to the place of accident	6–30 h 9–15 h
Basic Phases of Medical Assistance Organization **(At Specific Times after the Chernobyl Accident)**	
4. Admission of patients to clinic	30–38 h
5. Establishment of dosimetry checkpoints and structural adjustments	2–6 days
6. Diagnosis and therapy of patients, training of temporary staff, providing of information to different organizations	2–90 days
Reporting of Data and Analysis	
7. Preparation of clinical section of the report to international organizations; report at WHO-IAEA-UNSCEAR meeting (Vienna, 1986)	90–120 days
8. Clinical pathology analysis of fatality structure; additional analysis of accidental situation materials vs. clinical experience; informing of international community; publications	1–12 years

neutron exposure played a very small part in the accident. Data on internal exposure are presented in Table 12.3.

Serial blood counts during the first 3 days were obtained for analysis of a number of factors, but particularly for the presence and severity of lymphopenia. This was of the greatest medical prognostic value when combined with the time of occurrence of symptomatology such as nausea, vomiting, and diarrhea.[14] Cytogenic dosimetry was also obtained from blood samples. During the

TABLE 12.2
Doses, Number, and Outcome of 134 Patients with ARS

Degree of ARS	Dose Range (Gy)	No. of Patients	No. of Short-Term Deaths	No. of Survivors
Mild (I)	0.8–2.1	41	0 (0%)	41
Moderate (II)	2.2–4.1	50	1 (2%)	49
Severe (III)	4.2–6.4	22	7 (32%)	15
Very severe (IV)	6.5–16	21	20 (95%)	1
Total	0.8–16	134	28	106

TABLE 12.3
Doses External and Internal Exposure of Lungs and Thyroid of 23 Patients Who Died at Early Times after the Chernobyl Accident[a]

Personal Code	Absorbed Dose (a) (mGy)		External Exposure Dose (Gy)
	Thyroid	Lungs	
25	21	0.26	8.2
18	24	2.8	6.4
22	54	0.47	4.3
5	62	0.57	6.2
9	71	0.77	5.6
21	77	0.68	6.4
8	130	1.5	3.8
2	130	2.2	2.9
19	210	3.5	4.5
23	310	2.3	7.5
1	340	8.7	11.1
15	320	27	6.4
16	470	4.1	4.2
3	540	6.8	7.2
17	600	120	5.5
4	640	34	6.5
7	780	4.7	10.2
10	890	9.4	8.6
11	740	29	9.1
14	950	20	7.2
20	1900	19	5.6
24	2200	21	3.5
13	4100	40	4.2

[a] Internal doses are accumulated to the moment of death and doses of external exposure are evaluated using chromosomal analysis of peripheral blood lymphocytes.

first 7 to 10 days, the depth and persistence of bone marrow depression became more evident, as well as the presence or absence of gastrointestinal symptoms. Less informative and more difficult to evaluate for prognostic determination was the radiation damage as a result of beta dermatitis and epithelial damage of the upper digestive and pulmonary tracts.

Bone marrow allogenic transplantation was considered based upon the clinical and laboratory data. Indications for patient selection were developed. These criteria were later found to be too broad. Allogenic bone marrow transplantation was performed on 13 patients, and implantation of human fetal liver cells was performed in six additional patients as a result of the absence of appropriate donors.[15]

All expected major clinical symptoms of ARS and their combinations were observed in personnel involved in the accidents, who had total-body gamma exposures of more than 1 Gy. As mentioned earlier, bone marrow depression was seen in 134 patients with ARS. The gastrointestinal syndrome was observed in 15 patients and radiation pneumonitis was detected in 8 patients. Combinations of these syndromes with severe widespread beta dermatitis occurred in 19 patients (Figure 12.4).[16] Skin doses exceeded bone marrow doses by a factor of 10 to 30 in some patients, and in these patients some had estimated skin doses in the range of 400 to 500 Gy. This local radiation damage to the skin resulted in significant aggravation of existing pulmonary and hepatic or renal abnormalities. Beta burns were the primary cause of death in a number of patients and significantly increased the severity of ARS. When skin injury exceeded 50% of the body surface area, this was a major contributing cause to morbidity and mortality.

In the early period (14 to 23 days postexposure, 15 patients died of skin or intestinal complications and 2 patients died of pneumonitis. In the period 24 to 48 days after exposure, there were 6 deaths from skin or lung injury and 2 from secondary infections following bone marrow transplantation. A patient who had severe ARS developed acute diffuse interstitial pneumonia with rapid development of hypoxemia, incompatible with life. Bacterial and fungal pneumonia was not confirmed at autopsy, and it appeared that there was acute radiation pneumonitis with possible cytomegalovirus being present. Two deaths at relatively late periods (days 86 to 96) were related to infectious complications of local radiation injury of the skin and renal insufficiency. One female patient died at 112 days from brain hemorrhage. Underlying bone marrow failure was the major contributor to all the deaths during the first 2 months.

In addition to utilizing blood counts as an assessment of dose, lymphocytes were also cultured. The exact dose the patient received was difficult to assess since estimates based on clinical symptomatology, marrow depression, and cytogenetics often yielded somewhat different values. Patients ultimately were followed with biochemical and hematological indices twice a day if they had acute radiation syndrome grade I to II and daily evaluation in the more severe patients. These serial counts were very important for the selection of supportive therapy as well as assessment of the effectiveness. Bacteriological tests were also important for effective organization of antibiotic or antifungal therapy. In the absence of signs of active healing of the skin at days 50 to 60, a number of patients received surgery with grafting. Leg amputation was performed on one patient more than 200 days after the accident.[15–17]

THERAPY AND OUTCOMES OF PATIENTS WITH ARS

Basic components of ARS therapy included:

- Prophylaxis and therapy of infectious complications;
- Detoxification;
- Parenteral nutrition;
- Transfusion therapy (allogenic transplantation of bone marrow and human hepatic fetal cell infusion);
- Topical therapy of damaged skin areas;
- Correction of secondary toxic metabolic disturbances.

All ARS patients who had grade II or higher ARS were placed in single rooms, adjusted for aseptic regimen. This was done by air sterilization utilizing ultraviolet lamps and thorough hand washing by the medical staff as well as obligatory use of lab coats, masks, and an aseptic solution

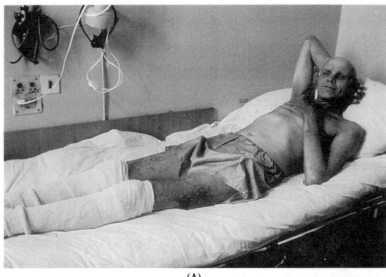

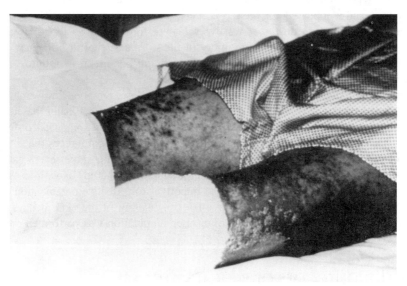

FIGURE 12.4 (A) Chernobyl worker with ARS. Note epilation and beta burns on the legs. (B) Closeup view of the beta burns.

for washing of shoes. Patients' clothes were changed daily. Microbial contamination indices were periodically monitored. Air microorganism concentration of below 500 colonies/m^3 was maintained.

All patients with grade II or higher ARS received prophylaxis against endogenous infections utilizing biseptol and nystatin when fever occurred. Patient received intravenously administered broad-spectrum antibiotics including aminoglycosides (Gentamicin, Amicacin), cephalosporins (Kefzol, Cefamizin, Cefobid), and hemisynthetic penicillins (Carbenicillin, Pipracil). In more than half the cases, this usually terminated fever. If the fever was not gone within 24 to 48 h, the patients received intravenous injection of gamma globulin (Sandoglobulin) given with four to five injections of 6 g each every 12 h. Acyclovir was widely and successfully applied for herpes infections for the first time in patients with acute ARS. About one third of patients manifested herpes on the face, lips, and oral mucosa.

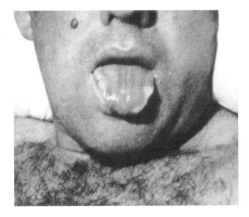

Chapter 11, Color Figure 1
Mucositis of the tongue and lips 12 days postexposure in a patient who was fatally involved in a criticality accident.

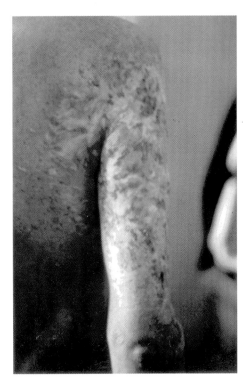

Chapter 12, Color Figure 1
Healed beta burns of the shoulder in a Chernobyl ARS (Grade III) survivor 5 years postexposure.

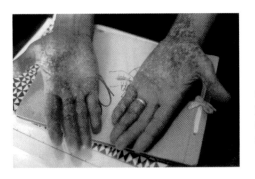

Chapter 12, Color Figure 2
Healed beta burns of the hands with multiple telangiectasias in the same patient.

Chapter 17, Color Figure 1
Patient who placed an industrial radiography source in the back pocket of his pants. Four days postexposure, there is a 4 x 4 cm blister and surrounding erythema and swelling.

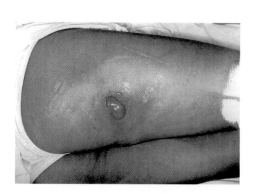

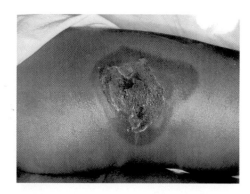

Chapter 17, Color Figure 2
The same patient 10 days postexposure.

Chapter 17, Color Figure 3
The same patient 29 days postexposure at which time there is a 2 cm deep and 10 x 10 cm ulceration.

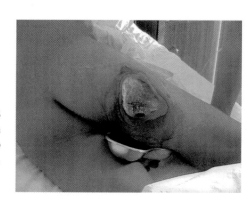

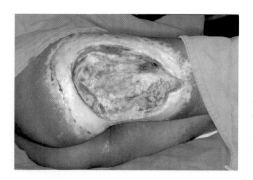

Chapter 17, Color Figure 4
The same patient 73 days postexposure. There is massive ulceration, necrosis, and infection. Amputation was ultimately required.

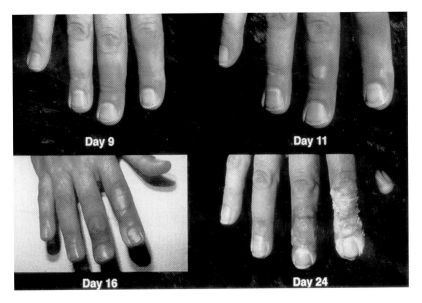

Chapter 18, Color Figure 1
The left fingers of a patient involved in an X-ray diffraction machine accident at a university chemistry department. Days 9–24.

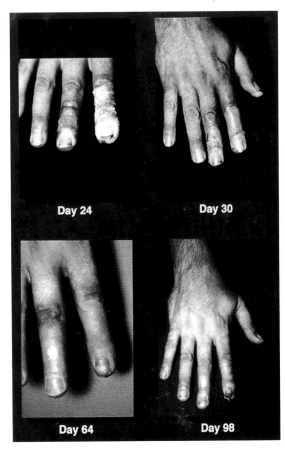

Chapter 18, Color Figure 2
Same patient. Days 24–98.

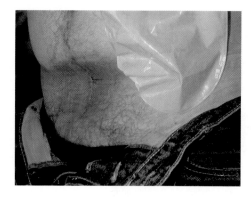

Chapter 21, Color Figure 1
Anterior lower abdomen of a patient overexposed in a radiotherapy accident. There is marked contraction, induration, and erythematous fibrosis. The patient has a colonostomy bag present after suffering from intestinal complication due to overexposure.

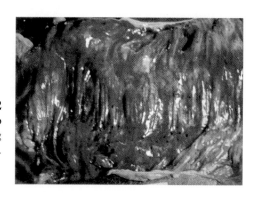

Chapter 21, Color Figure 2
Hemorrhagic intestine from a patient who died of intestinal complications following radiotherapy overexposure.

Chapter 22, Color Figure 1
Necrotic ulcer over the back in a patient who had been overexposed during cardiac catheterization and cardiac angioplasty procedure. Approximately 11 months postexposure.

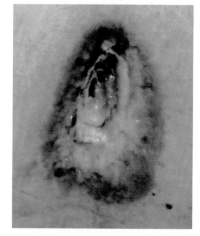

Chapter 22, Color Figure 2
Closeup of the lesion in the same patient.

Many of the patients received multiple transfusions with fresh donor thrombocytes. The efficacy of these transfusions was confirmed, not only by the absence of life-threatening bleeding in patients with prolonged (more than 2 to 4 weeks) of thrombocytopenia (below 5000 to 10,000/μl), but also by the absence of any visible signs of increased bleeding in the majority of the patients. On the average, three to five thrombocyte transfusions per patient were necessary for successful therapy of grade III ARS.

Red cell transfusions were not necessary for therapy of agranulocytic infectious complications. Red cell transfusions were needed in a number of patients with grade II to III ARS who also had significant injury. Evaluation of myelodepression and potential need for additional measures was done according to the scheme previously elaborated by Baranov and others.[10-12] Additional data from the blood lymphocytes indicating a dose over 6 Gy also was utilized. Bone marrow sampling was done from both patient relatives who were identical (six cases), HLA haploidentical (four cases), or haploidentical plus one common antigen in second haplotype (three cases). Typing was only done for A, B, and C loci because of the urgency of the situation. The cases of haploidentical bone marrow transplantation were done with elimination of T lymphocytes.

Application of allogenic bone marrow transplantation in these radiation accident victims has demonstrated that:

- In radiation accidents, the percentage of victims having the absolute indication for allogenic bone marrow transplantation and who can get a definite benefit from such transplantation is very small.
- In the case of bone marrow damage resulting from total-body gamma exposure of 6 to 8 Gy, transplant survival is possible; however, the transplantation may be life-threatening because of secondary disease development and graft-vs.-host disease.
- Recovery of myelopoiesis and survival is possible following whole-body exposures of 6 to 8 Gy, and this was found after rejection of HLA haploidentical transplant (three cases) as well as in patients who were not transplanted due to absence of an appropriate donor (four cases).

All patients who had severe multiple organ damage were treated by modern detoxification techniques, anti-infectious and symptomatic therapies. Hemoabsorption, plasma absorption, and plasmapheresis were applied. Direct anticoagulation (heparin) was used, as well, as a means to improve microcirculation (Repoliglukin, Neogemodez, Troxevasin, Trental, Solcoseril). The major feature of intestinal syndrome therapy was total parental nutrition with correction of volume deficiency with nutritive liquids and electrolytes. This therapy had high efficiency.

Each patient who had bone marrow syndrome, grade III to IV, usually also had radiation skin damage and required 24-h nursing provided by highly qualified personnel. Therapy effectiveness was judged as satisfactory since there were no fatalities in the ARS grade II (2 to 4 Gy doses), excluding the one female patient who died from brain hemorrhage in the late term. There were 27 patients in the clinic who had ARS grade III to IV. The fatal outcomes in this group basically resulted from acute severe cutaneous injuries, from lung damage, and from a combination of skin and intestinal damage combined with a bone marrow depression. Three deaths were felt to occur unnecessarily as a result of inappropriate bone marrow transplantation. Bone marrow transplantation in patients with doses below 9 Gy only worsened the ARS therapy results, due to the development of side effects.

FOLLOW-UP OF THE ARS SURVIVORS

Within the first 5 years after the accident, ARS survivors were observed in only one medical center. Subsequently, the ARS survivors have been observed near their place of residence, usually by the

Ukrainian Center for Radiation Medicine,[17] and only 13 survivors with the highest severity of acute damage have been followed at the Institute of Biophysics (Figure 12.5). At least 17 of the survivors have developed radiation cataracts. All of these patients (excluding one) had gamma radiation doses over 2 Gy. The cataracts formed 3 to 8 years postexposure. Surgery with artificial lens implantation was effective and noncomplicated. In addition to the cataracts, the major consequence is management of severe local skin radiation injuries (eight patients, see Color Figures 1 and 2*). Of the 20 survivors with various degrees of cutaneous injuries that were treated in Germany; many of those with cutaneous fibrosis have been treated with low-dose interferon. Results of this treatment are mixed. Three other survivors developed oncological diseases.

Within 12 years after the accident, 13 additional ARS survivors of grade I to II have died from different causes. These are shown in Table 12.4 with the exception of two who died in 1999–2000. Clarification of their deaths is incomplete, because in some cases an autopsy was not performed. Some authors have referred to the "significant rate" of hypertension, ischemic disease, and atherosclerosis found in ARS survivors and in the Chernobyl accident recovery workers. These authors usually ignore the aging of the population and increases in disease incidence with age. In fact, there has been a similar rate of increase in these diseases in persons with lower doses who did not develop ARS.

Sexual behavior and fertility among ARS survivors was investigated up until 1996. In the majority of cases, functional sexual disturbances predominated, but fertility has recovered in persons who planned to have children; 14 normal children were born to ARS survivor families within the first 5 years of the accident.

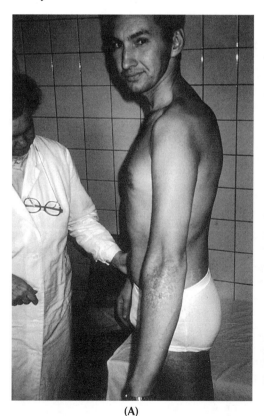
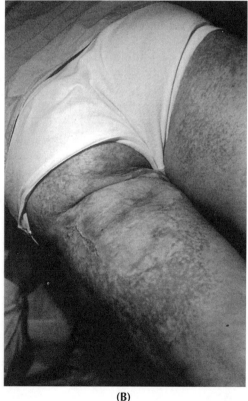

(A) (B)

FIGURE 12.5 (A) Survivor of ARS 5 years later. The subject has fathered normal children and has had eye surgery for cataracts. Note healed beta burn on elbow. (B) Healed beta burn of the posterior left thigh in the same subject.

---

* Color figures follow page 202.

TABLE 12.4
Late Lethality of Chernobyl ARS Survivors (1987 to 1998)

Patient Code	Name Abbreviation	ARS Severity Grade	Year of Death	Cause of Death	Age at Death (Years)
2024	VMJa	II	1987	Lung gangrene	80
1123	KjaF	II	1990	Ischemic cardiac disease	68
1087	VMP	III	1992	Ischemic cardiac disease	66
1083	PVO	I	1993	Ischemic cardiac disease	42
1068	BGV	III	1993	Myelodysplastic syndrome	52
	VOE	I	1995	Lung Tbc	
1096	BVI	II	1995	Liver cirrhosis	46
1048	KAP	I	1995	Fatty embolism	62
1042	DAO	II	1996	Myelodysplastic syndrome	64
1037	ShIP	II	1998	Myelomonoblastic acute leukemia	36
1101	GMU	II	1998	Liver cirrhosis	45

Source: Kovalenko, O.M., Ed., *Acute Radiation Sickness (Medical Consequences of Chernobyl Disaster)*, Kiev, 1998, 137 (in Ukrainian).

Patients with grade III to IV ARS were initially severely immunocompromised. While hematopoietic recovery in the survivors occurred within a matter of weeks, or at most months, future reconstitution of functional immunity may take at least half a year and may not be normal for several years. Studies of the immune status have revealed abnormalities in T-cell immunity for patients who received high doses of radiation. These abnormalities, however, have not been clearly associated with clinically manifest immunodeficiency.

EVALUATION OF PEOPLE WITHOUT ARS

Evaluation and characterization of people who did not develop ARS but who may have had doses up to 1 Gy represent a serious difficulty, both initially and at later phases of accident management. Recovery operations at Chernobyl have involved several hundred thousands of people, and significant radionuclide fallout (area of strict control) was observed in areas where there were approximately 272,000 people residing.

For purposes of characterization, these subjects are often divided into patients with ARS and others who were exposed during the so-called "iodine period" (April to June of 1986, group 1). Group 2 usually refers to those recovery workers engaged in work at or near the plant during 1986 and 1987. For these workers, there is incompletely recorded gamma radiation dose information. The majority of recovery workers appear to have received between 0.1 and 0.25 Gy. Subsequent assessment of the early health changes in these two groups has been very contradictory. Some authors[17] correlate every identified subclinical change to the effects of accidental exposure, and then make a monofactorial analysis and ignore other causes. They occasionally see some dose dependence but usually over a very narrow dose range and not over the wider dose range experienced by the workers.[15]

Based upon the vast experience in the observation of large group of radiation workers, when these data are examined, it is necessary to analyze the potential sources of error. Most scientific reviews of these studies have revealed aggravation of preexisting diseases, psychosomatic, or emotional changes. In both groups 1 and 2, there may be an increased risk of cancer, although, with the exception of childhood thyroid cancer, this is unlikely to occur within 10 years postexposure. At 2 years postexposure and subsequently, there may have been an increased risk of leukemia, although this has not yet been found.

Psychological effects have occurred in the exposed population. These psychological reactions are not directly related to ionizing radiation but rather social factors surrounding the accident. The accident did cause long-term changes in the lives of people living in contaminated districts as a result of resettlement, changes in food supplies, and restrictions upon individual and family activities. Individuals and families often had to make difficult decisions about relocation, and people did not trust scientific, medical, and political authorities.

Recovery workers who worked in 1988 and the following years (group 3) actually form a good control group for comparison with groups 1 and 2, particularly with regard to radiation effects. By 1988, the specific features of work at the power plant site included better organization and improved dosimetry monitoring. Even in this group, however, legislation that rewards disability forces people to "find and to aggravate diseases." As a result of this, there can be development of pathological personalities and, if obvious disease causes are absent, rehabilitation measures are usually ineffective.

Group 4 is composed of the population of the regions where relocation from contaminated areas was delayed and the people did not receive adequate recommendations regarding contamination in the food chain, appropriate precautions, or iodine prophylaxis. Since relocation, these people often have suffered adaptation problems. People in this group often have children who are at high risk for thyroid cancer. This issue is discussed more later in this chapter. Due to relatively small effective doses (usually less than 100 mSv), only large epidemiological studies will have the statistical power to evaluate possible radiation effects. Unfortunately, the prevalence, frequency, and changes of disorders in this large population vary so much that small radiation effects might be obscured.

The last group (group 5) are persons who have the minimal level of radiation exposure as a result of the accident and essentially have always lived in "clean" areas. Differences between this latter group and the general public are the result of social and economic complications. This may be the result of mass media claims and legislation, which provides compensation for ill-defined or nonradiation-related diseases and findings.[18,19]

CANCER AFTER THE CHERNOBYL ACCIDENT

The Chernobyl accident released a large amount of iodine-131, as well as other short-lived radio-iodines. Over the last decade, there has been a marked increase in the number of thyroid cancers among children and adolescents.[20–22] Among those less than 18 years of age at the time of the accident, over 1400 cases of thyroid cancer were diagnosed between 1990 and 1997. The total number of thyroid cancer cases in the different republics by year of diagnosis is shown in Figure 12.6. A corresponding increase in thyroid cancer among those exposed as adults has not been identified. The number of childhood cases began to increase in 1990, four 4^1/$_2$ years after the accident. Most of the cases occurred in the severely contaminated portions of the three affected republics. Approximately 40 to 70% of the cases have been found through screening programs, and the majority of the remaining cases have been detected either by parents or through standard physical examinations.

The risk of leukemia has been shown in other epidemiological studies to be increased by radiation exposure. However, as of 1999, no increased risk of leukemia linked to ionizing radiation has been described in children, recovery workers, or in the general population as a result of exposure from the Chernobyl accident.[23–26]

PRINCIPLES OF ORGANIZATIONAL DECISIONS

The unique experience of the large-scale accident at the Chernobyl Nuclear Power Plant was initially reported in August 1986 by Legasov, Ilyin, and Guskova. One can not only analyze the lessons of this experience, but also make some recommendations on the organizational decisions for future accidents of this type. Organizational decisions for such situations require clear coordination of

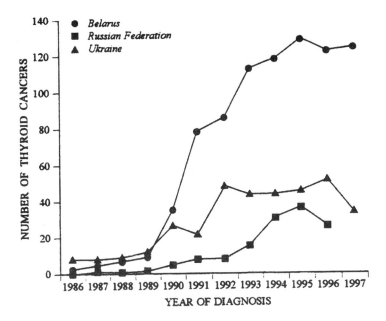

FIGURE 12.6 Increase in thyroid cancer cases since the accident.

the actions of the nuclear power plant personnel, all regional authorities, the medical staff, and the local population. The character of these decisions is determined by the potential radiation doses due to the radioactive sources as well as by the clinical signs that are expressed. Prognoses should be formed for separate groups of people, for example, the nuclear power plant staff and critical population groups, such as children and pregnant women.

From the first moment, it is urgent to gain an approximate understanding of dose levels, which can result in development of typical deterministic radiation effects. Decisions to keep dose levels below 1 Gy and to avoid acute deterministic effects is an essential principle that should be noted by nuclear power plant personnel and responsible authorities. Dose levels below 1 Gy usually will not require special therapy, although iodine prophylaxis may be considered. Triage of those who have received more than 1 Gy should be the focus of urgent measures and is important for proper utilization of medical resources. Systemic radiation monitoring is carried out at all nuclear power plants, and with this information, it should be possible to make a rapid assessment of the quantity and structure of radioactive environmental releases. This also gives information on approximate localization and scale. Utilizing this to forecast levels of internal and external exposure and geographic mapping of predicted levels allows evaluation of possible health effects in different groups.

The stages of information accumulation and utilization with particular reference to medical purposes in the case of a reactor accident can be conceptualized in the following time frames. Phase I covers the initial period of 2 days. During this time, urgent measures are required to deal with life-threatening trauma and gamma dose rate levels requiring immediate removal of people from dangerous areas. During this time, it should be clear to various authorities that the major part of the radiation dose to patients and population can be accumulated within a very short time period (hours to days). Typically, values of external and internal exposure have been specified in most countries to provide protection and are below the doses that result in early damage or ARS. Measures considered during this time period include (1) evacuation, (2) sheltering, (3) limitation of contaminated foodstuff, particularly milk for children, (4) administration of stable iodine, and (5) potential administration of methods to accelerate excretion of internal radionuclides and removal of surface and skin contamination. Discussion of decisions regarding evacuation is presented in Chapter 32. Evacuation decisions also need to take into account nonradiation circumstances, such as availability of transportation, distance to place of resettlement, number of people to be evacuated, etc.

Medical needs during the first phase also include changing of clothes for power plant personnel, showering and provision of emergency aid, medical examination to include blood counts, assessment of initial clinical symptoms, and findings and determination of those patients who need urgent admission to a hospital, particularly with grades ARS II to IV or severe local radiation injuries.

Phase II covers the days 2 to 7. During this time, there is clarification of the different radiation sources, and levels of therapy and prophylaxis, particularly by evaluation of blood counts and lymphocytopenia. The presence of neutron activation products in blood should be done to exclude accidental neutron exposures. Measurements of internal contamination, particularly the thyroid, can also be performed during this time. Evaluation of fallout and changes needed in the food chain in terms of restriction and distribution also need to be established. In general, indications for hospital admission during the first week of an accident include those who have an estimated whole-body gamma dose of more than 1 Gy.

Phase III is an intermediate phase between the accident and normal situation, and the duration of this phase depends on the scale of the accident. During this time, therapy will be carried out according to the expected health effects in the different groups of people. Determination is made of what outpatient surveillance and future therapy will be required for the beginning stages of rehabilitation of ARS survivors. The mid- to long-term risks of ARS survivors are based on both whole-body and organ dose, and both of these should be recorded. Utilizing standard risk factors published in the literature, estimates can be made of the future incidence of neoplasms and what particular plan, if any, needs to be adopted in this regard. Taking into account the spontaneous morbidity level for such diseases, it is unlikely that whole-body radiation doses of less than 0.5 Gy will change the natural rate by more than 1%. Special population groups such as those children who have thyroid cancer will require special medical programs.

CHERNOBYL ACCIDENT LESSONS

There have been a number of lessons learned from the Chernobyl accident and several unique features, as follows:[27]

1. There was a massive source of relatively uniform gamma radiation and a heterogeneous source of beta radiation resulting in 134 cases of ARS and 28 acute and subacute radiation deaths. This one accident accounts for about 40 to 45% of all accidental cases of ARS.
2. The ratio of persons involved to those significantly exposed and to those with major injury was about 1000:100:1.
3. Basic clinical manifestations included ARS of various grades that in many patients was aggravated by widespread beta radiation dermatitis requiring specialized skin care.
4. Bone marrow transplants were of very limited use. In two or three patients transplantation complications were felt to be the cause of death. Those who received bone marrow transplants and survived had very heterogeneous doses and recovered their own marrow.
5. There was a dramatic increase in the incidence in thyroid cancer among those who were very young or *in utero* at the time of exposure. There has been no demonstrated increase in either leukemia or thyroid cancer among adults.
6. The accident caused important unfavorable global and local social, economic, and psychological effects. These, as well as radiation exposure, influenced the perception of risk and health consequences.
7. Information was provided to the victims in a better way than it was presented to their relatives and to the world community.
8. National legislation regarding compensation was adopted by the former U.S.S.R. that is in conflict with the actual medical and scientific findings. This has complicated the social and psychological issues by discrediting the medical efforts.

The Chernobyl accident has also highlighted the need for international cooperation both in assessment and in management of large-scale radiation accidents.

REFERENCES

1. *Manual for Organization of Medical Care in Persons Who Have Undergone Ionizing Radiation Exposure*, Ilyin, L., Ed., Energoatomizdat Publisher, Moscow, 1986 (in Russian).
2. *Manual for Organization of Medical Care in Case of Radiation Accidents*, Energoatomizdat Publisher, Moscow, 1989 (in Russian).
3. International Chernobyl Project. Technical Report. Evaluation of Radiological Consequences and Protective Measures. Report of International Committee to IAEA, Vienna, 1992 (in Russian).
4. Medical aspects of Chernobyl accident, in *Proceedings of Scientific Conference*, May 11–13, 1988, Zdorovie Publisher, Kiev, 1988 (in Russian).
5. Ilyin, L., Kirillov, V., and Korenkov, I., *Radiation Safety and Personnel Protection Handbook*, Medicina Publisher, Moscow, 1966 (in Russian).
6. Ilyin, L., *Realities and Myths of Chernobyl*, Alara Ltd. Publisher, Moscow, 1994.
7. Barabanova, A., Baranov, A., Guskova, A. et al., *Acute Effects of Human Radiation Exposure*, TchiiAtomInform Publisher, Moscow, 1986 (in Russian).
8. Mettler, F.A. and Upton, A.C., *Medical Effects of Ionizing Radiation*, W.B. Saunders, Philadelphia, 1995.
9. Guskova, A.K., Nadejina, N.M., Moiseev, A.A. et al., Medical assistance given to personnel of the Chernobyl NPP after 1986 accident, *Sov. Med. Rev.* (Gavrilov, A.K., Sect. Ed.), 7(1), 29–102, 1996.
10. Guskova, A.K. and Baranov, A.E., Hematological effects in people exposed to radiation resulted from Chernobyl Accident, *Med. Radiol.*, 36(8), 31–37, 1991 (in Russian).
11. Konchalovsky, M.V., Baranov, A.E., and Soloviev, V.Ju., Dose Curves of neutrophils and lymphocytes in case of total body relatively uniform exposure (Chernobyl accident materials), *Med. Radiol.*, 34(6,) 52–56, 1989 (in Russian).
12. Piatkin, E.K., Nugis,V.J., and Chirkov, A.A., Evaluation of absorbed dose from the results of cytogenetic counts of lymphocyte culture in Chernobyl NPP accident victims, *Med. Radiol.*, 34(6,) 52–56, 1989 (in Russian).
13. Sevan'kaev, A.V., Lloyd, D.C., Braselman, H. et al., A survey of chromosomal aberrations in lymphocytes of Chernobyl liquidators, *Radiat. Prot. Dosimetry*, 58, 85–91, 1995.
14. International Atomic Energy Agency. Summary report on the post-accident review meeting on the Chernobyl accident, Safety Series No. 75, INSAG-1, IAEA, Vienna, 1988.
15. Guskova, A.K., 10 years after the accident at the Chernobyl NPP (retrospective evaluation of clinical events and countermeasures for consequences mitigation), *Clin. Med.*, 3, 5–8, 1996 (in Russian).
16. Barabanova, A.V. and Osanov, D.P., The dependence of skin lesion on depth-dose distribution from beta-irradiation of people in Chernobyl Nuclear Power Plant accident, in *Proceedings of the 1st Int. Conf.*, Minsk, Belarus, March, Karaoglu, A., Desmet, G., and Kelly, G.N., Eds., EUR-16544, 1996.
17. Bebeshko, V., Kovalenko, A., and Belyi, D., Long-term follow-up of irradiated persons: rehabilitation process, in *Radiation Consequences of the Chernobyl Accident, Proceedings of the 1st Int. Conf.*, Minsk, Belarus, Karaoglu, A., Desmet, G., and Kelly, G.N., Eds., EUR-16544, March 1996.
18. Guskova, A.K., Radiation and human brain, in *Proc. of the Int. Conf. on the Mental Health Consequences of the Chernobyl Disaster: Current State and Future Projects*, Kiev, Ukraine, May 1995,
19. Chinkina, O.V., Chernobyl NPP accident: clinic psychological results of examination of clean-up participants, in *Proc. of the Int. Conf. on the Mental Health Consequences of the Chernobyl Disaster: Current State and Future Projects*, Kiev, Ukraine, May 1995.
20. Astakhova, L.N., Ed., Thyroid of Children: Chernobyl Consequences, Ministry of Health of the Republic of Belarus, Minsk, 1996 (in Russian).
21. Likhtarev, I.A., Shandala, N.K., Gulko, G.M. et al., Ukrainian thyroid dose after the Chernobyl accident, *Health Phys.*, 65(6), 594–599, 1993.
22. Demidchik, E.P., Tsyb, A.F., and Luchnikov, E.F., *Thyroid Cancer in Children*, Medicina Publisher, Moscow, 1996 (in Russian).

23. Njagu, A.I. and Soushkevitch, G.N., Eds., *Proceedings of 2nd Int. Conf. on Long-Term Health Consequences of the Chernobyl Disaster*, Chernobylinterinform, Kiev, 1998, 655.
24. One Decade after Chernobyl: Summing up the Consequences of the Accident, International Conference, Book of Extended Synopsis, Vienna 08-12.04, EC-IAEA-WHO, 1996.
25. Ivanov, E.P., Tolochko, G.V., Shuvaev, L.P. et al., Childhood leukemia in Belarus before and after the Chernobyl accident, *Radiat. Environ. Biophys.*, 35, 75–80, 1996.
26. Ivanov, V.K., Tsyb, A.F., Konogorov, A.P. et al., Analysis of leukemia morbidity in recovery workers living in Russia with care control technique, 1986–1993. *Radiat. Risk*, 8, 110–115, 1996 (in Russian).
27. Guskova, A.K. et al., Medical assistance given to personnel of the Chernobyl nuclear power plant after the 1986 accident, in *Soviet Medical Reviews*, Harwood Academic Publishers, March 1996, vol. 7, part 1, pp. 29–99.

13 Accidents at Industrial Irradiation Facilities

Fred A. Mettler, Jr.

CONTENTS

Introduction 211
Whole-Body and Partial-Body Irradiation at the Commercial Irradiation Facility
    in Brescia, Italy 214
Overexposure at an Industrial Irradiation Facility in Kjeller, Norway...........................214
Whole-Body and Local Radiation Injury at the Industrial Irradiation Facility
    in San Salvador, El Salvador 214
Whole-Body and Local Radiation Injury from a Commercial Irradiation Facility
    at Soreq, Israel 216
Whole-Body and Localized Injury at an Industrial Irradiation Facility in China.........218
Whole-Body and Localized Radiation Exposure after an Accident in the Irradiation
    Facility at Nesvizh, Belarus...220
References 222

INTRODUCTION

Extremely high doses of ionizing radiation are used to sterilize agricultural products as well as medical supplies. Currently, there are between 150 and 200 large gamma irradiation facilities throughout the world and more than 600 electron beam irradiation facilities. The gamma facilities have been involved in accidents that have resulted in the most fatalities. The general design of these facilities is a heavily shielded room with a maze entrance and multiple interlocks and alarm systems. The highly radioactive source usually is kept in a pit or water-filled pool when not in use, and the objects being irradiated are typically sent in on a conveyor belt system. The activity of the radioactive sources is very high, since typical sterilization procedures require tens of thousands of gray. In most accidental situations, there have been multiple failures, both of equipment and operator technique. Often, the operator is faced with conflicting instrumentation and chooses to believe that the radioactive source has been placed in a safe position when it, in fact, has not. With the source exposed, fatal doses of radiation can be received in only a few minutes. Fatal accidents have occurred in San Salvador in 1989, at the Sor-Van Facility in Israel in 1990, in Brescia (Italy) at the Stimos Plant, in Kjeller (Norway) in 1982, and in Nesvizh (Belarus) in 1991.

A number of other accidents involving irradiation facilities have occurred and have resulted in significant exposures but not fatalities. Those accidents that have included fatalities are reviewed in the following sections, and for comparative purposes the clinical data are presented in Table 13.1.

TABLE 13.1
Summary of Medical Data for Patients Involved in Fatal Accidents at Commercial Irradiator Facilities

Site	Brescia	Norway	San Salvador	San Salvador	San Salvador	Soreq	Shanghai	Shanghai	Nesvizh
Year	1975	1982	1989	1989	1989	1990	1990	1990	1991
Case ID	1	1	A	B	C	1	S	W	1
Whole-body dose	12 Gy	10–22 Gy	8.1 Gy	3.7 Gy	2.9 Gy	10–20 Gy	12 Gy	11 Gy	11 Gy
Incapacitation							No	No	
Early hypotension							90/60 mmHg	98/60 mmHg	
Nausea (onset)	<30 min	<30 min	<1 h	<3 h	<3 h	<15 min	20 min	10 min	<10 min
Vomiting (onset)	<30 min		<1 h	<3 h	<3 h	<15 min	20 min	50 min	<10 min
Diarrhea (onset)		Began day 6	Began day 8			1 h	48 h	50 min	<1 h
Initial headache			Yes			Within minutes			<30 min
Weakness			Yes						<30 min
Initial fever	40.2 C	38.8 C				40.7 C		No	38.5 C
Numb/tingling hands				Painful feet 9d					
Edema			Legs at day 3	Legs at day 3		Days 13–21			11 days
Blistering						Days 13–21		day 16	15 days
Epilation			Yes				Day 13		11 days
WBC × 10E6/l									
1d		7800				19100 at 3h	15000 at 4h	14800 at 4h	13000 at 2h
2d	800 at day 3	6000				23000	28400	17200	8000
4d	500	5100	2900 at day 6			22000	18400	20000	2500
8d	200	0	900 at day 10			19000	5000	1500	300
16d		0 at day 13				0	800	200	20
24d			200	700 at day 26		4000	200	0	0
32d						9000	100	500	80
40d						9000			
Lymphocytes × 10E6/l									400
1d	70 at day 3	200	500 at day 3			1150 at 3h	738 at 4 h	1184 at 4h	900 at 2 h
2d	200	100				900	398	241	100
4d	50	50				700	258	0	40
8d		0				0	132 at 3 days	55	20
						0			10

Accidents at Industrial Irradiation Facilities

16d		0 at day 13		0			0
24d				250			40
32d			2300 at day 33	200			100
40d							300
Thrombocytes 1d ×10E6/l	110000	180000		290000	190000	150000	300000
8d	80000	180000			100000	80000	
16d	26000 at day 10	30000		30000	30000	70000	30000
24d		50000 at day 13	20000	54000 at day 26	10600	60000	
32d			35000 at day 33	20000	4000	5000	20000
40d						8000	10000
							7000
Transplant	No	No	No	BMT day 4	3 FLC days 1–3	BMT day 4	No
Death	12 days	13 days	197 days	36 days	25 days	90 days	133 days

WHOLE-BODY AND PARTIAL-BODY IRRADIATION AT THE COMMERCIAL IRRADIATION FACILITY IN BRESCIA, ITALY

The accident occurred in Northern Italy on May 13, 1975.[1] The irradiation facility was used for irradiation of cereal. The source was cobalt-60. The operator entered the room and was not wearing a film badge. Of particular note was the rapid drop in white blood cells and lymphocytes and the onset of nausea and vomiting in less than 30 min. Details of the medical treatment have not been reported in the literature. After an initial fever, the patient experienced a latent period for approximately 6 days, after which time fever rapidly rose and the patient died 12 days postexposure. The terminal event was listed as dramatic deregulation of the cardiac rhythm with extreme tachycardia, very high central temperature oscillations, and a Cheyne–Stokes rhythm.

OVEREXPOSURE AT AN INDUSTRIAL IRRADIATION FACILITY IN KJELLER, NORWAY

The accident occurred at the Institute of Energy Technology on September 2, 1982.[2] A cobalt-60 source was being used to sterilize medical equipment. A 64-year-old worker entered the sterilizing room, assuming that the radiation source was in a safe position. He became ill after a few minutes and began having chest pain. He did have a previous history of hypertension and angina pectoris. With the potential diagnosis of myocardial infarct, the man was admitted to an intensive care unit.

After a few hours, it was discovered that the warning lamp and the automatic lock on the sterilizing room were defective, resulting in the patient being exposed to a large dose of gamma radiation. He did have a film dosimeter, which had been damaged and was useless. Dosimetry was somewhat uncertain. Chromosome analysis indicated that the whole-body dose was likely to be at least 10 Gy. Electron spin resonance was done on nitroglycerin tablets that the patient carried in his trouser pocket. This indicated a dose of approximately 40 Gy to the pelvis. The physicians felt that the mean bone marrow dose was approximately 21 Gy, and that the dose to the brain was 14 Gy. In retrospect, the fact that the thrombocytes did not reach a nadir until 8 days suggests that the bone marrow dose was likely to be in the range of 10 to 15 Gy. Initially, the patient had a fever. The patient was placed in isolation and he was treated with penicillin and gentamicin. Partial gut sterilization was also done with neomycin and Nystatin. The patient received a white cell transfusion on days 8, 9, and 12 postexposure. At 6 days after exposure, the patient started having diarrhea with two to three stools per day. The patient became gradually weaker, and on day 11, there was a rise in serum creatinine. On day 13, the patient became oliguric and then anuric. Blood pressure was normal and the patient was drowsy. He died rather abruptly on day 13. Autopsy showed hypocellular bone marrow and lymph nodes. There was marked atrophy of the small intestine and total atrophy of the glands in the large intestine. The kidneys were enlarged and had interstitial edema. Overall, the autopsy findings were less marked than physicians expected as compared with similar reports in the literature. The cause of death was not clearly identified.

WHOLE-BODY AND LOCAL RADIATION INJURY AT THE INDUSTRIAL IRRADIATION FACILITY IN SAN SALVADOR, EL SALVADOR

The accident occurred on February 5, 1989, at an industrial irradiation facility near San Salvador in the Republic of El Salvador.[3] Prepackaged medical products were sterilized at the facility by passing them on a conveyor belt next to a cobalt-60 source. The cobalt was arranged in pencil configuration in a flat source rack. At the time of the accident, the activity of the cobalt-60 was 0.66 PBq (18 kCi). When not in use, the source was stored in a 5-m-deep water pool. At approximately 2:00 A.M. on Sunday, February 5, 1989, the operator (Patient A) noticed a source transit alarm ringing, indicating that the source was neither fully up nor down. The worker then climbed to the roof and manipulated both the source hoist and the cable. This did not solve the problem. A fixed radiation monitor, which normally would have been in the room, had been removed more than 5 years earlier and not replaced. At approximately 2:30 A.M., he managed to open the door, switched off the power supply, and entered the irradiation room with a flashlight. He removed two of the five boxes that contained medical supplies, and this took several minutes. Since he was unable to free the source rack containing the cobalt, he left the room. At approximately 3:00 a.m., he returned with two other workers (Patients B and C). The three men raised the source rack, assuming that there was no danger since power to the machine was switched off. When they returned the source rack to the water, they saw the blue glow of the Cerenkov radiation. When this was seen by Patient A, he advised everybody to withdraw immediately. All three workers began to vomit within 1 h and were subsequently admitted to a local hospital. Dose rates were estimated to be between 1.5 and 80 Gy/min. The highest dose rate involved the feet (20 to 80 Gy/min), whereas the area of the torso received approximately 1.5 to 5 Gy/min.

The clinical data during the first 30 days is somewhat limited. Initially, at 2 h postexposure, Patient A was noted to have intense nausea, vomiting, erythema, weakness, and headache. No diarrhea was reported. He was misdiagnosed as having food poisoning and discharged on that day. Over the first 3 days, weakness and pain in the feet also became evident. Mucositis and esophagitis developed on day 4 postexposure, and diarrhea, vomiting, and pain occurred on day 8. By day 3, severe lymphopenia was noted. By day 20, thrombocytes had decreased to approximately 20,000/µl. From day 4 to day 14, the skin lesions caused severe pain with edema of the feet and lower extremities with ultimate development of ulceration. Dose to the feet probably exceeded 200 Gy, and the total midline air dose had been as high as 15 Gy.

Patient A was transferred to a hospital in Mexico City on day 24 postexposure, and he was severely ill with gastrointestinal and hematopoietic radiation syndrome. He had extensive burns to both legs and feet and edema of the hands. He was placed in isolation and received transfusions. He also began a 20-day course of treatment with granulocyte/macrophage colony–stimulating factor (GM-CSF). There was a question whether this administration did or did not expedite bone marrow recovery, although there were side effects of tremors and weakness noted as a result of the administration. The patient was removed from isolation on day 47; however, the leg burns were not recovering and on day 132 postexposure, his right leg was amputated above the knee. By day 173, he was able to return to El Salvador. Patient A contracted pneumonia on day 191 and then developed a pneumothorax after placement of a jugular catheter. After 1 week in intensive care, the patient died on day 197 postexposure, $6^1/_2$ months after the accident. Cause of death was attributed to residual radiation damage of the lungs complicated by pneumothorax.

Patient B was not seen initially at the hospital and returned to work on day 4 postexposure. By day 9, he was having pain in the feet and was admitted to the hospital. Patient C was seen at the hospital on day 2, when nausea and vomiting continued. He was admitted with a diagnosis of food poisoning. Patient B was transferred to Mexico City on day 26, also with gastrointestinal and hematopoietic syndrome as well as severe burns to the legs and feet (Figure 13.1). He received a 10-day course of GM-CSF. Again, it was not clear whether this was particularly effective in promoting recovery, but it was felt also to be an important psychological support. Aggressive necrosis of the toe and changes to the lower extremity necessitated the amputation of the left leg above the knee on day 161 postexposure. After this, he returned to San Salvador. On day 202, Patient B had his right leg amputated.

Patient C refused to remain in the hospital and was discharged on day 5, but returned on day 8 and then left again on day 11. He subsequently was admitted to the hospital in Mexico City on day 33, with mild hematopoietic syndrome and burns to the left feet. He received a 9-day course of GM-CSF beginning on day 34 without side effects. He was released on day 55 postexposure.

None of the workers in this accident had been wearing radiation dosimeters. For all three patients, the administration of GM-CSF (rHuGM-CSF) was a daily dose of 240 µg/m^2 of body

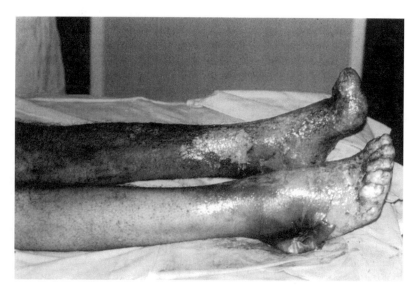

FIGURE 13.1 Burns of the feet on day 26 postexposure in Patient B in the San Salvador accident. (From IAEA.[3])

surface area by intravenous transfusions. This was continued until the total neutrophil count had increased at least to 1500/μl.

WHOLE-BODY AND LOCAL RADIATION INJURY FROM A COMMERCIAL IRRADIATION FACILITY AT SOREQ, ISRAEL

The accident occurred on June 21, 1990 at a commercial irradiation facility used to sterilize prepackaged medical products and spices.[4] The radioactive source was cobalt-60 metal, and the total activity of the source elements at the time of the accident was 12.6 PBq (340 kCi). The cobalt-60 elements were in the configuration of pencils, which were placed in a rack and stored when not in use at the bottom of a water pool. To be used, the racks of sources were lifted by a pneumatic hoist and cable system. A microswitch indicated that the source was in a down position, and the cartons undergoing irradiation on a conveyor belt jammed. A gamma radiation alarm was activated, but in the face of conflicting signals the operator disconnected the cable from the alarm system and entered the irradiation facility.

The operator went down a maze into the irradiation room, noticed the damaged cartons on the conveyor belt, and then left the irradiation room to fetch a cart, then, he reentered the room. After working for a minute or so, he began to feel a burning in the eyes and have a headache. He left the irradiation room and informed the radiation safety officer. Within 30 min, he felt nauseous and began to vomit. The patient was admitted to the hospital $2^{1}/_{4}$ h postexposure. Estimated dose was between 10 to 20 Gy to the whole body, and the exposure was estimated to be 1 to 2 min.

The patient, upon initial admission was noted to have erythema of the anterior abdomen, palms of hands, upper chest, and face. This persisted on both hands and face for 8 h. There was no evidence of initial hypotension; however, there was a fever. The patient was placed in a laminar airflow room and was treated with antibiotics (cephazolin sodium) and fluid support. He was also given acyclovir (500 mg three times a day), as well as GM-CSF (rhGM-CSF) to stimulate residual marrow (Figure 13.2). Blood was drawn for chromosome analysis; however, the yield of metaphases was inadequate. Many chromosomes were abnormal, and there were many translocations and fragments present. Dose estimation on this basis could not be done. Vomiting continued at 8 h and again on day 3. By day 4, no lymphocytes were observed, and a decision was made to perform a

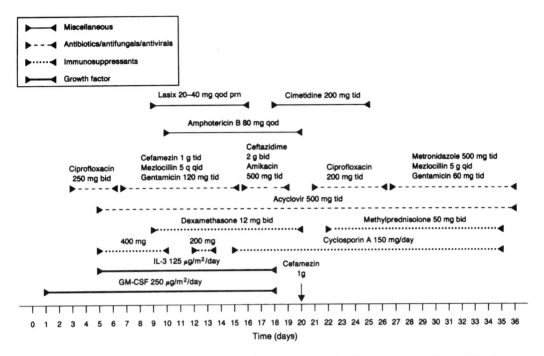

FIGURE 13.2 Medical treatment and medications used in the Soreq accident. (From IAEA.[4])

bone marrow transplant. This was done utilizing the patient's brother for a haploidentical bone marrow, T lymphocyte depleted. For prevention of graft-vs.-host disease, cyclosporin-A (6 mg/kg/day) was given. After the transplant, hematopoietic stimulation was attempted through administration of recombinant human hematopoietic growth factors including rhGM-CSF and interleukin-3 (rhIL-3). The rhIL3 was given as a continuous infusion of 250 μg/day. Platelet transfusions were given as needed to maintain a platelet count above 20,000. rhGM-CSF and rhIL-3 were discontinued on day 18.

On days 5 through 12, white blood cell and lymphocyte count remained extremely low, watery stools persisted, and the patient developed a grade III mucositis (Figure 13.3). On day 14, 10 days after bone marrow transplantation, the patient began to develop renal insufficiency with rising creatinine levels and bilirubin and gamma glutamine transpeptidase (gamma GT) rose consistent with veno-occlusive disease of the liver. Chest radiographs remained normal. Persistent fever caused the ciprofloxacin to be replaced with gentamicin, meslocillin, and cephazolin sodium. Amphotericin-B was also added.

On days 13 to 21, the patient continued to have nausea, vomiting, and diarrhea with fever persisting. Small vesicles appeared on the hands, and there was patchy hair loss on the skull, face, and pubis. On days 13 to 21, marrow transplant graft was documented but the clinical condition did not improve. On day 15, the patient's mental condition began to deteriorate, and he was restless during the daytime and had difficulty sleeping at night. Liver function continued to deteriorate and there was hypoalbuminemia, which required albumin administration. On days 22 to 34, the patient was jaundiced with right upper abdominal tenderness and hepatomegaly. On day 24, endoscopy revealed diffuse and severe edema with hyperemia and infiltration as well as widespread ulceration of the upper and lower gastrointestinal tract. L-Glutamine (40 g/day) was added in parallel with total parenteral nutrition solution. Massive bloody diarrhea continued. The patient began to confuse names, and, by day 27, he was totally confused. Clonazepam was initially prescribed, but this was replaced later with haloperidol. On day 35, the patient became confused and disoriented, and there was evidence of respiratory failure, hypoxia, and metabolic acidosis. Chest radiographs, which had

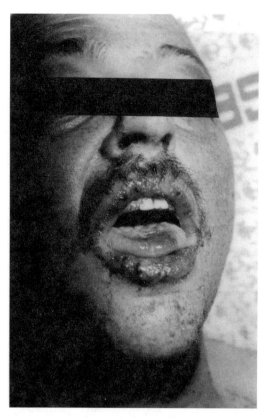

FIGURE 13.3 Mucositis occuring during the third week postexposure to the patient in the Soreq accident. Also note patchy epilation of the moustache. (From IAEA.[4]).

been predominantly normal up until this time, now revealed bilateral interstitial infiltrates. The patient died on day 36 postexposure. An autopsy was performed. There was marked depletion of various lymphatic tissues, and the expected aspermatogenesis. With regard to the gastrointestinal system, there was severe erosive esophagitis and gastritis. There was complete loss of crypt anatomy and complete denudation of the epithelial layer of the small bowel and secondary infection with cytomegalovirus. The colon demonstrated intimal thickening, edema, and thrombosis with pseudomembrane in the lumen of the colon. The liver was enlarged with necrosis of hepatocytes and changes of veno-occlusive liver disease with central lobular necrosis. The lungs revealed severe radiation pneumonitis with obliteration of the alveolar spaces, thickening of alveolar septa, and infection by cytomegalovirus. Graft-vs.-host disease could not be entirely excluded.

This accident is quite similar to the criticality accident in Tokaimura, Japan. Even though there was bone marrow transplant with significant hematological therapy and successful engraftment, the patient ultimately died from gastrointestinal and pulmonary complications. Hepatic and renal disease also complicated matters.

WHOLE-BODY AND LOCALIZED INJURY AT AN INDUSTRIAL IRRADIATION FACILITY IN CHINA

The accident happened on June 24, 1990.[5] A cobalt-60 source with an activity of 8.5×10^{14} Bq was being used to sterilize medicines and cosmetics. Four workers (S, L, J, and W-1) entered the room without carrying a personnel dose alarm and without checking the location of the source. At 9:08, 9:20, and 9:23 A.M., additional workers (W-2, J-2, and G) came into the room to help. At

9:40, worker S came back to the control room and noticed the source was still positioned at the working level. The estimated average whole-body dose for the victims was as follows: S: 12 Gy; W-1: 11 Gy; L: 5.2 Gy; J-1: 4.1 Gy, W-2: 2.5 Gy; G: 2.4 Gy; and J-2: 2.0 Gy. Dose distribution in most of the works was quite uneven with the maximal dose occurring approximately at the waist level anteriorly (Figure 13.4). Due to the penetrating nature of the radiation dose, the exit dose was approximately half of this, and dose to the head was approximately half of the maximum. Cytogenetic dosimetry as well as dose reconstruction was attempted. On the two most highly exposed individuals, the cultures failed to grow.

Patient S had some minimal early hypotension as well as nausea and vomiting. The patient received three fetal liver cell suspension infusions during the first 3 days. There were transfusions of whole blood on day 2, 6, and 22, platelet transfusions were given on days 8, 14, 22, and three transfusions on day 23. The patient was initially treated with antibiotics including penicillin and gentamicin as well as glucocorticoids and was placed in a laminar airflow room with skin sterilization as well as oral cavity and intestinal disinfection. Patient S received a bone marrow transplant on day 11. Epilation occurred from day 13 to day 21 with almost complete epilation by day 21. On day 20 and 21, there was a fever, bloody sputum, microhematuria, and probable gastric bleeding. Patient S was intubated on day 22 and, by day 23, had decreased blood pressure, oliguria, anuria, which failed to respond to a large dose of furosemide. Blood bilirubin was also elevated. On day 25, the patient had a cardiac arrest and died. Autopsy showed hemorrhage in multiple organs and massive hemorrhage in the lungs with mycotic septicemia and adult respiratory distress syndrome.

Patient W received five fetal liver cell suspension infusions during the first 48 h and a bone marrow transplant on day 4. During the course of treatment over 90 days, the patient received approximately 45 platelet transfusions and 7 transfusions of whole blood. The patient also received penicillin, gentamicin, carbenicillin, antifungal agents, immunoglobulin, and glucocorticoids for most of the treatment. Epilation began to occur in day 11. Blisters were seen over arms and upper abdomen beginning on day 16. Healing of the skin was almost completely by day 56 with the exception of local desquamation. Gastrointestinal symptoms included diarrhea with significant

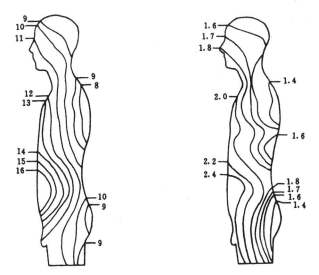

FIGURE 13.4 Isodose curves of two patients (W and J) in the Shanghai accident. Note the inhomogenous exposure even though this is very penetrating gamma radiation. (From Liu, B. and Ye, G., Eds., *Collected Papers on Diagnosis and Emergency Treatment of the Victims Involved in a Shanghai, June 25, Cobalt-60 Radiation Accident*, Military Medical Science Press, Shanghai, China, 1986.)

occult blood in the stool and pain. Gastrointestinal symptoms subsided by day 30. Peripheral HLA converted to the bone marrow donor's type at 24 h post-transplant, and at 60 days post-transplant the bone marrow had also converted to the karyotype of the donor. The patient's bilirubin was raised at day 22 post-transplant and at day 29 postexposure, and the patient became icteric. Various erythema areas were noted, and it was difficult to differentiate this from graft-vs.-host disease. Skin biopsy suggested that graft-vs.-host disease was indeed present. At day 57 postexposure and 50 days post-transplant, chest radiographs became abnormal, and the patient had a dry cough, increased respiratory rate, and decreased oxygen saturation. By day 62 postexposure, tracheotomy and respirator were necessary with a cough that was resistant to most therapy. Alveolar lavage showed a culture positive for cytomegalic inclusion virus. Patient died of respiratory failure on day 90, and the autopsy indicated the diagnosis of radiation pneumonitis, complicated by cytomegalovirus infection and diffuse fibrosis of the lung.

All the remaining patients in the accident were given blood transfusions and fetal liver cell infusions over the first 10 days of the treatment. This was true even for the patients receiving doses as low as 2 Gy. Use of cytokines such as GM-CSF or IL-3 and erythropoietin (EPO) were not available to the physicians at the time of this accident. No adverse effects were identified and the physicians concluded that timely use of fetal cell liver transfusions can strengthen immune function and stimulate hematopoiesis.

WHOLE-BODY AND LOCALIZED RADIATION EXPOSURE AFTER AN ACCIDENT IN THE IRRADIATION FACILITY AT NESVIZH, BELARUS

This accident occurred on October 26, 1991 at a facility located approximately 120 km from Minsk, Belarus.[6] The facility was used to sterilize agricultural and medical products. The source was cobalt-60 metal in the form of metallic rods. At the time of the accident, the cobalt activity was 28.1 PBq (760 kCi). This source was stored in a shielded dry storage pit and was raised when irradiation of products was desired. There was a jam in the product transport system, and the operator entered the irradiation room. He thought the source was in a safe position and bypassed a number of safety features. Estimated whole-body dose was 11 Gy with localized areas up to 20 Gy. The patient died 113 days postexposure.

After approximately 1 min in the irradiation room, the operator developed an acute headache and pain in the joints and gonads. He also felt unwell and had difficulty breathing. The majority of the time the operator was in the room, the source was directly in front of him at waist level. Nausea and vomiting occurred within 5 to 6 min. The patient was admitted to the local hospital within 20 min and transferred to a hospital in Minsk 4 h after exposure, and then within 16 h, he was admitted to the Institute of Biophysics in Moscow (Figure 13.5). At that time, he had swelling of the parotid glands and increased amylase. His body temperature had returned to normal, and at this time there was no nausea and vomiting. The patient was placed in isolation, and blood samples taken for HLA typing and cytogenetic analysis. GM-CSF was begun on day 1, and IL-3 on day 6. Due to the high dose and the low level of circulating lymphocytes, dose analysis from lymphocytes was not possible.

On day 6, the latent period ended, and mucocytis was evident in the mouth with pain in the esophagus and diarrhea resumed. Erythema was seen initially, then disappeared and recurred on day 11. Dry desquamation occurred on the left side of the face, ear, and neck on day 24 to 25. By the end of the first month, there was almost total erythema of the entire body. Severe pain began in both feet around day 20 and persisted for 1 week. Chest radiographs were essentially normal during the first month, but became abnormal on day 38 and a localized fungal pneumonia was suspected. Treatment with Amphotericin-B was then started.

IL-3 was given from day 6 to day 34, and GM-CSF was given from day 1 to 8 and then again from day 16 to day 40 postexposure. Platelet transfusions were necessary at approximately day 9, and continued until day 110.

During days 40 to 70, neutrophil counts remained between 400 and 1000, and lymphocytes and thrombocytes also remained low. Platelet transfusions were necessary. Gastrointestinal manifestations decreased somewhat after day 40, but anorexia was persistent, and there were occasional episodes of vomiting and biochemical signs of hepatitis. During days 50 to 100, there were occasional pulmonary parenchymal densities; however, the cause was not obvious, and there were no classical signs of radiation pneumonitis. No bacterial or fungal agent could be identified.

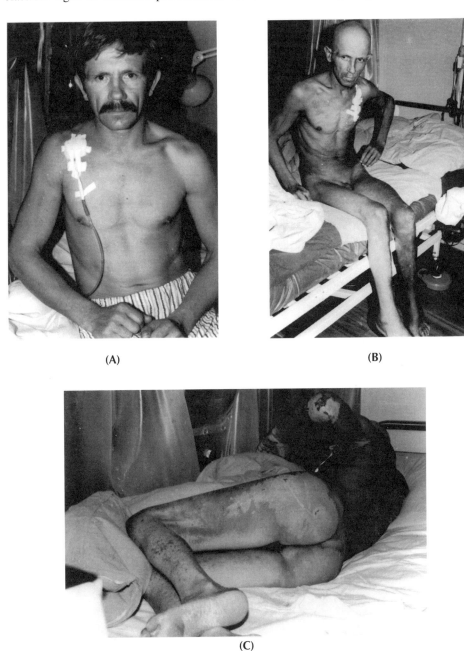

FIGURE 13.5 Patient involved in the Nesvizh accident initially (A) and at 74 days postexposure (B). The patient has epilation, weight loss, and healing skin lesions on the arms and legs (C).

Approaching 100 days, signs of renal failure appeared. From days 100 to 113, the patient's respiratory condition suddenly worsened with what appeared to be acute adult respiratory distress syndrome. The respiratory insufficiency was accompanied by hypoxia, chest pain, and slight cough. Artificial ventilation was ineffective, and a pneumothorax and severe pneumonia appeared, as well as a hyperosmolar state and increasing renal insufficiency. The patient's blood pressure decreased on day 112, and he died the following day in a hypoxemic coma from respiratory distress.

Initial treatment was with the classical antibiotics as well as antiviral and antifungal agents. Additionally, he was given total parenteral nutrition with 2500 kcal/day. A bone marrow transplant was considered, but it was decided not to perform this, either from the haploidentical sister or from a donor found in France, because of the hazards. There were classical transfusions of red cells and platelets (T leukocytes depleted). Before any decision was made whether or not to carry out bone marrow transplants, two growth factors were used to stimulate hematopoiesis. These were GM-CSF (slow intravenous infusion 11 μg/kg/day) was started on day 1, however, this was interrupted on day 6 from potential side effects of fever, edema, pain, arthropathy, and thrombophlebitis. At this point, the GM-CSF was replaced by IL-3 injected slowly intravenously (10 μg/kg/day) from day 6 to 31. GM-CSF was again used from day 16 to 39.

An autopsy was performed. This demonstrated hyperpigmentation of uneven distribution, epilation, and atrophic radiation dermatitis. Examination of the lungs demonstrated both microbial and fungal infection, edema of the blood vessel walls with severe hemorrhage, and general alveolar epithelial damage with desquamation and disseminated foci of intra-alveolar sclerosis. This appeared to correspond only slightly to typical radiation pneumonitis.

Examination of the gastrointestinal tract showed almost complete denudation of the mucosa of the distal small bowel and some punctate hemorrhages in the mesentery. The rest of the gastrointestinal tract was almost normal, except that the mucosa was significantly thinner than usual. It was concluded that partial recovery of the gastrointestinal system had taken place. The liver demonstrated some focal necrotic areas of parenchyma.

The patient received a number of other drugs including heparin 5 to 24×10^3 international units/day. This was given from the first day of her exposure for the first 2 months. Steroids were also administered including prednisolone 0.03 to 0.06 g/day from 2 days postexposure for the first 2 months, and during the same time the patient was also given methylprednisolone 0.06 to 1.00 g/day. Additional other drugs were given, including sodium bicarbonate, metronidazole, Nandrolone, nituroxazide, norfloxacin, and a number of other antibiotics.

REFERENCES

1. Jammet, H., Gongora, R., LeGo, R., and Doloy, M.T., Clinical and biological comparison of two acute accidental irradiations: Mol (1965), in Brescia (1975), in *The Medical Basis for Radiation Accident Preparedness*, Hubner, K.F. and Fry, S.A., Eds., Elsevier-North Holland, New York, 1980, 91–104.
2. Stavem, P., Brogger, A., Devik, F. et al., Lethal acute gamma radiation accident at Kjeller, Norway: report of a case, *Acta Radiol. Oncol.*, 24, 61–63, 1985.
3. IAEA, The Radiological Accident in San Salvador, STI/PUB/847, International Atomic Energy Agency, Vienna, 1990.
4. IAEA, The Radiological Accident in Soreq, STI/PUB/925, International Atomic Energy Agency, Vienna, 1993.
5. Liu, B. and Ye G., Eds., *Collected Papers on Diagnosis and Emergency Treatment of the Victims Involved in a Shanghai, June 25, Cobalt-60 Radiation Accident*, Military Medical Science Press, Shanghai, China, 1986.
6. The Radiological Accident at the Irradiation Facility in Nesvizh, STI/PUB/1010, International Atomic Energy Agency, Vienna, 1996.

14 Local Radiation Injury

Anjelika V. Barabanova

CONTENTS

Introduction 223
Conditions of Accidental Localized Exposure 223
Radiobiology of Local Radiation Injuries 225
The Role of Physical Dosimetry 226
Clinical Course and Classification of Local Radiation Injury..226
Local Radiation Injury of the Hand 228
Local Radiation Injury to Other Parts of the Body 230
Treatment of Local Radiation Injuries 231
References 239

INTRODUCTION

Radiation accidents that involve localized irradiation to small parts of the body are much more frequent than those that result in whole-body radiation.[1-4] Archives of the Institute of Biophysics of the Ministry of Health in Moscow include about 300 cases of local irradiation injuries (LRI). In addition, in about half of the cases where there is significant whole-body radiation, there is usually enough nonuniform distribution that not only is the acute radiation syndrome (ARS) present, but there is also significant LRI (sometimes called the cutaneous syndrome) that complicates the course of ARS.

Most cases of localized overexposure (and the doses can be very high) are usually compatible with life because of the small volume of tissue irradiated; however, highly penetrating LRI to vitally important organs, such as the heart and brain, can lead to death. The treatment of LRI is difficult and takes a long time. The issues of diagnosis, prognosis, and treatment are very important. There is no one single methodology, since there is a wide variation in LRI accidents, both with regard to conditions of exposure and the tissues involved.

CONDITIONS OF ACCIDENTAL LOCALIZED EXPOSURE

The clinical course of LRI in a specific case depends upon the following:

- The kind of radiation (beta, gamma, X ray), and especially upon the energy of the radiation or its penetrating ability;
- Type of source (sealed, unsealed, irradiation device);
- Dose of radiation including dose rate characteristics;
- Duration of exposure (this is often difficult to ascertain);
- Distribution of dose within the tissue exposed;
- Part of the body and size of the area exposed.

Knowing all these parameters is very important for the physician. However, receiving complete dosimetric information in a reasonable amount of time to facilitate treatment is almost impossible. In addition, some patients present long after the time of exposure, preventing early medical intervention, and patients often provide very poor histories of the accident itself.

Many years of experience with LRI allow summarization of some information of importance. The general character of LRI accidents is presented in Table 14.1. It can be seen from the table that industrial radiography accidents are the most frequent type to result in LRI, and since the radioactive source itself is quite small, it can be picked up and easily handled. As a result, most frequently there are injuries to the hand and tissues that are near pockets of the clothing.

TABLE 14.1
General Character of the Most Frequent Radiological Accidents (RA) That Cause LRI

Area of Use	Sources	Exposure	Part of Body Exposed	Victims, No.	% in General Number of RA
Industry:					
Sterilization	^{60}Co, ^{137}Cs	External	Whole body, hands, other	Professionals, 1–3	2–3 40–45 1–2
Industrial radiography	^{137}Cs, ^{192}Ir, ^{137}Cs	External	Hands, other parts		
Medicine:					
Therapy	^{60}Co, ^{137}Cs, X-ray machine accelerators	External	Whole body, other parts	Patients, 10s; professionals 1–2	5–10
Diagnostic	X-ray machine, radionuclides	Internal	Same	Same	0–1
Science: Research	Broad spectrum of sources	External Internal	Hands, face, other parts, whole body	Professionals, 1–3	5–10
Atomic energy	Reactors, radio-chemistry	External Internal	Whole body, hands, other parts	Professionals, 1–5	10–15
"Wasted" sources	^{60}Co, ^{137}Cs, ^{192}Ir, and others	External Internal	Hands, other parts, whole body	Individuals from public, children	15–20

Highly intense radioactive sources are sometimes listed as "spent" or "wasted," but in spite of this, their activity can be very high. Persons who find them not only may have significant doses to the whole body, but often have very high doses to the extremities. A number of case reports of this type exist in the literature[5–8] (see Chapters 16 through 21).

The cause of such accidents is usually linked to some technical defect of the machine or to a violation of standard radiation protection policies and procedures.[9] A number of cases have been reported in which such metallic sources are found by nonprofessionals, persons in the public, or even children. Often they look at it for a long time, transfer it from one pocket to another, and even bring it home.[10–13] In this situation, many people can be exposed and they can have several lesions or even whole-body exposure. Occasionally, the capsule surrounding the radioactive material can be breached, and significant internal contamination with the radionuclide can also result. Such an accident occurred in Goiânia (Brazil) and is discussed in Chapter 26.

Radiation accidents with LRI also occur with X-ray devices used for X-ray defraction, spectrometry, and crystallography. These often involve injury to the dorsal surface of the hand. These accidents usually occur while manipulating a sample near the beam of the machine while the X-ray beam is turned on. These accidents are not considered very severe because of the low-energy X ray used. Sometimes, not only the hands, but also the face and head are exposed, and under these circumstances, the consequences may be more serious.[14-16]

Accidents involving accelerators of high energies often occur in research and medicine. While these may be with an electron beam of substantial energy, additional accidents with proton beams and other forms of energy have been described. In many of these accidents, the reason has been exposure to so-called dark current, which occurs at the moment the accelerator current, is "off," but the voltage remains "on."

LRI as a result of medical uses of ionizing radiation was once very common, particularly in the early 1900s. Significant accidents, however, continue to occur with radiation therapy. Recent accidents described elsewhere in this book include large accidents occurring in the United States, Spain, Costa Rica, and the United Kingdom (see Chapters 20 and 21). The number of patients who are significantly overexposed in radiation therapy accidents may be as small as one, but may be as high as several hundred.[20-23]

There have been some rather unusual circumstances related to LRI where people have exposed themselves to sources of beta radiation such as strontium or tried to commit suicide utilizing high-intensity radioactive sources. Significant local skin injury has been described in the literature as a result of beta burns from metallic bomb testing, as well as in the nuclear power plant accident at Chernobyl.[24,25]

RADIOBIOLOGY OF LOCAL RADIATION INJURIES

The visible clinical changes in LRI relate to the skin, and, therefore, knowledge of radiobiology of the skin is very important. The most recent complete description of radiation effects on the skin has been published by the International Commission on Radiological Protection.[26] This chapter includes only the most important aspects necessary for medical management of LRI.

Massive death of the stem cells of the skin is the basic process underlying the main clinical manifestations that are seen, particularly dry and moist desquamation. The threshold doses for these effects are 8 to 12 Gy and 15 to 20 Gy, respectively. As the area of injured skin increases, the less is the threshold dose necessary for the same effects. Death of skin cells is not the only process responsible for all signs of injury. Early and secondary erythema depend on the functional changes in the blood vessels and the appearance of ulcers may be due to necrosis, but also injury of blood vessels and underlying connective tissue elements. The radiosensitivity of epidermal cells, other than the basal layer, is not known exactly; however, their destruction after doses in excess of tens of gray is clear. At higher absorbed doses, more cells and other elements are destroyed and, thus, the injuries are seen earlier postexposure. The time of appearance of different effects depend on the renewal time of the cells of those tissues. Obviously, the more energetic the radiation, the deeper the injury. With exposure to X rays of approximately 20 keV, only skin damage is observed, and this is true in some cases of beta ray exposure. However, in all cases with gamma radiation, there can be damage to subcutaneous structures including muscle, cartilage, and even bone. Large blood vessels and nerves are quite radioresistant.

Data on the radiosensitivity of various tissue elements and the time of appearance of clinical effects are presented in Table 14.2.

The depth of structures that are critical for some effects listed in Table 14.2 are the following: basal layer of the epidermis of the skin 70 to 100 μm; skin, blood, and capillary 200 to 1000 μm (but on the palmar surface of the hand and foot these structures are significantly deeper). The dose to muscles, bone, and cartilage obviously also varies with the depth, but this depends on the particular portion of the body involved.

TABLE 14.2
Threshold Dose for the Most Important Effects in Locally Irradiated Tissues

Tissue Structure	Threshold Dose (Gy)	Clinical Effect	Time of Appearance
Skin	10–15	Erythema	18–20 days
	20–25	Moist desquamation	20–25 days
Blood capillaries	8–10	Dilatation	15–18 days
	25–30	Alteration	2–3 months
Arterial vessels	70–80	Sclerosis	3–5 years
Cartilage	20–30	Radionecrosis	6–12 months
Bone	35–40	Osteoporosis	12–20 months
Muscles	30–35	Radionecrosis	6–7 months
Nerves	>100	Destruction	3–5 years (?)

For the process of reepithelialization, especially in the case of low-energy X-ray or beta ray exposure, the undamaged state of epithelial cells of hair follicles is very important. Depth of the hair follicles varies somewhat between individuals, as well as from one part of the body to another.

Complete healing of the skin is possible after dry desquamation. Moist desquamation results from having significantly more cells killed, and healing then depends on the size of the injury. As early as 1942, Ellis[27] showed that an area of skin 6 × 4 cm would reepithelialize after 20 Gy, but an area of 8 × 10 cm would repair only after doses up to about 15 Gy. Whether radiogenic ulcers will heal is more difficult to say. Small ulcers may heal by scar formation, but even this depends upon the depth of radionecrosis and the energy and dose of the incident radiation.

Late effects in locally overexposed tissues are characterized by skin atrophy, alteration in pigmentation, and fibrosis development. Telangiectasia is also typical.

THE ROLE OF PHYSICAL DOSIMETRY

The role of physical dosimetry in cases of accidents would seem to be important, although in practical terms, access to this information is very limited.[17,28] Neither in the literature nor in practice has the author ever come across a victim of LRI who has carried a dosimeter located near the place of maximum exposure. Doses of radiation in these situations have to be established by accident reconstruction and a description of the accident by the patient or witnesses. Technical documentation of exact type and strength of the source is important for the dose calculation.

Accident reconstruction and dose estimation is a widely used procedure; however, correct calculations require, as a minimum, knowledge of the type of radiation, its energy, dose rate at a given distance, and duration of the exposure. Sometimes accident reconstruction with phantom and special dosimeters is helpful. In spite of all this, the results of such calculations are usually not available for some time, and they usually also contain significant uncertainty. A more precise dose evaluation can be made by using electron spin resonance for dosimetry.[20,21] This can be performed on cloth, any personal belongings, or biological substances exposed at the same time as the victim. In practice, all the above methods should be used together. Although there is necessarily a delay in getting this information, and it is not particularly helpful for early diagnosis or prognosis, it can be helpful later in making surgical treatment decisions.

CLINICAL COURSE AND CLASSIFICATION OF LOCAL RADIATION INJURY

Local radiation injuries progress in a certain temporal sequence, and it is useful throughout this process to try to assess the grade of severity of the injury. Grading is typically done from I to IV.

The first phase of localized radiation is initial erythema. Skin reddening may occur in the first minutes or hours after exposure and is usually observed for at least 1 to 2 days. Observation of this is important for determination of the tissues irradiated. Erythema gives little prognostic evaluation for long-term effects. Occasionally, erythema is not present, but the patient may complain of a sense of heat or itching as the only symptom.

The latent phase occurs after the initial erythema. Usually, nothing can be clinically identified in the region of the exposed tissue. The duration of the latent phase in general is longer as the dose is decreased, although this dependence is different for various body parts. It is shorter for skin of the face, neck, and chest, and longer for palmar surfaces of the hands and feet. Some authors have used infrared techniques, including thermography, to look for areas of raised temperature in the skin during the latent phase.[29] These techniques are not widely available, and recently some authors advocated the use of diagnostic radionuclide with images of the exposed body parts in the arterial and particularly blood pool phases of vascular flow. Such intravenously injected radioisotopes can indicate local changes in tissue before clinical signs appear. Cutaneous laser Doppler also has been used for similar purposes. A complete review of the modern possibilities for laboratory diagnosis of LRI has been presented recently by Lefaix and Daburon.[30] The presence of the latent phase is notable for radiation injury, because this can be regarded as an important sign differentiating radiation burns from burns of other types.

The latent period ends when the second (or main) erythema appears. The time of its appearance corresponds to the renewal of the epidermal cells at about 2 to 3 weeks. In practice, the second erythema appears in a shorter time with significant overexposure or at longer times with milder damage. The bounds of the secondary erythema conform to the zone of overexposure. Second erythema changes somewhat in time beginning with redness of the skin, a sense of heat, and slight edema, and in many cases the color of the skin then becomes somewhat brown. After 1 to 2 weeks, dry desquamation then develops. This is grade I of LRI.

If edema occurs, not only of the skin but also of subcutaneous tissues, and blisters develop with resultant moist desquamation, this is characterized as grade II LRI. At later times, epithelialization can occur.

If secondary erythema occurs at 8 to 14 days and is followed by erosions and ulceration, as well as severe pain, this is grade III in severity. The healing of ulcers formed with this type of injury is very difficult and takes a long time. If the ulcer is small enough, it can be replaced with scar tissue.

With any grade of injury, the third (or late) wave of erythema takes place between 10 to 16 weeks postexposure. This is most notable after beta exposure and relates to injury of the blood vessels.[31] It is accompanied with edema and increasing pain. At this time, even if epithelialization had taken place, it may stop or new ulcerations and necrotic changes may appear during this time.

Early necrosis can occur after very high doses and local exposure. When the dose of gamma radiation (or other highly penetrating radiation) from 800 Gy and higher, there is an early erythema accompanied by swelling, no latent phase occurs, and a secondary erythema and blisters appear within day 3 or 4. For this type of injury, there is substantial pain, and tissues become necrotic within the first week. In most severe cases, there is early ischemia of tissue; the tissue turns white and then dark blue or black with substantial pain. This is a grade IV injury.

Late effects of LRI depend upon the degree of severity in the early stages, and the late effects can vary from slight skin atrophy to constant ulcer recurrence and deformity. In the late period, there may be atrophy of the skin and epidermis as well as occlusion of small vessels with subsequent disturbances in the blood supply, destruction of the lymphatic network, regional lymphostasis, and increasing fibrosis and sclerosis of the connective tissue. At much later times, of course, formation of skin cancer can occur as a result of acute localized radiation, although most radiation skin cancers occur following chronic exposures.

LOCAL RADIATION INJURY OF THE HAND

Particular attention to LRI of the hand is important for several reasons: (1) hands are the most frequently involved body part in radiation accidents, (2) the hand has major functional significance for daily life, (3) the anatomical features are unique.

In most radiation accidents involving small but highly radioactive gamma sources, the palmar surfaces of the fingers and palms usually receive the highest exposures. In contrast, with accelerators and X-ray devices, the dorsal and lateral aspects of the hand tend to be more involved (Figure 14.1). As a result of this, it is important to keep in mind that there are significant differences between the palmar and dorsal aspects of the hand. The dorsal surfaces have much thinner skin than on the palmar surface. This is predominantly due to differences in thickness of the corneal layer of epidermis (7 and 50 mg/cm, respectively). More subcutaneous cellular tissue and sweat glands are

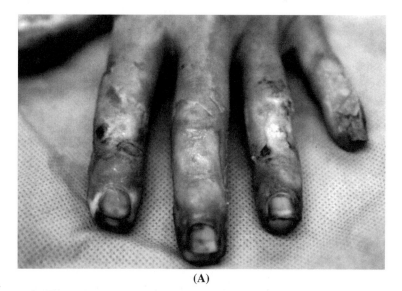

(A)

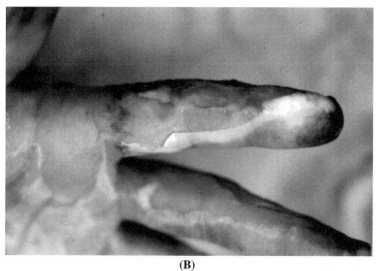

(B)

FIGURE 14.1 Local injury to the hand and fingers on the dorsal (A) and lateral surfaces (B) incurred when repairing a low-energy X-ray source while it was turned on.

Local Radiation Injury

also present on the palmar surface of the hand. Hair follicles are found on the dorsal surface only, and renewal of the cells in the thin skin of the dorsal aspect of the hand is more rapid than on the palmar surface. This is important for reepithelialization. Rich blood supply is a characteristic feature of fingers, especially in the distal phalanges. The same is true relative to the presence of nerve endings. On the dorsal surface, bones and joints are very close to the skin. Tables 14.3 and 14.4 demonstrate the time of onset of the various clinical phases of LRI involving the hand following a gamma exposure. In practice, the time of appearance of the signs has significant variation. Nevertheless, the data presented in Tables 14.3 and 14.4 are helpful for prognostic evaluation.

The most typical late effects involving highly penetrating radiation are gross deformities with significant functional disruption as well as amputation defects. With penetrating radiation, osteoporosis and osteolysis also may occur. With mild to moderate LRI of the palmar surface of the hand, erythema often is absent or faint. Sometimes, there is only an intermittent feeling of pain or other strange feeling. The time of the main erythema depends not only on the dose, but also upon the size of the area exposed. Swelling and pain can occur with the second erythema. With necrotic injuries of the hand following penetrating radiation, the presence of unrelenting pain is often a decision point for early amputation. Injuries to the fingers may heal faster and better than injuries to the palmar surface.

The typical course of injury following exposure to penetrating cesium with a dose of about 25 Gy (250 rad) is shown in Figures 14.2A through D. Injury was classified as a grade II to III and was treated conservatively using DNA solution for application; satisfactory healing occurred in 3 months. However, 3 years later, the amputation of one right index phalanx was performed because of recurrent necrosis and infection. More extensive and higher-dose lesions lead to more severe consequences as shown in Figures 14.3 and 14.4.

With injuries involving low-energy X-ray exposure to the dorsal surface of the hand, either from X-ray defraction, spectroscopy, or crystallography accidents, there is usually a very short latent period, but healing tends to be more complete and earlier than that seen with more-penetrating radiation. In the late period, there will be skin atrophy, depigmentation, and telangiectasias. The more severe cases develop hyperkeratosis and superficial erosions. Figures 14.5A and B show the typical clinical findings of grade II to III injury.

TABLE 14.3
Time of Onset of Clinical Phases of LRI to Hand (Palmar Surface) Following Gamma Exposure Depending on the Dose to Skin

Dose, Gy (grade of severity)	Early Erythema	Second Erythema	Blisters	Erosion and Ulcer	Necrosis	Healing, Character	Late Effects, Character
10–12 (I)	Not seen	20–24 days	No	No	No	35–40 days, dry desquamation	Slight skin atrophy
15–20 (II)	Day 1	15–20 days	20–25 days	No	No	45–50 days, moist desquamation	Expressed atrophy, late ulcer
25–50 (III)	Day 1	8–14 days	10–18 days	20–30 days	No, or 3 months	Scar formation	Late ulcers, deformation
>50 (IV)	4–6 h	4–6 days	6–8 days		10–12 days	No	Amputation defects
>200 (V)	1–2 min	1–2 days	4–6 days		5–7 days	No	Amputation defects

TABLE 14.4
Time of Onset of Clinical Phases of LRI to Hand (Dorsal Surface) Following Low-Energy Radiation, Depending on Dose to Skin

Dose, Gy (grade of severity)	Early Erythema	Second Erythema	Blisters	Erosion and Ulcer	Necrosis	Healing, Character	Late Effects, Character
8–15 (I)	12–24 h or not seen	12–20 days	No	No	No	28–35 days, dry desquamation	No consequences
18–30 (II)	6–12 h	6–14 days	10–15 days	No	No	40–45 days, moist desquamation	Slight atrophy
35–70 (III)	4–6 h	3–7 days	5–10 days	12–18 days	No	50–70 days, epithelialization	Skin atrophy, depigmentation
>70 (IV)	1–2 h	1–4 days	3–5 days	6–8 days	7–10 days	60–80 days, scar formation	Atrophic scar, depigmentation, ulceration

As mentioned previously, dose estimation in the case of accidental hand exposure can be difficult. When there are accidents involving unusual types of beams, such as proton beams, the accidental situation can sometimes be relatively precisely reconstructed with the use of a hand phantom and multilayered tissue equivalent dosimeter. These occasionally will reveal unexpected doses at various depths, and in one case of 40 MeV proton beams, the dose at a depth of 1000 to 1500 μm can be three times higher than on the skin surface due to the Bragg effect[20] (Figure 14.6). As a result, there are more severe late effects.

LOCAL RADIATION INJURY TO OTHER PARTS OF THE BODY

Unfortunately, it is quite typical that people who find a small but highly radioactive source would handle it and then put it in their pocket. As a result, radiation injuries of the thighs, buttocks, abdomen, or chest are relatively common. There are a few cases in which individuals aiming to harm or even kill somebody have placed radioactive sources in a chair. LRIs of the face and head also are observed, but they are typically caused in radiation therapy accidents and less commonly by accelerators.

LRI to the thigh or buttocks usually takes place with essentially direct contact of the source with the skin. Two types of exposure can take place: (1) the source is fixed in a small narrow pocket or the individual has been sitting on it for some time, and (2) the source was moving in a large pocket and its position relative to body part changed several times. In the first case, the size of the area exposed conforms to the size of the source, and significant decrease of the dose with depth and distance is distinctive. In the second case, the size of the injury is larger and the type of depth or distribution is more complicated. These differences need to be considered in each particular case.

Clinical healing of these thigh and buttocks injuries differs from LRI to the hand since there is less blood flow and more delayed healing. In almost all cases of LRI to the thigh or buttock, surgical treatment is required (Figure 14.7). Damage to muscle and bone is typical for radiation injury of the thigh in such accidents. Osteoporosis develops in 3 to 4 years, and fracture with relatively slight trauma can occur. A number of LRIs to the buttock also involve injury to the rectum, bladder, and genital organs, and they often become infected. A graphic example of this type of injury is discussed in Chapter 17 on an industrial radiography source accident in Peru.

LRI to the abdomen is very serious because of the high risk of intestinal damage. Even a relatively small injury to the skin of the abdomen with a dose above 15 Gy can lead to pain and episodes of diarrhea within 8 to 10 days postexposure. Higher doses above 30 Gy often cause deep

Local Radiation Injury

injury to the intestine with perforation and peritonitis, even several months after exposure (Figure 14.8). In cases where there is a large amount of intestinal damage, the patient may die, as was the case in Figure 14.8. In cases in which there is less intestinal damage, resection or diversion may be successful.

LRI to the chest can result in damage to the ribs, heart, lungs, and even spinal cord, depending on the dose distribution. A number of cases are very severe. One of these cases occurred in Bulgaria about 20 years ago when a radiographer kept a highly radioactive cesium-137 source in his chest pocket for several hours with the intent of committing suicide. Estimated dose in the center of the lesion was 250 Gy and 12 Gy at a distance of 4 cm. The dose to the heart apex was estimated to be 20 to 25 Gy. Necrosis of the heart apex developed with acute cardiac insufficiency, and the patient died. Autopsy revealed sclerotic changes in the pleural and pericardium. Multiple other injuries related to radiation therapy have been reported, and a number of these are discussed in detail in Chapters 20 and 21. These often involve injury of the head and neck, thorax, abdomen, and pelvis.

LRI to the head and face has been observed with accidents involving X-ray machines as well as accelerators. Three cases that the author has treated that involved low-energy X rays of about 20 keV ended without severe consequences. In these cases, there was only slight skin atrophy and minimal deformity. Two more severe cases merit detailed discussion. In the first of these, irradiation of the face and frontal part of the head with 30 Gy of 50 keV X rays resulted in severe skin and eye injury in the early period followed by almost complete blindness, osteonecrosis and osteomyelitis of the frontal bone, and some psychiatric disorder 3 to 4 years later. The patient died 7 years after exposure as a result of an inflammatory process of the brain. In the second case, exposure was due to highly penetrating radiation from a very narrow 600 MeV proton beam, which went from the back of the head to the nose. In the early phase, injury of the left facial nerve and the exit wound to the side of the nose were evident as well as signs of injury to the middle ear. There was osteonecrosis of the bones that were in the path of the beam, and 4 years later, the patient developed petit mal seizures and deformity of the occipital lobe. In spite of this, the patient has continued to work for 20 years postexposure (Figures 14.9A to C).

TREATMENT OF LOCAL RADIATION INJURIES

Patients with LRI need special medical treatment. Often a combined team approach is necessary with health physicists and physicians who have knowledge of radiopathology. Careful observation with clinical photographs and/or video cameras as well as description of the skin reactions can help in evaluation of the severity and choice of therapeutic modalities. Overall, two main approaches are considered: (1) conservative and (2) surgical.[33] In the author's experience, both approaches are used, sometimes together. Conservative methods are only utilized in cases of superficial damage to the skin, which typically occurs with accidents of low energy such as X-ray radiation less than 30 keV and beta radiation not higher than 1 MeV.

Conservative therapy methods include a number of agents that are anti-inflammatory, inhibit proteolysis, analgesic, regeneration stimulators, and those which improve circulation. In the case of widespread and deep injury, anticoagulative agents are also useful. In all situations, the therapy should be correlated with laboratory data and detailed clinical observation. Thus, in the first stage, early erythema, and in the latent phase, anti-inflammatory medicines such as corticosteroids, as well as creams and sprays, and desensitizing drugs are used. In the middle of the latent phase, proteolysis inhibitors (Gordox) are indicated. There are a number of solutions that can stimulate regeneration of DNA, which are applied to the injured surface. One of these agents is Leoxasol. Biogenic drugs, such as Actovegin and Solcoseril, can be used later when regeneration has started. Stimulation of the blood supply should be started in the third or fourth week, and at this time Pentoxifylline (400 mg 3 times a day) is probably the most effective. This latter drug is systemic and is contraindicated in patients with atherosclerotic heart disease.

Treatment of late effects such as radiation-induced fibrosis and late radiation ulcers includes stimulation of vascularization, anti-infectious agents, and any agents that may reduce fibrosis. Typically, with most LRIs, surgical treatment earlier is much better than later. Surgical treatment is based upon three main principles: (1) operative intervention should be taken as early as possible, (2) resection must be made in the zone of healthy tissue or at least on the borderline, and (3) full-thickness graft and microsurgery techniques usually provide the best results.

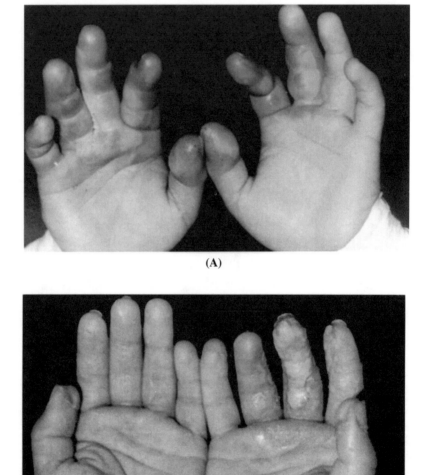

FIGURE 14.2 (A) Patient VS. LRI to both hands, grade II to III of severity, 21 days after gamma irradiation (^{137}Cs). (B) The same case, 42 days after irradiation. (C) The same case, 70 days after irradiation. (D) The same case, 2 years later — unguinal panaritium of the right index finger that was amputated.

Local Radiation Injury

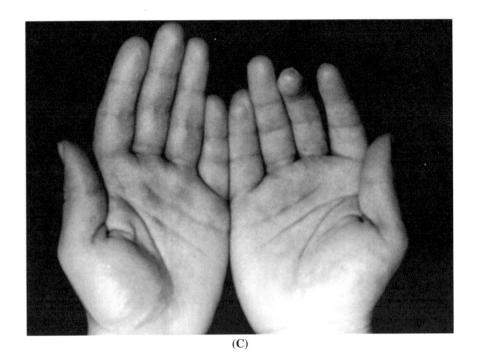

(C)

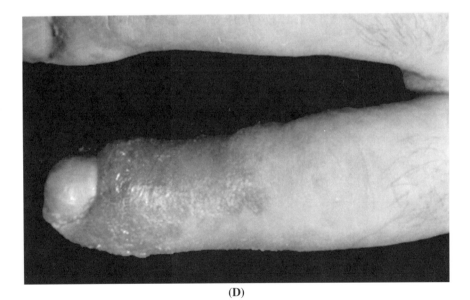

(D)

FIGURE 14.2 (Continued)

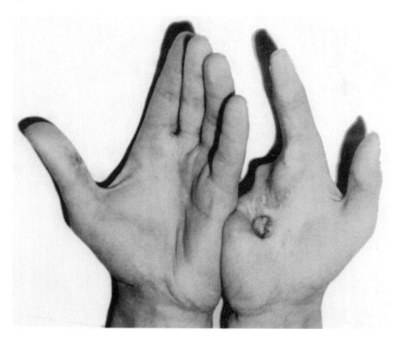

FIGURE 14.3 Patient AK. Late effect of LRI to left hand of grade II and to right hand of grade III to IV, 5 years after gamma irradiation (dose >40 Gy).

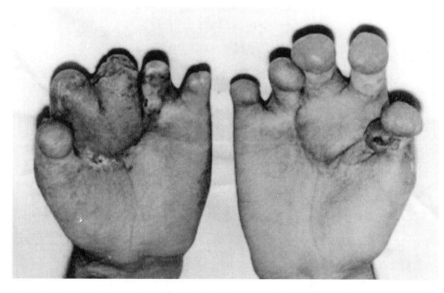

FIGURE 14.4 Patient VL. Late effect of LRI to both hands, grade IV, 2 years after gamma irradiation (dose >50 Gy).

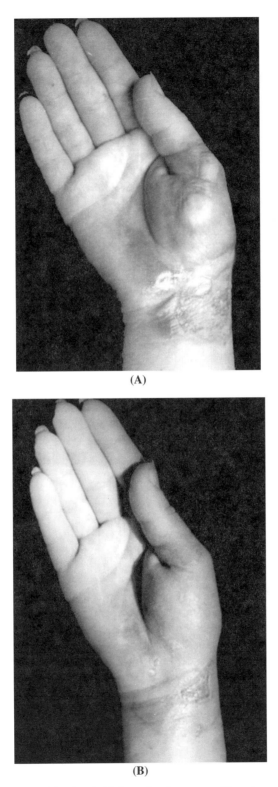

FIGURE 14.5 (A) Patient TC. LRI to hand, 12 days after low-energy X-ray beam irradiation. (B) The same case, 48 days after irradiation.

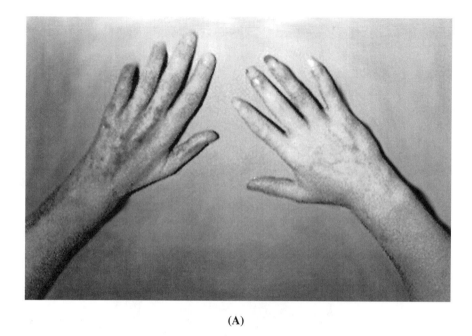

(A)

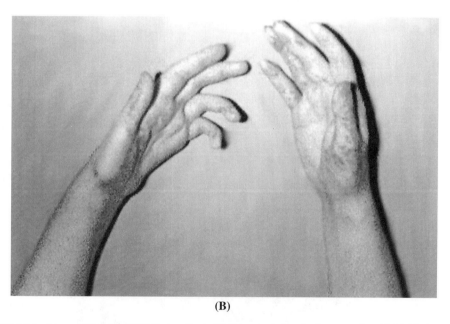

(B)

FIGURE 14.6 (A and B) Patient VS. Late effect of LRI to both hands, 2 years after 40 MeV proton beam irradiation.

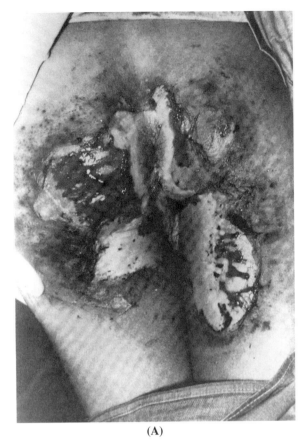

(A)

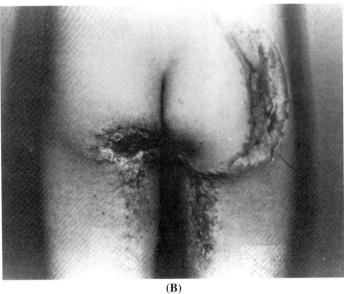

(B)

FIGURE 14.7 Injury to the buttocks (A) from carrying an industrial radiography source in the back pockets. (B) Same patient after grafting.

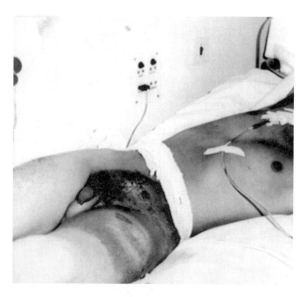

FIGURE 14.8 Patient N. LRI to low part of the abdomen and to the left thigh, grade IV of severity, 10 days after gamma irradiation (^{137}Cs); the dose to the thigh = 900 Gy, to the left low abdomen about 50 Gy.

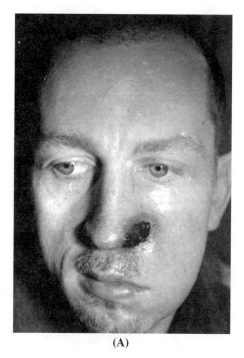

(A)

FIGURE 14.9 Case of 600 MeV proton beam irradiation through the head. (A) The point of beam entry. (B) The point of beam exit, left facialis paresis. (C) The same case, 3 years later.

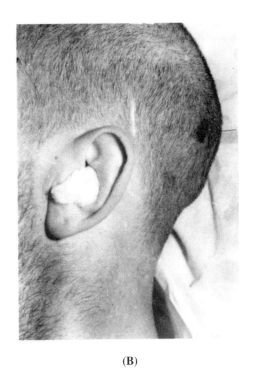
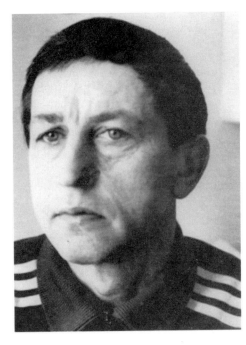

(B)   (C)

FIGURE 14.9 (Continued)

REFERENCES

1. Lushbaugh, C.C., Fry, S.A., Ricks, R.C. et al., Historical update of past and recent skin damage radiation accidents, *Br. J. Radiol.*, 19 (Suppl.), 7–12, 1986.
2. Gongora, R. and Magdelinar, H., Accidental acute local irradiations in France and their pathology, *Br. J. Radiol.*, 19 (Suppl.), 12–15, 1986.
3. Cosset, J.M., Perdereau, B., Gongora, R. et al., La Radiopathologie L'Institut Curie: analyse preliminaire d'une cohorte de 952 patients vus de 1951–1994, *Radioprotection*, 30, 119–122, 1995 (in French).
4. Ilyin, L.A., Soloviov, V., Baranov, A. et al., Historical analysis of direct medical consequences of radiological incidents taking place in the former USSR, in *Radioecological and Medical Consequences of the Chernobyl Accident, Proceeding of the All-Russia Conference*, Galicino, Moscow, 1995 (in Russian).
5. Jacobson, A., Wilson, B.M., Banks, W.T. et al., ^{192}Ir over-exposure in industrial radiography, *Health Phys.*, 32, 291–293, 1977.
6. Jalil, A. and Molia, M.A., An overexposure in industrial radiography; a follow-up study, *Health Phys.*, 57, 117–119, 1989.
7. Chone, B., Schneider, G.J., and Fehrentz, D., ^{192}Iridium-kontactbestrahlung und Folgeerscheinungen, *Strahlentherapie*, 140, 113–122, 1970 (in German).
8. Milanov, N.O. and Shilov, B.L., *Plastic Surgery Treatment of Radiation Injury*, National Research Centre of Surgery, RAMS, Moscow, 1996.
9. International Atomic Energy Agency, Lessons Learned from Accidents in Industrial Irradiation Facilities, IAEA, Vienna, 1996.
10. Hirashima, K., Sugiama, H., Ishihara, T. et al., The 1971 Chiba, Japan accident: exposure to iridium-192, in *The Medical Basis for Radiation Accident Preparedness*, Hubner, K.F. and Fry, S., Eds., Elsevier North Holland, New York, 1980, 179–195.

11. Jammet, H., Gongora, R., Jockey, P., and Zucker, J.M., The 1978 Algerian accident: acute local exposure of two children, in *The Medical Basis for Radiation Accident Preparedness*, Hubner, K.F. and Fry, S., Eds., Elsevier North Holland, New York; 1980, 230–240.
12. International Atomic Energy Agency, The Radiological Accident in Goiânia, IAEA, Vienna, 1988.
13. Ruwei, A., Guang, B. et al., Eds., China Nuclear Science and Technology Report: Selected Compilation of Clinical Cases for Over-Exposure of Workers in the Chinese Nuclear Industry in the Past 30 Years, China Nuclear Information Centre, 1989.
14. Barabanova, A.V., Sokolina, L.L., and Novikova, L.V., Clinical–dosimetrical correlation in local irradiation from sources of different energy, *Med. Radiol.*, 10, 46–50, 1974 (in Russian).
15. Barabanova, A., Treatment of late radiation injury to skin, in *Advances in the Biosci.*, 94, 241–247, 1994.
16. Berger, M.E., Hurtado, R., Dunlap, J. et al., Accidental radiation injury to the hand; anatomical and physiological considerations, *Health Phys.*, 72, 343–348, 1997.
17. Barabanova, A., The use of dosimetric data for the assessment of the prognosis of the severity and outcome of local radiation injuries, *Br. J. Radiol.*, 19 (Suppl.), 73–74, 1986.
18. International Atomic Energy Agency, An Electron Accelerator Accident in Hanoi, Vietnam, IAEA, Vienna, 1996.
19. Schauer, D.A. et al., A radiation accident in an industrial facility, *Health Phys.* 65(2), 131–140, 1993.
20. Alekhin, I.A., Babenko, S.P., Kraitor, S.N. et al., Experience from application of radioluminescence and electron paramagnetic resonance to dosimetry of accidental irradiation, *Atomnaya Energ.*, 53(2), 91–95, 1982 (in Russian).
21. Kraitor, S.N., Kushnereva, K.K., Kalmanson, A.E. et al., Reconstruction of dosimetrical picture of an accidental irradiation, *Atomnaya Energ.*, 43(3), 196–197, 1982 (in Russian).
22. Mettler, F.A., *Medical Effects of Ionizing Radiation,* Saunders, Philadelphia, 1996.
23. International Atomic Energy Agency, Accidental Overexposure of Radiotherapy Patients in San Jose, Costa Rica, IAEA, Vienna, 1998.
24. Bond, V.P., Cronkite, E.P., and Dunham, C.L., Some effects of ionizing radiation of human beings. A report of the Marshallese and Americans accidentally exposed to radiation from fallout and a discussion of radiation injury in the human being, United States Atomic Energy Commission, New York, July, 1956.
25. Barabanova, A.V. and Osanov, D.P., The dependence of skin lesions on the depth–dose distribution from β-irradiation of people in the Chernobyl Nuclear Power Plant accident, *Int. J. Radiol. Biol.*, 57(4), 775–782, 1990.
26. International Commission on Radiological Protection, Biological Base for Limitation of Dose to Skin, Publ. 59, 1992. *Ann. ICRP*, 22:2, 1991, Pergamon Press, Oxford, U.K.
27. Ellis, F., Tolerance of skin in radiotherapy with 200 kV X-rays, *Br. J. Radiol.*, 15, 348–350, 1942.
28. Permentier, N. and Luccioni, C., Local overexposure: the role of physical dosimetry, *Br. J. Radiol.*, 19 (Suppl.), 66–72, 1986.
29. Jammet, H. and Gongora, R., Radiolesions aigues localisees: interetde la dosimetrie physique et biologique; etude clinique, in *II Sistema Tegumentariao e la Radiozoni Ionizzant*, Strambi, E., Ed., Roma, 1981, 9–39 (in French).
30. Lafaix, J.L. and Daburon, F., Diagnosis of acute localized irradiation lesions: review of the French experimental experience, *Health Phys.*, 75 (4), 375–384, 1998.
31. Leluk, V.G. and Filin, S.V., Possibilities and first results of quantitative blood flow evaluation in subcutaneous vessels in patients with LRI, in *Method of Flowmetry Set of Articles*, Echography J., Moscow, 1997.
32. International Atomic Energy Agency, Diagnosis and Treatment of Radiation Injuries Safety Rep. Series, No. 2, IAEA, Vienna, 1998.
33. Guskova, A.K., Basic principles of the treatment of local radiation injury, *Br. J. Radiol.*, 19 (Suppl.), 122–124, 1986.

15 Accidental Radiation Injury from Industrial Radiography Sources

Fred A. Mettler, Jr. and Jean-Claude Nénot

CONTENTS

Introduction 241
Causes and Characteristics of Industrial Radiography Accidents 243
Local Exposure 244
    A Case of Child Abuse 244
    Accident in Texas, U.S.A. 246
Local and Whole-Body Exposure 246
    Accident in Iran, 1996 246
    Accident in Algeria, 1978 248
Whole-Body Exposure 253
    Accident in Morocco, 1984 253
    Accident in the Ukraine, 1988 to 1991 257
Summary 258
References 258

INTRODUCTION

Industrial radiography should not be confused with the very large, fixed industrial sterilization facilities that usually use cobalt-60, which have already been discussed in Chapter 13. Industrial radiography devices are small and portable. They are used to make "X rays" or radiographs of metallic objects. They most commonly are used to look for defects in pipe welds. As such, they are common on oil and gas pipelines and in any type of construction site. The device has a small but very intense radioactive source that is housed in a portable metal-shielded container. The radioactive material is usually iridium-192, but cesium-137 and cobalt-60 also have been used. The activity of such sources is usually in the range of 1.85×10^{11} to 3.7×10^{12}, Bq (5 to 100 Ci). The radioactive material itself is often in a shiny, metallic capsule and with its attachment is about the size of a pencil (Figure 15.1). Most sources do not have any warning label or indication that they are either radioactive or hazardous.

    The entire device is often called a "camera." In addition to the shielded housing, there is a tube attached to each end (Figure 15.2). The operator places the housing within a meter or so of the weld to be examined. Film is placed on the other side of the weld. The operator places the source tube end next to the weld and then unrolls the operator tube, which has a crank on the end. After the operator has extended enough of the operator tube to be a safe distance from the housing, he turns the crank, which drives a cable forward inside the tube. The cable is attached to the source and the source is pushed out the other side of the shielded housing into the source tube. The length

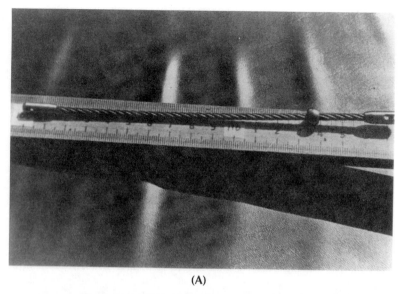

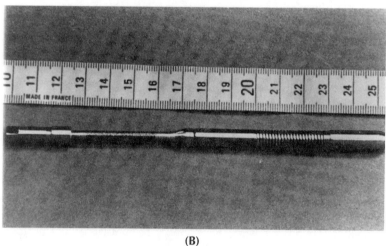

FIGURE 15.1 Typical ^{192}Ir industrial radiography sources (A and B). These sources can become unhooked from the drive cable. (From Collins, B.P. and Gaulden, M.E., in *The Medical Basis for Radiation Accident Preparedness*, Hübner, K. and Fry, S.A., Eds., Elsevier/North Holland, New York, 1980, 198. With permission.)

of time the source remains out of the housing is dependent upon the thickness of the metal weld, but exposures are usually several minutes. When the exposure is complete, the operator reverses the crank and the cable is supposed to pull the source back into the housing. The operator is supposed to check that the source has been returned to the shielding by using a Geiger counter and making radiation measurements.

The dose rate from industrial radiography sources can be extremely high. For example, the surface dose rate from a 3.7×10^{11} Bq (10 Ci) iridium-192 source is 81.3 Gy/min, and at 1 and 3 cm deep in tissue the dose rates are 4.3 and 5.5 Gy/min, respectively. The surface dose rate is not only due to the radionuclide emissions themselves, but also to electron production in the stainless steel capsule wall. The number of such devices worldwide is unknown, but is at least in the tens of thousands. In the United States alone there are at least 200 reports annually of stolen or lost radioactive sources. There also appears to be an illicit trade in these cameras and

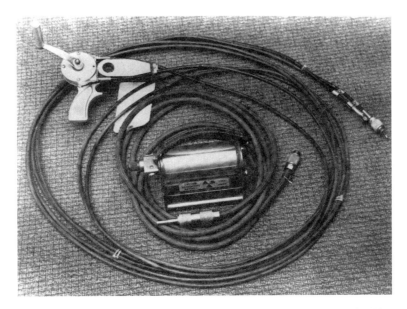

FIGURE 15.2 Typical industrial radiography "camera." (From Collins, B.P. and Gaulden, M.E., in *The Medical Basis for Radiation Accident Preparedness*, Hübner, K. and Fry, S.A., Eds., Elsevier/North Holland, New York, 1980, 198. With permission.)

their radioactive sources. Many governments have no idea how many of these devices exist in their countries.

CAUSES AND CHARACTERISTICS OF INDUSTRIAL RADIOGRAPHY ACCIDENTS

Industrial radiography accidents have several typical causes:

1. Operator error. The source becomes detached from the end of the cable and remains in the source tube and the operator does not check with a Geiger counter (Figure 15.3). In other cases the operator may knowingly pick up a disconnected source thinking that if the time of contact is short that there will be no harm (Figure 15.4).
2. Removal or loss of a source. In these accidents the source is stolen or lost and often not reported. Such sources are often found by persons who are interested in the "shiny, interesting" object and are not aware that it is radioactive.
3. Purposeful placement of sources with intent to cause harm. In these cases dissatisfied employees place sources in chairs of employers, and the sources have been used to commit suicide[1] (albeit slowly). In at least one 1979 French case, an executive of a nuclear fuel treatment plant found three radioactive sources under his automobile seat.

Clinical manifestations of industrial radiography accidents fall into three categories:

1. Local injury only. These accidents occur when a source is handled or is in very close proximity for a short period of time (several minutes). Typically these injuries are to the hands.
2. Local with whole-body injury. This occurs when a source is in close proximity to the body for an extended period of time (usually one to several hours). In these accidents, the source is usually placed in a pants or shirt pocket and remains there long enough to

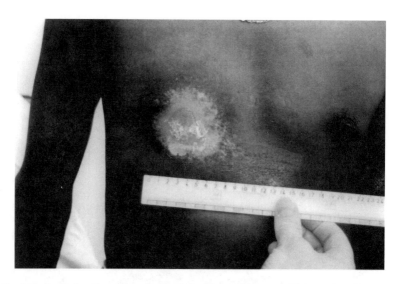

FIGURE 15.3 Localized chest burn from industrial radiography source. This worker did not realize that the source had become disconnected or that it remained in the source tube. He hung the source tube around his neck for 15 min while climbing down from a construction site. At that time, he experienced nausea and vomiting. This picture is approximately 30 days postexposure. Skin grafting was required.

cause a very severe local injury and enough whole-body exposure to cause bone marrow depression and symptoms such as local pain, nausea, vomiting, and sometimes diarrhea.
3. Whole-body exposure. This type of accident results from placing an unsuspected source in a desk or somewhere in the home and remaining there for days or weeks. Persons in the vicinity who have never handled the source receive high dose chronic exposure and often develop bone marrow depression. They typically present with fatigue, bruising, petechiae, bleeding, and, sometimes, gastrointestinal complaints.

Several cases of each type of accident are presented below and two accidents with severe local and whole-body injury are discussed in detail in Chapters 16 and 17. A number of other such accidents in China are discussed in Chapter 8.

LOCAL EXPOSURE

A Case of Child Abuse

A case of child abuse involving industrial radiography sources has been reported by Collins and Gaulden.[2] In this particular instance, a divorced petroleum engineer had intermittent custody of his two sons. He had possession of at least a 37 GBq (1 Ci) cesium-137 source used for oil and gas well logging. The dose rate at contact for such a source is approximately 5 Gy/min. One of the engineer's sons was subjected to various occasions in which "shiny silver pellets" were in the earpieces of headphones that he was told to wear, in a pillow he was told to use, and in a sock he found on his bed. It was also assumed that while under sedation, he was exposed at other times of which he was unaware.

He was first seen by a family physician for what appeared to be bruises and reddish-brown blisters. These were assumed to be infections, but over succeeding weeks and months, new lesions appeared on the medial aspects of the thighs, right ankle, right hand, and left side of his forehead. He was seen again by the family physician because epilation was noted on the left side of his head.

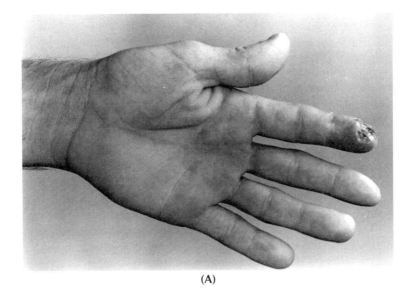

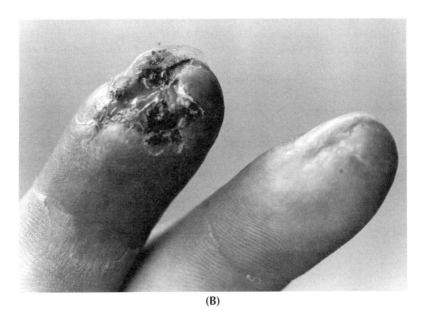

FIGURE 15.4 (A) Long-term radiation effects on the left hand as a result of picking up an industrial source for about 1 min. This was a late ischemic and infected lesion that occurred 18 months postexposure after the initial lesion had healed. Amputation of the distal phalanx was necessary. (B) Closeup shows deformity of third distal phalanx as well with atrophic skin and loss of the normal fingerprint pattern.

Over the next 6 months, persistent, ulcerating lesions of the right thigh kept the child out of school. A psychiatrist considered the diagnosis of neurodermatitis as a result of the conflict between the parents. Finally, after more than a year, a plastic surgeon recognized the lesions as radiation necrosis. Both testes had been effectively destroyed, and the boy was functionally castrated. Ultimately, the father was prosecuted.

Accident in Texas, U.S.A.

A 32-year-old industrial radiographer presented with skin changes involving the distal aspects of the first three digits of both hands. There was deformity of the left distal third digit and ulceration of the distal second digit. The patient had been an industrial radiographer for approximately 10 years.

Approximately 2 years prior to presentation, the patient had knowingly handled an industrial radiography camera in which the 3.1×10^{12} Bq (85 Ci) iridium-192 source had become disconnected from the cable and remained in the source tube. He knew the source was there, but elected to pick it up and reconnect it to the cable, thinking that if time were short there would be no hazard. He noted erythema and blistering of the first three digits of the left hand 2 to 4 weeks postexposure. His fingernails came off 4 to 5 weeks post exposure. He did seek medical attention, but was told by several physicians that this was not a radiation injury. Healing occurred over the next 1 to 3 months.

Approximately 18 months after exposure, the distal second digit became ulcerated and did not heal over the next 6 months. Finally, the patient sought medical care again. The ulceration was clearly visible as were skin thinning and loss of the normal fingerprint pattern (Figure 15.4). A radiograph of the hand revealed a lytic destructive lesion of the bone in the distal phalanx. Three-phase radionuclide bone scanning was performed and demonstrated little blood flow to the area. As a result, amputation of the distal phalanx was performed and pathological examination revealed both osteonecrosis as a result of radiation injury and concurrent osteomyelitis. The lesion healed satisfactorily after surgery. The main issue in such cases is to determine where the blood flow remains adequate for a satisfactory surgical margin. This unfortunately is a rather common example of initial misdiagnosis and late presentation of a local radiation injury.

LOCAL AND WHOLE-BODY EXPOSURE

The scenario that corresponds to this type of accident is stereotyped:

1. An iridium source belonging to a foreign company disappears in a country where safety regulation is weak or nonexistent.
2. The source stays in a house for several weeks and delivers protracted doses to various family members.
3. The injuries are not recognized as related to the source.
4. Some individuals die at home and/or are hospitalized without any causal recognition of the diseases.
5. And, finally, by chance the radiological origin of the injuries is evoked and results in discovery of the source.

Therefore, the reported number of accidents with similar causes is probably much smaller than the real number. This fact is rather serious, since this kind of accident often results in severe effects to several individuals.

Accident in Iran, 1996

The accident occurred on the night of July 23, 1996. Industrial radiography was being performed on the welds of a boiler using a 1.85×10^{11} Bq (5 Ci) iridium-192 source. The radioactive source became detached from the cable, fell to the floor, and was left unnoticed. The next morning, a worker saw the metallic object, picked it up, and put it in the right breast pocket of his coveralls. Several times he took it out to look at it. An hour and a half later, he began to experience dizziness, nausea, weakness, and a burning feeling in his chest. He related the symptoms to the source in his pocket and went back and put the source on the floor. A summary of the clinical findings is shown in Table 15.1.

The patient spent 2 days at home, during which the dizziness and nausea improved, but the burning sensation in his chest remained. He then was transported to a medical facility and was noted to have erythema on the right side of his chest and upper abdomen. Over the next few days, the chest lesion continued to expand with erythema, and a 30 × 15 cm area of moist desquamation appeared. By day 6, there was erythema over the right elbow, and by day 10, erythema and blistering

TABLE 15.1
Patient Z Iran Accident; Estimated Whole-Body Dose 2 to 5 Gy

Findings	Postexposure	Value
Initial incapacitation	No	
Initial hypotension	No	
Nausea	1½ h, <24 h duration	
Vomiting	No	
Diarrhea	No	
Headache	No	
Weakness	1½ h, <24 h duration	
Fever	No	
Edema		
Blistering	Yes, day 6–10 hand	
White blood cells		
	1 day	18,300
	2 days	
	4 days	6,500
	8 days	2,800
	16 days	3,500
	24 days	800
	32 days	2,600
	40 days	4,900
Lymphocytes		
	1 day	NR
	2 days	NR
	4 days	260
	8 days	600
	16 days	490
	24 days	300
	32 days	670
	40 days	1,000
Thrombocytes	1 day	222,000
	2 days	NR
	4 days	232,000
	8 days	204,000
	16 days	79,000
	24 days	15,000
Epilation		
Death	No	

Note: NR = not reported.

on the palm of the left hand. By day 18, there was a tense bulla on the palm of the left hand, and note was made of decreasing white cell and platelet count. Cytogenetic dosimetry was consistent with a whole-body dose of 4 to 5 Gy, while the patient's symptomatology would suggest a somewhat lower value. On day 24, the patient was transferred to Paris for further management at the Curie Institute. The patient had severe pain from the skin lesions as well as total loss of epidermis in a 30 × 15 cm area of the right anterior chest wall with necrosis at the edge. Chest radiograph was normal. The patient was treated in a reverse isolation room with platelet transfusions, intravenous antibiotics, and intravenous morphine. He was also given 300 g of granulocyte colony–stimulating factor (G-CSF) subcutaneous daily for 10 days beginning on day 25. The marrow subsequently recovered with this therapy.

On day 66, there was reepithelialization at the edges of the chest lesion, but none within the lesion itself, and the size was 23 × 15 cm. A graft was applied from the thigh to the chest lesion. The hand lesion healed with some scarring, but without functional impairment. The patient was transferred back to Tehran on day 94 postexposure. The graft remained in good condition $8^1/_2$ months after the accident.

Initial prodromal symptoms of nausea and fatigue suggested an average whole body dose in the range of 3 to 4 Gy. The lack of vomiting indicated that the dose was probably less than this. Results of the blood picture indicate a whole-body average dose of 2.5 to 3.5 Gy. The dose to the lesion on the chest is uncertain, but the fact that the graft was successful suggests the possible presence of a large component of superficial and only mildly penetrating radiation. The bulla that developed on the hand is suggestive of a skin dose in the region of 60 to 80 Gy.

Accident in Algeria, 1978

The Algerian accident was not the first related to an iridium source irradiating a whole family for several weeks before the source of the accident was recognized. In fact, the first such accident happened in Mexico City in 1962; a whole family died as a result of a 2×10^{11} Bq (5.4 Ci) cobalt-60 source, which caused the death of four people, including two children aged 3 and 10 years.[4]

In Algeria, on May 5, 1978, an iridium source of about 1×10^{12} Bq (27 Ci) for industrial gammagraphy fell from a truck on the road from Algiers to Setif. It was found 2 or 3 days later by two boys aged 3 and 7. The children played with the pencil-like object for a few hours. The 47-year-old grandmother confiscated the source in order to avoid any altercation and hid it in the kitchen. The source remained in the house for 5 to 6 weeks, where five members of the family were exposed under various conditions depending on time spent and location. In general, the men of the family were not exposed since they spent long periods of time outdoors and entered the kitchen only occasionally, while the grandmother and four young females, 14 to 20 years old, spent most of their time busy at home. The female victims stayed for many days at some distance from the source. Two of them (a pregnant 20-year-old and her sister of age 19) regularly frequented the kitchen and stayed at distances of between 0.80 and 1.50 m from the source; exposure lasted about 6 to 8 h/day. Two younger sisters, 17 and 14 years old, usually spent some time in the kitchen doing their homework. After 4 weeks, the eldest sister suffered malaise and decided to leave the house and go somewhere else. She was replaced by the two youngest, who were irradiated for 5 to 8 h daily. Moreover, the grandmother came frequently into the kitchen and often leaned against the shelf where the source had been hidden; thus she was very close to the source and her back almost in contact with it. It seems that none of the women touched the source. The dose rate was around 70 mGy/h at 1 m. Figure 15.5 shows the place in the kitchen where the source was stored and the dose rates as they were measured later when the dose reconstruction was performed on the site.

The two boys, who handled the source for several hours, rapidly exhibited skin injuries, localized on the mouth and both hands for the youngest one, and on both hands, buttocks, and

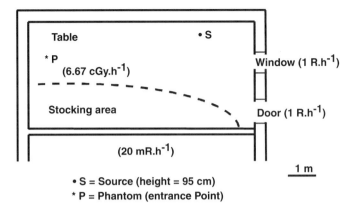

FIGURE 15.5 Map of the kitchen, showing the reconstruction of the accident. Dose rates are shown at places where victims were irradiated during their work in the home.

thighs for the oldest one. They also had a whole-body exposure, which was delivered in a short period of time and was not life-threatening, since it was at a moderate level and very heterogeneous.

When the operator reported the loss, the Algerian authorities decided to look for the missing source. Information was rapidly disseminated among regional medical authorities so that they could recognize potential radiological burns and/or radiation-induced hematological syndrome. Fortunately, a country physician heard of a family presenting clinical signs that might be associated with radiation. The local authorities were alerted and the source was located on June 12, i.e., 38 days after it fell from the truck. The victims were hospitalized successively in Setif and Algiers, and then transferred to Paris, to the Institute Curie, after various delays from 2 to 20 days. The grandmother, the 19-year-old girl, and the two boys came first on June 14, then the pregnant sister on June 18, and the two youngest sisters of 17 and 14 on July 2 and 5.

When they arrived in Paris, the clinical and biological findings since the onset of the exposure were unknown. The five whole-body-irradiated patients (the grandmother of age 47 and her four grandchildren) were in a bad general state, with prostration, anorexia, and nausea. They exhibited hemorrhagic and digestive syndrome, with severe mucous bleeding, ecchymotic suffusion, and purpura. In addition, the grandmother, who had her back close to the wooden basket where the source was hidden for several hours, had severe radiation skin burns over a large area.

The five whole-body-irradiated patients had profound hematological changes. For the four sisters, blood lymphocytes were 15 to 20×10^7, granulocytes 0 to 1×10^8, platelets 7 to 30×10^9, and reticulocytes 0 to $20 \times 10^7/l$.[5] The minimal values that the lymphocytes reached in the early period remain unknown. The bone marrow examinations from various areas, such as sternum and iliac spines, showed zero cellularity.

The grandmother showed a progressive deterioration of her general clinical state and a rapid aggravation of her skin lesions with extensive necrotic lesions on her thoracic and abdominal walls. She died on June 27, 2 weeks after the source had been found. Her death seems to have been caused by an hemoptysis related to both bone marrow aplasia and lung exposure at very high doses, complicated by extensive superinfected burns.

The two boys, who did not present signs of acute radiation syndrome and were in good general condition, had severe disseminated skin lesions.[6] The 3-year-old showed lesions of the mouth with lip and tongue ulceration, demonstrating that he had sucked the source, and had lesions of both hands with deep ulceration (2 cm in diameter) at the hypothenar area of the right hand and a much less severe lesion on the left hand. This boy had initially been playing with the source holder using it as a drumstick. The other boy, 7 years old, had also severe lesions on the hands, which were more symmetrical than those of his brother and affected the metacarpals and fingers. In addition, he presented with lesions of both buttocks and thighs, probably because he had placed the source in his school satchel, on which he sat from time to time.

To assess the severity of the exposure and its distribution within the body, biological dosimetry based on chromosome analysis as well as a physical reconstruction of the accident were performed. The chromosome analysis was difficult because of the lack of reference curves for protracted whole-body exposures. It was meaningless for the two boys who only received localized exposure. An aggravating factor for interpreting the chromosome analysis was related to the fact that the three youngest girls were given a total blood transfusion in Algiers. Even after the introduction of corrective factors taking into account the transfused lymphocytes, there was discrepancy between the final results and the severity of the hematological syndrome. It was concluded that the estimated doses could only be considered as the lowest values of the real exposures received by the victims. In addition, these estimates were expressed in terms of "mean dose," which has a limited value in the case of heterogeneous exposures. The preliminary evaluations based on dicentrics plus ring counting were expressed in "equivalent to acute homogeneous single dose": 3.7 Gy for the grandmother and around 4 Gy for the four sisters. On the basis on new experimental data on the effects of protracted exposure compared with acute exposure, a reevaluation 10 years later was performed and showed more realistic dose values for the four sisters: around 10 Gy for the oldest, nearly 20 Gy for the 19-year-old, and around 5 Gy or more for the two youngest ones (after correction for low-dose rate effect).[7] Abnormalities were found on the electroencephalograms: general disorganization of the alpha rhythm, spindles of diffused scattered waves, and graphoparoxystic abnormalities for the youngest girl. These findings favored the hypothesis of a global cumulative exposure of 6 to 10 Gy, combined with a heterogeneous exposure of the head higher to the right side.

As in any protracted whole-body exposure, the physical dosimetry was difficult and tainted with large uncertainties. These uncertainties included: the day the source was introduced at home, the source–victim geometry, which varied according to the housekeeping and homework activities of the girls, the postures and orientation toward the source (the grandmother was squatting for long periods with the source to her back while the girls were often standing, with the anterior part of their bodies facing the source), duration of presence in the kitchen throughout the day, and finally possible shadowing by other family members. A simulation was performed by a team of physicists, which permitted mapping of the doses for various distances and positions. Isodoses were then established according to the most likely positions and length of presence near the source. Figure 15.6 shows isodose mapping after the reconstitution in a phantom for two different positions, standing and squatting. For a mean distance of 1.25 m the total skin dose was about 25 Gy. The total mean bone marrow dose was estimated around 11 to 14 Gy.

Since nothing was known about the geometry and duration of exposure, the dosimetric estimation for the two boys' injuries was based on relative dosimetry weighted by clinical observation.[6] The shapes of the lesions provided information on the source position. The relative physical dosimetry for hands was obtained by measurements of dose rates to the surface of a molding obtained from a glove of adequate size. The depth doses were calculated on the basis of energy absorbed in tissues. Finally, on the basis of clinical experience (dose threshold for wet epithelitis and necrosis) and evolution of the lesions, dose estimation could be derived, and isodose curves could be constructed. Figure 15.7 shows the surface dose estimates for the youngest brother's right hand. These values are approximate and their interest relies more on the dose distribution in space rather than on absolute values. They were of some help for the surgical interventions that were performed later.

Despite the fact that each whole-body-overexposed patient was given several bags of freshly isolated cells of red cells and platelets daily, the critical period lasted for a period of between 30 and 60 days after the end of the exposure.[5] During about 3 weeks, the blood cell counts remained at levels as low as 0 to 4% of normal for granulocytes, 8 to 15% for platelets, and 0 to 0.1% for

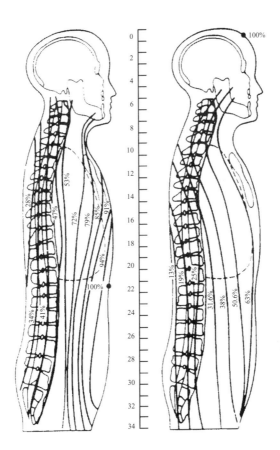

FIGURE 15.6 Isodoses obtained in a phantom after the physical reconstruction of the accident for two positions. On the left, facing and standing; on the right, facing and squatting. Source: iridium-192, 1 TBq. Distance source to phantom: 1.25 m.

reticulocytes. In contrast to the experience of acute exposures, the critical period in this accident was prolonged and necessitated a constant, long-term therapeutic effort. Maintenance of fluid and electrolyte balance was important. Liquid compensation often exceeded 5 l/day. One patient received a total of 222 l of various sera and another received a daily dose of about 500 mEq of Na^+, 120 mEq of K^+, and 650 mEq of Cl^-. In general, it was difficult to maintain potassium at a normal level. Nutritive requirements were satisfied by the administration of a daily total of 2000 calories.

Intensive care, anti-infectious treatment, and daily balance of the hematological deficiency were applied. The patients were isolated for 7 weeks in sterile rooms and asepsis controlled daily. Nevertheless, the four daughters developed local infections and septicemia, which necessitated major antibiotic and antimycotic treatment. They received hormonal therapy to compensate the adrenal deficiency induced by blocking the ovarian functions to inhibit menstrual flux, which was likely to trigger hemorrhage. One patient had a retinal hemorrhage; another presented a cataclysmic buccal bleeding due to a vessel ulceration. In addition, the patients presented aphthoid or ulcero-necrotic lesions of mouth and lips, leading in one case to severe feeding difficulties and inability to speak. For two patients (the 19- and 17-year-olds) the question of a bone marrow transplantation was raised, since the compensation treatment reached its limits of efficiency after a few days. Bone marrow donors were typed and kept on call. Because of a slight positive response, indicated by the reticulocyte counts, the procedure was not carried out. A major problem was raised by the pregnancy of the eldest. Before any decision about therapeutic treatment was made, the death of

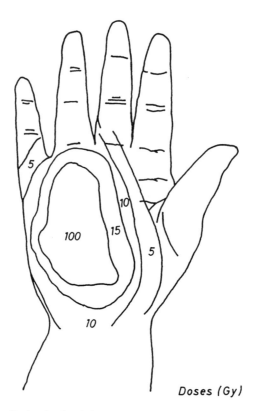

FIGURE 15.7 Isodose distribution in the right hand of the 3-year-old child. Doses were evaluated on the bases of (1) measured dose rates on the surface of a molding from an iridium source of little activity and (2) clinically evaluated doses at delineation lines of wet epithelitis and necrosis.

the fetus occurred during the hematological recovery period and its spontaneous evacuation occurred 2 weeks later.

The therapeutic problems raised by the two boys were surgical.[6] All efforts were devoted to avoid amputation as far as feasible. The clinical and biological findings were in favor of a limited amputation of the three last fingers of the right hand for the youngest boy, with a pair of pincers kept from the thumb and the forefinger. A more conservative approach was chosen and a graft was performed with a thick abdominal flap; amputation was limited to the fifth right finger. Results were satisfactory and the boy could use his hand a few months later. Some aesthetic surgery was still required. Similar treatment was given to the eldest brother, with abdominal flaps for both hands. His thigh lesions healed rapidly, but his buttocks and upper parts of his thighs showed necrotic evolution. Therefore, a local flap was inserted by rotation on the right buttock, which needed secondary successful intervention. On the left buttock a conventional skin graft covered adipose tissue of sufficient quality. Further evolution and results were good, except for a decrease in comfort on the left side.

The hematological recovery period started late with myelocytes and metamyelocytes appearing in the peripheral blood and progressed slowly before stabilizing at levels below physiological values, indicating the persistence of a long-term defect in hemopoiesis. The stabilized levels were only reached after 4 to 5 weeks. Reticulocytes showed a peak, reaching 140 to 280% of control. The eldest sister and her two brothers were able to return home after their hematological recovery and the complete healing of the surgically treated local injuries, which took more than 1 year. The long-term follow-up of the three other patients was possible since they stayed in France. One got married a few years later and gave birth to three normal children, the latest reported birth in 1995. Today, this patient is in good state, except for a previously diagnosed thyroid nodule. A medical consultation for the two boys was planned in the 1980s; unfortunately, in spite of a careful administrative preparation, they were rejected at the border because parental authorization was missing.[7] Since then, there has been a total lack of information on their health state, which might have been improved by specialized care.

WHOLE-BODY EXPOSURE

ACCIDENT IN MOROCCO, 1984

The accident in Morocco in 1984 illustrates the difficulties of accident recognition and of patient management, where exposure is unrecognized for long periods of time.

An industrial 6×10^{11} Bq (16.3 Ci) iridium source, used for evaluation of welding, disappeared in the night of March 18–19, 1984, and was rediscovered on June 26, i.e., 80 days later, which corresponds roughly to the radionuclide physical half-life ($T_{1/2}$ = 74 days). A man who worked at the site had taken the source and brought it home, probably because he found it attractive and potentially valuable. His house was situated in the Casablanca suburbs; it contained three small bedrooms. The first room, of about 10 m² (3.1 × 3.3 m) was used as a bedroom by the couple and their four children, 4, 5, 7, and 8 years old, who slept on mats; the second room was the grandparents' bedroom, and the third was reserved for visiting relatives. Figure 15.8 shows the places where the various members of the family slept in their bedrooms. A small kitchen and a hall were adjacent to these three bedrooms.

When the father brought the source at home, he placed it on a shelf near his bed. It seems that the source was not moved during the whole period before the accident was recognized. The first individual who exhibited signs of irradiation was the father, who was closest to the source and was directly exposed during his sleeping time. He was not exposed during daytime, except during weekends, since he was working outside and was away from 6:00 A.M. to 8:30 P.M. The oldest child was at school from 8:00 to 12:00 in the morning and from 2:00 to 5:00 in the afternoon, and stayed in the parents' room for his school work. During the day, the three other children stayed home or nearby and took care of animals; it is likely that they spent quite a lot of time playing outside the house.

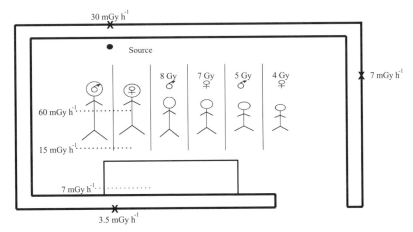

FIGURE 15.8 Map of the bedroom where the two parents and the four children slept. Dose rates are shown at various points in the bedroom. Dose rate values are calculated for a strength of the source of 500 GBq. Same calculations were performed at different periods to take into account the decrease in activity of the source.

On April 17, i.e., 1 month after the source was introduced into the house, the father started to have nosebleeds, nausea, vomiting, and diarrhea; he stopped working and stayed at home. Rapidly, he exhibited alopecia, limited to the head, and erythema of his right thigh; the skin lesions worsened within a few days and later on were described as necrotic by his relatives. He consulted a physician, to whom he did not show his skin lesions, and he was prescribed symptomatic drugs. The situation worsened until he was so weak that he had to stay in bed 24 h/day. He died 2 weeks later on May 3, i.e., 44 days after the beginning of his exposure. It seems that the main cause of his death was sudden and massive pulmonary bleeding, although this could not be confirmed.

The whole family was rapidly decimated.[8] Two children were seen by physicians as outpatients for vomiting, fever of 39°C, papular skin rash, and alopecia. Finally, the mother and her children were hospitalized in Casablanca on May 12 and 13 and were treated with antibiotics for an assumed typhoid state. The mother was the first one to complain about the loss of her hair. Rapidly confronted with the deep aplasia in all the children, resulting in frequent bleeding, the physician prescribed blood transfusions, which were unsuccessful. The youngest daughter died on May 14, the mother (who was pregnant) on May 19, and the three remaining children (two boys and one girl) on May 21, 23, and 24. All deaths occurred after voluminous bleeding.

During the course of the father's illness the rest of the family — staying permanently in the house but not sleeping in the room where the source had been displaced — consisted of the grandfather of 71, the grandmother of 66, and a cousin of 32. The grandmother spent a few hours per day in the source room, while she was taking care of her son when he was in bed in poor condition. The cousin, who was unemployed, spent many hours per day with his relatives, sitting on the bed near the source. After the father's death, two relatives, another cousin, and his mother came for the funeral and stayed in the house for a significant period. An aggravating factor for the latter cousin was that, because of a lack of beds, he slept in the deceased's bed. It is known that he died on June 25 and his mother later on, after they had returned home. The circumstances in which this woman had been lethally exposed remain unexplained. Consequently, the total number of reported deaths attributable to this accident is eight, but it cannot be excluded that some other individuals may have exhibited symptoms without attribution to their real cause.

Following an autopsy performed on the youngest girl (4 years old), several tissue samples were analyzed, such as bone from scapula and iliac crest, gut, liver, and trachea. The autopsy report concluded a possible poisoning. The cause of all these deaths was then reported to the Minister of Interior by the hospital management because a criminal origin was suspected, especially since a powerful rat poison had been bought by the grandmother some time earlier. It was only 2 weeks after the last child's funeral that the possibility of a radiological origin was considered. The national authorities requested help from France, and a team of physicists was dispatched. The source was located and put back under control on June 8, more than 11 weeks after it was introduced into the house.

In the meantime, the three surviving members of the family (the grandfather, grandmother, and cousin) were hospitalized in Casablanca, and another request for medical assistance was addressed to French authorities. Consequently, the three were sent on June 15 (8 days after the source was discovered) to Paris for medical care and hospitalized at the Curie Institute. At the time of hospitalization, the 66-year-old grandmother's physical status was relatively good (Karnovski index: 80), but with deep and persistent asthenia. She presented clinical symptoms of aplasia, paleness, and hematomas. In addition, she had a total alopecia, which indicated an overexposure of her head. Her hematopoiesis was significantly depressed, with less than 5000 reticulocytes, 100 polynuclears, and 30,000 thrombocytes/µl. She did not present with any infection or hemorrhage. She was placed in an isolated room with filtered and sterilized air. The 71-year-old grandfather was in good general state (Karnovski index: 100) and did not present any clinical and biological signs that could be related to irradiation; his blood counts were subnormal with a discrete thrombopenia at 100,000 to 150,000/µl. At the time his overexposure was questionable.

The 32-year-old cousin had scars from nasal herpes. His general state was very slightly impaired (Karnovsky index: 80). The hematological findings showed signs of moderate hypoplasia with slight anemia and neutropenia at 850/µl; platelets were normal at 200,000 µl. He did not show any skin lesions or digestive or neurological signs.

On the night of June 25–26, i.e., 17 days after the end of her exposure, the grandmother had a sudden, high-fever episode, which was due to a severe bacteremia, proven by blood culture and probably related to a central venous line.

As soon as the patients arrived in Paris, dose assessment was undertaken to evaluate the severity of their exposures and their distributions within the body. Distribution in time was more difficult to reconstruct, and the only reliable data were the total length of the exposure. Mean doses to the whole body were evaluated by cytogenetics and electroencephalographic examinations. The chromosome analysis was difficult because of the lack of reference curves for such protracted exposures. In any case, it was concluded that the estimated doses should be considered with caution. In addition, these estimates were expressed in terms of "mean dose," which is of limited value in cases of heterogeneous exposure. From cytogenetics, after corrections for low-dose-rate exposure, it was found that the grandmother had received a dose between 6 and 8 Gy, and the cousin between 1.5 and 2 Gy. Cytogenetics findings were difficult to interpret for the grandfather because of confounding factors including his frequent use of drugs such as hashish. From encephalographic responses the whole-body doses were evaluated between 3 and 5 Gy (prolonged heterogeneous exposure) for the grandmother and around 1 Gy for the two others; the cephalic dose was much higher, around 8 to 10 Gy, for the grandmother and grandfather. These results illustrate the difficulties of dose assessment when the exposure is prolonged and fractionated over long periods of time.[9]

The reconstruction of the various phases of the exposures received by these three persons could explain the differences in severity.[10] The most exposed person transferred to Paris was doubtless the grandmother. The duration of her exposure could be split into three parts, according to the severity of her exposure. She was moderately exposed during two periods of time: before her son got very ill and after he died, since she went in the room only for housework. In contrast, she was highly exposed when she looked after her son actively, providing him with food and taking care of his skin injuries. It was assumed that during the total duration of her exposure (82 days) she was standing up at a distance of 1.50 m (from source to entrance point) 4 h/day, most of the time facing the source; this led to an entrance dose of 8.3 Gy. During the 17 days when she took care of her son, she was sitting on the bed with her left shoulder at 0.75 m from the source; this led to an entrance dose of 5.2 Gy. Finally, during the same period, she was leaning over the bed with the back of her head at 0.30 m for 1 h/day; this led to an entrance dose of 10.8 Gy.

The cousin, who spent time in the room only when he sat on the bed during the critical 17 days, was assumed to be at 0.75 m from the source for 6 h/day; this led to an entrance dose of 10.4 Gy. The grandfather, who was involved neither in housework nor in visits to his son, was exposed only occasionally and his dose could not be evaluated.

Subsequently, the bone marrow doses were computed on the basis of these doses. The mean bone marrow doses were then evaluated, weighting each territory by the marrow percentages present. It was shown that 90% of the grandmother's bone marrow received more than 3 Gy with a mean dose of about 7 Gy and a cephalic dose of 12 to 14 Gy. Since distribution of exposure within the various bone marrow areas is determinative of prognosis and treatment strategy, a dose evaluation was performed for the main regions, based on the knowledge of age-related bone marrow distribution in the various parts of the skeleton. It was then expressed in terms of percentage of bone marrow in given dose ranges. Table 15.2 shows the dose range distribution for this woman. Schematically, 38% of her marrow had received doses between 6 and 12 Gy, and 62% between 3 and 6 Gy. The highest dose was to the cranium and the lowest to her left hip. It should be recognized that these data are only indicative, since the reconstruction was uncertain and the data on age-related marrow distribution in the skeleton vary from one individual to another. In any case, it was demonstrated that the overall exposure had been highly heterogeneous.

TABLE 15.2
Doses to the Grandmother's Bone Marrow
(in terms of bone marrow distribution)

Dose Range (Gy)	% of Bone Marrow
12–14	8
10–12	2
8–10	8
6–8	21
5–6	39
4–5	14
3–4	8

Note: These data were obtained by the theoretical reconstruction of the accident, taking into account (1) the time spent in the room where the source was located, (2) the various distances from the source, (3) the various positions of the victim, (4) the distribution of the bone marrow in the skeleton, and (5) distances from entrance points to bone marrow. The doses were expressed as doses at time of hospitalization, taking into account the physical half-life of iridium.

The cousin had much lower doses, with a mean dose around 3 Gy. The reconstruction was not feasible for the grandfather because of uncertainties about his behavior during his son's illness.

For the two patients who presented signs of bone marrow aplasia or hypoplasia, i.e., the grandmother and the cousin, conventional hematological parameters were complemented by bone marrow punctures, bone marrow cultures, ferrokinetic studies, and bone marrow scintigraphies, to evaluate the restoration capacities.[11] The punctures were chosen taking into account the dosimetric reconstitution. In bone culture assays, some colonies were selected for appreciation of the differentiation and maturation pattern in the clones. The results of the first punctures made on the grandmother were the following: the sternum, with an assessed dose of 8 to 10 Gy, showed a totally aplastic bone marrow, and the left iliac crest with 3 to 4 Gy showed for granulocytic and erythroid series a significantly higher colony-forming ability and a significantly lower number of progenitor cells than the normal range. The second punctures showed that the two territories had a higher colony-forming ability than normal and that the number of progenitor cells was still lower than the normal range in the sternum, whereas it was normal in the iliac crest. For the cousin, the results were lower than the normal range, but at a level that was not too disquieting for future prognosis. Studies on pluripotent hemopoietic progenitors showed that CFU-GEMM cloning ability was normal in all cultures. In the grandmother, committed progenitor cells were not detectable.

Ferrokinetics studies as well as scintigraphies were done 34 days after the end of exposure for the grandmother. The plasma iron turnover was slightly decreased, whereas the red blood utilization was normal. The erythropoietic activity was within the normal range in the pelvic area and lower in the sternum and dorsal vertebrae, which received 8 to 10 Gy and 5 to 6 Gy, respectively. Analogic scintigraphies with iron-59 did not reveal any extramedullary erythropoiesis.

On the basis of these clinical and biological findings, the prognosis was thought to be rather optimistic for the cousin and more reserved for the grandmother. The good clinical condition of the cousin, together with the results of the physical reconstruction and the bone marrow smears, indicated a spontaneous repair soon after his hospitalization. On the contrary, for the grandmother many parameters such as her age combined with the clinical conditions and the severity of aplasia did not allow a clear prognosis. Bone marrow cell cultures provided some argument in favor of spontaneous repair. This prognosis proved to be realistic, since restoration appeared slowly in the peripheral blood.

Platelet transfusions (60 units from day 12 to day 17 after the end of exposure) were required for the grandmother, who also received six units of red blood cell concentrates. Signs of bone marrow repair appeared on June 25 when fever decreased. Hematopoiesis was stabilized on day 50, although at a level lower than normal average. For the cousin, whose state raised no major problems, peripheral reticulocyte and neutrophil counts improved a few days after hospitalization. An increase in eosinophil count was then observed. However, 2 weeks later hematological repair was still incomplete.

The three patients were able to return to their country on July 13, i.e., 1 month after their arrival in Paris. At this time, their marrow was in a full restoration phase. Unfortunately, follow-up by the team involved in the medical management in France could not be performed; therefore, the history of these three patients is unknown, as well as the real number of victims, lethally exposed or not.

ACCIDENT IN THE UKRAINE, 1988 TO 1991

In the late 1980s a new apartment complex was built about 200 km southeast of Kiev. A family moved into a three-bedroom apartment. The mother and father slept in one bedroom, an older son in the second, and a younger son and daughter in the third bedroom. After living in the apartment for several months, the older brother began to develop petechiae and bruising. He was admitted to a hospital and found to have bone marrow depression. The cause was not identified, but after several weeks in the hospital he recovered somewhat and returned home. Over the next year, the same scenario was repeated several times and the boy always recovered when he was hospitalized for several weeks. The boy also developed an ulcerated lesion on his foot that did not heal well. About a year or so later he developed an osteosarcoma of the foot. Osteosarcomas in children almost always occur about the knee or shoulder, and this was a very unusual location. He subsequently developed metastatic disease and died. The osteosarcoma almost certainly was radiation induced.

The younger 9-year-old brother was then allowed to move into the bedroom. Within several months he also developed bruising and was hospitalized with severe bone marrow depression. Since the older brother had a similar picture, the physicians thought this might be an unusual hereditary form of aplastic anemia. Like his brother, he recovered when he was hospitalized and he also developed a necrotic lesion on his foot.

At the time, the children's mother thought that the problem might be attributable to Chernobyl, so she contacted the local health authorities. They pointed out that the Chernobyl plant was about 350 km away and that no fallout or elevated radiation levels had ever been reported in the area of the apartment during or after the Chernobyl accident in 1986. In spite of this, the mother kept insisting that radiation was the cause and, to placate her, authorities went to the house with a Geiger counter.

At the entrance to the apartment, elevated radiation levels were apparent. Ultimately, a 2.6×10^{12} Bq (70 Ci) cesium-137 industrial source was found embedded in the wall of the boy's bedroom located near the foot of the bed, about 0.3 m off the floor and about 1 to 2 cm deep in the concrete wall. How the source got there was never clear, but presumably it was dropped into the wall during construction and never reported or recovered.

The child was seen at the Department of Radiation Medicine at Hospital 6 in Moscow. His bone marrow had recovered somewhat and he was treated with a full-thickness graft for the foot ulcer. Several months later he had additional hematological problems and ultimately died from radiation-induced leukemia. This tragic accident shows that even if patients survive high acute effects from doses of chronic exposure, there is still a very real risk of subsequent radiation-induced neoplasms.

SUMMARY

Many of the thousands of portable industrial radiography sources are in the hands of people with minimal or no training. The sources in these devices are intensely radioactive, small in size, and commonly metallic in appearance. When the sources are lost, they often affect unsuspecting members of the public. The injuries from these sources are commonly misdiagnosed as insect bites, thermal burns, or marrow depression from drugs or unknown causes.

If the sources come into contact with the hands or skin a local burn with blistering and necrosis can result from only a few minutes of exposure. If they are kept for a few hours in pockets, there can be not only severe local injuries but also enough whole-body exposure to cause bone marrow depression. If the sources are not recognized and are kept at some distance for a period of weeks or months, they act as uniform irradiation sources and result in bone marrow depression, sometimes with fatal results. Dosimetry in many of these cases is a problem. The very heterogeneous exposure in these instances limits the use of biomarkers since they tend to give estimates only of average whole-body dose. Recently, computer programs using Monte Carlo code have been developed and have proved useful in local radiation injury accidents.[12]

REFERENCES

1. Vassileva, B. and Kruschkov, I., Suizid mit caesium 137, *Psychiat. Neurol. Med. Pyschol.*, 30, 116–119, 1978.
2. Collins, B.P. and Gaulden, M.E., A case of child abuse, in *The Medical Basis for Radiation Accident Preparedness*, Hübner, K. and Fry, S.A., Eds., Elsevier/North Holland, New York, 1980, 198.
3. Mettler, F.A., Monsien, L., Davis, M. et. al., Three-phase radionuclide bone scanning in evaluation of local radiation injury, *Clin. Nuc. Med.*, 12(10), 805–808, 1987.
4. Martinez, R.G., Cassab, G.H., Ganem, G.C., Gutman, E.K., Lieberman, M.L., Vater, L.B., Linares, M., and Rodriguez, H.M., Observations of the accidental exposure of a family to a source of cobalt-60, *Rev. Med. Inst. Mex. Seguro Soc.*, 3, 14–68, 1964.
5. Jammet, H., Gongora, R., Pouillard, P., Le Go, R., and Parmentier N., The 1978 Algerian accident: four cases of protracted whole-body irradiation, in *The Medical Basis for Radiation Accident Preparedness*, Hübner, K.F. and Fry, S.A., Eds., Elsevier/North Holland, New York, 1980, 113–129.
6. Jammet, H., Gongora, R., Jockey, P., and Zucker, J.M., The 1978 Algerian accident: acute local exposure of two children, in *The Medical Basis for Radiation Accident Preparedness*, Hübner, K.F. and Fry, S.A., Eds., Elsevier/North Holland, New York, 1980, 229–245.
7. Doloy, M.T., Personal communication, 1984.
8. United Nations Scientific Committee on the Effects of Atomic Radiation, Report to the General Assembly, Sources, effects, and risks of ionizing radiation. Annex G, Early effects in man of high doses of radiation, United Nations, New York, 1988.
9. Jammet, H.P., Problèmes posés par les irradiations accidentelles prolongées, *Bull. Acad. Nat. Med.*, 163(2), 48–160, 1970; Masson Ed., Paris, 1979.
10. Nénot, J.C., Surexposition accidentelle prolongée. Problèmes diagnostiques et pronostiques, in *Proceedings of a CEC Seminar on Medical Treatment Applicable to Cases of Radiation Exposure*, Luxembourg, February 19–21, 1986.
11. Parmentier, N., Nénot, J.C., and Parmentier, C., Two cases of accidental protracted overexposure: aspects of an extensive bone marrow study, in *The Medical Basis for Radiation Accident Preparedness II*, Ricks, R.C. and Fry, S.A., Eds., Elsevier, New York, 1990, 29–51.
12. Bottollier-Depois, J.F., Gaillard-Lecanu, E., Roux, A. et al., New approach for dose reconstruction: approach to one case of localized irradiation with radiological burns, *Health Physics*, 79(3):251–256, 2000.

16 Accident Involving Abandoned Radioactive Sources in Georgia, 1997

Ralf U. Peter, Hervé Carsin, Jean-Marc Cosset, Krishna Clough, Patrick Gourmelon, and Jean-Claude Nénot

CONTENTS

Introduction 259
Circumstances of the Accident 259
Initial Response 260
Clinical Course after Accident Recognition 262
    Clinical Findings 262
    Surgical Treatment 264
    Clinical Evolution, 1998 to 1999 265
Dose Assessment 265
    Local Exposures 265
    Whole-Body Exposure 266
Conclusions 266
References 267

INTRODUCTION

When Georgia was a republic that belonged to the former U.S.S.R., the Soviet Army had training camps in the country where troops were taught how to react in case of nuclear, biological, or chemical war. One of these centers was in Lilo, situated in a remote area about 25 km east of the capital, Tbilisi. This center covered approximately 0. 15 km^2 and was used for civil defense training, focused particularly on nuclear war or radiological accident. Soldiers were trained with radioactive sources, mainly for the purposes of calibration of survey equipment, radiological monitoring, and detection of radioactive material on a battlefield. When Georgia became independent in 1992, the center was transferred to the Georgian Army. It then became the Lilo Training Detachment of Frontier Troops where recruits received a 3-month course before being assigned to frontier surveillance. This course did not include any training in the radiological field.

CIRCUMSTANCES OF THE ACCIDENT

Review of the events shows that the Soviet Army left behind several radioactive sources when its troops left the site. On July 2 1996, a Georgian recruit exhibited skin reactions on the abdomen and a fever. Since this individual had received antidiphtheria and antitetanus vaccinations 2 days before, an allergic reaction to the vaccination was diagnosed. However, further lesions appeared on his hands and thighs, associated with general symptoms. The patient was admitted to a local hospital (Dmanisi hospital) on July 10; on July 17 (1 week later) he was transferred, without any preliminary diagnosis, to the Russian Military Hospital in Tbilisi.[1] The diagnosis "serum disease" was confirmed. Unfortunately, the patient's condition worsened and he was transferred in August to the National Antiseptic Center because of anaerobic abcesses of both thighs and both hands. He was discharged from this specialized hospital in December 1996 with skin and soft tissue defects of both thighs and finger contractures of both hands. In May 1997 he was readmitted in the Russian Military Hospital for a skin graft of the thigh lesion, which was unsuccessful. When he was discharged in August with a skin defect, the physicians considered a radiological etiology. Consequently, in October 1997, i.e., more than 15 months after exposure, he was sent to the National Antiseptic Center where the radiological origin was highly suspected.

In December 1996, i.e., 6 months after the first clinical manifestation exhibited by this patient, five other soldiers were hospitalized in the Research Institute of Skin and Venereal Diseases in Tbilisi. Since the relationship between the previous case and these patients could not be established, the origin was not detected. The patients, when transferred to the Russian Military Hospital, were diagnosed in April 1997 with a "polyform exudative erythema." They exhibited nausea, vomiting, weakness, and anorexia. There was then a severe deterioration of the skin conditions, leading to ulceration and necrosis. All presented with ulceration of their thighs or calves; in addition, one presented with multiple lesions, maculae-type, of the abdomen, back, arms, legs, and buttocks. Several local treatments were ineffective.

In May 1997, two additional soldiers, who suffered from nausea, headache, and weakness, presented with an erythema of the right thigh, which evolved toward ulceration and necrosis. At this time, their injuries did not justify hospital care; the patients were treated at home. Two other patients were admitted in June 1997 to Clinic No. 1 of the Tbilisi State Medical University, where they were thought to have a suprainfected "toxic dermatitis." One presented with an ulceration of the right thigh, while the other one had an erosion of the left calf and multiple macular-type lesions located on his left shoulder, thorax, abdomen, and back. The symptomatic treatment partially succeeded and the patients were discharged from the hospital, but because of relapses, they were readmitted in August 1997.

Although the role of radiation exposure in the development of the clinical signs and symptoms exhibited by these two patients was proposed in June 1997, the patients continued to be treated symptomatically. In August 1997, medical assistance was requested from the Institute of Biophysics, Moscow. Two senior officials from this institute went to Georgia at the beginning of September 1997, confirmed the diagnosis of radiation injuries, and provided the Georgian health authorities with advice on the medical care. It became evident that the exposure was fractionated and had lasted several months. The Georgian authorities started to search for radioactive sources and discovered a hot spot at the Lilo Center near the underground shelter with a dose rate of 45 mGy/h. An eleventh patient, who presented his first symptoms in October 1997, was hospitalized at Clinic No. 1 in Tbilisi with an ulceration of his right thigh.

In summary, 11 young recruits suffered from general and local signs of radiation injuries, which were reported to various physicians between July 1996 and October 1997. Since their medical care was the responsibility of different hospitals in Georgia, the link between them and the recognition of the cause were difficult to ascertain. Their exposure duration varied from one individual to another and some of them presented with multiple skin lesions.

INITIAL RESPONSE

When the radiological nature of the accident was recognized, the survey of the facility discovered several sources. Ten cesium-137 sources were detected with high dose rates ranging from 1.5 to

13,000 mGy/h at 1 m, corresponding to activity from 10 MBq to more than 150 GBq; two cesium-137 and one cobalt-60 source were also found, but the dose rates were very low since the sources were still inside their lead containers. In addition, about 200 night shooting guides with radium-226 were discovered at various sites at the center.[1] The cesium sources were normally locked onto a source holder, placed inside lead containers, and then in metal boxes. Although both the containers and the carrying box were sealed, nine sources were found outside their containers either fixed on the source holder or on their own.[2] This demonstrates that the metal box and the container had been forced open to remove the source holder. For the purposes of the military exercises the sources were buried at a depth of a few tens of centimeters (currently 10 to 30 cm). Apparently, some of these sources were found by young Georgian recruits and not identified as radioactive material. The first identified source was removed from a soldier's winter jacket; this source was the cause of the most severe injuries.

Following the medical examinations of the patients by the physicians from the Russian Institute of Biophysics, Georgia requested the International Atomic Energy Agency (IAEA) in Vienna to assist in the treatment of the victims at the beginning of October 1997. The World Health Organization (WHO) was then officially informed by the IAEA and asked to assist Georgia under the International Convention on Assistance in Case of a Nuclear Accident or Radiological Emergency. After numerous contacts among the Institute for Protection and Nuclear Safety, the Curie Institute in France, and the Georgian authorities, four of the most severely injured victims were transferred to Paris on October 22, 1997; two of them were admitted to the Curie Institute (Radiotherapy and Radiation-Pathology Department) and the two others to the Percy Hospital (Army Instruction Hospital, Burns Treatment Center).[2] A French medical mission went to Tiblisi on October 27 to assess the overall severity of the accident and reconstruct the circumstances and temporal distribution of the exposure. On October 29, the remaining seven patients were transferred to Germany, and admitted at the Dermatology Department of the University of Ulm (Armed Forces Hospital).

Detailed monitoring of the total area started on September 11, 1997, which was difficult because of lack of information about the sources. On September 13, three sources were found: one 22 m from the headquarters building on the soccer field, a second close to an open-air smoking area, and a third inside the left pocket of a winter jacket found in the storage room. The sources found on the soccer field and the smoking area were buried 25 cm, and the source holders were very corroded. The source removed from the pocket was a 12 mm cylinder with a 6 mm diameter. From the measurements made at different distances with and without a lead screen (no gamma spectrometer was immediately available), the presence of cesium could be determined. Other sources were found at a distance from the base, on or near the surface; a complete container was found close to the rubbish bins. A total of 250,000 m^2 was monitored.

Historical reconstruction of the accident was difficult because of lack of cooperation from the victims concerned and is therefore uncertain. The source found in the pocket was probably secondarily lost or neglected, then found again and placed in the pocket by the victim who exhibited the first injuries. The source was kept in its source holder for some time. The cesium capsule was then extracted and lost. After a delay, the duration of which is difficult to evaluate (related to the interval between the complaints of the first patients and the others), the source was found again by another guard and placed in the pocket of the coat. This coat containing the source was borrowed by several soldiers, who were exposed with different patterns. For example, the owner of the coat frequently wore it, and his left thigh, not far from the hip, was irradiated. Since these coats are long and wide, they are commonly used as blankets, especially during cold nights or when watching television. The coat was regularly borrowed by all other individuals of the group, which explains the very variable position of the lesions, even though the source remained for quite a long time in the same pocket.

CLINICAL COURSE AFTER ACCIDENT RECOGNITION

CLINICAL FINDINGS

When the victims (between 18 and 23 years old) were hospitalized in West Europe, their medical checkup showed that all 11 patients presented skin injuries at different stages (Figure 16.1), although the type and, particularly, the localization differed significantly from patient to patient and even in a single patient.[2] This difference applied as well for the whole-body exposure, which was expected to be heterogeneous in all cases. At the time of the checkup, none of the patients complained any longer of general signs and symptoms, as they did between the end of 1996 and the spring of 1997. Nevertheless, they complained about often intolerable pain that was localized around every radiation skin injury. Two patients, hospitalized in Paris, had extremely severe pain due to lesions situated on the hand, the left thigh, and the lower part of the thorax, and on a deformed hip, respectively. Most of the victims were in acceptable general condition. Since the injuries were related to a close contact between source and clothes, the lesions were not extensive; even when there were several lesions on the same patient (33 different lesions in one patient and 17 in another), the percentage of irradiated skin remained below or around 10%.

The patient who presented with 33 different lesions including necrotic lesions (3 to 4 cm in diameter) on an upper arm, the back, and a thigh constituted, by himself, a complete demonstration of various clinical cases of radiation injury. He was treated at the Curie Institute in Paris. The victim who first exhibited radiation lesions in July 1996 was more severely injured and was also hospitalized at the Curie Institute. He suffered from two necrotic lesions of both thighs, 10×6 cm and 8×3 cm, respectively, as well from several sequelae on the fingers (including necrosis of the distal part of the thumbs), which were blocked, and deep fibrosis (6×4 cm) on the lower anterior part of his thorax.[2] The two other victims treated in Paris were hospitalized at the Percy Hospital. They presented with the most extensive injuries. They presented their first signs at various periods, from December 1996 to May 1997, which implies that the evolution of their injuries lasted for different lengths of time. One of these patients, who had severe necrotic lesions of the right thigh, had been treated in Georgia with necrotomies without covering and presented with lateral necrosis 12 cm in diameter and an anterior one 2×3 cm; he also had three retracted fingers on his right hand. The fourth patient had a necrotic lesion 5 cm in diameter on his thigh. One injury, localized in the knee region, raised difficult functional problems.

The seven remaining victims, who were treated in Ulm, Germany, were less severely injured from the point of view of the number of lesions, their extent, and the degree of severity. Most of the lesions were ulcerous. Four patients had their lesions localized at the thigh level with ulcers varying from less than 2 cm in diameter to 5×6 and 7×2 cm; the ulcers of the three others were localized at the malleolus (3×2 cm), the upper arm (1.5×1 cm), the lower thoracic vertebra (2.2×2 cm), and the gluteal region (0.5 cm in diameter). Various diagnostic investigations such as magnetic resonance imaging (MRI), telethermography, ultrasound, X-ray, and bacteriological examination were performed.

MRI is a good means for appreciation of the musculoskeletal system since it allows detection of changes such as edema, inflammation, and necrosis. In 7 of the 11 patients, muscles and muscular fascia showed signs of impairment. For several patients, it was shown that lesions involved deep tissues. Modification of the bone marrow structure was found in one of the patients hospitalized in Ulm, whose irradiation was diagnosed only in May 1997.[1] In all patients, the lesions delineated by MRI were much larger than those that were clinically obvious. The MRI pictures, which were disquieting when the patients arrived in Paris, changed considerably after excision of the necrotic tissues; muscular lesions, attributable to fibrosis, improved notably. Telethermography, which was performed in the two patients hospitalized in the Curie Institute, demonstrated inflammatory processes and could pinpoint the extent of necrosis. Ultrasound (high-frequency 20-MHz sonography) was performed on the seven patients hospitalized in Ulm. It showed skin thickening with

Accident Involving Abandoned Radioactive Sources in Georgia, 1997

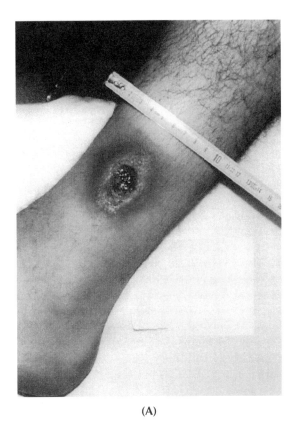

(A)

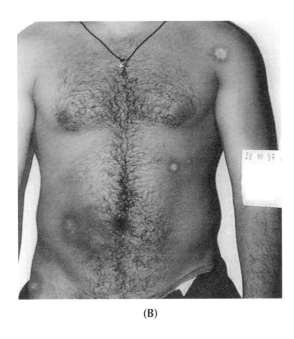

(B)

FIGURE 16.1 Localized skin lesions on the ankle (patient 2) and on the anterior chest and abdomen (patient 7) from carrying the abandoned sources.

fibrosis and/or the extent of injury to the subcutaneous tissues in three patients. Conventional X-ray examination was done in patients who presented with a possible bone involvement because of the depth of the ulcerous lesions; all patients exhibited normal pictures. However, the 11 patients were suprainfected, most of them with *Pseudomonas aeroginosa*, 7 of them with *Staphylococcus aureus* and some with various other bacteria. Antibiotic treatments were applied to the individual patients using conventional antibiotics.

Since the distribution of exposure was highly heterogeneous and many lesions were located near the pelvis, an exploration of reproductive capacities was done in all these young men. Azoospermia was found in seven victims with increased levels of follicle–stimulating hormone (FSH). Spermogram could not be performed in the first patient, but the increased FSH level in six of these patients suggested irreversible testicular damage. The seventh with azoospermia had a low FSH level, which favors a reversible injury. One other patient presented with oligospermia, which had probably developed before the accident (bilateral undescended testis complicated with sperm duct infection). The last patient, in spite of a large ulcerous lesion of the thigh, had a normal testicular function with normospermia and normal FSH level. All other hormonal findings were normal in all patients.

Although the exposure was highly nonhomogeneous, some hematological disturbances were found. Cell counts in peripheral blood were normal when the patients were admitted to the Paris and Ulm hospitals. These results demonstrated an amelioration when compared with the findings performed in Georgia, some time before their transfer to West Europe. At that time five patients showed moderate leukopenia and six developed lymphopenia of less than 50% of the normal value. Bone marrow explorations indicated a normal cell production and maturation of all cell lineages. However, there was a significant "dyshematopoeitic" cell proliferation and maturation activities, which demonstrated the hematopoietic recovery. No other abnormality was found.

The exploration of systems and individual organs, such as the cardiovascular and digestive systems, liver, lungs, and thyroid, did not reveal any abnormalities, except discrete goiters found at the ultrasound examination in two patients, who presented with skin injuries lesions on the upper arm and thigh, respectively.

SURGICAL TREATMENT

Topical and systemic treatment was applied to the patients but was not sufficient to solve the local injury. All had to be surgically treated to varying degrees. The four victims in Paris, after excision of the necrotic tissues, were treated with various techniques for skin grafting, depending on the severity of the cases: flap, autograft, xenograft, amplified skin autograft, and/or nonamplified skin autograft. For the first patient, a surgical reconstruction of the two thumbs and the left medial finger was performed.

The main issue, since radical amputation was not considered and all attempts were made to keep the legs, became the question of covering the lesions. Experience shows that physicians face two choices, either (1) a prompt graft, currently using a flap, may avoid severe and life-threatening suprainfection; however, the risk of graft rejection is extremely high and, in the most severely injured victim in this case, the size of one lesion forbade multiple successive grafts; or (2) a decision can be made to wait for all short- and medium-term radiation-induced processes to be stabilized before considering any grafting; however, a lesion cannot be left open for an extended time without unacceptable risks. A new technique, developed recently for the treatment of thermal burns using temporary covering of the lesions with artificial dermis with a silicon layer (INTEGRA technique), resolves these apparently contradictory conditions. The system allows the underlying tissues to recover and the fibroblasts to colonize the artificial dermis, to synthesize the intercellular matrix proteins, and to reconstruct the capillary system. It also provides a shelter against infection and moisture. It can be repeated as many times as necessary, and the transparency of the material allows direct visualization of the evolution. Since specialized units of the Percy Hospital are familiar with this technique in the case of severe thermal burns, it was used in the specific case of these radiation injuries. Only after everything seemed stabilized were autografts performed. This was the first time that this technique was used in the medical management of radiation injuries. Results were particularly good, in both avoiding complications and surgical results. The functional results were also better than expected, especially after grafting.

The seven victims in Ulm were treated with more or less extensive debridements and five of them received grafts; one had plastic surgery with synovectomy and muscle translocation (vastus lateralis). Six patients of the seven were able to return to Georgia at the end of 1997, i.e., about 2 months after admission. The seventh could not be released before June, i.e., 8 months after admission, because of radiation-induced synovitis and associated complications; he has since been free of any sequela.

The case of the four patients in Paris was more complicated; the patient with 33 lesions was released after almost 15 months of treatment. His last surgical intervention took place in January 1998; he underwent a total of 24 surgical steps, which included seven general anesthesias. He has exhibited a complete functional recuperation. Another patient had to stay after surgery for rehabilitation reasons, and the two others also remained because their lesions were still evolving and required further specialized medical care.

Clinical Evolution, 1998 to 1999

After their treatment in West Europe, the lesions of the 11 radiation victims could be considered cured, or at least consolidated. The latest news from Georgia, in summer 1999, i.e., 3 years after the initial exposure, does not fully confirm this optimistic prognosis. Since their discharge from French and German hospitals, almost all of the patients presented either recurrences or new ulcerous lesions.

The two patients previously hospitalized at the Curie Institute required additional operations. The patient with 33 lesions exhibited a new radiation ulcer on the right thigh, which was operated on in Obninsk, Russia, in July 1998; another new ulcer developed on his right shoulder, and will probably need surgical intervention. These events led to psychological depression. The second patient needed additional surgery (October 1998 to January 1999) because of new necrotic lesions in the inguinal region and on several fingers.

The two other patients treated in France at the Percy Hospital exhibited new lesions as well. The victim who had required the most intensive care had partial finger amputations (right hand) in Tbilisi in September 1998; afterward, a new ulcer appeared on his forefinger, which may require amputation in the future. The second patient developed an ulcerous lesion on his grafted area on his right thigh; this lesion was excised in Obninsk in April 1999.

Three of the seven patients previously treated in Ulm exhibited new or recurrent lesions after their return to Georgia. The recurrent ulcers required surgical intervention in July 1999: on the left malleolus for the first patient, on the right thigh for the second patient, and on the left shoulder for the third patient (previously treated in a conservative way). In addition, the first patient exhibited a new ulcer on the right malleolus. The four other patients treated in Germany showed neither recurrence nor new lesions. The psychological status of the seven patients was considered normal.

DOSE ASSESSMENT

Local Exposures

The local doses could not be estimated by means of a physical reconstruction with source and phantom because of the lack of information on the time and spatial distribution of the exposure in each individual. Nevertheless, a reconstruction was carried out by coupling the photon transport simulation with the clinical observations, on the assumption that the borders of the necrotic lesions had received about 25 Gy. Since distances between source and skin surface remained unknown, different values (3, 10, and 20 mm) were introduced in the model. The source dimensions were taken from the source found in the pocket: 6 × 12 cm. For example, the Monte Carlo method of dose reconstruction showed that, for one patient who presented a necrotic lesion, 5 cm in diameter, on the right thigh (Percy Hospital, Paris), the dose was estimated to be 150 Gy at the center of the lesion for a distance of source to skin surface of 1 cm.[2] The skin dose drastically decreased with the distance, and the deep dose gradient was very steep. The bone dose fell to approximately 4 Gy; the dose to the femoral artery was around 2 Gy. With the same hypothetical parameters, the surface dose decreased very quickly with distance: at 7 cm from the source, the dose was reduced by a factor of about 10 to 40, and the dose to the region of the hip joint by a factor of about 1500, resulting in a dose of about 25 mGy. This calculated reconstruction allowed the lesions shown by MRI imaging to be put into perspective. It demonstrated that doses were in fact lower than suggested by MRI. Consequently, surgery was directed more by clinical findings than by MRI images.

In accidents that are recognized only after long periods of time when lesions are in their ultimate phases of evolution, this type of reconstruction is not of major interest to the clinician who deals with skin and immediately underlying tissues. In contrast, it may be of great significance for some long-term injuries of deep essential tissues, such as big arteries (in the above-described case, prognosis on the femoral artery was fundamental).

WHOLE-BODY EXPOSURE

For all patients, the evaluation of the total-body dose is also of little value since the source was always at a short distance from the victim's body surface, resulting in nonuniform exposures. All exposures were also highly protracted, and the length of exposures varied from one patient to another. The first victim who exhibited injuries probably had the shortest exposure: from May to June 1996. The ten others were exposed from December 1996 to April 1997, at different degrees, as shown by the tentative historical reconstruction. Dose assessment based on cytogenetic investigations such as scoring unstable chromosome aberrations can only provide a "mean dose" and reference curves related to acute exposures. A weighing factor that is difficult to evaluate must be introduced for extrapolation from acute to prolonged exposure. Even so, scoring chromosome aberrations was performed by French and German biologists using the same techniques. At least 500 metaphases were analyzed, depending on the number of aberrations (dicentrics, rings, and excess acentrics) found. Recomputation was done to account for the protraction of exposure. Mean doses, after this correction, range from less than 1 Gy to near 6 Gy, received during several weeks for a few hours per day.[1] From the distribution of the aberrations, which follows Poisson's law only when the exposure is homogeneous, it was possible to confirm that exposures were nonuniform, especially for three patients, i.e., the two patients in the Curie Institute and one who was treated in Ulm (lesions in the back and buttock).

Electron spin resonance (ESR) dosimetry provides valuable information on the distribution of exposure, when performed at various sites. In these cases, ESR was performed on tooth enamel of eight patients at the Institute of Biophysics, Moscow; therefore, the dose could only be assessed at the head level and did not provide any information on the spatial distribution of exposure. Results were corrected from data obtained from radiological examination of the head and background levels. Doses were estimated between 0.1 and 4.5 Gy, the higher value being for the second patient hospitalized at the Curie Institute.

CONCLUSIONS

Although there is a lack of detailed information on the real history and chronology of the exposure, it may be certain that all patients, except the first one who exhibited lesions in May and June 1996, developed skin reactions of varying severity between April and August 1997. Most of the patients had been in the army since November 1996, except the first, who has recruited in November 1995. Consequently, it can be assumed that duration of exposure lasted from a minimum of 2 months to more than 300 days in a single case. When the skin injuries started to develop, the patients additionally complained of general signs such as nausea, vomiting, anorexia, weakness, which can be related to whole-body exposure. After a few months these general symptoms vanished without special treatment, but the skin symptoms worsened severely, reaching a critical point in October 1997.

When the patients were hospitalized in France and Germany in October 1997, the time elapsed since the patients' removal from the radiation exposure was between 2 and 14 months. The only remaining clinical signs of their whole-body exposure was azoospermia for 8 of them; elevated FSH indicated a severe impairment of their reproductive systems.

It cannot be excluded that other individuals have been exposed. For instance, the mother of one of the patients who presented up to 33 radiation lesions confirmed that she cleaned her son's jacket, while the son categorically denied having taken the jacket home with him. Since he was not cooperative during the military inquiry that followed the recognition of the accident (for example, he denied having picked up any object resembling a radiation source and refused to put on the jacket during the reconstruction of the accident), the question of the possible participation of sources other than the one found in the pocket is impossible to answer. Nevertheless, the accident sequences and the lesion localizations are not inconsistent with a unique source in a coat worn and/or used as a blanket by several soldiers.

In addition, it is not possible to be certain that all sources — hidden, buried, or lost — have been found and put in a safe position. Other sources could be hidden and remain unknown in neighboring villages or in a family of any one of the frontier guards who spent time at the center since 1992.

The main lessons learned from this accident and its management are the following:

1. This accident can be considered as a reference accident: for the first time, radiation accident victims received acute, fractionated (during a long period of time), and multiple exposures.
2. For the first time, MRI was used as a diagnostic and prognostic means for radiation injuries and could delineate deep lesions; it demonstrated that this technique provides a realistic picture of inflammatory processes, but shows lesions that cover a larger volume than the ones with a severe long-term evolution.
3. It was also the first time that artificial skin was used to cover lesions caused by radiation temporarily; it proved that it not only helps the favorable evolution of the injuries, providing the best conditions for further grafting, but it also has a favorable influence on the functional impairment especially when joints are involved.
4. In this accident, where victims were treated in foreign countries, a real and beneficial follow-up has not been feasible, probably because of communication difficulties. This deficiency in follow-up is detrimental both for the patients and for the lessons that can be derived from this exceptional event and that would be beneficial for other patients. It may be hoped that the situation will improve in the future to the benefit of patients and of knowledge.

REFERENCES

1. International Atomic Energy Agency, The Radiological Accident in Tbilisi, in press, 2000.
2. Gourmelon, P., Multon, E., Cassagnou, H., and Bottolier-Depois, J.F., Preliminary Report on the External Irradiation Accident of the Lilo (Georgia) Training Center, Report DPHD/9705, Institut de Protection et de Sûreté Nucléaire, France, 1997.

3. Gourmelon, P., Dose assessment in the Georgian accident and new therapeutic approach in the treatment of the cutaneous syndrome, in *Diagnosis and Treatment of Radiation Injuries, International Conference Organized by EC, DOE, IPSN and EUR*, 30 August–3 September, Rotterdam, the Netherlands, 1998.

17 Localized Irradiation from an Industrial Radiography Source in San Ramon, Peru

Mayer Zaharia, Luis Pinillos-Ashton, Ceasar Picon, and Fred A. Mettler, Jr.

CONTENTS

Introduction 269
Medical Care during the First 30 Days 270
Dose Estimates 270
Later Medical Care 273
Summary 273

INTRODUCTION

The accident took place on February 20, 1999 at the Yanango hydroelectric power plant, which is located in the jungle of the San Ramon district, Junin Department approximately 300 km east of Lima. At approximately 3 P.M. on February 20, 1999, a welder (Mr. C) picked up a radioactive iridium industrial radiography source with his right hand and placed it in his back right pants pocket. He was wearing loose-fitting denim jeans. He indicated that he continued to work, spending much of the time in a 2 m diameter pipe and claims that he was sitting for at least 3 of the next 6 h. About 9:00 P.M. he felt pain in the back of his right thigh. He left work at approximately 10:00 P.M. and took a minibus home. The ride lasted about 30 min.

At home he complained to his wife about the pain and she looked at his posterior right thigh and noted erythema. He took off his pants and placed them on the floor. He sought the advice of a local doctor who told him he had an "insect bite" and to put hot compresses on the area. His wife meanwhile spent about 20 to 30 min squatting/sitting on his pants while she breast-fed their 1½-year-old child. Two other children were at home, a girl of 10 and a boy of 7.

After discussing his pain with his wife, Mr. C indicated that he remembered the source in his pants pocket and took it with his right hand and carried it to the bathroom, which was outside the house. At the hydroelectric facility, radiographers noted that their camera was no longer taking pictures of the welds and noted that the source was missing. They initiated a search and went to the houses of the workers to search for the source.

Mr. C indicated that he noted some mild nausea at about 9:00 P.M. but that he never vomited. He had a normal stool at 10:00 P.M. and a slightly loose stool at 11:00 P.M. He never had what he would describe as diarrhea. At approximately 1:00 A.M. on February 21, 1999, plant staff came to Mr. C's house and questioned him about a "dangerous" radioactive source. He told them that he had the source and he went to the outside bathroom, wrapped the source in a piece of paper (since he had been told it was dangerous and he should not touch it) and carried it with his right hand to the front door. He estimated that in total he had handled the source with his right hand for about 4 to 5 min. The staff of the plant notified the Peruvian nuclear regulatory authorities, which had Mr. C transferred by vehicle to Lima. He was admitted to the National Institute for Neoplastic Diseases, which is the national center for treatment of radiation accidents.

MEDICAL CARE DURING THE FIRST 30 DAYS

The patient was initially examined at the National Cancer Institute Hospital on February 21 at 6:00 P.M. (approximately 18 to 20 h postexposure). At that time, he was noted to have an area of discrete erythema on his right upper posterior thigh. There was no evidence of lesions on his right hand. He was immediately begun on a course of Ciprofloxazin (500 mg/12 h) and dexamethasone (4 mg/4 h). He also received a Naprosyn-like compound for pain.

A drastic reduction in lymphocyte count (from 4000 down to $120 \times 10^6/l$) was noted by day 3 postexposure (Table 17.1). A blistering 4×4 cm lesion was noted on day 4 postexposure (Figure 17.1). The patient was switched to Clindamycin (800 mg/8 h), and the Ciprofloxazin dose was increased to 750 mg/12 h. By day 7, there was marked swelling of the thigh and edema of the cutaneous tissues visualized clearly on a computed tomography scan (Figure 17.2). This swelling almost completely resolved on day 9 postexposure, but there was progressive denudation and necrosis of the lesion (for complete temporal progression of the lesion, see Color Figures 1–4).*

On day 10 the superficial erosion extended and was surrounded by a hyperpigmented area. By day 15 there was a clear $10 \times 10 \times 2$ (deep) cm ulceration. The patient also had mild bone marrow depression. On day 27 postexposure the leukocyte count was 4100, neutrophils 3854, lymphocytes 205, and the platelet count 147,000. On day 23, the patient began to complain of numbness in the outer thigh and hypersensitivity of the inner part, and on day 25 the patient began for the first time to complain of some changes in his right fingertips. He described a change in sensation. By day 27, the patient had lost approximately 7 kg in weight. There was a 10×10 cm lesion that was about 2 cm deep (Figure 17.3). The subcutaneous fat had undergone necrosis and the underlying muscle was faintly visible. The lesion did not appear to be infected. The edge of the lesion was firm and dark. Hair was present on both legs. The hair was firm at 14 cm and farther from the lesion. There was only a little hair closer to the lesion. Whether the hair loss was due to radiation epilation or to the adhesive bandages was unclear. The patient's right hand showed only minor, if any, skin changes. There may have been minimal edema or swelling, but there was no desquamation or necrosis. Throughout the first 27 days postexposure he did not have a fever or evidence of petechiae or bleeding. By day 34 postexposure the neutrophil count had dropped to $1440 \times 10^6/l$ and the lymphocytes to $30 \times 10^6/l$, and the patient was given granulocyte colony–stimulating factor (G-CSF, Neupogen^R).

The patient's wife had apparently sat on the source that was in her husband's pants at home. She was examined and noted to have a 4×4 cm area of dry desquamation with 2×2 cm moist central desquamation over her sacrum (Figure 17.4).

DOSE ESTIMATES

Dose estimates were made by INEN (Peru) and IPEN (France) personnel. These were based upon the assumptions that (1) the source was 1.4×10^{12} Bq (36.75 Ci), (2) it was in contact with the skin, and (3) the contact time was 6 h. Patient-specific distances were measured from a computed tomography scan that was done on the patient on February 26, 1999. Since there was significant edema of the right thigh at that time as a result of the radiation injury, surrogate measurements were made of the left leg images. The provided calculations are shown in Tables 17.2 and 17.3.

---

* Color figures follow page 202.

TABLE 17.1
Hematological Evolution[a]

Day Postexposure	Leukocytes	Lymphocytes	Neutrophils	Platelets
1	7600	1500	6000	250000
2	7100	1064	5822	248000
5	6000	120	5880	252000
8	4200	42	4074	294000
10	3800	304	3420	280000
11	3700	111	3515	
13	5000	200	4650	239450
15	5200	312	4784	240000
17	6000	300	5580	232000
20	5200	52	5096	
22	5800	290	5220	
26	4100	205	3854	147000
31	3100	310	2759	
34	1500	30	1440	99900
35	2500	175	2275	152000
36	2000	340	1580	157000
37	4000	160	3720	109000
38	4200	420	3696	210000
39	3600	540	2988	156000
40	7900	474	7347	
41	8200	410	7708	112000
42	6100	854	5002	164000
43	8500	425	7990	187000
44	13200	792	11748	326400
45	18100	1810	15385	238500
46	11400	1368	9234	360000
47	7300	1460	5356	272000
49	8800	1584	6512	343000
50	25700	771	24158	377000
51	20000	2000	17400	469000
52	12100	1210	9922	562000
56	8000	1840	5840	685000
59	13400	1340	11524	666000
61	15900	1431	12879	698000
62	11800	118	11682	582000
66	13400	670	11524	520000
70	13900	556	12232	
72	13500	540	12555	696000
75	11200	1120	9856	759000
82	7100	1278	5467	629000
87	8300	581	7470	
91	8700	348	8178	468000

[a] Values of cells in 10^6/l.

As a result of these calculations, amputation by hemipelvectomy was being considered. The source strength ultimately was measured and the activity was found to be 9.6×10^{11} Bq (26 Ci). Scientists at the Institute of Biophysics in Moscow performed electron spin resonance dosimetry on the patient's pants. The preliminary result was that the dose was about 80 Gy to the thigh and

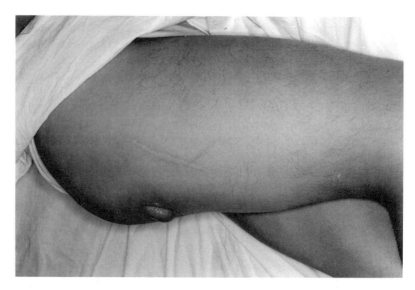

FIGURE 17.1 Blister formation on right posterior thigh at day 4.

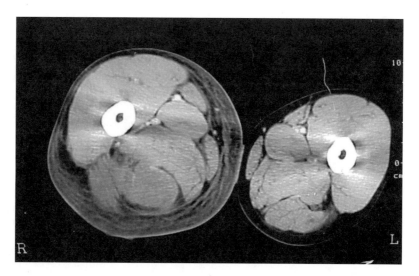

FIGURE 17.2 Computed tomography scan of upper legs showing marked swelling of right thigh with subcutaneous and fascial edema.

30 to 40 Gy to the lower part of the leg. The French Radiation Protection Institute (ISPN) also did computer reconstruction of local doses. Doses at the center of the lesion were estimated to be about 400 Gy, 30 Gy at 5 cm, and 2 Gy at 14 cm. At depth the calculated doses were 25 to 30 Gy at the sciatic nerve, 10 to 15 Gy at the femoral artery, and 0.5 to 1.5 Gy at the femoral head.

The biological findings based upon the size the initial blistering, the size of the current ulcer, the location of intact hair, and the hematological profile suggested that the actual dose may have been as much as five to ten times lower than calculated. The hematological parameters shown in Table 17.1 indicate mild/moderate bone marrow depression and suggest an average whole-body dose in the range of 1 to 3 Gy. As a result of these findings and because the patient was at the expected nadir of his hematological profile, it was recommended that surgery be postponed for several weeks and a full-thickness graft be considered prior to doing a hemipelvectomy amputation.

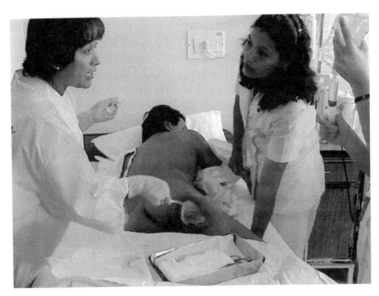

FIGURE 17.3 Ulcerated lesion on day 27.

LATER MEDICAL CARE

Although the patient had continued pain during the first several weeks, he had never needed narcotics, but after this, the pain became intense and was unrelieved by narcotics. Ultimate care of the patient depended very much on the local tissue doses. This was extremely complicated by uncertainties in source skin distance and duration of exposure.

By day 40 the patient's mild bone marrow depression was recovering, but the wound became infected. After terminating the systemic steroids the thigh lesion immediately became much larger and lesions on the hands with swelling became obvious (Figure 17.5). Desquamation was also now noted on the inner aspects of the thighs and the perineum. By day 80 the infection persisted, anemia necessitated transfusion, and the ulcerated area was 32 to 15 cm.

On day 91 postexposure, the patient was transferred to Paris for a "three-step" graft procedure. This involved ablation of the necrotic tissue so the sciatic nerve and femur were exposed and a porcine graft. Unfortunately, the wound became infected with methicillin-resistant staphylococcus, and the only remaining alternative was amputation of the right leg. The tissue from the right leg was discarded, and it was not possible to retrieve samples for electron spin resonance dosimetry to compare biodosimetry results with the initial dose estimates. After the amputation was performed, the patient returned to Peru. Approximately 7 months postexposure the patient was still having difficulties with radionecrosis of the perineum, scrotum, and testicles as well as fistula formation.

SUMMARY

There are a number of unusual aspects of this accident. While the calculated doses were higher than the biological and clinical indicators suggested, there were uncertainties in source location (especially with regard to movement of the source in the pocket) and there were uncertainties in the duration of exposure. In spite of this, there were major discrepancies in the calculated doses and the biological and clinical indicators. For example, a patient with an acute average whole-body dose of 15 to 20 Gy would have been expected to have diarrhea initially, possibly a fever, and much more significant bone marrow depression. One good explanation for the difference is the location of the source over the thigh and the marked inhomogeneity of the exposure. The bone

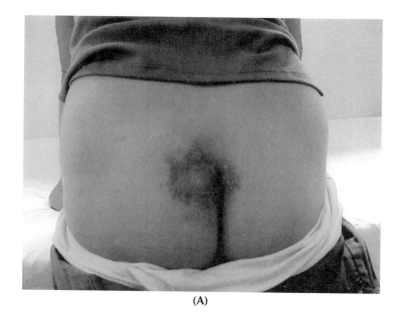

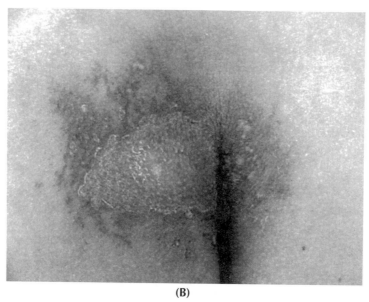

FIGURE 17.4 (A) Lesion over sacrum of patient's wife as a result of sitting on source for about 20 min. Photograph taken 27 days postexposure. (B) Closeup view.

marrow in the skull, cervical spine, and upper thorax would likely have had enough stems cells to prevent severe marrow depression. Another unknown factor is whether the exposure spread out over several hours substantially reduced the clinical effects.

The local tissue reaction also was less than expected. Of interest is that the patient was on dexamethasone until approximately day 30 postexposure. It was stopped at that time due to infection of the wound and the necrosis and radiation changes around the wound, perineum, and hands became much more intense. Dexamethasone appears to have played a role in decreasing the early clinical effects, but it does not seem to have affected long-term outcome. It is not clear whether

TABLE 17.2
Doses Calculated by INEN (Peru)

Organ	Distance (cm)	Dose (Gy)
Skin	1	9966
Soft tissue	2	2508
	3	1110
	4	617
	5	388
	6	265
	7	191
Femur and femoral artery	8	143
Soft tissue	9	111
	10	88
Gonads	18	23
Rectum and bladder	20	18

TABLE 17.3
Doses Calculated by IPEN (France) Using a Computer Phantom

Organ	Distance (cm)	Dose (Gy)
Skin	1	11752
Femur/femoral artery	8	188
Gonads	18	28.5
Bladder/rectum	20	21
Whole body		19.5[a]

[a] Inhomogeneous dose gradient.

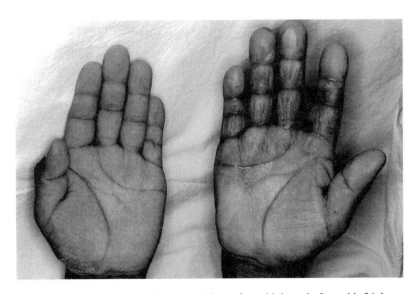

FIGURE 17.5 Changes of the hands that became obvious after withdrawal of steroids 34 days postexposure.

early hemipelvectomy would have affected the outcome, although it would have saved the patient a long, painful, and expensive hospital course.

This is the second case of local radiation injury in which cytokines were used. Most cases of local radiation injury do not have significant bone marrow depression. G-CSF was given at day 34 postexposure, but whether this had a beneficial effect is unclear. The bone marrow did improve, but this was at a time when spontaneous recovery would have been expected.

18 Exposure Analysis and Medical Evaluation of a Low-Energy X-Ray Diffraction Accident

Jerrold T. Bushberg, Thomas Ferguson, David K. Shelton, Gerry Westcott, Victor Anderson, and Fred A. Mettler, Jr.

CONTENTS

Introduction 277
Description of the Accident 278
Exposure Assessment 279
Clinical Evaluation 281
    Days 1 through 7 281
    Days 8 through 14 282
    Weeks 2 through 12 282
    Months 5 through 12 282
    Years 2 through 4 282
    Diagnostic Imaging Results 283
Recommendations for Evaluation and Treatment of Extremity Radiation Exposure 285
Key Findings and Recommendations 286
    Procedural Changes 286
    Training Enhancements 286
    Safety Audit Modifications 287
References 287

INTRODUCTION

X-ray diffraction units are widely used to examine and characterize the microstructure of materials for a variety of applications in industry, medicine, research, law enforcement, and many other areas. Accidents are rare. They do occur, however, and are primarily attributed to one or more of the following causes: failure to follow established safe work practices, lack of adequate training, unauthorized repair, or distractions in the work environment.

    This chapter will describe the sequence of events that led to an X-ray diffraction accident, the exposure assessment, the clinical evaluations of the radiation injuries, and recommendations for the evaluation and treatment for extremity exposures. Finally, key findings and recommendations to minimize the potential for future accidents are presented.

DESCRIPTION OF THE ACCIDENT

On the day of the accident, two graduate students were analyzing samples with a 6-year-old water-cooled Enraf-Nonius X-ray Diffraction Unit (Model FR-582). The X-ray tube utilizes a copper anode and a 0.2 mm beryllium window. At the time of the accident the unit was operating at 45 kVp, 25 mA, with the timer mode set at "continuous." The bright red warning light/X-ray production indicator on top of the X-ray tube column was illuminated (Figure 18.1).

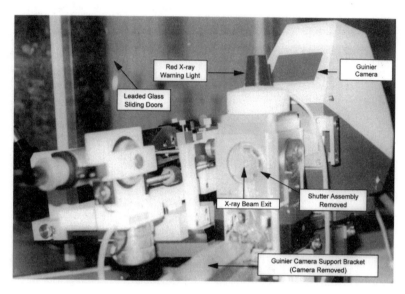

FIGURE 18.1 The Enraf-Nonius X-ray Diffraction Unit (Model FR-582) involved in the accident.

The students observed that the shutter status indicators (two small light bulbs connected in series) located beneath the X-ray tube column exit port were not illuminated, indicating that the primary shutter was not opening. The students informed the faculty member responsible for the unit of the situation. On two previous occasions the faculty member and students solved this problem by dismantling the unit to clean corrosion that had built up between the X-ray tube column exit port and the primary shutter. The first step in this procedure, as indicated in the manufacturer's instructions and the departmental safety protocol, was to turn off power to the unit. Given that the students had performed this cleaning operation before, the faculty member allowed them to clean the unit themselves. It is important to understand that, contrary to the manufacturer's instructions and the departmental safety protocol, the students had adopted the practice of expediting sample changing by bypassing the cabinet door safety interlock rather than shutting off power to the unit.

This practice may have led to a critical mistake when the students began the cleaning operation by bypassing the safety interlock using the key switch in the back of the unit. The Guinier camera was then pulled back from the secondary (outer) shutter. The secondary shutter then automatically closed. If the primary (inner) shutter had been open, it also would have closed at this point. During the removal of the Guinier camera, the warning light (X-ray production indicator) on top of the X-ray tube column was still illuminated and X rays were still being produced. However, the closed primary and secondary shutters were shielding the X rays and no significant radiation field was present.

Still inattentive to the X-ray production warning light, or that X rays were being produced, one of the students (Student A) proceeded to dismantle the secondary shutter, inner casing, filtration disk, and primary shutter checking for corrosion and cleaning each step of the way. Upon removing the primary shutter, the X-ray beam passed through the exit port (unshielded) creating an intense radiation field near the opening. Student A left the room to show the faculty member the corrosion on the primary shutter, while the remaining student (Student B) proceeded to vigorously remove the corrosion from the outer edges of the X-ray tube column exit port with a 3M scrub pad.

When Student A returned, Student B had finished the cleaning, and Student A began to reassemble the primary shutter to the exit port. While reassembling the unit, Student A inadvertently engaged the mechanical lever that connects the primary shutter to the shutter status indicators (two light bulbs) and the bulbs illuminated. Illumination of these bulbs indicates that the primary shutter is open and the X-ray tube is energized. At this point, both students thought they might have been exposed to the X-ray beam during the shutter disassembly and cleaning operations. The students consulted the faculty member, and they determined that there had indeed been an exposure. Shortly thereafter Student B informed the campus Radiation Safety Officer that an accidental radiation exposure had taken place.

EXPOSURE ASSESSMENT

Direct measurement of the exposure rates to the accident victims' fingers was not possible because of the extremely high X-ray beam intensity at the exposure site. Film badge and thermoluminescent dosimeter (TLD) studies could not be used because the vendors of that equipment did not have their dosimetry calibrated for the low-energy range (average energy of approximately 8 keV) of the photons encountered. Estimate of the skin entrance exposure rate required several steps including:

1. Measurements of X-ray beam exposure rates at varying amperages and distances from the X-ray beam port.
2. Defining the geometry of the X-ray beam at several locations using X-ray film.
3. Calculation of exposure rate at locations close to the exit port based on X-ray production theory and the use of correction factors determined from the exposure measurements.

The exposure rate along the central axis of the beam as a function of distance from the exit port is shown in Figure 18.2.

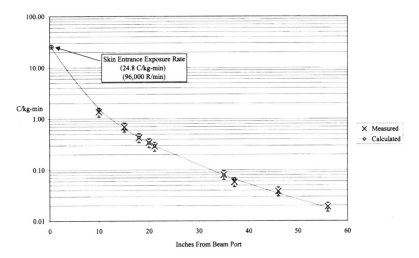

FIGURE 18.2 Measured and calculated X-ray exposure rates along the central axis of the X-ray beam as a function of distance from the X-ray port with the shutter assembly removed. Error bars are the 20% instrument measurement error. Divide C/kg-min by 2.58×10^{-4} to obtain R/min.

Kodak Type XV diagnostic film was used to define the area of the beam at various distances from the beam port with the shutters removed. The films showed that the beam was a well-defined rectangle whose area did not increase as the square of the distance from the exit port. At low electron energies, the generation of photons follows a severe angular dependence. The generation and directionality of X rays from a target is dependent on the target atomic number, target thickness, direction of electron beam, the electron energy (i.e., kVp), tube current, and the beam port construction, among other factors. At low energies, the X-ray beam is scattered over a wide angle with the peak intensity at approximately 90° to the direction of the electron beam.

The next step in dose rate determination was to determine the quality of the X-ray beam as it entered the skin. The X-ray output spectra for this system was available from the manufacturer. However, interviews with the accident victims revealed that the X-ray diffraction tube port had been cleaned while the individuals were holding a 3M scrub pad. The scrub pad was between the X-ray beam and the student's fingers. Therefore, the attenuation and beam hardening effects of the scrub pad had to be considered. The scrub pad composition was nylon fiber coated with aluminum oxide. The total density thickness of the scrub pad was measured and found to be 0.071 g/cm^2. Measurements showed that the scrub pad attenuated the X-ray beam by 45.5%.

It was determined that the position of the maximally exposed finger was 0.5 cm from the beam port (the approximate thickness of a moderately compressed scrub pad). The exposure rate at this distance was calculated without the attenuation of the scrub pad. The exact proportions of aluminum oxide and nylon were not available from the manufacturer (3M products). The reduction of photon flux by the scrub pad is dependent on the mass attenuation coefficients of nylon and aluminum oxide and the energy of the photons passing through the scrub pad. The density (g/cm^3) of the each of the above chemical compounds was multiplied by the mass attenuation coefficient (cm^2/g) to yield liner attenuation coefficients (cm^{-1}) and thus photon energy-specific flux reduction. The proportions of nylon and aluminum oxide were adjusted (while maintaining the total density thickness at 0.071 g/cm^2) until a mathematical model was obtained that produced an attenuation of 45.5%.

The dose rates at various depths in the finger were calculated using a reference model of the human finger[1] and a computer program to transport the X-ray spectra emerging from the scrub pad into the finger. Figure 18.3 shows the dose rate profile within the finger model. Because of the low effective energy of the beam (8 keV), the majority of the radiation was absorbed in the epidermis,

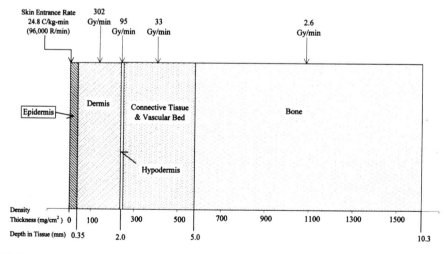

FIGURE 18.3 Dose rate estimates for the maximally exposed finger of Student A, calculated as a function of depth in tissue using a reference model of the human finger.

dermis, and hypodermis. By the time the beam reached the tissue–bone layer, it had been attenuated to about 1% of the skin entrance dose rate of 24.77 C/kg-min (96,000 R/min). This substantial attenuation accounts for the lack of more severe radiation-induced injuries. The effective energy of the radiation has been a critical element in determining the clinical consequences of other local radiation accidents,[1-6] where the higher effective X-ray energy led to much higher depth doses. Total dose estimates could not be calculated because it was impossible to determine accurately the location of their fingers relative to the exit port or the duration of exposure at any given location during the accident.

CLINICAL EVALUATION

Only Student A, who received the highest radiation exposure, will be presented in this chapter. An occupational medicine physician evaluated the student shortly after being exposed. The student described the accident but was not sure how long his hands and body had been in the X-ray field. He denied any pain and his physical exam on the day of exposure was normal.

DAYS 1 THROUGH 7

The day following exposure he complained of tightness and paresthesias in his fingers. He denied any gastrointestinal symptoms. His physical examination revealed mild diffuse swelling and very slight erythema of his fingertips. A complete blood count revealed normal leukocyte counts. He was prescribed piroxicam and arrangements were made for consultation with a hand surgeon. Three days following the exposure, he continued to deny systemic symptoms but his right index finger appeared swollen and slightly darker in color than the other fingers. On day 4 postexposure his paresthesia had improved except for the distal right index finger. His complete blood count continued normal and cultured lymphocyte analysis by Dr. Gayle Littlefield at Oak Ridge National Laboratories estimated a whole-body dose of 40 mGy (95% CI = 10 – 110 mGy). Photographs of the student's hands were obtained several times during the first 14 weeks following the accident (Figure 18.4; see Color Figures 1 and 2).*

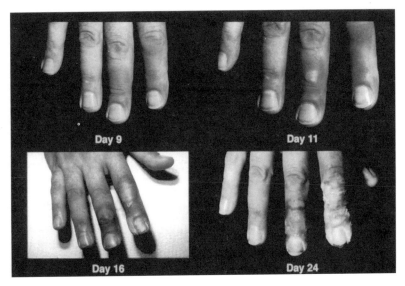

FIGURE 18.4 Photographs of Student A's hands at day 9, 11, 16, and 24 following the exposure. (See also color figures.)

---

* Color figures follow page 202.

Days 8 through 14

On postexposure day 8, the student complained of a swollen sensation over the right index and long fingers. His exam was remarkable for darkness under the fingernail of the index finger. He was prescribed pentoxyfylline, and piroxicam was continued. Blood counts remained normal and a consulting ophthalmologist reported normal slit lamp examination. On day 9 he reported progression of right index symptoms with moderate pain over the distal fingertip. On exam he had a 1-cm-diameter dry-appearing area at tip of right index finger. There were multiple raised erythematous areas on the fingers of both hands. He was started on oral hydrocodone and acetaminophen for increasing pain. On day 10 he reported continued progression of symptoms over the tips of his fingers. Punctate lesions resembling telangiectasias were noted in the subungual region of the right index finger. Examination on day 11 revealed bulla formation over the distal right index finger. By day 14 the patient had progression of bullae over the index and long fingers. He had difficulty flexing his right index finger past 30° at the DIP joint because of swelling. He was prescribed oral cephalexin and referred to the regional burn center to assist in burn care. Home nursing visits were arranged to assist in activities of daily living and to assist dressing changes.

Weeks 2 through 12

Desquamation continued over the next 2 weeks. At 4 weeks postexposure limited debridement was performed to the index fingertip. Dilaudid was added for additional pain control. Wound cultures were negative for bacteria. At 5 weeks postexposure the burns were healed with the exception of the right index fingertip. At 6 weeks postexposure he exhibited improvement of most areas except the distal index fingertip. At 8 weeks postexposure he was still with pain during dressing changes and debridement of the distal index finger. At 12 weeks postexposure he was having continued pain over the fingertip with a dysmorphic appearing fingernail. Based on the time course and extent of the injuries observed, it was estimated that superficial skin doses in the highest areas exposed to the central beam were in excess of 25 Gy (Figure 18.5).

Months 5 through 12

At 20 weeks postinjury, the patient had the nail and a hyperkeratotic cap of skin removed from his right index fingertip with significant relief pain. Approximately 7 months postexposure, the fingernail was growing back slowly and he had returned to much of his usual function. He reported sensitivity to pressure but could not sense temperature. Range of motion was normal. The skin over the index fingertip was susceptible to injury from shearing forces and he could not grasp objects tightly with the index finger because of pain. Approximately 1 year following the injury he returned for evaluation of chronic skin changes over the dorsum of his index and long fingers. His exam was remarkable for hyperkeratotic cuticles and atrophic and hypopigmented areas on the dorsum of both index and long fingers of the right hand. He was referred for dermatology consult for consideration of biopsy and skin grafting at 18 months postexposure, but declined surgical skin grafting.

Years 2 through 4

The student developed a rapidly progressive cellulitis over the right thumb approximately 2 years following exposure. He was hospitalized and treated successfully with intravenous antibiotics. He continued to have chronic hyperkeratotic regions over the dorsum of his exposed index and long finger as well as continuing hypersensitivity over the index fingertip and thumb tip. There were scattered telangiectasias over the dorsum of the fingers. At 3 years postexposure he continued to have hypersensitivity and pain with minor trauma to the right index fingertip. He was offered full-thickness skin grafting but declined. Approximately 4 years following exposure he returned for

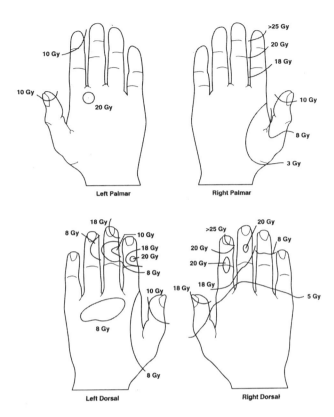

FIGURE 18.5 Dose estimate of Student A's hands based on clinical evaluation of radiation-induced injuries.

evaluation of fingernail changes. He had radiographs taken of bilateral hands, which were interpreted as showing decrease in soft tissue over the right hand suggestive of avulsion injury. He had progression of the hyperkeratotic region over his index fingertip as well as elongated hyperkeratotic plaque-like areas over the dorsum of the right middle and long fingers. The hyperkeratotic areas were biopsied to rule out squamous cell carcinoma. The skin surrounding the plaque-like areas appeared thin, erythematous, and atrophic. He continued to require occasional oral narcotic analgesics to control pain in the right index finger following minor trauma. Skin grafting vs. elective amputation of the distal index finger was offered because of ongoing hypersensitivity and dysfunction.

DIAGNOSTIC IMAGING RESULTS

A three-phase bone scan is considered the imaging method of choice for evaluating acute soft-tissue injuries such as radiation injury, frostbite, electrical burn, or infection. The three-phase bone scan is also considered the noninvasive imaging method of choice for imbalances in the peripheral circulation such as reflex sympathetic dystrophy or, as in this case, radiation-induced alteration in the blood flow. Plain films would be considered insensitive to these types of acute changes and would not be capable of detecting changes in the blood flow or evaluating erythematous-type soft-tissue injuries. On the other hand, MR angiography was also utilized in this case to evaluate noninvasively the arterial blood flow to the areas of the injured extremities.

The three-phase bone scan was accomplished utilizing approximately 740 MBq of technetium-99m methyenediphosonate (MDP) on days 4, 14, 35, and 52 after the accident (Figure 18.6). On day 4, arterial flow increased in the right hand involving the right second distal digit and the thumb.

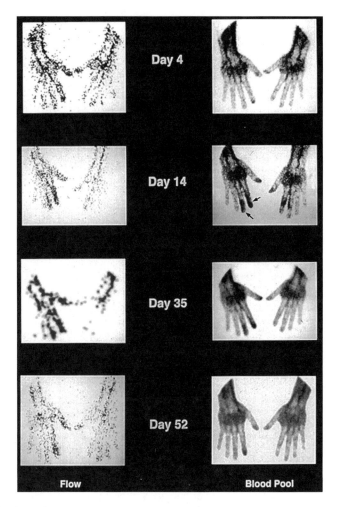

FIGURE 18.6 The three-phase bone scan images acquired utilizing approximately 740 MBq of technetium 99m MDP on days 4, 14, 35, and 52 after the accident. Arterial flow images are shown on the left and blood pool images, acquired 3 to 5 min after injection of the radiopharmaceutical, are shown on the right.

The distal area of the left thumb also showed increased blood flow. Blood pool images were acquired 3 to 5 min after injection, and reflected radiotracer activity within the blood volume as well as accumulation of the radiotracer in the extra cellular space. Blood pool information may be thought of as reflecting soft-tissue edema or cellulitis. The blood pool images from day 4 showed increased blood pool over the distal right second digit and thumb, as well as the distal left thumb. On day 14, blood flow images again demonstrated increased flow to the distal right thumb, but there was a marked increase in flow to the right second and third digits. Blood pool images reflected similar changes but more so in the right second and third digits. Blood pool images also reflect significantly marked increased radiotracer in the middle phalanx of the left second and third digits, reflecting injury in these areas as well.

On day 35, there was increased blood flow in the distal right thumb, right second, and right third digits. The blood pool images remained positive only in the tips of the right thumb and right second and third digits. Blood pool images of the left digits were essentially normal. On day 52, blood flow remained only slightly increased in the distal right thumb and distal second digit, reflecting a more marked degree of injury to the thumb and second digit. Blood flow in other areas was normal. Blood pool images on day 52 were essentially normal except for slight increased blood flow and blood pool radiotracer in the distal tip of the first and second digit.

MR angiography was also accomplished on day 17 and day 34. Increased arterial caliber and blood flow were demonstrated in the same areas of the right thumb, right second and third digits, as well as the left second and third digits. However, the significance of the blood flow changes, while being more detailed for the large vessels, was not as readily interpretable and did not demonstrate the more distal injuries, which were readily apparent on the blood pool images.

RECOMMENDATIONS FOR EVALUATION AND TREATMENT OF EXTREMITY RADIATION EXPOSURE

This case illustrates the importance of serial examination of patients who have sustained exposure to radiation. While exposures from a radiation source such as an X-ray diffraction unit may be expected to be focal, the actual exposure may in fact be quite inhomogeneous and difficult to assess fully based on initial exposure history. This case demonstrates the phases of radiation-induced injury reported for other radiation exposure cases. The initial quiescent phase showed few symptoms or physical findings. After 7 to 10 days erythema was evident over the exposed areas and by 10 to 14 days blister formation and desquamation occurred, which was similar to changes observed in thermal burns. Subsequently, the most severely irradiated tissue continued to be sensitive to shearing forces, and episodic pain control was problematic.

It is critical for the treating clinician to obtain as much information as possible surrounding the circumstances of exposure and to consult with local and regional radiation safety personnel. A knowledgeable radiation safety specialist (health physicist) can assist the treating physician in estimating the magnitude of the exposure, in describing the typical biological effects associated with such exposures, and in referring the physicians to other clinicians who have cared for such unusual injuries. As noted above, classic radiation injury follows a sequential pattern, and the physical findings and time course of the changes can be useful in estimating exposure dose. It is important to document examination findings with photography. If the whole-body dose is unknown and circumstances indicate possible whole-body exposure, then laboratory data including lymphocyte chromosomal analysis may be useful in estimating exposure.[7] Radionuclide imaging for assessment of degree of vascular compromise has been suggested by others.[8] In this case, the nuclear scans assisted in evaluating vascular supply and helped assess the need for surgical intervention.

There is very little accumulated medical literature regarding management of acute localized radiation injuries. Therefore, treatment recommendations are for the most part empiric. In the initial quiescent phase it is reasonable to avoid trauma to the exposed tissue. The skin should be protected from extremes in temperature, caustic materials, and direct trauma. The moist desquamation phase has been associated with skin breakdown and infection. Dressing changes should be performed in a fastidious fashion to prevent bacterial infection. Visiting home nurses can assist in care for burns, and other in-home assistance may be necessary if both hands are affected. Infection should be treated aggressively with antibiotics and debridement. Pain control should be achieved through use of nonsteroidal anti-inflammatory (NSAI) medications as well as opiate analgesics titrated to patient comfort and at times of dressing changes. The use of NSAIs may afford other benefits since in animal models indomethacin has been reported to reduce some radiation-induced organ injury.[9] Since the majority of radiation-induced injury is thought to be secondary to vascular injury, it has been postulated that a pharmacological approach to improve blood supply might be effective in preventing or reducing radiation-induced tissue injury. The results of one study suggest that pentoxifylline, which has a hemorheological effect on red blood cells and platelets, may provide some protection against radiation exposure.[10] Full-thickness skin grafting or even amputation of affected digits may be necessary to control pain and infection. Vascular compromise of the irradiated tissue may limit success of this technique. When attempting to assess acute exposure and predict outcome, nuclear blood flow imaging may be useful in gauging clinical response. Finally, the clinician should recognize the severe psychological impact of potential loss of extremity function for the patient. Recognizing the patient's concerns and recommending psychological counseling to encourage movement through the grief process is an important aspect of caring for these patients.

KEY FINDINGS AND RECOMMENDATIONS

Several key findings and recommendations were made in order to minimize the potential for this type of accident in the future. They can be classified under the general headings of procedural changes, training enhancements, and safety audit modifications.

PROCEDURAL CHANGES

The most significant factor that led to this accident was that the students had adopted a practice of expediting sample changing by bypassing the cabinet door safety interlock rather than shutting off power to the unit as instructed in the manufacturer's operating instructions and the institution's General Safety Protocol. This practice was also thought to prolong the life of the X-ray tube by reducing the number of times it was turned on from a cold start. The manufacturer denies that this aspect of operating the equipment has any significant effect on tube life. The investigation also found that the interlock bypass key was easily accessible by anyone in the room.

Recommendations by the institution's radiation safety committee included reinforcement (both in writing and during laboratory safety audits) of the standing prohibition of using the interlock bypass key to change samples. Exception to this policy will only be considered when written requests detailing the necessity for a change in standard practice is provided along with a detailed safety protocol. The necessity for this variance should be compelling and all alternatives should be fully explored. The safety protocol should include additional safety precautions and monitors to ensure the safety of the operators adequately. In addition, a strict key control policy was required to be implemented by the responsible faculty members.

TRAINING ENHANCEMENTS

Both students had attended the institution's analytical X-ray safety course specifically designed for X-ray diffraction users. One of the students (Student A) had several years of experience, while Student B was just beginning to learn the specific operating policies and procedures for this particular unit.

When questioned about how this situation occurred, the students replied with an answer all too familiar in accident investigations — We were in a hurry. This no doubt explains why they failed to turn the unit off while performing maintenance on the unit and failed to notice the X-ray production indicator (red light) positioned on top of the X-ray column. Other violations of the existing safety protocol included failure to use a radiation survey meter and to wear dosimetry when working with the unit.

In addition to the standard X-ray diffraction safety course provided by the institution's Health Physics Department, the radiation safety committee required all responsible faculty members to develop and implement a formal (written), unit-specific, operations, maintenance, and radiation safety training program for the users of X-ray diffraction units. The committee also required each user to view the X-ray diffraction safety training film entitled "The Double Edged Sword,"[11] that, while somewhat dated (1970s), provides an excellent overview of safety precautions and depicts in graphic detail the consequences of an accidental exposure to an X-ray diffraction beam.

SAFETY AUDIT MODIFICATIONS

It was noted that the safety audits performed by the radiation safety personnel did not reveal the fact the interlock bypass key was being used to expedite sample changing. Changes were made to the audit procedures that included a detailed review of the faculty members' formal training program and interviews with the authorized users during routine audits to assure that the established safety protocols were being followed. How questions are asked during the safety audit can be as important as the questions themselves. For example, users are asked to describe or demonstrate how samples are changed rather than simply being asked if they turn off the power to the X-ray tube between samples. This approach is more likely to reveal weaknesses in existing procedures than simple yes or no answers to established compliance questions.

REFERENCES

1. Thomas, R.H., Ed., Report of the Investigation of the Accidental X-ray Exposure at the Donner Laboratory of the Lawrence Berkeley Laboratory on April 6, 1977, Lawrence Berkeley Laboratory, University of California, Berkeley, 1977.
2. Laur, W.E., Posey, R.E., and Waller, J.D., Industrial Grenz ray overexposure, *J. Occup. Med.*, 20(2): 118–120, 1978.
3. Nénot, J.C., Medical and surgical management for localized radiation injuries, *Int. J. Radiat. Biol.*, 57: 783–795, 1990.
4. Schauer, D.A., Coursey, M.B., Kick, C.E. et al., A radiation accident at an industrial accelerator facility, *Health Phys.*, 65: 131–140, 1993.
5. Sweet, R.D., Acute accidental, superficial X-ray burns. An interim report of eleven cases, *Br. J. Dermatol.*, 74: 392–402, 1962.
6. Hollander, M.B., *Ultrasoft X-rays: An Historical and Critical Review of the World Experience with Grenz Rays and Other Rays of Long Wave Length*, Williams & Wilkins, Baltimore, MD, 1968.
7. Littlefield, L.G. and Lushbaugh, C.C., Cytogenetic dosimetry for radiation accidents, in *The Medical Basis for Radiation Accident Preparedness II*, Ricks, R.C. and Fry, S.A., Eds., Elsevier Science, New York, 1990.
8. Mettler, F.A., Monsein, L, Davis, M. et al., Three-phase radionuclide bone scanning in evaluation of local radiation injury — a case report, *Clin. Nucl. Med.*, 12: 805–808, 1987.
9. Fose, P.G., Halter, S.A., and Su, C.M., The effect of indomethacin on acute radiation induced gastrointestinal injury, *J. Surg. Oncol.*, 49: 231–238, 1992.
10. Dion, M.W., Jussey, D.H., and Osborne, J.W., The effect of pentoxifylline on early and late radiation injury following fractionated irradiation in C3H mice, *Int. J. Radiat. Oncol. Biol. Phys.*, 17: 101–107, 1989.
11. Durrin Films, Inc., "The Double Edged Sword," Washington, D.C., 1970.

19 Local Irradiation Injury of the Hands with an Electron Beam Machine

Fred A. Mettler, Jr. and Charles A. Kelsey

The accident occurred sometime during November 1999. A machine had been manufactured and was being tested as a biological sterilizer for a medical equipment company. The operator had assembled a nested high-voltage generator electron beam machine and was irradiating samples known to contain viruses. Typically, samples were irradiated to 2500–3000 Gy for the sterilization procedure. The beam diameter was approximately 2×4 in. and operated at a maximum energy of 0.7 MeV.

The operator would place a sample on a stainless steel tray beneath the exit port, perform a timed irradiation, and then remove the sample. Unbeknownst to the operator, after the current was turned off, residual scattered electrons were detectable for approximately the next 60 s. The operator ran about 20 samples per day and had his hands in the residual beam for 3 to 10 s each time. No pain was felt while the hand was in the residual beam.

Toward the end of November of 1999, the patient noted some pain on the dorsal aspect of the second and third digits bilaterally, and 3 to 4 days after that, he began to notice blister formation. The patient was sent to a local physician who diagnosed a chemical burn and to another physician who gave him a diagnosis of herpes virus. The patient continued to have severe pain in the back of the fingers of both hands, and the lesions were nonhealing. In January of 2000, he was referred to another clinic that diagnosed radiation burns. At that time, the skin on the dorsum of both hands over the first through fourth digits was edematous, thin, and erythematous. There was associated epilation and dry desquamation peripherally with marginal pigmentation. The lesions were more severe on the right hand. The nail beds were raised, and the patient was having significant pain that required narcotics. The patient had also been on systemic antibiotics. These were discontinued and replaced with local antibiotics and standard wound care with limited physical therapy. The patient also was treated for 6 weeks with pentoxyfline (a peripheral vasodilator). There was rapid granulation of the denuded area and, as soon as granulation was complete, pentoxyfline was discontinued. The patient experienced some dizziness from the medication. At 4 to 5 months postexposure, the hands were generally well healed although the skin was sensitive, atrophic, and there was still limited range of motion in the distal interphalangeal joints.

The images associated with this accident are presented in Figure 19.1. Although the lesions appear quite severe, the electron beam was not very penetrating, and conservative treatment often has a successful outcome. Given the surface dose here, if the radiation had been significantly penetrating such as gamma rays, amputation of the distal aspects of the digits would likely have been necessary.

Dose to the hands is difficult to estimate. Acute doses causing blister formation, and moist desquamation would range from 15 to 25 Gy. Given the fractionated nature of the radiation over a period of 1 month, the skin dose likely was over 50 Gy.

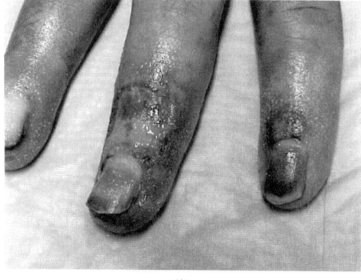

(A)

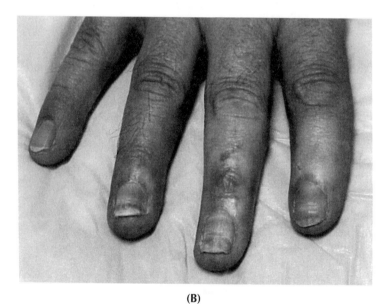

(B)

FIGURE 19.1 (A) Appearance of finger lesions at presentation approximately 30 days postexposure. There was erythema, swelling, and ulceration almost to the bone surface. (B) Healed lesions 5 months postexposure. There remained skin atrophy, some limitation of motion, and fingernail changes.

20 Accidents in Radiation Therapy

Fred A. Mettler, Jr. and Pedro Ortiz-Lopez

CONTENTS

Introduction 291
Examples of Radiotherapy Accidents...293
    Accident in Riverside, Ohio, U.S.A., 1974 to 1976 293
    Underexposure during Radiotherapy Accident in the United Kingdom, 1982 to 1990 293
    Accident at the Linear Accelerator in Zaragoza, Spain, 1990...294
    Overdose from Malfunction of High-Dose-Rate Brachytherapy Equipment in the
        United States, 1992 294
    Therac-25 Accidents 295
References 297

INTRODUCTION

Worldwide, there are millions of radiation therapy treatments each year. Radiation therapy typically involves localized radiation fields with the intent of eradicating a tumor. Since tumor cells are approximately the same radiosensitivity as nearby surrounding cells, technological means must be used to deliver a higher dose to the tumor than to normal surrounding cells. Typically, effects of killing normal cells are minimized by (1) centering and collimating the radiation beam on the tumor while including as little normal tissue as possible, (2) using multiple fields so the dose at the center where the beams intersect is higher than any point on the surface, and (3) dividing or fractionating a treatment into about 25 days. Usual fractionation schemes give doses of 1 to 2 Gy/day, 4 to 5 days/week. Even when these precautions are employed, complications occur in approximately 5% of cases, and this is usually considered acceptable practice. Obviously, if the radiation doses are lower, fewer if any complications arise, but also there will be fewer cures. There are well-known radiation tolerance levels for many normal tissues, and these have been published in a number of tables.

Typically, the prescribed dose delivered within a range of ±7% is considered acceptable. Deviation much beyond this will cause either a very high incidence of unacceptable complications or an unacceptably low tumor cure rate. Thus, in contrast to most of the other accidental situations related in this textbook, radiation therapy accidents involve not only overexposure but can also have significant consequences from mistakes involving underexposure. Fortunately, the large practice of radiation therapy and the large scientific literature have made it possible to predict the outcome of such accidents if the total dose and fractionation scheme is known. Of particular importance is that reducing the number of fractions and increasing the dose per fraction (as in many accidents) causes a disproportionate increase in chronic effects as compared with acute effects. Thus, one is not able to rely only on the acute presentation of overexposures in radiation therapy for the prediction of late effects. If this is done, it results in underestimation of the actual extent of late effects.

Most accidents involving radiation therapy involve specific body parts where the majority of tumors arise. These include head and neck, chest, and pelvis. When there is overexposure of these regions, the most radiosensitive tissues demonstrate complications first. Typically, these are the skin, bowel, mucosa, and spinal cord. The well-documented radiation therapy accidents[1] are shown in Table 20.1. This table is predominantly illustrative, and it should be realized that many radiation accidents involving radiotherapy have never been reported in the literature. Often, the symptoms involved from radiation overexposure are complicated or confused by the presence of tumor and often infection. Illustrative examples of some well-known radiotherapy accidents will be described briefly in this chapter, and a major accident in Costa Rica will be presented in detail in Chapter 21. Note should also be made that abandoned or stolen radiotherapy sources have been involved in accidents in which the public has been exposed. An example of one of these accidents is also included in Chapter 26 in this text, specifically the accident in Goiânia, Brazil. Another occurred in Thailand, in January 2000, and resulted in three fatalities.

Medical treatment of radiation therapy accidents is also somewhat different from most other types of accidents in that there are a high percentage of local injuries involving the trunk as opposed to local injuries of extremities in most other types of radiation accidents. Medical treatment of

TABLE 20.1
Major Reported Accidents Involving Radiotherapy Patients

Country	Year	No. of Patients Affected	Causes and Main Contributing Factors
U.S.A.	1974–76	426	^{60}Co dose calculations based on erroneous decay chart (varying overdoses)
			No independent verification of dose calculations
			More than 2 years without beam measurements
Canada and U.S.A.	1985–87	3 deaths	Old software used on new design accelerator
Germany	1986–87	86	^{60}Co dose calculations based on erroneous dose tables (varying overdoses)
			No independent determination of the dose rate
U.K.	1988	207	Error in the calibration of a ^{60}Co therapy unit (25% overdose)
			No independent calibration of the beam
U.K.	1988–89	22	Error in the identification of ^{137}Cs brachytherapy sources (–20 to +10% dosimetry errors)
			No independent determination of source strength
Spain	1990	27 (15 deaths from radiation)	Error in the maintenance of a clinical linear accelerator
			Fault in procedures for transferring machine from and to maintenance
			Conflicting signals and displays not analyzed
			Procedures for periodic beam verifications (QA) not implemented or insufficient
			Overdosage ranging from 200 to 700%
U.K.	1982–91	1045	Inappropriate commissioning of a computerized treatment planning system (5–30% underdosage)
U.S.A.	1992	1 (death from radiation)	High-dose-rate brachytherapy source left inside the patient
			Source dislodged from equipment
			Conflicting monitor signals and displays ignored
Costa Rica	1996	114 (17 deaths from radiation)	Error in calculation during the calibration of ^{60}Co therapy unit
			Lack of independent beam calibration and of quality assurance
			Recommendations of external audit ignored
			Overdosage about 60%

radiotherapy accidents is complicated by the presence of concurrent tumor, which in addition to the vascular changes due to radiation, limits the potential for reconstructive surgery. In addition, unusual forms of local radiation injury that are not typically identified in other accidents are present. Examples of this include focal stenosis or narrowing of large blood vessels, loss of mucosa of the trachea and esophagus resulting in infection and death, as well as central nervous system damage.

EXAMPLES OF RADIOTHERAPY ACCIDENTS

ACCIDENT IN RIVERSIDE, OHIO, U.S.A., 1974 TO 1976

The accident involved 426 patients treated on a cobalt teletherapy unit over a 16-month period from 1974 to 1976.[2] During this time, the dose rate had been underestimated by a factor ranging between 10 and 45% of the true value. The unit had been calibrated correctly at first, but subsequent dose calculations included an incorrect decay curve, and no periodic calibration of the output was made. The overdose was approximately 10% at 5.5 months and was as high as 50% at the end of 16.5 months. Of 183 patients who survived beyond 1 year, 34% had severe complications, some of which led to death. At the end of 5 years, 78 patients remained alive of whom 42% had severe complications. At 15 years after the accident, 10% of the patients remained alive with 41% having severe complications. In general, those patients who received target absorbed doses of 50 to 70 Gy had complication rates of approximately 15%, whereas those who received 70 to 90 Gy had a complication rate of close to 40%. The site of the complications was related to the original site of the tumor and the distribution of these tumors in the patient population. Crude complication rates indicated that for treatment of the head and neck, the complication rate was 12 to 13%, the thorax 16%, the abdomen 18%, and for the pelvis 29%. As will be seen in Chapter 21, in the Costa Rican accident complications included severe skin reactions with ulceration, mucosal reactions with necrosis, stenosis of the pharynx, and esophagus, as well as ulceration of the stomach and bowel, bone necrosis, and myelopathy.

UNDEREXPOSURE DURING RADIOTHERAPY ACCIDENT IN THE UNITED KINGDOM, 1982 TO 1990

This is probably one of the most difficult types of accidents to identify since underexposure does not cause any obvious radiation effects and the injury, as a result of this type of accident, causes increased cancer deaths. This type of accident can typically only be detected by examining outcome data.

At this treatment facility, only manual treatment planning was available before 1982. A computerized treatment planning system was then acquired, but the technologists continued to perform a manual distance calculation without realizing that the computer software already took into account the change in source–skin distance.[3] The adjustment was, therefore, duplicated. No quality control measurements were taken, and it was not until 1991 that the error was discovered. The result was that 1045 patients received a radiation dose lower than prescribed. The underdosage was between 5 and 35% with the distribution of patients as follows:

0–5%	5
6–10%	99
11–20%	255
21–30%	611
>30%	75

The major cancer sites involved were

Bladder	242
Cervix	162
Endometrium	104
Lung	206
Esophagus	134
Prostate	47
Rectum/colon	75
Others	75

After the error was discovered almost a decade after it began, an analysis of cancer sites and survival was performed and compared with published literature for the same sites and stage of disease. Overall, 492 patients of the 1045 were judged potentially to have had an adverse effect as a result of underexposure with a local recurrence, and there were an additional 189 in whom it was not possible to be sure whether the underdosage had an effect. The effect of underdosage was relatively tumor specific. For example, for lung cancer the survival rate is so poor with radiotherapy or other treatments that survival was not affected much; however, for patients with cancers of the bladder or prostate, a 20% reduction in dose appeared to result in a 50% reduction in the chance of being disease-free at 5 years. For patients with stage II cancer of the cervix, there was a reduction in the cure rate from the expected rate of 60 to 65% down to 46%.

ACCIDENT AT THE LINEAR ACCELERATOR IN ZARAGOZA, SPAIN, 1990

The accident began on December 5, 1990. Because of instability of the beam in a linear accelerator, the interlock system terminated treatment of the patient.[4] Over the following weekend, a maintenance technician was unable to identify the fault, but was able to generate a radiation beam by manipulating its energy. On Monday, treatment was resumed, and no postmaintenance testing was performed. The meter on the control panel permanently indicated 36 MeV, regardless of what energy the operator selected. The repair technician indicated to the operators that the meter must have been stuck at 36 MeV, not realizing that the beam had been adjusted to its maximum. The accident was not discovered until 10 days later. The increased energy resulted in more penetration with doses delivered to deeper tissues than intended, and the electrons were focused in a smaller cross section of the beam. This resulted in doses three- to sevenfold higher than intended. During the 10 days of the accident, 27 patients were treated with electrons. Ultimately, 15 patients died with radiation as a primary or major cause, and several others had major disabilities.[5] The clinical findings as of 1993 are summarized in Table 20.2. As can be seen, the majority of the deaths occurred within 2 years of the accident and most within 1 year. The majority of fatalities resulted from radiation injuries of the lungs and spinal cord.

OVERDOSE FROM MALFUNCTION OF HIGH-DOSE-RATE BRACHYTHERAPY EQUIPMENT IN THE UNITED STATES, 1992

High-dose-rate brachytherapy involves placement of intense radioactive sources inside the patient for short periods of time. This particular accident involved a 16 GBq (4.3 Ci) iridium-192 source. The prescribed dose was 18 Gy in three fractions. Five catheters were used and placed in the tumor, and there was difficulty placing the radioactive source wire into the fifth catheter. The source became dislodged and remained in the patient. The patient was transported to a nursing home and remained there for 4 days, at which time the catheter fell out. The patient was estimated to have received a dose of 16,000 Gy at 1 cm from the source instead of the prescribed 18 Gy. The source in the catheter that fell out was sent off with typical medical waste to be incinerated; however, it was

TABLE 20.2
Outcome of Overexposure in the Zaragoza Radiotherapy Accident

Patient	Age/Sex	Clinical Findings or Cause of Death	Death	Radiation Related
MV	35F	Radiation-induced respiratory insufficiency	May 20, 1991	Yes
BC	69F	Rupture of esophagus due to overexposure	May 8, 1991	Yes
PS	45F	Myelitis, paraplegic, esophageal stenosis		
DR	59F	Pneumonitis, hepatitis due to overexposure	March 26, 1991	Yes
JC	60M	Hypovolemic shock due to radiation-induced hemorrhage in neck	Sept. 14, 1991	Yes
FT	68M	Myelopathy due to radiation	April 15, 1991	Yes
MP	55M	Myelopathy, lung metastases, respiratory insufficiency possibly due to radiation	March 16, 1991	Possibly
IL	65M	Myelopathy postradiation	Dec. 25, 1991	Yes
JV	67M	Left thigh and groin fibrosis		
AS	67M	Ulcerated hypopharynx, cervical myelitis, radiation burn of neck		
JG	60F	Respiratory insufficiency due to overexposure	Sept. 7, 1991	Yes
AG	60F	Respiratory insufficiency due to overexposure	July 28, 1991	Yes
BG	50F	Healed skin burns of anterior chest		
CM	51F	Respiratory insufficiency due to overexposure	March 9, 1991	
AR	71F	Skin burns, esophagitis, femoral vein thrombosis	April 8 1992	Probably not
IG	68F	Paraneoplastic syndrome, metastases	Nov. 22, 1991	No
SA	45	Inguinal skin burns		
FS	59F	Pneumonitis and myelopathy	Aug. 29, 1991	Yes
JS	42M	Skin burns shoulder, fibrosis, necrosis		
TR	87F	Respiratory and renal insufficiency and encephalopathy due to overexposure	July 12, 1991	Yes
BF	39F	Respiratory fibrosis and metastases	May 20, 1992	Yes
NC	72F	Skin burns chest, pleural and pericardial effusion		
PS	42F	Respiratory insufficiency due to overexposure	Feb. 21, 1991	Yes
LS	72F	Generalized metastases	Jan. 9, 1991	No
JG	80F	Generalized cancer	Jan. 8, 1991	No
JS	56M	Myelopathy due to overexposure	Feb. 16, 1991	Yes
SM	53M	Myelopathy due to overexposure	Feb. 17, 1991	Yes

discovered when it tripped a radiation monitor at the incinerator. The patient died shortly after, and radiation was the major contributing cause of death. In all, 94 other individuals had been exposed to the source at the clinic, at the nursing home, and other areas.

THERAC-25 ACCIDENTS

The Therac-25 has been associated with at least five serious accidents in the United States and Canada[6] and three of the six patients subsequently died from radiation injuries. All accidents involved a problem of integration with the software and hardware of the system. In one particular case on April 7, 1986 in Tyler, Texas, the operator noted that the mode and energy of the accelerator was set for 25 MeV photon. She then used an edit key and edited the prescription to 10 MeV electrons. Unfortunately, once the original energy and mode were selected on the computer screen, it took approximately 8 s to reconfigure the magnets mechanically. During these 8 s, subsequent changes and edited entries were not noted by the computer. The results were an unscanned 25 MeV electron beam operating at a much higher photon beam current than expected. Dose estimates were approximately 165 Gy occurring in about 1 s with a beam size 1 cm diameter. The machine was designed with dosimetry to average the first few pulses. If the average was too high, the beam terminated or the system went into pause mode. At Tyler, the system tripped out, giving a "malfunction 54" message. The operator was allowed to restart the system at least three times. Not knowing what the message meant and thinking that no dose had occurred, the operator restarted the machine a second and third time.

In Tyler, Texas on March 21, 1986, a male patient came into the Cancer Center for his ninth treatment. The patient was to receive 60 Gy over 6.5 weeks to the upper back, a little to the left of the spine. The patient was placed facedown on the table. After the first attempt to treat him, the patient said he had felt like he had received an "electric shock or that someone had poured hot coffee on his back." He felt a thump and heat and heard a buzzing sound from the equipment. Since he had received treatments before, he knew this was not normal, and he began to get off the table. However, the operator pushed the button a second time. The patient said he felt like "his arm was being shocked by electricity and that his hand was leaving his body." He went to the treatment room door and pounded on it, and the operator opened the door and let him out. Immediate examination by a physician showed intense erythema over the treatment area. Simulations later indicated a dose of 165 to 250 Gy in less than 1 s over an area of about 1 cm. During the weeks following the accident, the patient continued to have pain in the neck and shoulder. He lost function of his left arm and had periodic bouts of nausea and vomiting. He was hospitalized for radiation-induced myelitis of the cervical spinal cord, resulting in paralysis of the left arm and both legs, as well as the left vocal cord. He also had neurogenic bowel and bladder, as well as paralysis of the left hemidiaphragm. He died 5 months later as a result of complications of the accident. The machine was shut down 1 day after the initial accident, but thorough testing could not reproduce the malfunction-54 error. The machine was checked to see whether electrical shocks may have caused the initial injury, and the calibration was checked. These were all found to be satisfactory, and the machine was put back into service on April 7, 1986.

On April 11, 1986, another male patient was to receive electron treatment for skin cancer on the side of his face. After the operator finished editing, she pressed the return key several times to place the cursor on the bottom of the screen and turned the beam on. The machine shut down, but made a loud noise. The operator rushed into the treatment room, and the patient was moaning and trying to take the tape off that held his head in position. She asked him what he felt, and he replied "fire" on the side of his face. The patient also indicated he saw a flash of light and heard a sizzling sound. The patient died 3 weeks after the accident following coma, fever, and neurological damage. Autopsy showed acute high-dose radiation injury to the right temporal lobe of the brain and the brain stem. Dosage at the center of the fields was estimated to be 250 Gy.

Additional accidents also were described involving a Therac-25. One accident occurred at the Kennestone Regional Oncology Center in Marietta, Georgia in 1985. The details are sketchy, but on June 3, 1985, a female patient was set for a 10 MeV electron treatment to the clavicle area. When the machine turned on, she described, "tremendous force of heat … this red hot sensation." The patient went home, but shortly afterward developed an erythema and swelling in the center of the treatment area. Pain increased to the point where her shoulder could not be moved, and she experienced spasm. Then, 2 weeks later, it was noted that there was a matching erythema on her back as though a through burn had occurred in the body. The swollen area in the clavicle region began to slough layers of skin, and the patient was in great pain. Estimated doses of radiation were 150 to 200 Gy. Eventually, the patient's breast had to be removed, and she lost use of her shoulder and arm and was in constant pain.

Another accident occurred with the Therac-25 at the Ontario Cancer Foundation in Hamilton, Ontario, Canada about 7 weeks after the patient in Georgia was overexposed. On July 26, 1985, a 40-year-old patient came to the clinic for treatment of carcinoma of the cervix. The machine shut down several times. The operators, who had become used to frequent malfunctions (and since the display showed "no dose") restarted the machine five times. After the treatment, the patient complained of a burning sensation described as "an electric tingling shock to the treatment area about the hip." The patient returned the next day complaining of burning pain and swelling. The patient died approximately 6 months later as a result of the cancer, but it was noted at autopsy that if she had not died, a total hip replacement would have been necessary as a result of radiation overexposure. The dose was later estimated to be between 130 and 170 Gy.

Two additional accidents happened with the machine at Yakima Valley Memorial Hospital in the State of Washington. During December 1985, a woman came in for treatment. She developed erythema in a parallel striped pattern at one port site over the right hip. It was determined that open slots in the blocking trays in the Therac-25 could have caused the abnormal pattern. Finally, the injury was attributed to a heating pad that the woman used. In the same hospital, approximately a year later, a second overdose resulted in a skin burn and a chronic skin ulcer with constant pain. This was surgically repaired. The reaction initially was less intense than in their earlier patient, and necrosis did not develop until 6 to 8 months postexposure. The patient died, and the death was alleged to be related to the overexposure.

REFERENCES

1. International Atomic Energy Agency, Accidental Overexposure of Radiotherapy Patients in San Jose, Costa Rica, IAEA, Vienna, 1999.
2. Cohen, L., Schultheiss, T.E., and Kennaugh, R.C., A radiation overdose incident: initial data, *Int. J. Radiat. Oncol., Biol. Phys.*, 33(1), 217–225, 1995.
3. Ash, D. and Bates, T., Report on the clinical effects of inadvertent radiation underdosage in 1045 patients, *Clin. Oncol.*, 6, 214–225, 1994.
4. The Accident of the Linear Accelerator in the Hospital Clinico de Zaragoza, Report of the Spanish Society of Medical Physics, Spain, August 1991.
5. *El Periódico*, Account of the court proceedings and verdict for the case of the accelerator accident in Zaragoza (Spain), reproduced in the newspaper of April 7, 1993, Madrid (in Spanish).
6. Leveson, N.G. and Turner, C.S., An investigation of the Therac-25 accidents, *Computer*, 26(7), 18–41, 1993.

21 A 2-Year Medical Follow-Up of the Radiotherapy Accident in Costa Rica

Fred A. Mettler, Jr., Torsten Landberg, Jean-Claude Nénot, Fernando Medina-Trejos, Roxana Ching, Ivette Garcia, Vincinio Perez-Ulloa, and Mayela Valerio-Hernandez

CONTENTS

Introduction 299
Records and Examinations...300
Dose Reconstruction 301
Results 301
    Number of Fractions 301
    Treatment Dose 302
    Deceased Patients..305
    Sites of Irradiation and Catastrophic Complications 307
        Central Nervous System Complications...308
        Tracheal, Laryngeal, and Bronchial Necrosis 308
        Bowel Perforation and Necrosis 309
Discussion 309
Acknowledgment..310
References 311

INTRODUCTION

An accident occurred with the Alycon II radiotherapy unit at San Juan de Dios Hospital in San Jose, Costa Rica. The cobalt-60 source was replaced on August 24, 1996. At that time an error was made by assuming the units on the timer were in seconds rather than in hundredths of a minute. As a result, the dose rate was underestimated by a factor of 1.66. The machine was used until September 27, 1996. In the spring of 1997, the Costa Rican government requested assistance from the International Atomic Energy Agency to help distinguish which health effects in the patients were due to overexposure and which were due to tumor. An expert team of physicians and physicists evaluated the accident in July 1997[1] and again in October 1998.

In the course of this accident, 114 patients were treated. There was a wide spectrum of how much overexposure actually occurred. A number of patients completed their treatments in late July and early August 1996, and these patients may have had only one or a few treatments with the miscalibrated source. Thus, their overexposure involved a 50% increase in dose for only one or two of the 20 to 25 treatments. These patients would have had a total overexposure for their entire treatment of only a few percent, and no major complications would be expected as a result of the accident.

In a similar fashion, there are patients who had only a few treatments before the error was discovered. These patients finished their therapy on a properly calibrated machine, and since the overexposure of the initial treatments was known, the subsequent treatment doses were reduced to compensate and achieve a correct final treatment dose.

A number of unfortunate patients began treatment at the time the miscalibration occurred in the last week of August and had most or all of their treatment before the end of September when the problem was discovered. These patients would have had total overexposures in the range of 50 to 60% higher than prescribed and have had a very high incidence of severe complications. Some patients fit between the above-mentioned groups. A few patients began therapy just before the accident was discovered and never finished their full radiotherapy treatment. Thus, they were underexposed as an indirect result of the accident, and they would be expected to have a lower-than-expected cure rate.

Very few accidents provide human data on complications and mortality from partial body exposure in this dose range. The total dose range and the dose per fraction in this accident extends higher than in the previously reported 1974 to 1976 accident in Riverside, Ohio[2] (see Chapter 20). Apparently, many patients in that accident suffered from similar complications, but the publications to date have concentrated only on long-term outcome. This report concerns acute and subacute complications by site and dose.

RECORDS AND EXAMINATIONS

The material for study included clinical files from the San Juan de Dios Hospital and from Calderon Guardia Hospital. The hospital charts of the latter were needed since patients from this hospital were sent to San Juan de Dios for radiotherapy. These charts included information on prior treatment, tumor stage, early reactions to the radiation, and clinical assessments since the accident. For patients who had died, clinical and autopsy records at the Office of the Medical Examiner were reviewed as well as available photographs of gross specimens, and in selected cases there was review of tissue histology.

The technical data (treatment charts) were of variable quality. They did list the date, field size, fraction number, and the assumed session dose and total dose. Some patients were treated with daily parallel-opposed fields, while others had been treated with a "one field on alternate days" technique. In general, there was no daily record of treatment time, nor an indication of how the treatment time was calculated. There often were no port films and a simulator was not available. In the charts of the Calderon Guardia Hospital there were diagrams showing the site of the fields and the blocks used.

The vast majority of patients were examined simultaneously by three physicians with experience in radiation accidents and radiation oncology. The prior findings, clinical charts, and available imaging studies were also reviewed at the same time. In addition to physical examination, the team also employed a suggested but untested grading system that has been proposed for evaluation of long-term effects (LENT). This system was useful in that it has detailed forms for various different tissues. This allowed a systematic and uniform assessment of the patients. A score can be derived for each patient, but the usefulness of this score is not known at the present time. Therefore, as in the previous report, and for consistency, the patients were assigned to one of five categories as follows:

- *** Severe or catastrophic effects due to overexposure from the accident
- ** Marked effects due to overexposure from the accident and at high risk for future effects
- * Radiation effects from the accident not severe at this time and at low risk for future effects

0 No radiation effects at this time are attributed to the accident; these patients may have radiation effects that would be expected from standard radiotherapy protocols
− Underexposure because radiotherapy was discontinued; at higher-than-expected risk for tumor recurrence

DOSE RECONSTRUCTION

Because of the limitations of the treatment charts, a simplified dose reconstruction was performed. The prescribed dose, the number of fractions prior to the source change, and the number of fractions after the source change, as well as other important parameters, were extracted from the charts. Calibration measurements made after the accident was initially discovered were checked and utilized. The tumor dose during the accident was reconstructed by multiplying the prescribed dose by an overexposure factor of 1.55. This was derived by taking a sample of the patient charts and correcting for a 2 cm SSD (source skin distance) error, including information on dose rate, field size factor, PDD (percent depth dose), the derived dose at the depth of the tumor, and the prescribed dose. A maximum entrance dose was calculated in those cases where it was evident that this would pose an unusual problem, for example, if there were only one field.

In addition to the approach of using a common factor of 1.55, specific calculations were made for 28 patients who showed medical evidence of extensive overexposure. For these patients, doses were calculated to specific organs at risk. To assess how the dose per fraction, as it was higher than normal, might influence late chronic effects, the biologically effective dose (BED) was calculated for a small sample of the patients using the linear-quadratic model for cell killing. The BED was then used to derive the dose that would be biologically equivalent, had it been delivered in fractions of 2 Gy. This is relevant for comparison to tissue tolerance doses.

RESULTS

A total of 114 patients were involved in this accident. Of these, 51 patients had received radiotherapy prior to the source change and 63 patients had not received any prior radiotherapy treatments.

NUMBER OF FRACTIONS

The 114 patients had a total of 152 irradiated fields. The percentage distribution of total fractions for both before and during the accident is as follows:

0–5	18%
6–10	21%
11–15	24%
16–20	18%
21–25	15%
>26	4%

For those patients who were treated after the source change, the average number of fractions was 10.7 (range 2 to 24). The percentage distribution is as follows:

21% received 0 to 5 treatments
26% received 6 to 10 treatments
29% received 11 to 15 treatments
20% received 16 to 20 treatments
4% received 20 to 25 treatments

TREATMENT DOSE

The total dose at the tumor was evaluated retrospectively. It varied widely from patient to patient. The average value for the whole of 114 patients was 40 Gy (range 4 to 92 Gy). About 27% of the patients received over 50 Gy and 15% received over 60 Gy. The percentage distribution of total doses both before and after the source change for all 152 irradiated fields was as follows:

0–10 Gy	4%
11–20 Gy	16%
21–30 Gy	10%
31–40 Gy	17%
41–50 Gy	24%
51–60 Gy	13%
61–70 Gy	9%
71–80 Gy	4%
80–90 Gy	<1%
91–100 Gy	<1%

The average dose per fraction after the source change was 3.5 Gy (range 0.5 to 15.5). For many patients the skin and superficial dose per fraction was twice this since, rather than being treated with anterior and posterior fields each day, they received one anterior treatment one day and one posterior treatment the next day. Each of these was twice the absorbed dose that would have been given if the patients were given anterior and posterior treatments each day.

In July 1997, the medical team examined 70 of the 73 surviving patients, and, in October 1998, the same team examined 51 of the surviving 53 patients (Table 21.1). One patient was removed from the list between the two examinations since it was determined that exposure did not occur during the accident period. Those surviving patients who were in the first three categories (***, **, and *) had injuries related to the specific body part irradiated and the sensitive tissues in that area. There were five general categories of effects as follows:

1. Nervous system:
   - Brain: Atrophy, necrosis, decreased cognitive function, headaches, mood alteration, seizures, decreased intellectual function.
   - Spinal cord: Paralysis, quadriplegia, paraplegia (Figures 21.1 to 21.3).
2. Skin: Fibrosis, atrophy, contraction, induration, edema, pigmentation, puritis, hypersensitivity, pain (Figures 21.3 to 21.7 and Color Figures 1 and 2*).
3. Lower gastrointestinal: Chronic or bloody diarrhea, bowel stenosis, stricture, fibrosis, obstruction, fistula perforation.
4. Bladder: Dysuria, hematuria, contracture, incontinence.
5. Vascular and lymphatic: Stenosis and premature atherosclerosis.

Over the time since the initial visit, many patients gained a significantly improved outlook on their situation. It was not possible to quantitate this specifically. Generally, they replaced anger and fear with acceptance and are attempting to cope with their problems. This is probably the result of a multifactorial process of natural psychological processes, psychological therapy, education, and more involvement with their physicians.

---

* Color figures follow page 202.

TABLE 21.1
Medical Assessment

	October 1998
	(25 months)
Total patients	114
Alive — Category	53 (51 examined)
***	2
**	12
*	22
0	13
–	2
Deceased — Category	61
Radiation related	13
Possibly related	4
Not related	35
Insufficient data	9

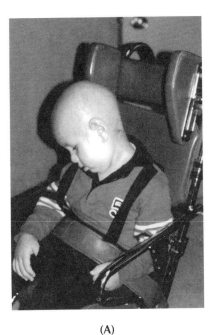
(A)

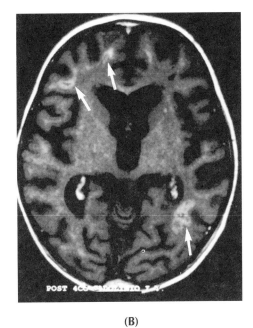
(B)

FIGURE 21.1 (A) Patient who received 58 Gy of cranial radiation in 20 fractions. The patient is somnolent, unable to speak, and confined to a wheelchair. (B) Computed tomography scan of the brain demonstrates central and cortical atrophy as well as mineralizing microangiopathy particularly in the right frontal and left parietal-occipital regions.

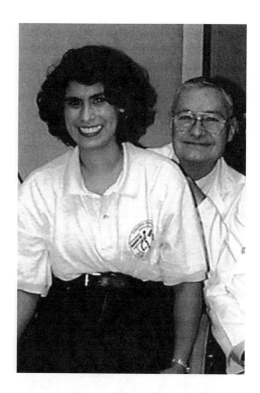

FIGURE 21.2 A young woman who received 51 Gy of mediastinal irradiation in 17 fractions and became paraplegic.

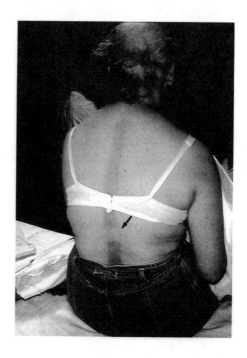

FIGURE 21.3 Pigmentation of linear treatment fields over the spine due to radiation. Note that this radiation effect allows visualization of a gap over the lower spine where the two fields should have been contiguous.

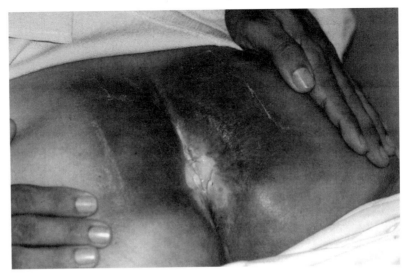

FIGURE 21.4 Marked hyperpigmentation over the sacrum and tissue breakdown as a result of overexposure.

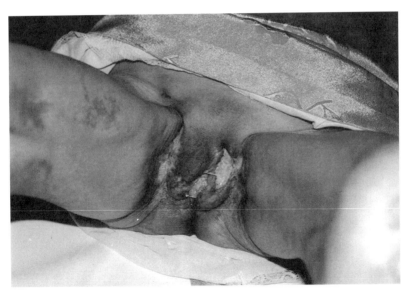

FIGURE 21.5 Necrosis of the perineum due to overexposure. Diagnosis is complicated by a recurrent tumor.

DECEASED PATIENTS

The team also reviewed the available autopsy and histological data on patients who had died. This was evaluated in light of prior clinical findings and exposure data. Autopsy data were available on 41 of 61 patients (67%) who had died. Where autopsy data were not available the clinical charts were reviewed to attempt to reach a conclusion about the possible role of radiation. Patients who had died were assigned to one of four categories, as follows:

1. Radiation overexposure may be the major cause of death
2. Radiation overexposure possibly a significant contributor to death
3. Death due to causes other than radiation overexposure
4. Insufficient data at this time to make an informed judgment

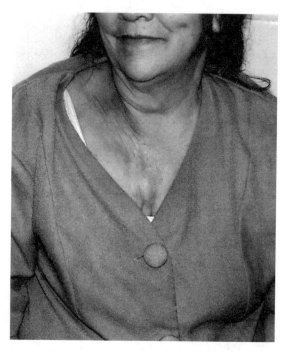

FIGURE 21.6 Overexposure of a treatment field in the right clavicular area resulting in marked fibrosis and limitation of motion.

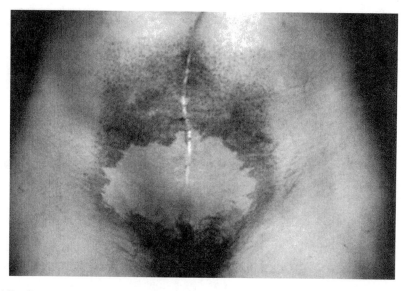

FIGURE 21.7 Overexposure of the pelvis resulting in hyperpigmentation, desquamation, and multiple underlying bowel and bladder problems.

It should be pointed out that this assessment was related to the cause of death only. In the third category (not radiation related) some patients had overexposure and radiation injury (for example, to an arm) but, in the authors' opinion, was not a cause of death. In this regard, some data were available on those patients who were initially clinically examined and who expired in the interval. The 17 patients for whom there were sufficient data to think that they died from radiation-related injuries can be divided into three general categories, as follows:

1. Central nervous system: Brain necrosis and complications of quadriplegia
2. Neck and upper mediastinal: Pharynx, tracheal, and bronchial necrosis, tracheoesophageal fistula
3. Lower gastrointestinal: Colitis, hemorrhage, obstruction, fistula, perforation, peritonitis

Data on patients who died are presented in Table 21.2.

TABLE 21.2
Summary Data on Deaths Thought to be Directly Radiation Related

Patient No.	Autopsy	Date of Death	Radiation Related?	Comments
8	Not Yet	08/30/98	Possibly	
18	Yes	10/19/96	Yes	Peritonitis, perforation
41	Yes	08/29/97	Possibly	Spinal cord, pneumonia
46	Yes	01/26/97	Yes	Pharynx, larynx necrosis
47	Yes	07/18/98	Yes	Pituitary necrosis
48	Yes	07/18/97	Yes	Tracheoesoph fistula
52	Yes	01/14/97	Yes	Tracheal necrosis
57	Yes	12/22/96	Yes	Bowel necrosis
59	Yes	10/28/96	Yes	Tracheal, bronchial necrosis
60	Yes	11/10/96	Yes	Tracheal, laryngeal necrosis
68	Yes	06/23/97	Yes	Fistula peritonitis
73	Yes	11/20/96	Yes	Intestinal necrosis + sponge
77	Yes	08/01/97	Yes	Bowel perforation
78	No	06/21/98	Possibly	
85	Yes	10/25/97	Yes	Bowel perforation
86	Yes	12/07/96	Yes	Tracheal, bronchial necrosis
108	No	10/13/96	Possibly	Colitis

SITES OF IRRADIATION AND CATASTROPHIC COMPLICATIONS

During the course of the accident, there were 125 different anatomical sites treated. The sites were as follows:

Head	23
Neck	18
Spine	15
Chest/shoulder	22
Abdomen	3
Pelvis	37
Extremity	7

The patients who either died as a result of irradiation or who have had severe complications demonstrate reactions that are consistent with the scientific literature.[3-7] In almost all the cases both the total dose and the dose per fraction was higher than that known to cause the complications observed in these patients.

Central Nervous System Complications

In the first 24 months there were severe central nervous system (CNS) complications in at least four patients, as follows:

Brain: The scientific literature indicates that radiation necrosis of the brain occurs with moderate probability when doses exceed 50 Gy in 20 fractions. Two patients with severe complications received doses substantially over 50 Gy.

1. Patient 47 received 69 Gy in 28 fractions. This would have been equivalent to a dose of 76 to 78 Gy in 2-Gy fractions. About 23 months after treatment, there was development of radiation necrosis of the pituitary gland resulting in death.
2. Patient 109 is a child who received cranial irradiation of 58 Gy in 20 fractions. Within 9 months, the patient lost all ability to speak and was confined to a wheelchair. Computed tomography scans of the brain show severe central and cortical atrophy, as well as mineralizing microangiopathy.

Spinal Cord: There is a 25 to 50% incidence of thoracic spinal cord myelopathy at dose levels of 60 Gy with 2-Gy fractions, 40 Gy with 3-Gy fractions, and 35 Gy with 4-Gy fractions. There are a number of patients whose fractions exceeded 3 Gy, and the total doses were well in excess of 40 Gy.

1. Patient 40 received 51 Gy in 17 fractions, or 3 Gy/fraction. The patient developed a T6-level paraplegia about 12 months after treatment.
2. Patient 41 received 57 Gy in 15 fractions, or 3.8 Gy/fraction. This is equivalent to 75 to 81 Gy if the fractions had been 2 Gy each. This patient was paralyzed within 9 months and died from pneumonia about 11 months after the accident. Pneumonia is a well-known cause of death following high spinal cord injury.
3. Patient 80 received 50 Gy in 16 fractions, or 3.1 Gy/fraction. The patient became quadriplegic within 9 months and has since regained some very slight sensory and motor function.

Since radiation necrosis of the brain and spine may occur up to 5 years later, three other patients in the same calculated dose ranges are still at high risk. In other words, five of the eight patients expected to have major neurological sequelae had developed them by 24 months.

Tracheal, Laryngeal, and Bronchial Necrosis

The literature on radiation effects on the pharynx indicate that doses in excess of 60 Gy in standard treatment fractions of 2 to 2.4 Gy each will result in denudation of the mucosa acutely and nonhealing ulcers later. Necrosis of the laryngeal cartilage can occur within 12 months. At least six patients died with neck and mediastinal complications. Five of these six had doses in excess of 60 Gy with about 3 Gy/fraction. All of these patients died within 10 months of the accident. There are no surviving patients in this category.

1. Patient 46 received irradiation to the face and neck with a dose of 62 to 70 Gy in about 20 fractions, or over 3 Gy/fraction. The patient died 4 months after the accident from necrosis of the pharynx and larynx.

2. Patient 48 received mediastinal irradiation of 62 Gy in 15 fractions, or 4.1 Gy/fraction. The patient died 10 months after the accident from a tracheoesophageal fistula.
3. Patient 52 received 92 Gy in 33 fractions, or 2.8 Gy/fraction. The patient died with tracheal necrosis 5 months after the accident.
4. Patient 59 received neck irradiation with a dose of 62 Gy in 20 fractions, or 3.1 Gy/fraction. The patient died with tracheal and bronchial necrosis about 6 weeks after the accident.
5. Patient 60 received 74.4 Gy to the neck in 24 fractions, or 3.1 Gy/fraction. The patient died about 2 months after the accident with tracheal and laryngeal necrosis.
6. Patient 86 received mantle irradiation of 44 Gy in 14 fractions, or 3.1 Gy/fraction. The patient died with tracheal and bronchial necrosis about 10 weeks after the accident.

Bowel Perforation and Necrosis

In the large bowel the incidence of severe complication is 40% at a dose of 60 Gy given in 2-Gy fractions. Six patients died from radiation-related bowel complications within the first 13 months after the accident. Only three patients remained alive with pelvic doses between 54 and 72 Gy.

1. Patient 18 received a dose of 60 Gy in 12 fractions, or 5 Gy/fraction. At 6 weeks after treatment, the patient died from bowel perforation and peritonitis.
2. Patient 57 received about 40 Gy in 22 fractions. This calculated dose seemed low for the observed clinical findings, and the patient died from bowel necrosis about 3 months after the accident. Pathological findings are consistent with radiation as the cause.
3. Patient 68 received 59 Gy in 19 fractions, or 3.1 Gy/fraction. The patient died about 9 months after the accident from bowel fistulas, perforation, and peritonitis.
4. Patient 73 received 68 Gy in 25 fractions, or about 2.7 Gy/fraction. The patient died from intestinal necrosis about 2 months after treatment.
5. Patient 77 received about 70 Gy in 25 fractions, or about 2.8 Gy/fraction. The patient died about 4 months after the accident from bowel perforation.
6. Patient 85 received about 50 Gy in 18 fractions, or about 2.7 Gy/fraction. The patient died about 13 months after the accident from bowel perforation.

DISCUSSION

There are a least three complicating factors in the medical evaluation of both the surviving and deceased patients. The first of these is the inadequate quality of the patient radiotherapy records at San Juan de Dios Hospital. This relates not only to evaluation of dose to the tissues but to the exact location of the radiation beam. In most cases, no films or drawings are available to show the location of the radiation treatment beam on the body. For some deceased patients, this poses a major problem in evaluation. For patients who were alive, the field location could almost always be ascertained by clinical examination of the subcutaneous fibrosis, skin pigmentation, and loss of hair. It is clear that some of the patients had skin changes indicating that the radiation fields were several inches from where they should have been.

A second complicating factor in evaluation of some of the patients is prior or subsequent treatment either with surgery or chemotherapy. Usually the complications and side effects could be distinguished by knowledge of the effects of the specific drugs, time the effect occurred, and knowledge of the type and timing of radiation effects relative to exposure.

The third complicating factor is that even though patients who received a few treatments at the beginning or end of the accident may not be expected to have radiation effects as a result of overexposure of a few treatments, they will have the "normal" incidence of radiation effects expected from standard radiotherapy.

The authors used the SOMA/LENT grading system proposed for evaluation of long-term effects.[8] The system was useful to provide a framework for evaluation of subjective, objective, management, and analytic findings; however, it had some limitations. In this patient population there were results of tests on some patients but not on others. It was felt that the resultant scores did not reflect the potential future consequences. For example, a high score relating to skin changes does not carry as serious an implication as a medium score relative to the CNS. The system also has no way of examining the dose and fractionation scheme to predict future effects, which is the important issue to both patients and their treating physicians. This could only be done on the basis of the dosimetry and clinical expertise.

The accident at San Juan de Dios Hospital was a very serious one. There have been many patients with marked radiation effects due to overexposure. Both morbidity and mortality have been increased. The accident remains unique. There have been accidents involving much higher exposures that have resulted in mortality, but there are none where the acute and subacute effects have been described in which the dose level is 10 to 50% above prescribed radiotherapy doses with fewer than the normal number of treatments.

Not all of the radiation effects noted in these patients can be attributed to the accident. There are patients who received treatment at the time of the accident who have radiation effects that would be expected as a consequence of accepted radiotherapy protocols. While effects on normal tissues are expected as a result of standard radiotherapy protocols, the incidence of serious and obvious radiation effects is much higher than expected.

Since many surviving patients received higher-than-prescribed doses, there is a theoretical possibility that the ultimate cure rate of the malignancies might be higher than otherwise expected. The team feels that with fewer than 55 patients, any such effect would be too small to detect reliably and certainly would not begin to approach the increase in mortality as a result of the accident.

Despite that there was little human data for much of the dose range in this accident, that the delayed and chronic radiation effects had yet not occurred, and that many patients who had died did not have finalized autopsies, the previous medical evaluation predicted the current findings with about 90% accuracy. By 2 years after the accident somewhat more than half of the patients had died. Of those cases in which there were sufficient data for evaluation, about one third of deaths were directly related to radiation and about two thirds were mainly related to the primary malignant disease. The deaths were primarily related to mediastinal, bowel, and CNS complications.

While there will continue to be delayed radiation effects and complications, which will appear over the next 5 years, the majority are felt to have manifested themselves at this time. In the remaining patients, the percentage of deaths that are radiation related will decrease. The ultimate percent of patients who will die as a result of overexposure in this accident will likely be between 15 and 30%.

Of the surviving patients, there are several predominant groups of radiation effects related to the body part irradiated. These include brain and spinal cord, lower abdominal, gastrointestinal, and bladder, vascular, and skin injuries.

Medical care and surveillance needs to continue to be provided for the surviving patients. The medical care should be provided in an interdisciplinary approach. Of particular importance are physiotherapy and infection prevention for those with CNS effects, dental care for those with neck and face irradiation, cardiac and vascular care for those with cardiac or large blood vessel irradiation, and gastrointestinal and urological care for those with pelvic irradiation.

ACKNOWLEDGMENT

The authors would like to acknowledge the help of J. Francisco Aquirre, Liliana Arrieta, Gerry J. Kutcher, Pedro Ortiz-Lopez, Patricia Mora-Rodriquez, Ronald Pacheco-Jiminez, Luis Bermudez-Jimenez, and Hugo Marenco-Zuniga.

REFERENCES

1. IAEA, Accidental Overexposure of Radiotherapy Patients in San Jose, Costa Rica, International Atomic Energy Agency, Vienna, 1998.
2. Cohen, L., Schultheiss, T.E. and Kennaugh, R.C., A radiation overexposure incident: initial data, *Int. J. Radiat. Oncol. Biol. Phys.*, 33(1), 217–224, 1995.
3. Mettler, F.A. and Upton, A.C., *Medical Effects of Ionizing Radiation*, Saunders, Philadelphia, 1996.
4. Gutin, P.H., Leibel, S.A., and Sheline, G.E., *Radiation Injury to the Nervous System*, Raven Press, New York, 1991.
5. Scherer, E., Streffer, C., and Trott, K., Eds., *Radiopathology of Organs and Tissues*, Springer-Verlag, Berlin, 1991.
6. Fajardo, L., *Pathology of Radiation Injury*, Masson Monographs in Diagnostic Pathology, Masson, New York, 1982.
7. Rubin, P. and Casarett, G., *Clinical Radiation Pathology*, Saunders, Philadelphia, 1968.
8. Pavy, J.J., Denekamp, J., Letschert, J., Littbrand, B. et al. Late effects toxicity scoring: the SOMA scale, EORTC late effects working group, *Radiat. Ther. Oncol.*, 35, 11–15, 1995.

22 Medical Accidents with Local Injury from Use of Medical Fluoroscopy

Chris Sharp

CONTENTS

Introduction 313
Accident Reports 314
Specific Cases 315
Contribution of Operational and Equipment Factors to Injury 316
    Equipment Factors 316
    Operational Factors 316
Postaccident Treatment of Skin Injuries 317
    Prediction 317
    Possible Treatments 317
        Early 317
        Later 318
Acknowledgments 318
References 318

INTRODUCTION

Medical fluoroscopy has been available for several decades and has been used, and still is in developing countries, instead of conventional film radiography. This is because once the capital cost of the equipment has been expended, operating costs are lower than film radiography, primarily those costs relating to film purchasing and processing costs. For most simple examinations, the doses delivered to the patient (and particularly the skin) are much higher than those seen in film radiography. Fluoroscopy continues to be used for more complex examinations, e.g., barium studies and other examinations of function, although many of these are being replaced by alternative techniques, e.g., endoscopy.

Since the late 1960s, medical practice has seen interventional procedures utilizing fluoroscopy increase significantly, with predictions of continued growth. The basic concept is of keyhole surgery using X-ray vision, with the vision provided by the fluoroscopy; although in today's practice the vision can also be provided by other modalities, e.g., ultrasound, magnetic resonance imaging (MRI), and computed tomography (CT). Interestingly, before the late 1960s attempts at interventional radiology had been curtailed, mainly because of the radiation hazards involved, primarily to those manipulating the fluoroscopy. As indicated by this concern, such procedures have the potential to deliver substantial doses to both staff and patients, and particularly to skin.

Most interventional techniques comprise procedures utilizing guided therapeutic and/or diagnostic interventions via percutaneous access, usually performed under local anesthesia and/or sedation, with fluoroscopic imaging used to localize the lesion/treatment site, monitor the procedure, and control and document the therapy. As these techniques often involve the passage of catheters into narrow and tortuous vessels deep inside various organs, the operative time can be extended, causing long fluoroscopy exposure to the patient, resulting in high localized skin exposures. Also, some procedures may need to be repeated, and often within short periods of time, e.g., percutaneous transluminal coronary angiography/angioplasty.

Interventional radiology offers to medicine in all countries, no matter the stage of development, the opportunity to treat a greater range of pathologies, in more patients, and at lesser cost. Interventional techniques reduce the need for expensive operating suites and extended hospital in-patient admissions. They also reduce most of the risks to the patient by the use of minimally invasive techniques and through lesser requirements for general anesthesia. Additionally, they may allow therapy of lesions not previously accessible, although with concomitantly greater risks.

Although originally developed by radiologists, early in the evolution of interventional techniques cardiologists entered the field and worldwide cardiology still represents, in numbers of procedures, the specialty with the highest activity. However, interventional radiology has been "discovered" by many other specialties and the list of nonradiologists using fluoroscopy is growing (e.g., urologists, gastroenterologists, orthopedic surgeons, vascular surgeons, traumatologists, anesthesiologists, pediatricians). It is likely that practitioners in most specialties will become "interventionalists" and increasingly use such techniques in the near future. Interventionalists have often received only minimal, or no, training in radiation effects, or may have forgotten or not be aware of the possible doses that their equipment may deliver. Consequently, there is growing evidence that many interventionalists have a less-than-ideal understanding of the risks of radiation-induced injuries from X rays. This has undoubtedly led to local injuries in many patients, some of which have had serious implications for the affected patients.

ACCIDENT REPORTS

Since the early 1990s,[1-4] reports of radiation-induced injuries to patients' skin have steadily increased, spanning the whole spectrum of skin injury from erythema to ulcers requiring major plastic surgery (see Color Figures 1 and 2*); these reports are likely to represent a small fraction of the actual cases, particularly as such problems are usually manifest after the patient has left the interventionalist's care — appearing from several days to months after the procedure. Many of these injuries are avoidable, certainly all of the severe ones. This is particularly important as the most severe lesions can lead to permanent disability and chronic, intractable pain. Most occur because interventionalists are not aware of the radiation doses that are delivered to skin. In neuroradiology, there is a particular risk to the eyes of cataract, if the radiation primary beam passes through the lens, and also to the hair, where loss may be temporary or permanent. Table 22.1 gives the range of threshold doses for skin injury. Typically, fluoroscopy equipment delivers skin doses of 20 mGy/min (low-dose-rate mode) to 200 mGy/min (high-dose-rate mode), although in some countries dose rates can be higher.

The initiation of skin injuries after repeated (fractionated) exposures is much more complex and is dependent, among other factors, on the time between exposures — the shorter the time, the more likely that effects will appear. It is also important to note that reports of injuries are not limited solely to the use of older equipment, but also to new and digital equipment, which can produce high dose rates. Skin radiation doses are also increased in proportion to the number of spot films taken, either digital or analog, in addition to those derived fluoroscopically. The number of digital image acquisitions can sometimes exceed 1000 in any one examination.

It is clear from most reports that monitoring of fluoroscopic system operational parameters was not a routine practice, and therefore skin doses had to be retrospectively estimated, based on typical

---

* Color figures follow page 202.

TABLE 22.1
Ionizing Radiation: Thresholds for Skin Effects (Single Doses)

Skin Response	mGy	Appearance
Erythema	2,000–6,000[a]	2–24 h (transient)
Desquamation		
Dry	3,000–5,000	3–6 weeks
Moist	15,000–18,000	~4–6 weeks[b]
Epilation		
Temporary	2,000–5,000	2–3 weeks
Permanent	>6,000	3 weeks[c]
Necrosis	>18,000	>10 weeks
Dermal atrophy	10,000	>12 weeks
Telangiectasia	10,000	>52 weeks
Fibrosis	Associated with any marked damage	>52 weeks

[a] Area dependent, > area = < dose.
[b] Dose dependent.
[c] Dose dependent, > dose = < time.

X-ray system technique factors or dose measurements using patient phantoms. This should provide a strong impetus to the provision of dose displays on equipment, so that interventionalists are aware when they are approaching the threshold for skin injury and other radiation effects.

SPECIFIC CASES

One example of skin injury attributable to X rays from fluoroscopy was illustrated by a 40-year-old man who acquired a substantial skin dose from a diagnostic coronary angiography followed by a coronary angioplasty and then a second angiography procedure due to complications. The complications led to a coronary artery bypass graft, all occurring on the same day. The skin where the X-ray beam had entered the body turned red about 1 month after the procedure and started to peel 1 week later. Then, 2 months after the procedures, the skin had the appearance of a second-degree burn, but 4 months later had healed, except for a small ulcerated area near the center. However, the skin showed progressive necrosis over the following months and eventually required a skin graft.[5] It is probable that the absorbed dose to the skin exceeded 20 Gy.

Interventional neuroradiological procedures requiring extended fluoroscopic exposure time have been described as leading to epilation. Temporary epilation of the right occipital region of the skull has been reported following transarterial embolization of a left paraorbital arteriovenous malformation performed in two stages, 3 days apart. The total absorbed dose was estimated at around 6 Gy. Regrowth occurred after 3 months, although the regrown hair was grayer than the original.

The injuries resulting from transjugular intrahepatic portosystemic shunt (TIPS) procedures have been described. In one, a 42-year-old male patient with diabetes mellitus and alcoholic liver disease had three different TIPS procedures separated by 2 and 9 days and a total procedure time of 12 h, 15 min. Then, 6 weeks after the first procedure, he presented with a 20 × 15 cm focally necrotic, ulcerating plaque on the mid-back of 2 weeks duration. He was treated conservatively and was left with a sclerotic plaque. In two other cases injuries resulted from 90 min of fluoroscopy (total procedure time of 4 h, 20 min) and from an unknown amount of fluoroscopy (total procedure time of 6 h, 30 min). Both injuries required split-thickness skin grafting.

There have been more reports of radiation injuries associated with radiofrequency catheter ablation of cardiac arrhythmias than for any other procedure. A 7-year-old girl developed radiodermatitis on the right arm following an ablation procedure 4 months before, which required an estimated 75 to 100 min of fluoroscopy with a horizontal X-ray beam. Several injuries have resulted or been made more severe when patients underwent repeated procedures, in some cases in different health care facilities, in attempts to obtain a successful outcome. A patient developed chronic radiodermatitis after two ablation procedures performed 13 months apart. A month following the second procedure the patient presented to the dermatology department with lesions on her right side; 2 years later, the patient had a 10 cm × 5 cm indurated plaque having both hyper- and hypopigmentation with multiple telangiectasia. Effects on the muscles in her right arm resulted in limited movement. Each procedure was reported to have lasted 5 h, but exposure times were not available. During the second procedure it was estimated that the horizontal X-ray beam was used during the procedure for 90 to 120 min. An exposure time of this length was estimated to result in a skin dose from the lateral beam of some 11 to 15 Gy/procedure. These instances illustrate the need for physicians to have information regarding radiation exposures associated with prior interventional procedures.

CONTRIBUTION OF OPERATIONAL AND EQUIPMENT FACTORS TO INJURY

Various factors influence patient and staff doses. These may be categorized into operational or equipment related. Some dose control measures are dependent on the equipment design for interventional radiology — if the equipment is not specifically designed it can deliver substantially higher doses. However, the way in which the equipment is operated, e.g., how the interventional procedure is performed, is usually the main determinant of the dose. Some examples are given below.

EQUIPMENT FACTORS

Dose reduction measures may be designed into the equipment at the outset. An example of an aspect of equipment design that may result in lower doses is the use of carbon fiber tabletops when the image intensifier is below the table. Reducing the attenuation between the exit surface of the patient and the image receptor directly reduces doses. Carbon fiber has excellent mechanical properties and strength, but has low attenuation. The provision of a display to show cumulative skin dose would help to maintain the interventionalist's awareness of when thresholds for skin damage are likely to be exceeded. Display of the dose rate being delivered to patients by fluoroscopic equipment utilizing automatic exposure rate controls (AERC) would also be very useful. Facilities for pulsed fluoroscopy, "last image hold," and "road-mapping" that are available with modem digital fluoroscopy equipment can be used to reduce the time that patients are exposed during fluoroscopically guided procedures.

OPERATIONAL FACTORS

If one area of skin is irradiated for extended periods, then, clearly, problems may occur. This can be avoided by changing the site of entry of the beam periodically, or in the case of repeat procedures perhaps reversing the tube and image intensifier between procedures. Most image intensifiers have at least two modes of operation. The first, the normal low-dose-rate mode, is normally used for the majority of the procedure. The second, or high-dose-rate mode, is used for more-complicated and difficult parts of the intervention, where improved image quality is required. It appears that many interventionalists are not aware that the high-dose-rate mode has a dose rate ten or more times higher than the lower, normal mode. Additionally, equipment may have a magnification mode, which operates using a reduced field of view (FOV); this typically increases the dose rate by a factor of 4, if the FOV is halved. Excessive periods of usage of both these facilities has been a common factor in reported accidents. Unexpectedly long, complicated procedures even in low-dose-rate mode can result in cumulative skin doses sufficient to cause damage. Patient size is also an important factor. As patient size increases, so does skin dose (Figure 22.1). The central message is that interventionalists need to take account of the possibility of excessive skin dose, as part of their operational technique.

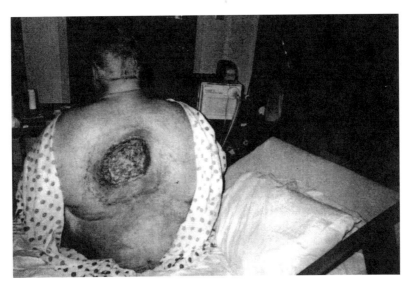

FIGURE 22.1 Case of a 166-kg patient approximately 9 months after coronary angioplasty and stenting. Ultimately, the procedure was teminated because of X-ray tube overheating. (Photograph courtesy of F. Mettler.)

POSTACCIDENT TREATMENT OF SKIN INJURIES

PREDICTION

Knowledge of the skin doses delivered in common procedures will allow prediction of whether skin or other local injuries are likely to occur. For departures from the "normal," and hence when skin doses are likely to have been high enough to produce injury, it is essential to have clinical protocols that identify the normal procedure. Patients falling outside these parameters need a personalized dose assessment if doses from often repeated procedures are >1 Gy or for other procedures are >3 Gy; clearly, recording of doses in patient notes for commonly repeated procedures are essential. For those procedures exceeding these parameters, the dose data provide a prediction of the effects expected and an indication of the follow-up required.

POSSIBLE TREATMENTS

Early

If a high-dose area is identified promptly, use of anti-inflammatory agents (locally and possibly systemically), e.g., steroids and antihistamines, will limit the damage done by the body's own inflammatory response, and consequently have the potential to limit the scale of subsequent surgery. Similarly, the use of agents that maintain blood flow (pentoxyfillin) and antioxidants (vitamin E and C), acting as free-radical scavengers, are first-line treatments. Concurrently, the prevention of superinfection is essential when the outer epidermal layer is lost, as the extent and severity of lesions can be significantly increased if infection supervenes — a limited lesion capable of self-repair can be converted into one requiring extensive operative intervention. Healing and repair of large ulcers can be facilitated by using animal (mainly porcine) and artificial skin for both temporary and, for the latter, permanent repair depending of the depth of radiation damage.

Later

In the later stages, the application of retinoids (vitamin A derivatives) can reduce unsightly keratoses (crusty, sore areas of skin) and may reduce longer-term skin cancer risk. Equally unsightly telangiectasia (dilated and tortuous surface blood vessels) can be treated with tunable dye lasers. However, the really serious long-term sequel of skin injury — fibrosis — is a significant problem for which no really lasting effective therapeutic agents have been identified. The process seems to be one of constant remodeling, but the mechanisms for this remain to be identified. Interferon has been injected subcutaneously to control the process, but it is expensive and the fibrotic process is only held in suspension until after treatment is terminated. A possible therapeutic agent is superoxide dismutase. The action of this bovine-derived liposomal substance appears to be to decrease the production of fibrotic cytokines (TGFbl) by myofibroblasts, which leads, in cellular models, to the reversal of radiation fibrosis and promotion of the regeneration of normal tissue. The availability of a human recombinant preparation is crucial to further clinical research, as bovine spongiform encephalitis — mad cow disease, or BSE — has compromised the use of bovine-derived material. Future improvements in treatment are likely to be linked to collaboration with those involved in wound-healing research, where evaluation of anti-inflammatory cytokines (IL-10 and IL-13) and selective inhibitors of radiation-induced signal transduction pathways are likely to be the most productive lines of research.

ACKNOWLEDGMENTS

The author wishes to acknowledge the assistance of Mr. Barry Wall, National Radiological Protection Board (U.K.), in preparing the equipment aspects of this chapter.

REFERENCES

1. Food and Drug Administration. Avoidance of serious X-ray-induced skin injuries to patients during fluoroscopically guided procedures. September 9, 1994.
2. Shope, T.B., Radiation-induced skin injuries from fluoroscopy, *Imaging Ther. Technol.*, September 1996.
3. Schmidt, T., Wucherer, M., and Zeitler, E., Grundlagen zur Abschatzung der Strahlenexposition bei interventionellen Massnahmer, *Aktuelle Radiol.*, 8(1), 11–17, 1998, (in German).
4. Vafio, E., Arranz, L., Sastre, J.M., Moro, C., Ledo, A., Garate, M.T., and Minguez, I., Dosimetric and radiation protection considerations based on some cases of patient skin injuries in interventional cardiology, *Br. J. Radiol.*, 7(1), 510–516, 1998.
5. Shope, T.B., Radiation-induced skin injuries from fluoroscopy, *RadioGraphics*, 16, 1195–1199, 1996.
6. Koenig, T., Wolff, D., Mettler, F.A., and Wagner, L., Skin injuries from fluoroscopy-guided procedures, *Am. J. Roentgenol.*, in press, 2001.

23 Assessment and Treatment of Internal Contamination: General Principles

George L. Voelz

CONTENTS

Introduction 320
Initial Priorities 320
Initial Evaluation 321
Biokinetic Models and Dosimetry 324
Basis for Treatment Decisions 328
Treatment 329
    Reduction of Gastrointestinal Absorption 329
        Stomach Lavage 329
        Emetics 329
        Purgatives 329
        Ion-Exchange Resins 330
        Prussian Blue 330
        Aluminum-Containing Antacids 331
        Barium Sulfate 331
    Blocking and Diluting Agents 331
        Iodides 331
        Strontium 332
        Calcium 332
        Phosphate 332
        Forced Fluids 332
    Mobilizing Agents 332
        Antithyroid Drugs 332
        Ammonium Chloride 333
        Diuretics 333
        Expectorants and Inhalants 333
        Parathyroid Extract 333
        Sodium Bicarbonate 333
    Chelating Agents 333
    Lung Lavage 335
References 335

INTRODUCTION

How does a physician become aware that his patient(s) may have an internal exposure to radioactive material? Usually, someone tells her. This someone may be the patient who suspects or knows that he has been in a contaminated area or accident. It may be a radiation monitor or a fellow worker who is familiar with details of the accident.

However the issue is raised, the physician is faced with finding means to evaluate the exposure. Medical history can develop preliminary details of the accident or situation, but signs and symptoms from an exposure are highly unlikely unless some corrosive or irritant chemical exposure is also present. There may be traumatic injuries that need attention. The usual clinical laboratory tests are not helpful in determining exposure and only a few radioactivity measurements may be available at the time the first decisions must be made.

Is treatment necessary? Is effective treatment available? These are the physician's questions to answer. If possible, early telephone consultation with a radiation specialist may be helpful. This chapter focuses on the assessment and treatment of internally deposited radionuclides to assist physicians in the medical management of these cases.

INITIAL PRIORITIES

The first priority in the care of the patient is to attend to any life-threatening condition. Attention to vital functions and control of severe hemorrhaging take priority. The presence of potential radioactive contamination should not deter the nature or rapidity of medical care. Even if radiation levels are not known and survey instruments are not immediately available, proceed with lifesaving assistance. Wear gloves and wrap the patient in a sheet or blanket if radioactive contamination is suspected to be a problem; this is done to reduce the spread of contamination. Accidental contamination levels are almost never a serious hazard to personnel for the time required to perform lifesaving measures. High-level radioactive contamination, such as that which occurred to the Chernobyl firemen and rescue personnel, will not be encountered without immediate recognition of the occurrence of an extraordinary accident. Hospital personnel will be alerted to such unusual high-contamination accidents.

As soon as it is practical, a determination should be made regarding the presence or absence of radioactive contamination on clothing and skin. If radioactivity is present, clothing removal and skin decontamination should be performed. Skin decontamination usually only requires washing thoroughly with detergent and water. If an individual has been exposed to neutrons, e.g., from an accelerator or criticality accident, induced radioactivity in the body masquerades as nonremovable contamination on skin. Early decontamination not only reduces exposure but also helps prevent contamination of other persons and the facilities. Contaminated clothing and wastes should be contained in plastic bags. Emergency medical plans for management of a radioactively contaminated patient should include written decontamination procedures.[1,2]

Another priority is to assess the potential of an internal deposition of radioactive material. An important first step is to take a preliminary history on facts concerning the accident. Table 23.1 lists questions and subject areas that assist in taking this history from the patient and other knowledgeable persons who may be available. If the accident occurred in a university or industry, the best information will probably be obtained from a health physicist, radiation safety officer, supervisor, or occupational physician familiar with the facility and accident details.

One of the more serious constraints on the physician is the limited time available for making a treatment decision. For maximum effectiveness, most treatments for internal radioactive nuclides must begin within about 3 h after exposure. With each additional hour, the effectiveness of most treatment regimens is reduced. Thus, an early decision is necessary based on meager, and often confused, information.

TABLE 23.1
Medical History Questions for Radioactivity Contaminated Persons

When did the accident occur? What are the circumstances of the accident? Are external radiation and/or internal contamination involved?
What injuries have occurred? What potential medical problems may be present besides radiation exposure or radionuclide contamination?
Are toxic or corrosive chemicals involved in addition to the radionuclides? Have any treatments been given for these?
Was the person exposed to penetrating radiation? If so, what doses were measured by personal dosimeters, e.g., thermoluminescent dosimeter, or pocket ionization chamber? If not yet known, when is the information expected?
What radionuclides are involved? What are the most likely pathways for exposure? Are preliminary dose estimates available?
What information is available about the chemistry of the radioactive compounds? Soluble or insoluble? Any information about probable particle size?
What radioactivity measurements have been made at the site of the accident, e.g., air monitors, smears, fixed radiation monitors, nasal smear counts, and skin contamination levels?
What skin decontamination efforts have already been attempted? What were the results? What are the radiation measurements at the surface?
Have any therapeutic measures, such as blocking or chelating agents, been given?
Have samples of the contaminant from the accident area, clothes, etc. been saved for nuclide and isotope analyses and particle size studies?
What excreta have been collected? Who has the samples? What analyses are planned? When will they be done?

INITIAL EVALUATION

Essential information needed to make immediate treatment decisions for possible internal exposure to radioactive material is identification of the radionuclide(s) involved, general level of potential exposure, and mode of potential intake. One should also find out if the patient may have received significant external radiation exposure. There may be few, if any, radioactivity measurements available at this early time.

The physician should determine the specific hazards and characteristics of the principal radionuclide(s) present in the exposure. Appendix 4 has several tables of information on selected radionuclides for use in early evaluation of an accidental exposure. The metabolic behavior of radionuclides must be understood. This subject is discussed briefly in the next section, entitled Biokinetic Models and Dosimetry.

For decontamination work, it is usually adequate to know simply whether one is dealing with a "beta-gamma" emitter or an "alpha" emitter. The key point is to ensure that the survey instrumentation being used can detect the radiation in question. For treatment decisions, it is necessary to know the exact nuclide(s) involved to determine its radiological and chemical properties, metabolic behavior, and the available treatment regimens. If the contaminating radionuclide(s) cannot be identified with confidence based on available information, samples of the contamination should be identified by gamma and/or alpha spectroscopy.

Information to appraise the extent of internal exposure will be limited at the early time when treatment decisions should be made, if possible within 1 to 3 h. At this time one should have an idea of the level of skin and clothing contamination, which is a rough indication of how much radioactivity is present. If the accident occurred in a facility where measurements are made, there should be contamination levels (floor, benchtops, equipment, etc.) and possibly air concentration levels to estimate potential levels of exposure. A rough estimate of inhalation potential can be made by using air concentrations times the occupancy time by the patient (without respirator) in the room.

Nasal swipe samples taken within a few minutes of the exposure can give a rough idea of inhalation potential. Swipe samples are taken from each nostril separately using a moistened cotton swab or moistened filter paper on a swabstick. The samples are dried and counted. These samples are subject to error because the individual's anterior nasal passage may have been contaminated with the patient's hands or from surrounding facial contamination. Nose blowing or swiping prior to sampling also invalidates the results. By the time the individual gets to a hospital, it is likely to be too late to obtain useful information from nasal swabs.

Nasal swabs have been used most often at facilities handling alpha emitters, such as plutonium or americium. Interpretations vary at different facilities, but one rule of thumb judgment is that counts over 500 disintegrations per minute (dpm) may indicate a significant exposure, while results less than 50 dpm suggest no more than a possible low-order exposure. High values in one nostril with low or no activity in the other are suggestive of contamination by means other than inhalation. In these cases, one should check whether there is reasonable nasal airflow through the low side. Mouth breathing can also cause nasal swab results in general to be low. High nasal counts can result from activity transferred from contaminated hands or face.

Radioactivity measurement of wounds potentially contaminated with plutonium, americium, or other alpha emitters should be made as soon as initial skin decontamination efforts are completed. Facilities with the potential of such accidents need to have the special wound counters required to make such measurements. Beta-gamma contamination often can be counted satisfactorily with conventional beta-gamma survey instruments, but good localization of the activity may be a problem. Small end-window probes or special detectors for wound monitoring are much better at locating the loci of activity in or near the wound.

The above information may be all that can be collected before making a timely treatment decision. There is always a question of to how much detailed monitoring and dosimetry information is needed before treatment is begun. Medical decisions are based on a professional judgment, not dose limits, and the fact that treatment will result in more good than harm. This decision can usually be rendered by assessing the limited early information outlined above. Simply estimating whether exposure potential is low, medium, or high and knowing the risks of the proposed treatment is sufficient to make such a decision. Once the decision to treat is made and treatment is started, the urgency of a time constraint is past and the detailed dosimetry studies can begin. This discussion of treatment decisions is expanded in a later section of this chapter.

The more definitive means of estimating internal deposition of radionuclides is by direct whole-body counts (Figure 23.1), chest counts, wound counts, and by excretion measurements in urine or fecal samples. Interpretation of direct counting is often complicated by residual surface contamination during the first hours after an accident. Whole-body counters are extremely sensitive, measuring total gamma activity of 37 Bq (1 nCi) or less. With this level of sensitivity, counts registered from skin contamination can be significant even though careful decontamination has been performed and conventional handheld survey instruments show little or no activity. The results are often more confusing than helpful in the first day or two because it may not be possible to distinguish clearly between activity from external and internal contamination. High sensitivity of a whole-body or chest counter also limits the capacity of these counters to measure very high levels of activity that could be involved in some exposures. Even though *in vivo* counters may be available nearby, it is usually not necessary to delay treatment decisions for an hour or more to make a whole-body or lung count. Identification of the specific radionuclides involved can be made by quick measurements of contaminated clothing, skin, or other contaminated objects. Counts of the individual can wait until after therapy has been started.

Some soluble radionuclides can be detected in urine within minutes after exposure. Notable examples are radioiodine, tritium (radioactive hydrogen), and radiocesium. Radioactivity levels present in urine are used to calculate the uptake in the body by means of excretion models appropriate for the specific nuclide.[3] For emergency estimates, spot urine samples are taken as a rough estimate of excretion and uptake. The patient should empty the bladder once after exposure before providing a spot sample. Precautions must be taken to prevent sample contamination if there is external skin contamination present.

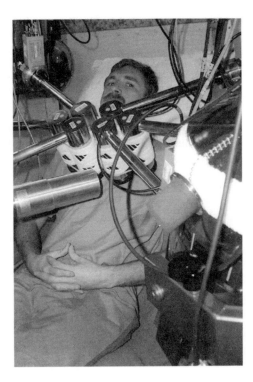

FIGURE 23.1 Current whole-body counter and new germanium detectors for plutonium and americium lung measurements at Los Alamos.

Uptake of *radioiodine* can be measured either by urine excretion measurements or by direct counts over the thyroid. Accident response usually involves thyroid counts within an hour or so of intake and, therefore, the results must be adjusted for time after exposure because the peak thyroid activity occurs at about 24 h after exposure. Measurement in urine samples has been found to be an efficacious method for detecting thyroid burdens within the first 12 h after exposure.[4,5] A three-compartment model,[4] using a 4-h integration period, predicts the percent of iodine intake to be excreted via urine at the following times after a single acute exposure: 0 to 4 h, 25% of iodine excreted in urine; 4 to 8 h, 16%; 8 to 12 h, 10%; 12 to 16 h, 6.1%; 16 to 20 h, 3.8%; 20 to 24 h, 2.3%. There are large uncertainties in the use of such model calculations as applied to an individual, but such estimates can be useful for early evaluation of exposures. Effective treatment of a radio-iodine exposure must be done as soon as possible, preferably in the first hour. The above data indicate that a single urine sample taken early will be useful for a rough estimate of the potential uptake of iodine. The first voiding after the uptake can have a falsely low value because of dilution with urine excreted by the kidney prior to exposure.

Tritium is a weak beta emitter that is not detectable by normal survey instruments or by whole-body counting. Detection of exposure is by urine samples, which show excretion immediately after exposure. The first voiding after exposure should not used because dilution by preexposure urine may cause a falsely low reading. The sample is counted by liquid scintillation techniques. A conservative rough rule of thumb, based on the peak urine concentration after a single acute exposure, is that 37 Bq (1 nCi)/l of tritium equates to a total integrated whole-body dose of about 100 µSv, if the person is not treated by forcing fluids.

Radiocesiums, cesium-134 and cesium-137, are gamma emitters that can be detected by whole-body counting techniques or by urine excretion. Whole-body counting in the first few hours may be complicated by the presence of external contamination. Careful collection of a urine sample should prevent contamination of the sample. Measurement by gamma spectroscopy will identify the activity due to the cesium nuclides. A rough estimate is that about 1% of the cesium activity in the body will be excreted in urine each day during the first 3 days after a single acute intake of soluble cesium.

All urine and feces should be saved in individual containers marked by patient name and time of collection until the health physicists have determined a specific sampling program. If there is transportable (loose) contamination on the patient, the samples must be collected in a manner that avoids contaminating them.

Reference materials, such as References 1 and 2, should be obtained for use during an emergency. They describe common radionuclides, their physical and biological properties, dosimetry information, and treatment options. The references are also helpful in developing emergency plans and procedures for nuclear facilities and hospitals.

BIOKINETIC MODELS AND DOSIMETRY

The success of the initial evaluation described above is dependent on the physician's knowledge of the modes of uptake, metabolism, excretion, and dosimetry of the involved radionuclide. In developing models for the behavior of radionuclides in humans, these various transfer rates are determined, estimated, or assumed for absorption, retention, internal distribution, and excretion of each nuclide. Standard models have been recommended and published by the International Commission on Radiological Protection (ICRP)[6,7] for calculating allowable limits of intake for workers. Figure 23.2 is a schematic representation of the principal routes of intake, physical and metabolic transfers in the body, and major excretion pathways.

The gastrointestinal (GI) tract, respiratory tract, and skin are the more common organ systems through which radionuclides enter the body. The quantity of radionuclide taken into the body is called the *intake* by health physicists and modelers. Intake should not be confused with *uptake*, which is the amount retained in the body either in the lung or absorbed systemically. The difference between intake and uptake is due to short-term clearance mainly by the lung and GI tract. The nuclide(s), if soluble in body fluids, will be absorbed in the extracellular fluids (lymph fluid and blood) of these entry organs. Distribution to other organs is made primarily via blood circulation. The radioactive nuclide deposited in organs via the systemic circulation is termed the *systemic deposition*. A small portion of the nuclide deposited in organs is reabsorbed later and recirculated

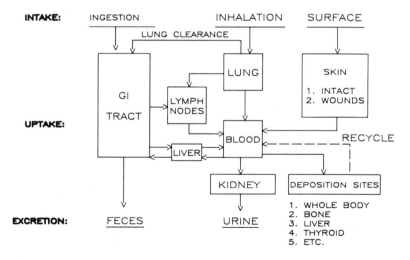

FIGURE 23.2 Diagram representation of intake, metabolism, and excretion of radionuclides.

via blood. Some of the recycling radionuclide is excreted through the kidney or GI tract, and the rest is redeposited in organs. It is a dynamic, rather than static, process.

Uptake from the GI tract depends upon the chemical characteristics of the element. The absorption of many radionuclides is small, 10% or less. Small GI uptake is found for radionuclides of chromium, manganese, iron, cobalt, zirconium, ruthenium, silver, antimony, cerium, inorganic mercury, uranium, plutonium, americium, curium, and californium. Elements with higher absorption from the GI tract are radium (20%), strontium (30%), and phosphorus (80%); tritium (radioactive hydrogen), iodine, and cesium are completely absorbed.

For the portion of radioactive material that is not absorbed by the GI tract, the highest radiation dose will be delivered to the lower large intestine because of the longer residence time in this segment of the tract. In the ICRP models, mean residence time to traverse the GI tract is taken to be 1 h for stomach, 6 h for small intestine, 13 h for upper large intestine, and 24 h for lower large intestine.

The schematic drawing on radionuclide uptake (Figure 23.2) indicates that material inhaled into the lung can be cleared in three ways: (1) lung clearance to the GI tract by means of the mucociliary escalator of the tracheobronchial tree and swallowing, (2) absorption and systemic distribution through blood, and (3) insoluble particulate transfer to lymph nodes by phagocytic cells. The type and rate of these transfers are influenced primarily by the chemical characteristics of the inhaled material and the particle sizes. Completely soluble material, such as tritium or iodine, will transfer immediately to blood. Lung clearance rates for less soluble particles depend on the rate of solubility in fluids of the respiratory tract and the distribution of particle deposition within the respiratory tract.

The rates of transfer of the radionuclide among entry organs, blood, and deposition organs are determined primarily by the biochemical properties of the radionuclide. Some ingested or inhaled radioactive particles may include radionuclides contained within a matrix of different materials. Solubility of the particle may be determined by the character of the matrix, which may be quite different from that expected for the radionuclide inclusion. This phenomenon is observed mostly in particles with induced radioactivity around nuclear reactors or accelerators. It is usually noted when the matrix is less soluble than the radionuclide; thus, the systemic uptake from the lung or GI tract is much slower or less than expected.

The principal excretion pathways from the body are through urine and feces. Lesser pathways are by perspiration and exhalation. Concentration of the radionuclide in urine often correlates with the concentration present in the blood. Fecal excretion of radioactive material consists of two components: (1) insoluble material from direct ingestion or lung clearance that passes unabsorbed through the GI tract and (2) excreted systemic material via bile and GI secretions.

Both the ICRP and the National Council on Radiation Protection and Measurements (NCRP) have developed models for the deposition, retention, and dosimetry of inhaled radionuclides.[8,9] They both arrive at remarkably similar mathematical assessments in general, although detailed calculations for specific radionuclides can be quite different in terms of the way they are handled. The ICRP respiratory tract model[9] divides the system into five regions: anterior nasal passage (ET_1), posterior nasopharynx and larynx (ET_2), tracheobronchial (BB), bronchiolar (bb), and alveolar-interstitial (AI). Deposition of inhaled particles is assumed to vary with the aerodynamic properties of the aerosol, as shown graphically in Figure 23.3. Inspection of this figure shows that larger particles (>5 μm) are mostly deposited in the extrathoracic regions (ET_1 and ET_2). The percent of deposition in the lung (BB, bb, and AI) increases with smaller particle sizes. General knowledge of particle size after an inhalation exposure may provide some notion on particle deposition in the respiratory tract. For example, radioactive particles from mechanical-type operations (filing, sawing, lathe work, explosions without fire) are often of a large size. Inhalation is likely to deposit such particles in the nasopharyngeal regions. If so, one might see significant clearance (sometimes essentially 100%) of insoluble particles within the first few days. A high proportion of the fine

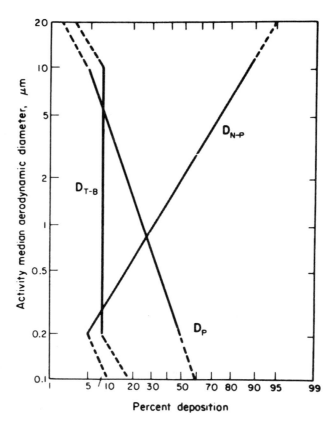

FIGURE 23.3 Fractional deposition in each region of the respiratory tract as a function of aerosol size for a reference worker (normal nose breather).

particles (<10 μm) from a fume, fire, or smoke are more likely to be deposited in the AI region, which is below the ciliated portion of the respiratory tract. In this case, relatively little lung clearance is likely and retention can be expected to be long term.

The ICRP recommends that material-specific rates of absorption should be used in the respiratory tract model for compounds for which reliable human or animal experimental data exist. But it also recommends three default parameters, which may be used for dosimetry calculations if specific information is not available, which is the situation in the majority of cases. The selection of default parameter to use is according to whether the lung absorption rate is considered to by fast (Type F), moderate (M), or slow (S). The approximate half-time for type F is 10 min for 100% absorption; for type M, 10 min (10%) and 140 days (90%); and type S, 10 min (0.1%) and 7000 days (99.9%). Gases and vapors are treated separately in three classes: highly soluble, partially soluble, or insoluble and nonreactive, depending on the chemistry of the compound.

A unique characteristic of relatively insoluble (Type S) alpha-emitting radionuclides inhaled into the lung is the nonuniform distribution of radiation dose that occurs (Figure 23.4). The penetration range of alpha particles is only 50 μm or less in tissue, or about 4 to 5 cell diameters. The subject of nonuniform radiation doses in lung raises a controversy about whether this phenomenon produces an elevated risk of lung cancer compared with a comparable intake of radioactivity but with uniform lung dose distribution. A committee of the NCRP[10] concluded, based on a substantial body of experimental animal data, that there is no greater hazard from particulate plutonium doses in the lung than from the same amount of plutonium more uniformly distributed throughout the lung. The NCRP concluded that averaging the dose from particulate alpha-emitting

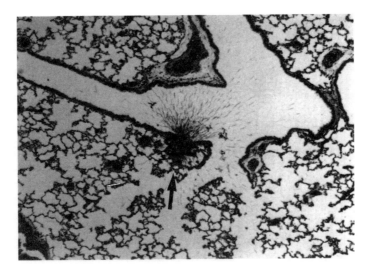

FIGURE 23.4 Autoradiograph of alpha particles from a plutonium particle deposited on the epithelial lining of an airway of hamster lung illustrates nonuniform radiation dose distribution within lung. Animal studies have not demonstrated a greater risk for induction of lung cancer from nonuniform dose distribution compared with the same total radioactivity distributed more uniformly throughout the lung. (Courtesy of Los Alamos National Laboratory.)

radionuclides over the entire lung is a defensible procedure. Nonuniform dose distribution by alpha emitters also occurs in other organs, i.e., skin (wounds), lymph nodes, and bone.

After uptake into the systemic circulation, radioactive compounds are distributed to and deposited in various organs depending on their biochemical properties. The ICRP model assumes systemic distributions to organs and tissues for specific nuclides in accordance with transfer rates described in Publication 78.[7] ICRP values have been incorporated into a variety of available computer programs used by dosimetry specialists to calculate organ and/or effective doses. Appendix 4 lists critical organs for various radionuclides. This designation is a simplified, and limited, method for indicating the organ expected to receive the highest dose or having the most significant potential biological effect.

Most models use coefficients specific for each radionuclide to determine the systemic biokinetics, two generic physiologically based models have also been developed.[7] One is applied for strontium, radium, and uranium; the other for thorium, neptunium, plutonium, americium, and curium. This type of generic model is designed to predict long-term retention in organs or tissues, which dominate the committed dose and may not yield reliable estimates of excretion values, especially at early times after an intake.

It should be noted that the models rely on many assumptions regarding uptake, absorption, transfer coefficients, organ distribution, and excretion. Variability in these functions among individuals is not known. As a result, there are large uncertainties in the answers derived from modeling. An NCRP scientific committee studied the reliability of models and parameters used to assess individual doses for risk assessment purposes.[11] For most radionuclides, it was estimated that the effective dose coefficients were expected in many cases to vary by a factor of 2 to 10 for groups of healthy adult males. For a special population (infants, people in bad health, etc.) the uncertainties were expected to be even greater, perhaps factors of 5 to 20.

This brief discussion on biokinetics and dosimetry of internal radionuclide depositions illustrates their complexities and characterizes the nature of these exposures. It is presented to help conceptualize the many parameters needed to try to understand this complex exposure and dosimetry problem. Models are primarily developed for radiation protection purposes, such as calculating allowable limits of intake or interpreting measurements of activity in the body for monitoring workers. In higher accidental exposures, the need for quick decisions obviates effective use of models. In these cases, medical decisions are simply professional judgments made to benefit the patient. Initial decisions will always be made on limited and inadequate information. A rationale for making these decisions is outlined in the next section.

BASIS FOR TREATMENT DECISIONS

The decision whether or not to treat a person exposed to internal radionuclides is a subjective judgment. Organ doses from internal emitters are hardly ever so high that they cause acute radiation effects. An exception to this statement is on that rare occasion when medical misadministration (unintended high dose) of therapeutic levels of radionuclides has occurred. When exposure to internal contamination is high enough for acute radiation effects, there is no problem making the decision to treat, but rather on deciding how to treat most effectively.

The usual treatment decision will involve concerns about the risk of a late health effect, primarily radiation-induced carcinogenesis. Our understanding of the dose/effect relationship due to radiation is limited, especially at low dose rates. Therefore, decisions will often be based on anticipated, but poorly understood, risk. The need for a medical treatment decision at the earliest time possible after an internal exposure makes assessing the risk even more tenuous.

Few studies or data are available to address the question of whether or not current treatment effectively reduces health effects due to internal radionuclides. The benefits of treatment are assumed to parallel the reduction in the quantity of radionuclide deposited in the body. Thus, the benefits of treatment are understood even less well than our imperfect understanding of radiation risk at low doses and low-dose rates. A reasonable decision for treatment is often based simply to achieve a lesser internal deposition and dose.

The physician will usually not have dose estimates at the time of decision. If the radionuclide is of a type that a direct *in vivo* measurement or immediate spot sample bioassay can be made, an early estimate of the quantity of radionuclide present in the body is possible. In this case, a quick but tentative assessment of organ dose can be calculated. Table A4.5 in Appendix 4 lists absorbed dose estimates in mSv/MBq for various radionuclides to estimate 50-year committed dose to critical organs and lung. Even if an early dose is derived, the result should be used as only one factor in making the treatment decision regardless of whether it is above or below some dose limit.

One way of judging the seriousness of a radiation dose, in terms of late effects, is comparison with doses that are known to cause some excess cancers in humans. In epidemiological studies of exposed human populations, excess cancers are usually not statistically evident unless lifetime doses of 0.5 Sv or more are present. Bone marrow and thyroid are more radiosensitive for late effects than other organs, and one may wish to reduce potential doses to these organs by an additional factor of 5.

By this comparison, it appears that doses less than about 0.1 to 0.5 Sv, depending on the organ systems involved, would be a point of diminished benefit for treatment of internal contamination. Another recommended occupational dose limit for internal emitters is the annual limits of intake for workers, which are based on a limit of effective dose of 20 mSv/year. Work histories in the industry indicate that workers are not involved in significant accidental internal intakes every year. This latter value is not a good measure for evaluating the need for therapy of internal radionuclides; it is intended for occupational radiation protection control programs. Fortunately, the risk from treatments used for internal exposure to radionuclides is mostly slight to negligible. If the treatment risk is small, one may decide to proceed even if the potential benefits appear to be limited. The physician must make this judgment concerning the possible ultimate benefit vs. the potential harm or side effects of the therapy — a type of judgment common to all medical practice.

Other considerations in the treatment decision are also important. Probably the most important is the age of the persons involved. Children have longer life expectancy and greater radiosensitivity that increases the potential benefits of treatment for them compared with an older person. Similarly, one may treat a young adult more aggressively than older individuals. A second consideration of importance is the general health of the individual. Persons with a significant health risk already from other disease will probably benefit less from treatment of internal radionuclides than a healthy person of the same age simply on the basis of shortened life expectancy.

With proper use of currently available treatment, it is possible to reduce the dose from some radionuclides taken internally by factors of about 2 to 10. The goal of reducing dose is a worthy objective. That health effects do result from internal emitters has been amply demonstrated in radium dial painters, uranium miners, thorotrast-injected persons, Marshallese Islanders exposed to radioiodines in fallout, and others. However, in all these cases there were high exposures that were orders of magnitude above those permitted by the regulatory guidelines applied to the radiation worker. The point is that the physician must keep in perspective the benefits and risks of treatment in each situation. The fact that the decision must be made very early after exposure places the physician at a great disadvantage. For therapy that involves essentially no risk, errors of therapy omission can be more serious than those of commission.

TREATMENT

Reduction of internally deposited radionuclides can be accomplished by means of two general processes: (1) reduction of absorption and internal uptake and (2) enhanced elimination or excretion of absorbed radionuclides. Both are achieved more effectively when treatment is begun at the earliest time after exposure, preferably in the first 3 h.

Skin decontamination and wound management are used to reduce uptake via the skin. Other chapters in this book should be consulted for discussion of these topics.

The next sections contain summaries of the main procedures and drugs available to treat internally deposited radionuclides. A quick reference to these sections for selected radionuclides is listed in Table 23.2.

REDUCTION OF GASTROINTESTINAL ABSORPTION

GI absorption can be reduced by removing radioactive materials before absorption can occur, or by speeding up gastrointestinal evacuation, or by changing the solubility of the radioactive material. The main procedures and drugs are summarized:

Stomach Lavage

A nasogastric or gastric tube may be used to empty the stomach in the unusual circumstance where a large quantity of radionuclide is present in the stomach.

Emetics

Stomach lavage is often the procedure of choice, but may not always be successful. Apomorphine hydrochloride or ipecac is the most likely emetic drug to consider in such cases.

Purgatives

Selection of a purgative to speed the elimination of GI tract contents depends largely on its speed of action. An exposure of concern might be a known ingestion of a large quantity of an insoluble radionuclide that may remain in the colon and rectum for many hours. A bisacodyl or phosphate soda enema will empty the colon in a few minutes and should be given primary consideration.

TABLE 23.2
Treatment Index for Selected Internal Contaminants

Contaminant	Therapy	Comments
Americium (Am)	Wound excision, DTPA	
Californium (Cf)	Wound excision, DTPA	
Cerium (Ce)	DTPA	Special FDA approval needed
Cesium (Cs)	Prussian Blue	
Curium (Cm)	Wound excision, DTPA	Special FDA approval needed
Fission Products		Depends on major isotopes present
Gold (Au)	BAL or penicillamine	No therapy for colloidal form
Ingested material	Stomach lavage, emetics, purgatives	
Inhaled insolubles	Lung lavage	Consider only for very high doses
Iodine (I)	Stable NaI or KI	
	Propylthiouracil or methimazole	
		1. Use iodides in first 12 h
		2. Consider use of antithyroid drugs from 12 to about 36 h
Lanthanum (La)	DTPA	Special FDA approval needed
Mercury (Hg)	Penicillamine	Gastric lavage with egg white solution or 5% sodium formaldehyde sulfoxide
Phosphorus (P)	Stomach lavage	Add parathyroid extract in severe cases
	Al-antacids	
	Phosphate	
Plutonium (Pu)	Wound excision, DTPA	
Polonium (Po)	Penicillamine or BAL	BAL has greater toxicity
Potassium (K)	Diuretics, oral K dilution	Al-antacids reduce GI uptake
Radium (Ra)	Magnesium sulfate	No useful therapy postabsorption
Rubidium (Ru)	Prussian Blue	Chemical properties similar to K
Strontium (Sr)	Al-antacids, barium sulfate, phosphate	Ammonium chloride and stable Sr or Ca to attempt removal from bone
Tritium (3H)	Force fluids, diuretics	Force fluids to tolerance
Uranium (U)	Sodium bicarbonate	Treat chemical nephrotoxicity
Zinc (Zn)	CaEDTA	Use oral zinc sulfate as diluting agent and zinc supplement

A bisacodyl suppository takes up to an hour for action. Purgative drugs taken orally, such as bisacodyl, castor oil, or phenolphthalein, require several hours before taking effect. Some purgatives may have special advantages because they produce a less soluble compound of certain radionuclides. Magnesium sulfate is a saline cathartic that produces insoluble sulfate compounds with some radionuclides, e.g., radium.

Ion-Exchange Resins

Strong cation or anion exchange resins can produce toxic side effects and are generally not recommended. While no studies are noted in the literature on the use of activated charcoal in cases of radionuclide intake, it would seem to be a potentially useful procedure to reduce uptake.

Prussian Blue

In animals, ferric ferrocyanide (Prussian Blue) has been found to be effective in accelerating the removal of cesium, thallium, and rubidium through feces.[1] Prussian Blue is not absorbed from the

GI tract and has low toxicity. Constipation is the most notable side effect. A dose of 1 to 3 g of Prussian Blue taken orally three times/day is well tolerated in adults. In humans, the compound reduces the biological half-time of cesium-137 to about one third of its normal value. It was used effectively on 46 persons internally contaminated with cesium-137 in the Goiânia (Brazil) accident. The average dose reduction in this group was 71%, ranging from 51 to 84%. Prussian Blue has FDA approval for pharmaceutical use in the United States as an investigational new drug. Prussian Blue is distributed by Oak Ridge Institute for Science and Education, Radiation Emergency Assistance Center/Training Site (REAC/TS), Oak Ridge, TN. A package insert and protocol for its use may be obtained by calling (423)576-3131.

Aluminum-Containing Antacids

These are effective agents in reducing intestinal uptake of strontium. A single oral dose of 100 ml aluminum phosphate gel given immediately after ingestion of radioactive strontium will decrease absorption by about 85%. A single dose of aluminum hydroxide, 60 to 100 ml, given immediately after exposure will reduce uptake by about 50%. Both drugs are nontoxic and well tolerated.

Barium Sulfate

This highly insoluble salt is used orally and in enemas as an X-ray contrast agent for GI tract examinations. Except for constipation, no adverse effects have been observed. A combination of barium sulfate and magnesium sulfate is often recommended. A possible use of this combination is oral administration shortly after ingestion of radioactive alkaline earth metals (barium, strontium, radium). Changing the chemical form of these elements to insoluble sulfates markedly decreases their absorption rates.

BLOCKING AND DILUTING AGENTS

A blocking agent, a stable isotope of a radionuclide, saturates a specific organ and reduces the quantity of the radionuclide that can be taken up by that tissue. Isotopic dilution is achieved by the administration of large quantities of a stable isotope of the radionuclide, thereby reducing organ uptake of it due to the dilution factor. Displacement therapy is a special form of isotopic dilution in which a stable element with a different atomic number successfully competes with the radionuclide for uptake in an organ.

Iodides

The administration of stable iodide before or shortly after an intake of radioiodine blocks much of its uptake in the thyroid. A dose of 390 mg of sodium or potassium iodide (300 mg iodide) achieves maximal blocking. Administration of a single dose of stable iodide within the first few minutes after exposure to radioiodine may limit uptake to about 1 or 2% compared with the normal 12 to 20% uptake. Only about half of the uptake is blocked if the iodide administration is delayed 6 h, and little effect is achieved if delayed by as much as 12 h. Daily administration of 100 mg of potassium iodide (KI) may be continued for a few days to prevent recycling of the radioiodine into the thyroid. The above dose schedule is recommended for individual exposures under medical supervision, but for general public use in emergencies an initial dose of 130 mg KI (100 mg iodide) is recommended.[5,9] Reported adverse reactions from daily 300-mg doses of iodide suggest a reaction rate of about 1 to 10 per 10,000,000 administrations.[12] Incidence of adverse reactions is related to dose and length of administration. After iodine administration usually for several weeks or longer, the reported iodine-induced reactions include thyrotoxicosis, iodide goiter, hypothyroidism with goiter, iodide parotitis, acneform skin eruptions, and even less frequent systemic manifestations (fever, arthralgia, inflammatory joint involvement, etc.). Because these reactions reverse within a few days after discontinuing the drug, monitoring for reactions need not be continued beyond a few days after the last iodide administration. The side effects problem is thought to be negligible for the dose schedules discussed here. Potassium perchlorate can be used in place of the iodide for a rare person known to develop angioedema due to significant iodide sensitivity.

Strontium

Stable strontium is useful as a diluting agent for radiostrontium. It is available as tablets (strontium lactate, 300 mg, to be given two to five times daily) or intravenous solutions (strontium gluconate, 600 mg strontium per day infused with 500 ml 5% glucose in water over 4 h). The tablets are well tolerated if given with meals and are nontoxic at this dosage. It can be given daily for several weeks.

Calcium

Orally administered calcium gluconate or calcium lactate increases the urinary excretion of radioactive strontium and calcium. Intravenous calcium gluconate can be used, but should not be given to persons receiving quinidine or digitalis preparations or to persons who have a very slow heart rate.

Phosphate

Phosphate can be used to decrease the intestinal absorption of radioactive strontium. It may also be useful as a diluting agent in case of medical misadministration of phosphorus-32. Oral phosphates can be given in inorganic (sodium or potassium phosphate) and organic forms (sodium glycerophosphate). Vomiting, diarrhea, or both may occur from phosphate administration in doses exceeding 2 g/day. Phosphate can also be used as a saline cathartic. Intravenous administration of phosphate is unlikely for treatment of radionuclide uptake. It must be done cautiously because rapid administration can cause severe hypotension, renal failure, and myocardial infarction. Serum calcium and electrocardiograms must be monitored during such infusion.

Forced Fluids

A high level of fluid intake by mouth will increase tritium excretion proportionately. The half-time of tritium in the body can be reduced from the normal 10 to 12 days to 6 days or less by forcing at least 3 to 4 l to 10 l or more of fluid per day. Forcing to tolerance should be continued for at least 1 week or until further dose reduction is judged to be insignificant. The dose may be reduced by a factor of 2 or more by early treatment and careful management.

MOBILIZING AGENTS

Mobilizing agents are compounds that increase a natural turnover process, thereby inducing a release of some radioisotopes from body tissues. This results in an enhanced rate of elimination from the body and a reduced biological half-time. These agents are more effective given soon after exposure, but some still produce an effect if given within about 2 weeks.

Antithyroid Drugs

The treatment of choice for reducing the dose from radioiodine is to block the thyroid by administration of an iodide as discussed earlier. If time since exposure is 12 h or more, the use of iodide has limited effectiveness because the radioiodine is already deposited in the thyroid. In this situation the use of an antithyroid drug, such as propylthiouracil or methimazole, may be considered. These drugs interfere with the oxidation of the iodide ion and block the formation of hormone. The response to these drugs is greatly reduced if the thyroid already has an ample supply of stable iodine, such as when stable iodide has already been administered. The risk of side effects is much higher than with stable iodides. About 2 to 8% of patients on these drugs develop a maculopapular rash, which does not usually require discontinuation of the drug. Much rarer but serious side effects are hepatocellular damage, vasculitis, and agranulocytosis (in less than 1% of patients). These side effects are usually reversible on discontinuance of the drug. The effective half-time of iodine-131 was reduced about 25% using methimazole in several human volunteers when given several days after radioiodine administration;[13] thus, the reduction of radiation dose is not likely to be great if treatment is started as late as several days after exposure.

Ammonium Chloride

This acidifying salt given orally (1 to 2 g four times a day) is effective in mobilizing radiostrontium deposited in the body. Its effectiveness can be enhanced by simultaneous use of intravenous calcium gluconate, 500 mg calcium in 500 ml 5% glucose in water over 4 h on 3 to 6 consecutive days. An estimated reduction in the body burden of radiostrontium between 40 and 75% may be obtained if started soon after exposure. Ammonium chloride frequently causes gastric irritation, nausea, and vomiting, and should not be used in persons with serious liver disease.

Diuretics

The value of diuretics is untested for treatment of internal radionuclide deposition. Enhanced excretion of sodium, chloride, potassium bicarbonate, magnesium, and water in the urine occurs with induced diuresis. Some corresponding radionuclides that could be involved in radiation accidents are sodium-22, sodium-24, chlorine-38, potassium-42, and hydrogen-3.

Expectorants and Inhalants

Studies on the effect of these agents on inhaled radioactive particles are disappointing. None provides effective action that would be dependable or particularly useful in treating persons after inhalation of radioactive particles.

Parathyroid Extract

Intramuscular injections of parathyroid hormone promote urinary excretion of phosphorus and have been used effectively to treat an overdose of radiophosphorus.

Sodium Bicarbonate

Sodium bicarbonate is the treatment of choice for kidney toxicity that results from chemical damage of acute uranium exposures. It converts uranyl ions to a uranyl bicarbonate complex in urine within the tubules of the kidney. This complex is less toxic to the kidney and also promotes migration of uranium to extracellular fluids and deposition in bone. Oral administrations or intravenous infusions of sodium bicarbonate are regulated to keep the urine alkaline as determined by frequent pH measurements. Administration of sodium bicarbonate by infusion requires monitoring of blood pH and electrolyte balance. Hypokalemia may occur and can be prevented or treated with supplementary potassium. If the kidney damage becomes severe enough, renal dialysis presumably would be useful because the damage to the proximal convoluted tubule is usually reversible and recovery is fairly rapid.

CHELATING AGENTS

A number of chemical compounds enhance the elimination of metals from the body by chelation, a process by which organic compounds exchange less firmly bonded ions for other inorganic ions to form a relatively stable nonionized ring complex. This soluble complex is excreted readily by the kidney. The excretion of certain radionuclides can be increased by means of a properly selected and administered chelating agent.

The principal drug used for treatment of radionuclides is DTPA, an acronym of its chemical name, diethylenetriaminepentaacetic acid. It is approved as an investigational new drug (IND) by the FDA for two salts of DTPA (CaDTPA and ZnDTPA) to chelate plutonium, berkelium, californium, americium, and curium. In addition to these transuranium metals, DTPA is also an effective chelator for some rare earths (cerium, yttrium, lanthanum, promethium, and scandium) and some transition metals (zirconium and niobium). The FDA approval of DTPA covers its use only for the above-listed transuranium metals; special permission would be needed for use in exposures to radioactive rare earths or other radionuclides.

DTPA is rapidly distributed throughout the extracellular fluid space. It does not cross cell membranes so chelation occurs only in extracellular fluid, such as blood. Chelation therapy is most effective when it is begun as soon as possible after exposure because it works only on the metallic ions in extracellular fluids and not on those already incorporated in cells. Almost the entire DTPA dose is excreted within about 12 h.

No serious toxicity has resulted in humans in a total of about 5500 administrations of either ZnDTPA or CaDTPA used in recommended doses. In high doses in animals, toxicity has occurred from CaDTPA due to chelation and excretion of trace metals, such as zinc and manganese. Animals given doses 200 times or more than that used in humans develop severe lesions of the kidneys, intestinal mucosa, and liver. Teratogenesis and fetal death occur in mice when similarly high doses are given throughout gestation. As a precaution, CaDTPA is contraindicated for persons with serious kidney disease or depressed myelopoietic function, e.g., leukopenia or thrombocytopenia. Discontinue DTPA therapy if diarrhea occurs.

Animal studies indicate that the ZnDTPA form is less toxic than CaDTPA. ZnDTPA is recommended for long-term treatment and for use in pregnant women, but CaDTPA is about ten times more effective than ZnDTPA for initial chelation of transuranium metals. For this reason, CaDTPA is preferred for use during the first day or two of treatment. By 24 h after exposure, ZnDTPA is about as effective as CaDTPA.

For plutonium exposures, the effectiveness of DTPA chelation is highly dependent on the chemical form of the plutonium and time of first administration. The efficacy of DTPA is good for internal contamination with the soluble plutonium salts, such as the nitrate or chloride, but is essentially nil for highly insoluble compounds, such as the high-fired oxide. Data from persons treated with CaDTPA within about 3 h of an inhalation exposure indicate that about 60 to 70% of soluble plutonium is removed compared with that excreted by untreated persons. Insoluble plutonium is absorbed slowly into the extracellular fluids over many years. As a result, the plutonium concentration in extracellular fluid is minute and chelation does not enhance urinary excretion significantly. However, the chemical form of inhaled plutonium is rarely known accurately so an initial therapeutic test dose of DTPA is often justified for determining therapeutic effectiveness even in cases where the exposure is thought to be to insoluble plutonium oxide. Effective chelation should raise urinary excretion of transuranics, i.e., plutonium, americium, or others, by a factor of 50 or more compared with initial baseline urinary excretion.

The recommended dose for both ZnDTPA and CaDTPA is a single 1 g dose per day. The dose should not be fractionated, i.e., divided into multiple administrations per day. It can be given either intravenously or by aerosol inhalation. The conventional procedure for intravenous administration has been to dilute 1 g DTPA in 100 to 250 ml normal saline or 5% glucose in water and give over a period of about 30 min and, in any case, less than 2 h. An alternative procedure, using a slow intravenous push of the undiluted DTPA solution over a period of 3 to 4 min, is preferred by some physicians. In either case, care should be taken to avoid extravasation from the vein. Aerosol administration is done with a nebulizer using the contents of a 1 g CaDTPA ampule diluted 1:1 with water or saline. The aerosol is inhaled over 15 to 20 min. It is prudent not to use the inhalation treatment in persons with preexisting pulmonary disease.

DTPA is not available commercially. Physicians with a potential need for DTPA or for package insert information should contact Oak Ridge Associated Universities, Radiation Emergency Assistance Center/Training Site (REAC/TS), Oak Ridge, TN, 37831-0117, phone (423)576-3131. Use of a prescribed treatment protocol and submission of follow-up reports are required under the terms of the IND agreement.

If DTPA is not available immediately, the calcium salt of ethylenediaminetetraacetic acid (otherwise known as CaEDTA, calcium disodium edetate, or Versenate) may be used. It is about ten times less effective than DTPA in enhancing the excretion of transuranic metals. Its primary use has been to treat lead poisoning, but it also chelates zinc, cadmium, chromium, and nickel. Other chelation drugs to consider for specific nuclides are dimercaprol (BAL) for mercury; penicillamine for copper or mercury; and deferoxamine for iron.

LUNG LAVAGE

Inhalation of radioactive particles is a common mode of intake from occupational exposures. If the particles are insoluble, a large proportion of the radioactive material is retained for many months or years in the lung. Chelation therapy is not effective in these cases.

In dog studies, lavage of the tracheobronchial tree removes about 25 to 50% of inhaled insoluble particles.[14-16] The procedure requires placement of an endotracheal tube into the trachea and major bronchi under general anesthesia. The airways are lavaged with isotonic saline. Experimentally, five lavages were performed on both right and left lung for a total of ten procedures. Treatment was started in the first week after exposure and each lavage was done about 3 days to a week apart. Radiation pneumonitis and early deaths occurred in only 25% of treated dogs in contrast to death of all untreated dogs. In baboons, 60 to 90% of the lung burdens of plutonium oxide was removed by ten pulmonary lavages.[17]

Use of this treatment requires a careful risk–benefit assessment. The risk lies primarily in the administration of a general anesthetic. This procedure risk is immediate, whereas radiation-induced cancer risk to the lung will be many years later. The use of this procedure should probably be limited to cases in which the radioactivity in the lung from insoluble particles of alpha emitters is sufficiently high (probably >37 Bq or 1 µCi of plutonium) to produce acute radiation damage to the lung. The decision for lung lavage to remove radionuclides may be appropriate for a young healthy person at a lower lung deposition than for an unhealthy and/or older individual.

REFERENCES

1. Management of Persons Accidentally Contaminated with Radionuclides, NCRP Rep. 65 National Council on Radiation Protection and Measurements Publications, Bethesda, MD, 1979.
2. Gerber, G.B. and Thomas, R.G., Eds., Guidebook for the treatment of accidental internal radionuclide contamination of workers, *Radiat. Prot. Dosimetry*, 41, 1–45, 1992.
3. Use of Bioassay Procedures for Assessment of Internal Radionuclide Deposition, NCRP Rep. 87, National Council on Radiation Protection and Measurements Publications, Bethesda, MD, 1987.
4. Broga, D.W., Berk, H.W., and Sharpe, A.R., Jr., Efficacy of radioiodine urinalysis, *Health Phys.*, 50, 629, 1986.
5. Ribela, M.T., Marone, M., and Bartolini, P., Use of radioiodine urinalysis for effective thyroid blocking in the first few hours postexposure, *Health Phys.*, 76, 11, 1999.
6. Dose coefficients for intakes of radionuclides by workers, International Commission on Radiological Protection, ICRP Publ. 68, *Ann. ICRP*, 24(4), 1994.
7. Individual monitoring for internal exposure of workers, International Commission on Radiological Protection, ICRP Publ. 78, *Ann. ICRP*, 27 (3–4), 1997.
8. Human respiratory tract model for radiological protection, International Commission on Radiological Protection, ICRP Publ. 66, *Ann. ICRP*, 24 (1–3), 1994.

9. Deposition, Retention and Dosimetry of Inhaled Radioactive Substances, National Council on Radiation Protection and Measurements, NCRP Rep. 125, NCRP Publications, Bethesda, MD, 1994.
10. Alpha Emitting Particles in Lungs, National Council on Radiation Protection and Measurements, NCRP Rep. 46, NCRP Publications, Bethesda, MD, 1975.
11. Evaluating the Reliability of Biokinetic and Dosimetric Models and Parameters Used to Assess Individual Doses for Risk Assessment Purposes, National Council on Radiation Protection and Measurements, NCRP Commentary 15, NCRP Publications, Bethesda, MD, 1998.
12. Protection of the Thyroid Gland in the Event of Releases of Radioiodine, National Council on Radiation Protection and Measurements Publications, NCRP Rep. 55, NCRP Publications, Bethesda, MD, 1977.
13. Tanaka, S., Mochizuki, Y., Yabumoto, E., Iinuma, T.A., Kumatori, T., Yamane, T., Akiyama, T., and Matsusaka, N., Protection of thyroid gland and total body from radiation delivered by radioactive iodine, in *Diagnosis and Treatment of Deposited Radionuclides,* Kornberg, H.H. and Norwood, W.D., Eds., Excerpta Medica Foundation, Amsterdam, 1968, 298.
14. Pfleger, R.C., Wilson, A.J., and McClellan, R.O., Pulmonary lavage as a therapeutic measure for removing inhaled "insoluble" materials from the lung, *Health Phys.,* 16, 758, 1969.
15. Boecker, B.B., Muggenburg, B.A., McClellan, R.O. et al., Removal of ^{144}Ce in fused clay particles from the beagle dog by bronchopulmonary lavage, *Health Phys.,* 26, 605, 1974.
16. Muggenburg, B A., Mauderly, J.L., Boecker, B.B. et al., Prevention of radiation pneumonitis from inhaled cerium-144 by lung lavage in beagle dogs, *Am. Rev. Respir. Dis.,* 111, 795, 1975.
17. Nolibe, D., Nénot, J.C., Metevier, H. et al., Traitement des inhalations accidentelles d'oxyde de plutonium par la vage pulmonaire *in vivo,* in Diagnosis and Treatment of Incorporated Radionuclides, IAEA Publ. STI/PUB/411, International Atomic Energy Agency, Vienna, 1976, 373.

24 Lifetime Follow-Up of the 1976 Americium Accident Victim

Bryce D. Breitenstein, Jr. and H. Earl Palmer

CONTENTS

Introduction 337
Initial Medical Care and Findings 337
Case Management 338
Medical Course, September 1976 to January 1977 338
Medical Course, 1977 to 1987 339
Radiation Dosimetry Evaluation 340
Effectiveness of DTPA Therapy 341
Conclusions 342
Acknowledgments 342
References 342

INTRODUCTION

On August 30, 1976, at 2:55 A.M., a 64-year-old nuclear chemical operator was injured by a chemical explosion of an cation exchange column in a glove box used for americium-241 recovery. This explosion occurred at Hanford, Washington, U.S.A., in a waste treatment facility. The primary materials in the resin column were concentrated nitric acid, exchange resin, and americium-241.[1,2] As a result of the accident, he was heavily contaminated with americium, sustained a substantial internal deposition of this isotope, was burned with the nitric acid, and injured by flying debris about the face and neck.

This report describes the immediate and long-term medical care, including decontamination procedures, chelation therapy, and routine and special clinical laboratory studies. The estimates of the operator's americium-241 deposition, postaccident and during the remainder of his life, and postmortem tissue analysis are reported. The special techniques and equipment used to make the estimates are described. He died of complications of chronic coronary artery disease on August 17, 1987.

INITIAL MEDICAL CARE AND FINDINGS

The nuclear chemical operator, Mr. McCluskey, injured primarily in the face and neck, was assisted from the accident scene by co-workers. His contaminated clothing was removed and decontamination was begun by flushing his face and eyes with water. An ambulance transported him 40 km (25 miles) to the Emergency Decontamination Facility (EDF)[3,4] in Richland, Washington, where he arrived about 2 h after the accident. Upon arrival at the EDF, 1 g of calcium diethylenetriaminepentate (CaDTPA) was administered intravenously and he was further decontaminated with soap and water in a shower. Removal of superficial foreign matter from the face and neck and irrigation of the eyes with normal saline were carried out by attending physicians and nurses.

The initial medical appraisal revealed nitric acid burns (redness and moderate tissue swelling without blister formation) of the face, eyes, neck, and upper back, with small lacerations and embedded foreign bodies on the face, neck, and upper back. These burns, lacerations, and foreign bodies permitted internal deposition of americium-241, in addition to the inhaled americium-241. He had a productive cough associated with the inhaled acid fumes. Mr. McCluskey's vital signs were normal and no significant systemic effects were evident. The patient was alert, cooperative, and able to walk with assistance, although his vision was markedly impaired by chemical eye burns. His occupational medical record revealed an acute myocardial infarction in October 1974 and surgical treatment in 1971 with a prosthetic graft for an abdominal aortic aneurysm. There were no significant current cardiovascular signs or symptoms. He was taking CardioquinR and ValiUMR, for control of premature ventricular contractions. A hospital facility bed care unit was set up in the EDF. The patient was confined to a radiation zone established and controlled by radiation monitor technicians. Round-the-clock nursing care was instituted. During the first day he was seen by a surgeon, an ophthalmologist, and other medical members of the Hanford Environmental Health Foundation (HEHF) staff.

CASE MANAGEMENT

Decisions regarding treatment and the patient's care after discharge were made by team approach. The team, which consisted of the patient, attending and consulting physicians, radiobiologists, a staff psychologist, health physicists, nurses, and radiation monitors, met frequently; the procedures and methods used were a consensus of the assembled group. The case aroused worldwide interest in the scientific community and the communications media. From the beginning, public relations professionals worked effectively with the professional and technical staff. The importance of carefully organizing the public relations aspects of such an emergency cannot be overemphasized.

MEDICAL COURSE, SEPTEMBER 1976 TO JANUARY 1977

The daily description of the patient's care during this time period has previously been published.[5] The following is a summary of the medical care and evaluation during his stay at the EDF and his transition discharge. Administration of DTPA continued, with several doses daily for the first month. The DTPA was given undiluted by intravenous injection over 3 to 5 min and the dose titrated against urinary americium-241 excretion to maintain a high excretion rate. The maximum dose was 1 g every 8 h. Since long-term DTPA therapy was anticipated, it seemed advisable to switch promptly from CaDTPA to ZnDTPA.[6-11] ZnDTPA had been used clinically in Europe, but was not approved for human use in the United States. The U.S. Food and Drug Administration gave permission to use ZnDTPA in this case.

Decontamination was undertaken twice daily for the first week after the accident and then once a day until the time of discharge in January 1977.[12]

Fluid intake was encouraged to promote urinary excretion. Liquid and solid intake and output were recorded, and all urinary and fecal specimens were collected separately for radiobioassay. The chemical burns on the face, neck, and right shoulder were left exposed; no dressings or external medications were used. A principal medical problem was the patient's eyes, which had corneal nitric acid burns with superficial corneal and conjunctival foreign bodies; the latter were excised or spontaneously extruded over a period of months. Initially, he received prolonged irrigation of both eyes with normal saline. Ophthalmic steroid–antibiotic ointment was instilled in his eyes several times daily. Surgical removal of some of the larger and more deeply embedded foreign bodies in the face was attempted during the first week. This effort proved unsuccessful because the foreign bodies identified by radiograph were no more radioactive than the surrounding skin and subcutaneous tissue. For the first 4 months, daily superficial debridement of the face and neck was performed without anesthesia to remove scales, crusts, scabs, and extruding foreign bodies. The frequency of debridement was then decreased. Over several months, metallic, plastic, cloth, and glass foreign bodies measuring up to 0.5 cm were extruded spontaneously or removed with forceps.

Laboratory studies were conducted daily during the first 3 months and less frequently thereafter. These included a complete blood count, urinalysis, blood chemistry tests, and fecal occult blood. The results were normal except for a decline in the peripheral lymphocyte count from 1860/mm^3 on the day of the accident to 530/mm^3 1 week later; it remained depressed for several months. Previous lymphocyte counts were 1520 in January 1976, 2332 in 1973, 2805 in 1970, and 3151 in 1967.[13] Serial chest radiographs, pulmonary function tests, and electrocardiograms were normal.

Special studies included analyses of peripheral lymphocyte chromosomes, a facial skin biopsy, and a bone marrow aspiration. Radiation-induced cytogenetic lesions in lymphocytes were observed and have been the subject of publication.[14] The skin biopsy revealed scattered alpha "gistars" using autoradiography; all other changes were compatible with the patient's age.[15] The bone marrow was examined 2 weeks after the accident and was normal. None of these studies indicated a change of therapy.

The HEHF staff psychologist was involved in the early care of the patient and continued to advise the staff, the patient, and his family.[16,17]

After 2^1/$_2$ months of treatment in the EDF, the patient was transferred to a 9 m (30-ft) travel trailer adjacent to the EDF, which provided a controlled transitional environment before discharge. While the patient, his wife, and their dog lived in the trailer, wastes were collected and measured for radioactivity, and routine environmental surveys were made. From mid-November 1976 until discharge in late January 1977, no unexpected americium-241 contamination was found in the trailer.

MEDICAL COURSE, 1977 TO 1987

After discharge to his home in Prosser, Washington (35 miles from Richland), the patient received daily DTPA intravenous therapy by local medical professionals and follow-up care by HEHF. In the spring of 1977, he was treated for acute prostatitis with a 6-day hospitalization and antibiotic therapy. In the summer, he developed acute iritis. Both of these conditions subsided with therapy. A 90% mature left cataract was removed in February 1978; it contained 0.019 Bq (0.5 pCi) americium-241. The ophthalmologist felt the cataract was traumatic in origin and not induced by ionizing radiation.

During the winter of 1978–79, the patient was evaluated by an internist for recurrent episodes of chest discomfort and weakness. He was diagnosed by coronary arteriography to have seriously compromised coronary artery circulation, but he was not recommended to be a candidate for coronary artery bypass surgery. He was treated with an oral beta blocker (Inderol^R) and experienced a significant improvement in exercise tolerance and abatement of angina pectoris.

A right cataract was extracted surgically in 1979, along with five small foreign bodies from the cornea and conjunctiva. In late 1980, the patient was evaluated for asymptomatic thrombocytopenia, first observed in September 1979. A hematologist concluded that impaired platelet production was probably related to an aplastic syndrome from the americium-241 exposure or the development of a myeloproliferative syndrome. No specific therapy was recommended.

The patient was hospitalized for 11 days in early 1981 for treatment of acute thrombophlebitis of the left calf. He was treated successfully with intravenous heparin and bed rest. He was discharged on the oral anticoagulant warfarin. Coincident with starting the heparin, the platelet count returned to normal and remained normal with the oral anticoagulation. The reason for the reversal of the thrombocytopenia by the anticoagulant therapy was not known.

He was stable during the remainder of 1981 and 1982. During monthly visits to HEHF, he was interviewed, examined clinically, screened with laboratory tests, evaluated by an ophthalmologist, and had external body counting to estimate the americium-241 deposition.

In January 1983, drainage occurred for 1 month from his right forehead. An uneventful left eye corneal transplant was performed in December 1983.

In the summer of 1984, leukopenia was evaluated by a hematologist. Diagnoses of a possible hypoproliferative, myeloproliferative, or myelodysplastic syndrome was considered. Observation and serial follow-up were recommended.

The last corneal transplant sutures were removed in the spring of 1985. At this time, bilateral glaucoma was diagnosed; medical therapy reduced the intraocular pressure to normal.

He was hospitalized in early 1986 for an acute genitourinary infection that resolved on antibiotics. In the summer, he was rehospitalized for several days for treatment of left leg traumatic phlebitis. He fell at home in the autumn, sustained fractured ribs with secondary internal hemorrhage and was hospitalized for 1 month. Oral anticoagulation was discontinued at this time. Less than a week after discharge, he was rehospitalized for exhaustion, nausea, and a cardiac arrhythmia. He was transfused for blood loss anemia and treated in a coronary care unit for the arrhythmia. He fell again at home in January 1987 and was hospitalized for several weeks.

In March 1987, he developed left upper lumbar herpes zoster, was hospitalized, and treated with Acylovir[R]. The medication produced hallucinations and disorientation; treatment was discontinued, he improved, and was discharged after 2 weeks. He was readmitted for a few days in early April and the long-term quinidine preparation (Cardioquin[R]) was discontinued. He was rehospitalized in late April to mid-May with a respiratory infection, cardiac arrhythmia, and probable myocardial infarction. From May to August 1987, he received home care. In mid-August, he was hospitalized with progressive cardiac deterioration and died in a coma on August 17. His widow consented to a U.S. Transuranium Registry-sponsored autopsy that revealed chronic coronary artery disease and congestive heart failure. Postmortem tissue for radiochemical analysis was obtained.

RADIATION DOSIMETRY EVALUATION

Detailed external measurements of the internally deposited americium-241 were made on the patient.[18] Quantitative measurements of the lung, liver, and bone began on day 3 after exposure and the rate of excretion and accretion by these organs was determined by daily measurement for the first few weeks. These were diminished to monthly intervals until several months before death when measurement was not possible. The americium-241 embedded in the skin of his face and head were carefully mapped periodically over the 11-year period. The body distribution was determined periodically with gamma camera and linear scanning devices.

In a previous paper,[19] the results of many of these *in vivo* measurements were listed and estimates of absorbed dose were made on those organs that received the highest dose using whole-body and organ measurements up to the time of death and also measurements made on organs removed at autopsy soon after death. The organs included lung, liver, bone, and some of the most highly contaminated skin of the right face and neck. Since that time several papers have been published on the dosimetric and related aspects of this case.[20–25]

Radiochemical analysis of 18 different soft tissues and five types of bone were performed at Los Alamos National Laboratory.[22] From the results of these analyses and the previous *in vivo* and excretion measurements,[19] the accumulated absorbed doses were calculated and a summary of those tissues containing the highest percentage of the total-body burden is shown in Table 24.1. Similar results presented 10 years ago have been changed in this table to reflect the difference between the *in vivo* measurements before death and the radiochemical analysis of the autopsy samples with the assumption that the radiochemical results are more accurate.

The absorbed dose for the bone shown in Table 24.1 was calculated assuming the americium-241 was uniformly distributed throughout the bone mass. Alpha particle spectrograms of bone samples

TABLE 24.1
Summary of Accumulated Absorbed Dose

Organ	Organ Wt., g	Absorbed Dose, Gy, Postexposure	
		5.3 Years	11 Years
Bone	7,000	7.4	18
Liver	1,270	2.4	8.1
Lungs	900	1.3	1.7
Muscle	15,000	—	4.4
Skin	20 (right side of face and neck)	8,800	10,300

taken at autopsy from the patient were performed.[23] These showed that essentially all the americium-241 was deposited directly on the exposed bone surfaces and only a very small amount had been translocated to within the bone volume. The estimated cumulative bone surface dose for the few bone samples ranged from 120 to 210 Gy. Another calculation of surface bone dose gave an estimate of 510 Gy.[21] Some redistribution of americium-241 and some pathological changes were observed in another study of the autopsied bone samples.[24] The greatest redistribution occurred in the vertebra, suggesting that this bone area had the largest rate of turnover.

The dose rate to the lungs varied from 0.12 Gy per day for the first day of exposure to 0.0001 Gy per day at death. The liver rate varied from 0.36 Gy per day to 0.0017 Gy per day at death with even lower rates between 300 and 900 days postexposure before DTPA therapy was discontinued. The bone dose rate was initially 0.011 Gy per day, rapidly dropping to 0.0038 Gy per day until 900 days postexposure when it gradually increased to 0.0051 Gy per day.

After DTPA therapy, most of the activity in the skin translocated to the liver and bone. During years 6 to 10, the skin lost about 93 kBq (2.5 µCi) of americium-241, the bone gained about 67 kBq (1.8 µCi), the liver gained about 7.4 kBq (0.2 µCi), and about 30 kBq (0.8 µCi) were excreted in the urine and feces.

The dose to the skin is an estimate of the average dose to approximately 20 g of tissue that contained most of the radioactive debris embedded in the skin. Specific small areas of skin, such as the area about the right eye that initially contained more that 740 kBq (20 µCi) in a 2-cm area, received a dose significantly greater than 10^4 Gy.

EFFECTIVENESS OF DTPA THERAPY

The total americium-241 excreted from the body was 41 MBq (1.1 µCi). Of this amount, almost half was excreted in the first 3 days. This large quantity of radioactivity was transferred to the blood from the material inhaled in the lungs and from the chemical burn and debris embedded in the skin of the face and neck. DTPA was very effective in preventing americium-241 deposition in the bone and liver. Without this therapy, the resulting deposition of approximately 18.5 MBq (500 µCi) of americium-241 in the bone and liver would have produced life-threatening doses of 0.07 Gy/day, 25 Gy/year to the bone and 1 Gy per day to the liver. DTPA was also effective in reducing the clearance half-time of the liver activity to about 20 days as compared with the 20 years estimated by ICRP Rep. 48[26] for unchelated americium-241. Essentially all of the americium-241 initially deposited in the liver was cleared by day 400; significant liver redeposition occurred after termination of the DTPA injections.

The americium-241 clearance from the lung may have been enhanced by DTPA therapy, but this effect was not measurable since the clearance rate agreed with the 50-day half-time predicted by ICRP Rep. 48[26] for the class W oxide form of material.

The clearance of americium-241 from the bone was not affected by DTPA, except for a small possible effect during the first week of treatment.

CONCLUSIONS

The only clear radiation effects were seen in the circulating blood, where lymphocytes, platelets, and neutrophils were variously depressed; lymphocytes also demonstrated cytogenic effects. None of these findings was associated with observable clinical effects on health. The large radiation doses to extensive areas of facial skin may have contributed to slow healing of the nitric acid burn, and a sensation of tenderness. The acid burns (especially in the eyes) and trauma from blast and debris had the most serious medical consequences for the patient.

Prompt and intensive chelation therapy proved extremely effective. The fact that radiation effects played a minor role in this case must be credited to the chelation treatment. ZnDTPA was as effective as CaDTPA in removing americium from the body and preventing its translocation. No DTPA toxicity was observed following the intravenous administration of 583 g from 1976 to 1980. This was the first patient in the United States in which ZnDTPA was used. As a direct consequence, ZnDTPA is now generally available for investigational DTPA therapy in the United States.

Reasonably accurate *in vivo* measurements of internally deposited americium-241 were achieved and were consistent with the transfer of americium-241 from facial and lung deposition sites to bone, liver, and excreta, and with postmortem measurements in tissue.

A team approach to decision making in this case was highly successful and helped surmount the many uncertainties encountered. The patient was an important member of this team.

The initial care of this heavily contaminated worker was greatly simplified by the availability of the Emergency Decontamination Facility (EDF). The use of transitional discharge (EDF–trailer–home) during the acute phase of treatment was very beneficial. These measures assured adequate contamination control and provided radiation protection for the staff.

Careful coordination of public and media relations under the stress of an emergency was well worth the effort.

ACKNOWLEDGMENTS

An earlier version of this report, "Lifetime Followup of the 1976 Americium Accident Victim" was published in *Radiation Protection Dosimetry* in 1989.[19]

REFERENCES

1. McMurray, B.J., 1976 Hanford americium exposure incident: accident description, *Health Phys.*, 45 847–853, 1983.
2. Energy Research and Development Administration, Investigation of the Chemical Explosion of an Ion Exchange Resin Column and Resulting Americium Contamination of Personnel in the 242-Z Building, August 30, 1976, ERDA 76, 1976.
3. Norwood, W.E. and Quigley, E.J., *Experimental Radiosurgery for Care of Injured Radiating Patients*, Excerpta Medical Foundation, Amsterdam, 1968, 608–613.
4. Berry, J.R., McMurray, B.J., Jech, J.J, Breitentein, B.D., and Quigley, E.J., 1976 Hanford americium exposure incident: decontamination and treatment facility, *Health Phys.*, 45, 883–892, 1983.
5. Breitenstein, B.D., 1976 Hanford americium exposure incident: medical management and chelation therapy, *Health Phys.*, 45, 855–866, 1983.
6. Sullivan, M.F., Mahoney, T.D., Ragan, H.A., Lund, J.E., Hackett, P.L., Beamer, J.L., and Smith, V.H., Toxicity of Continuously Maintained Levels of Chelating Agents in the Rat and Miniature Swine, PNL Annual Report for 1973 to USAEC, BNWL-1850, 114–117, 1974.

7. Taylor, G.N., Williams, J.L., Roberts, L., Atherton, D.R., and Shabestari, L., Increased toxicity of NA₃CaDTPA when given by protracted administration, *Health Phys.*, 27, 285–288, 1974.
8. Ohlenschlager, L., Efficiency of Zn-DTPA in removing plutonium from the human body, *Health Phys.*, 30, 249–250, 1976.
9. Planas-Bohne, F., and Olinger, H., On the influence of Ca-DTPA on the Zn and Mn concentrations in various organs of the rat, *Health Phys.*, 31, 165–166, 1976.
10. Lloyd, R.D., Mays, C.W., McFarland, S.S., Taylor, G.N., and Atherton, D.R., A comparison of Ca-DTPA and Zn-DTPA for chelating ^{24}Am in beagles, *Health Phys.*, 31, 281–284, 1976.
11. Volf, V., Should Zn-DTPA replace Ca-DTPA for decorporation of radionuclides in man?, *Health Phys.*, 31, 290–291, 1976.
12. Jech, J.J, Berry, J.R., and Breitenstein, B.D., 1976 Hanford americium exposure incident: external decontamination procedures, *Health Phys.*, 45, 873–881, 1983.
13. Ragan, H.A., Mahaffey, J.A., and Breitenstein, B.D., 1976 Hanford americium exposure incident: hematologic effects, *Health Phys.*, 45, 923–932, 1983.
14. Littlefield, G., Joiner, E., Dufrain, R.J., Colyer, S., and Breitenstein, B.D., Six year cytogenetic study of an individual heavily contaminated with Am-241, in *Proceedings of the 7th International Congress of Radiation Research*, Section E 3-05, Broerse, J.J., Brendsen, G.W., Kal, H.B., and Van der Koyle, A.J., Eds., Martinus Nijhoff, Amsterdam, 1983.
15. Hampton, J.C., 1976 Hanford americium exposure incident: histologic and autoradiographic observations on skin, *Health Phys.*, 45, 933–935, 1983.
16. Brown, W.R., 1976 Hanford americium exposure incident: psychological aspects, *Health Phys.*, 45, 867–871, 1983.
17. Breitenstein, B.D., The Hanford accident: psychological effects on the patient, his family and caregivers, in *The Medical Basis for Radiation Accident Preparedness, The Psychological Perspective*, Ricks, R.C., Berger, M.E,. and O'Hara, F.M., Jr., Eds., Elsevier Science, New York, 1991, 193–198.
18. Palmer, H.E., Rieksts, G.A., and Icayan, E.E., 1976 Hanford americium exposure incident: in vivo measurements, *Health Phys.*, 45, 893–910, 1983.
19. Breitenstein, B.D. and Palmer, H.E., Lifetime followup of the 1976 americium accident victim, *Radiat. Prot. Dosimetry*, 26, 317–322, 1989.
20. Robinson, B., Heid, K.R., Aldridge, T.L., and Glen, R.D., 1976 Hanford americium exposure incident: organ burden and radiation dose estimates, *Health Phys.*, 45, 911–921, 1983.
21. Toohey, R.E. and Kathren, R.L., Overview and dosimetry of the Hanford americium accident case, *Health Phys.*, 69(3), 310–317, 1995.
22. Mcinroy, J.F., Kathren, R.L., Toohey, R.E., Swint, M.J., and Breitenstein, B.D., Jr., Postmortem tissue contents of ^{241}Am in a person with a massive acute exposure, *Health Phys.*, 69(3), 318–323, 1995.
23. Schlenker, R.A., Toohey, R.E., Thompson, E.G., and Oltman, B.D., Bone surface concentrations and dose rates 11 years after massive accidental exposure to ^{241}Am, *Health Phys.*, 69(3), 324–329, 1995.
24. Priest, N.D., Freemont, A., Humphreys, J.A.H., and Kathren, R.L., Histopathology and ^{241}Am microdistribution in skeletal USTUR case 246, *Health Phys.*, 69(3), 330–337, 1995.
25. Filipy, R.E., Toohey, R.E., Kathren, R.L., and Dietert, S.E., Deterministic effects of ^{241}Am exposure in the Hanford americium accident case, *Health Phys.*, 69(3), 338–345, 1995.
26. ICRP, Phantoms and Computational Models in Therapy, Diagnosis and Protection, Rep. 48, 1992.

25 Two Los Alamos Plutonium Accidents

George L. Voelz

CONTENTS

Introduction 345
Accident Involving Inhalation Exposures..345
    Nose Swipes..346
    DTPA Chelation Decision...346
    Lung Counts..347
    Urine Bioassays...348
    Fecal Samples 348
    Discussion 350
Accident Involving a Plutonium-Contaminated Wound..350
    Initial Wound Counts and Excision..351
    Second Tissue Excision 351
    Chelation Therapy...351
    Urine Bioassay Results 352
    In Vivo Measurements 352
    Discussion 352
References 354

INTRODUCTION

Every occupational plutonium exposure nowadays is considered to be an accidental exposure because elaborate protective systems and operating procedures are designed to prevent even minimal exposures. Almost all such exposures are minor and are followed with urine bioassays and *in vivo* chest counts, but they do not require treatment. Nevertheless, more serious accidents that require treatment can and do happen. Two accidents, one an inhalation exposure and the other a contaminated wound, are described here, including the methods and judgments used in evaluating and managing these cases. A brief critique on the lessons learned with regard to the medical responses to these accidents is also given.

ACCIDENT INVOLVING INHALATION EXPOSURES

On February 10, 1977, five employees were exposed, via inhalation, to plutonium-239 particles from an explosion that occurred in a glove box. The explosion resulted from a failure of a metal gasket that sealed a reduction vessel operating at a high temperature. The plutonium release involved plutonium oxyfluorides of unknown stoichiometry and perhaps some plutonium oxides. Two gloves were torn off the glove box and approximately 5 g of plutonium was released into the room. No one was working at the involved glove box at the time of the accident. There were no physical injuries to the employees and no release of plutonium outside the facility.

Technician 1 was sitting at a desk with his back to the glove box. After the explosion, he went the length of the room, turned off electrical power, and exited to the outside of the building. He reentered an adjacent room without respiratory protection to close the door. The other four employees — Technicians 2 and 3, a supervisor, and a health physics surveyor — left the room immediately. Contaminated clothing was removed and areas of more highly contaminated skin were decontaminated with detergent and water. Showers were taken, and repeated as necessary, until the remaining alpha contamination appeared to be fixed in place. Doorways and any wall penetrations were taped shut until a decontamination crew went in later and cleaned up the room.

NOSE SWIPES

All five employees had nasal swipes taken immediately after leaving the room. The results are listed in alpha disintegrations per minute from the left and right nostrils: Technician 1 (12759/13385), Technician 2 (801/1849), Technician 3 (611/1193), Supervisor (1091/1193) and BP Surveyor (226/577). These counts were available within an hour of the accident.

In a plutonium facility, the health physicists and technicians should be trained to take nose swipes immediately from individuals potentially exposed to contaminated air. Using a moistened cotton swab, the anterior chamber of each nostril is swiped separately with a clean swab. The cotton swabs are placed in separate clean containers, dried in the laboratory, and then counted for alpha activity. Each facility will develop its own interpretation, but one rule of thumb is that levels of 500 disintegrations per minute (dpm) or less suggest a relatively low inhalation potential, which may not require treatment. Persons with 2000 dpm or higher in each nostril are good candidates for treatment. Results of nasal swipes are only a crude indicator of the potential amount inhaled. Differences in particle sizes significantly influence the retention in the anterior nasal region. If there is a gross disparity between the counts from the right and left nostril, e.g., 50 on one side and 2000 on the other, this suggests that the contamination may have come from nearby facial contamination or a contaminated finger. Much less trust is put in such results. An obstructed nasal passage from a severely deviated septum or polyps may also cause these findings. Results from nasal swipes taken an hour or more after the accident are not reliable as a result of possible nose blowing, snuffling water in the shower, and normal clearance from the anterior nares. Nonetheless, early nasal swipes do have some useful, even if rough, predictive value.

At Los Alamos, irrigation of the mouth, nose, and the nasopharynx is not normally done in treating inhalation cases. This material will be swallowed in the normal course of events and evacuated with feces. Because of the very low uptake of plutonium from the gastrointestinal tract, the passage of plutonium through it does not add significantly to the internal deposition.

DTPA CHELATION DECISION

The supervisory staff held preliminary discussions for over an hour with the men about their knowledge of events and shutdown status of the equipment. Then discussions with the employees were held with the physician-in-charge on the need for treatment.

The immediate objective was to come to a decision whether or not some or all of these men should be treated by chelation. For greatest effectiveness, the treatment should be started within the first 3 h after exposure, or sooner if possible. At this early time, the decision should be made on the circumstances of the accident, the length of exposure time, plutonium air concentrations in the room at the time of the accident (if available), levels of contamination in the accident area, levels of contamination on the patient's clothing and skin, previous plutonium exposure histories of the men, their age, and early nose swipe results. Information on the chemical forms of plutonium and particle sizes are not usually known this soon after an accident, which was the case in this accident. Plutonium air concentration measurements were also not available in this case, but were obviously high.

At the meeting with the exposed men, it was recommended that chelation therapy should be started immediately on Technician 1. The nasal swipe results played a major role in coming to this decision. The details about DTPA and the purpose of chelation therapy were explained to Technician 1. Although the chemical form of plutonium was unknown, it seemed likely that plutonium oxides were present. Chelation is not effective in enhancing the excretion of insoluble plutonium oxide, so the recommendation to treat was considered a therapeutic trial of the efficacy of CaDTPA for this specific exposure. He agreed with the recommendation. A gram of CaDTPA was given intravenously within 3 h after the accident (day 1) and again on days 2, 6, and 9. The treatment of Technician 1 with DTPA was the first use of this chelating agent in the history of the Los Alamos National Laboratory.

A different decision concerned the Supervisor, who had significant previous plutonium exposures with an estimated systemic deposition of 1.31 kBq (35.4 nCi) before this accident. [Note: Recent dosimetry models have revised the Supervisor's preaccident deposition down to 692 Bq (18.7 nCi).] It was thought, based mainly on the nose swipe results, that the additional uptake from this accident would probably not add significantly to his total plutonium deposition. It was determined much later that this accident added about 0.28 kBq (7.7 nCi) to his total deposition. No chelation treatment was given to him or to the other three men.

Lung Counts

In vivo chest (lung) counts would seem to be an ideal way to determine the quantity of plutonium inhalation. Plutonium measurements made by these very sensitive counters (phoswich detectors in 1977) shortly after an accident are often confounded by an inability to discriminate between plutonium that remains on the skin from that taken internally in the lungs. The importance of getting this type of measurement in the first few hours after a plutonium accident is overrated. After this accident, no time was wasted in making these counts before the important initial medical treatment decisions were made. An initial count, made on Technician 1 the day after the accident (day 2), showed "obvious" surface contamination, which interfered with reliable determinations of either plutonium or americium uptake. Due to the surface contamination, no further counts were taken during the next 2 days. Chest counts were done daily from day 5 through day 9 on all five exposed men. Technician 1 had the highest average plutonium-239 activity 1.2 kBq (33 nCi), but it was possible that surface contamination contributed to the count. The counts on the other four were above background, but were not statistically above the minimum detection limit.

Chest counts were done twice each week for the next 5 weeks, and then weekly for another 5 weeks. The chest counts for plutonium-239 for all five men from day 18 through day 73 were not significantly elevated. The americium-241 activity in the chest counts was less than 37 Bq (1 nCi) for all five individuals. The highest americium-241 activity 24 Bq (0.65 nCi) was present in the supervisor, who had several known inhalation exposures prior to this accident.

Chest counters have better sensitivity for americium-241 than for plutonium itself. Measurement of americium is often useful after an accident because this transuranium element is usually present up to 10 or even 15% of the total radioactivity present in plutonium contamination cases. The plutonium/americium ratio of the specific material involved in the accident is measured so that the plutonium deposition can be calculated from the americium data. The relative isotopic abundance (% activity) involved in this accident was plutonium-239, 240 96.3 %, plutonium-238 3.0%, and americium-241 0.7%. This low americium-241 content accounts for finding little americium that was attributable to this intake in chest counts.

Urine Bioassays

Plutonium excretion in urine is the principal and most sensitive method of estimating the deposition of plutonium in the body. Urine levels reflect the plutonium concentration in the blood. The blood level soon after an inhalation is dependent on the solubility of the inhaled plutonium particles. After inhalation of high-fired, insoluble plutonium oxide, the urine excretion may be below minimum detection levels or at a low level for weeks to months before it starts to rise. Thus, early urine sample results may be misleading. Furthermore, the collection of a 24-h sample plus a long processing time means that urine bioassay results are not available at the time of early medical decision making. However, this information becomes valuable later in determining if continued treatment is needed or not.

Technician 1 collected all his urine starting February 10 (day 1) until April 15 (day 65). After April 15, a 24-h urine sample was collected weekly for several more months. This comprehensive sampling was scheduled to obtain data on plutonium excretion after CaDTPA chelation that might be useful in assessing future accidental exposures and to evaluate his plutonium uptake. The untreated men provided three 24-h urine samples in the first 12 days followed by one sample per month for a year.

Urine bioassays for plutonium normally take several weeks to complete. With special effort, the radiochemistry laboratory was able to provide some preliminary data on Technician 1 from direct counts on his samples within 24 to 48 h. These data indicated that the plutonium excretion was high, suggesting that chelation therapy was effective. Subsequently, the definitive data indicated that he excreted 490 Bq (13.3 nCi) during the first day. The second day's urine samples contained only 30 Bq (0.8 nCi). During the first 65 days after this accident, when Technician 1 was collecting all his urine for analysis, he excreted a total of 840 Bq (22.7 nCi) of plutonium-239 plus 30 Bq (0.8 nCi) of plutonium-238. The excretion curve for plutonium-239 in urine for Technician 1 is shown in Figure 25.1. About 57% of the plutonium excreted in urine during the first 65 days occurred in the first 24 h after the accident, following the initial chelation treatment. This finding emphasizes the importance of starting chelation therapy as soon as possible after the accident. The excretion curve for plutonium in the urine of Technician 1 was elevated for about 120 days and it parallels very closely the Hall model for urinary excretion after a single 1-g DTPA dose soon after an accidental intake.[1]

Table 25.1 summarizes the plutonium deposition for the systemic burden before and after the accidental exposure, estimated from urine bioassays. The cumulative effective dose from plutonium depositions in these men through 1998 is also listed. There were no significant plutonium uptakes to any of these men after the 1977 accident. The listed doses come principally from plutonium exposures prior to and from this accident.

Fecal Samples

After this accident, daily fecal specimens (not total samples) were collected for the first 7 days from all exposed men. A direct count with a phoswich detector, which had a detection limit of 37 Bq (1 nCi)/sample, was used to get rapid results. The highest values were observed in samples collected on day 2 and 3. Technician 1 had the highest values with 2.9 and 5.7 kBq (78 and 155 nCi)/sample on days 2 and 3, respectively. The other men had from 70 to 2000 Bq (2 to 54 nCi)/sample on these days. By day 6, all samples were below 37 Bq (1 nCi)/sample. Samples were also collected from all exposed persons on day 10, 30, and 60, but none of these later samples had detectable activity above 37 Bq (1 nCi). More sensitive, but less timely, radiochemistry results were used to confirm measurements on many samples. The phoswich results were shown to be reasonable at levels above 37 Bq (1 nCi)/sample.

Activity measured in fecal samples is sometimes used to try to make a rough estimate of the amount of plutonium inhaled. The plutonium particles are cleared from the lung to the pharynx by

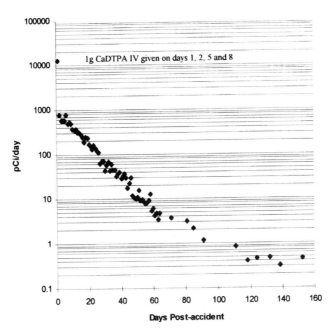

FIGURE 25.1 Plutonium-239 urinary excretion curve of Technician 1, who was treated with CaDTPA, after an inhalation exposure.

TABLE 25.1
Summary of Plutonium Systemic Depositions prior to and after the February 10, 1977 Accidental Inhalation (calculated from urinalysis data on ^{239,240}Pu plus ^{238}Pu[a])

Person	Preaccident Deposition kBq (nCi)	Postaccident Deposition kBq (nCi)	Attributable Deposition kBq (nCi)	Total Dose through 1988 (Sv)
Technician 1	0.14 (3.8)	0.48 (13.0)	0.34 (9.2)[b]	0.31
Technician 2	0.03 (0.9)	0.28 (7.5)	0.24 (6.6)	0.26
Technician 3	0.05 (1.5)	1.36 (36.7)	1.30 (35.2)	0.71
Supervisor	0.69 (18.7)	0.98 (26.4)	0.29 (7.7)	1.04
HP Surveyor	0.09 (2.5)	0.13 (3.4)	0.03 (0.9)	0.13

[a] Depositions and total effective (whole-body) dose were calculated by Dr. Guthrie Miller of the Dosimetry Group, Los Alamos National Laboratory.
[b] CaDTPA chelation therapy removed 0.85 kBq (~23 nCi) of plutonium.

mucociliary action of the bronchial mucous membrane and then swallowed. The total activity in fecal samples for the first several days is used to estimate the lung intake under the assumption that lung clearance is related to the initial lung deposition. These sample collections and measurements are not available at the time the initial medical decisions are made. They may help the dosimetry specialist ultimately, but are of little value to the medical management of the accident.

DISCUSSION

Chelation treatment of Technician 1 was effective in removing about 0.85 kBq (23 nCi) of plutonium. It resulted in removal of 71% of his overall uptake of 1.2 kBq (0.85 plus 0.34 kBq) [32.2 nCi (23 nCi plus 9.2 nCi)] attributable retention, Table 25.1. Activity on nasal swipes was an important piece of data used to decide who to treat, but obviously these data are crude and can be misleading. Nasal swipes from Technician 1 had ten times greater activity than any of the other men. Nevertheless, Technician 3 had an attributable deposition of 1.3 kBq (35.2 nCi), slightly more than the uptake of 1.2 kBq (32.2 nCi) of Technician 1. The uptake by Technician 3 was higher than was expected by the initial evaluation of the accident or was calculated by 1977 dosimetry models 0.3 kBq (8.1 nCi attributable retention) based on the first bioassay results. Technician 2 and the supervisor had nasal swipe results essentially identical to that of Technician 3, but had much smaller attributable depositions of 0.29 and 0.24 kBq (7.7 and 6.6 nCi), respectively.

In retrospect, a decision to administer DTPA to four of the five individuals immediately may have been appropriate rather than just treating the one person. The lack of information about individual intakes and solubility of the plutonium particles at the time of decision should not deter the administration of an initial therapeutic trial of the drug as soon as practicable. DTPA is a safe drug that has been given to hundreds of people without significant side effects or toxicity, provided it is given in accordance with the recommended dose (1 g given intravenously or by aerosol inhalation one time per 24 h). After a major accidental release, the use of chelation therapy as soon as possible in persons with a suspected significant exposure is better than its omission. This advice is not intended to imply that everyone who has potential for a plutonium exposure should receive DTPA. An evaluation of the accident circumstances and early information should be made before proceeding with DTPA therapy.

The cumulative effective doses through 1998 listed in Table 25.1 are the result of many years of plutonium deposition in these men. The average period of time from their first, preaccident plutonium uptakes to 1998 is 34 years, ranging from a low of 27 years and a high of 46 years.

All five men were restricted from working with plutonium until enough samples were measured to make a good dose assessment. Technician 2, Technician 3, and the health physics surveyor were permitted to resume their normal duties about 2 months after the accident. Technician 1 returned to his normal duties about 6 months after the accident. The supervisor was assigned to other supervisory work and was restricted permanently from doing plutonium work. The vital status of these men was checked through 1990. All of them were alive as of that time. Technician 1 was 67 years old in 1990, and the ages of the others ranged from 59 to 74 years.

ACCIDENT INVOLVING A PLUTONIUM-CONTAMINATED WOUND

On April 17, 1981, a 25-year-old technician employed in the Chemical Operations Section of a Plutonium Chemistry and Metallurgy Group injured himself with a paring knife contaminated with isotopes of plutonium and americium. The primary cause of the accident was the presence of a pointed knife in the glove box. The injury occurred in a glove box when the technician attempted to make a vent hole in the plastic cap of a 2 l plastic bottle, which resulted in a cut in the flesh web between his left index finger and middle finger. The wound was about $1/2$ in. long and less than $1/4$ in. deep, with very little immediate bleeding. A health physics technician monitored the hand and external clothing. He established that contamination was limited to the left hand. Initial counts of the area with an alpha survey instrument showed 80,000 dpm. Decontamination of the intact skin around the wound was carried out for 20 to 30 min with soap and water, a surgical scrub brush, and, finally, with sodium hypochlorite (household bleach). The contamination was reduced to 30,000 dpm. The exposed technician was then taken to the laboratory's occupational medicine facility for evaluation and treatment.

INITIAL WOUND COUNTS AND EXCISION

An initial wound count, using a Los Alamos wound counter, gave an activity of 24 kBq (645 nCi). The wound counter detects uranium L X rays that accompany plutonium alpha decays. This count was estimated to be low by a factor of 3 to 12, reflecting uncertainties due to geometry effects and tissue absorption of X rays. It was obvious that a serious wound contamination was present. Excision of the wound was performed immediately at the occupational medical facility.

Using the wound counter, an initial count suggested the excised tissue contained 14 kBq (390 nCi). Counts over the wound area suggested that about 60% of the deposited activity had been removed by the excision. Because of considerable bleeding, the surgeon decided to suture the wound and forgo any further tissue excision. A subsequent radiochemical analysis determined that 23 kBq (629 nCi) was present in the excised tissue. The contaminant contained 80.4% plutonium-239, 9.4% plutonium-238, and 10.2% americium-241.

SECOND TISSUE EXCISION

After the first excision wound had healed without complication, it was possible to achieve better counting geometry with an Si(Li) detector. By day 19, it was apparent that about 22 kBq (600 nCi) remained at the wound site. On day 26 (May 12, 1981), a second excision of the wound was performed by a hand surgeon, supported with wound counting equipment operated by laboratory health physicists. Examination of the excised tissue showed 21.8 kBq (590 nCi) was removed. Wound counts indicated that a residual of 16 kBq (42 nCi) remained at the wound site after the second excision.

Two or more debridement procedures have been necessary after other serious plutonium-contaminated wounds. The history of this accident is similar in this respect to a number of other accidents. For example, Lagerquist et al.[2] reported on an accident that embedded about 5.3 MBq (144 µCi) of plutonium in an employee's hand. Surgery was performed on the day of the accident and again 12 days, 11 months, and 17 months after the accident. Schofield et al.[3] managed a contaminated puncture wound that was also in the web between the index and middle fingers. Initially, 0.53 MBq (14.2 µCi) of plutonium was in the wound and was reduced to about 66 kBq (1.8 µCi) with surgical excisions about 1 h after the surgery and again on day 15. Both of the above cases were also treated with DTPA.

CHELATION THERAPY

Immediately after the first excision procedure, the benefits and small risk of DTPA chelation were explained to the exposed technician. About 3½ h after the accident, the first CaDTPA treatment (1 g intravenously) was given. A second CaDTPA dose was given the next morning. After that he was treated with ZnDTPA given intravenously three times per week.

By the end of the third week of treatment, the patient complained about the number of intravenous injections required, especially in view of the recommendation to continue treatment for a long period. He was placed on aerosol administrations of 1 g CaDTPA three times per week and maintained on that schedule for 11 weeks. By then, his excretion of plutonium was relatively small and stable at about 74 to 111 Bq (2 to 3 nCi) per month, so his aerosol treatment schedule was reduced to once a week and maintained at that rate for 9 months. His chelation therapy extended over a period of 1 year after the accident. The only complaint during this long treatment period was a poorly defined sense of nausea, tension, nervousness, or uneasiness during and for a short time after aerosol administrations. No other side effects were observed. Serum zinc level was normal.

Urine Bioassay Results

For 4 weeks after the accident, daily 24-h urine samples were collected. After that, two collections per week (one day before a DTPA treatment and one day after) were taken. The plutonium measurements on these samples were used to project an estimated total excretion for each week.

The bioassay results for the first weeks are shown in Figure 25.2A. The contaminant contained plutonium-239 80.4%, plutonium-238 9.4%, and americium-241 10.2% by activity. On day 1, 0.93 kBq (25 nCi) of plutonium-238,239 and 8.4 kBq (22.8 nCi) of americium-241 were excreted in urine. By day 2, the day's excretion had already dropped to 0.6 and 0.2 kBq (16 and 5.2 nCi), respectively. During the first week, 2.8 kBq (75 nCi) of plutonium-238,239 and 1.4 kBq (37 nCi) of americium-241 were excreted in urine. This first week's total activity of 4.1 kBq (112 nCi) is 51% of the total 8.1 kBq (220 nCi) excreted in urine during the first 15 months after the accident. The importance of administering the first chelation treatment soon after the accident is obvious here. This chelation efficacy in the early time period is even more impressive in the monthly excretion data shown in Figure 25.2B.

The isotopic distribution within urine during the first week contained 33% americium-241, much higher than the 10.2% americium-241 found in the wound. This increase is due to the greater solubility and speed of transport of americium compared with plutonium. Chelation therapy in the first few days removes a proportionately higher percentage of americium because of its availability in the blood. By week 8, the excretion in urine contained only 5% americium-241. Figure 25.2A shows the more rapid removal of americium from the body compared with plutonium over the first 8 weeks of chelation.

In Vivo Measurements

Direct radioactivity measurements at the wound site, chest, liver, and skull were made repeatedly for several years after the accident. The 60-keV gamma ray from americium-241 was the only detectable activity by direct counts. About 150 Bq (4 nCi) of americium-241 was in the wound after the second excision. The radioactivity declined steadily over the next 9 months, during the chelation treatment period. By then, the americium-241 activity was down to 48 Bq (1.3 nCi) and remained at that level for the next 3 years. There was a gradual buildup of americium-241 in liver to 18.5 Bq (0.5 nCi) and in bone (skull) to 30 Bq (0.8 nCi) during the first 3.5 years. Plutonium and americium have different rates of transport within the body so plutonium/americium ratios change significantly over time. Therefore, the use of plutonium/americium ratios to estimate the plutonium depositions by americium measurements is unreliable within months after an accidental intake, and the changes in the ratio are accelerated by DTPA chelation therapy.

Discussion

A summary of the bioassay results and dosimetry is listed on Table 25.2. The systemic deposition several years after the accident was estimated to be 7.15 kBq [193 nCi (174 nCi plutonium-239 and 19 nCi americium-241)]. The residual radioactivity in the wound after the excisions was 1.6 kBq (42 nCi). The initial radioactivity in the wound is estimated to have been about 61 kBq (1637 nCi). This estimate is derived from the sum of the measurements of activity in excised tissues and urine bioassays plus the estimates for retention in the wound and body. It does not include a factor for fecal excretion so this total may be slightly low. The treatment regimen, excisions plus urinary excretion, removed about 86% of the initial radioactivity in the wound.

Early excision of the wound is recommended, but there might be some advantage to waiting on excision until the administration of DTPA is started. A time delay would occur because the details of the DTPA treatment need to be explained to the patient, and a permission slip must be read and signed. There is also a requirement under the IND protocol to do a clinical urinalysis and certain blood tests prior to DTPA administration. No scientific data are available to indicate whether

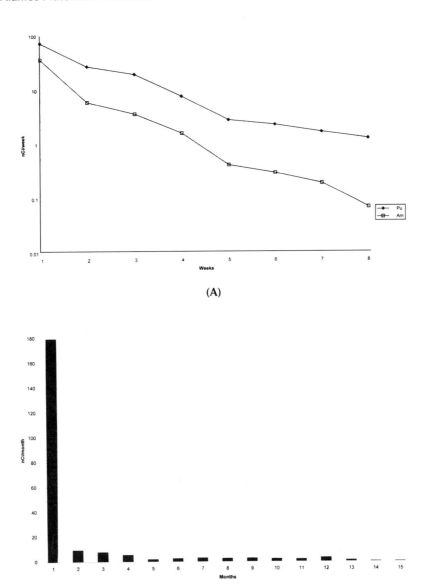

FIGURE 25.2 (A) Weekly plutonium-238,239 and americium-241 excretion in urine during DTPA treatment. (B) Monthly plutonium-238,239 excretion in urine. DTPA discontinued after 12 months of treatment.

the order of implementation of these procedures is important or not. NCRP Rep. 65 recommends immediate chelation therapy with CaDTPA, prior to surgical excision of the wound, to prevent possible systemic absorption.[4]

Consideration has been given to the therapeutic effect of using DTPA five treatments per week rather than three per week as used in this case. Five treatments per week was the maximum DTPA dose recommended at the time.[4] By interpolating plutonium excretion rates for the days on which DTPA was not given, an estimate of urinary excretion for treatment five times a week was made. This procedure estimated an increased excretion of 1.7 kBq (47 nCi), which would have raised the plutonium/americium excretion during the first month from 6.6 to 8.4 kBq (179 to 226 nCi), an increase of 26%. This benefit must be balanced against the increased number of intravenous infusions of the medication. Increasing the number of daily treatments in the first few weeks after

TABLE 25.2
Summary Information on Plutonium-Contaminated Wound Case

Description	Radioactivity
Date of injury: April 17, 1981	80.4% ^{239}Pu; 9.4% ^{238}Pu; 10.2% ^{241}Am
First excision: April 17, 1981	23.3 kBq (629 nCi) removed, chemistry on tissue
Second excision: May 12, 1981	20.5 kBq (553 nCi) removed, spectroscopy of tissue
Residual in wound: May 25, 1981	1.6 kBq (42 nCi) by spectroscopy
Total excretion in urine to April 23, 1982	8.5 kBq (229 nCi) ^{239}Pu + ^{241}Am
Systemic deposition: January 1, 1994	6.4 kBq (174 nCi) ^{239}Pu and 0.7 kBq (19 nCi) ^{241}Am
Total initial wound radioactivity	60.6 kBq (~1637 nCi)
Effective dose to December 31, 1998	4.09 Sv

a serious accident has a definite therapeutic advantage compared with a similar number of treatments at a later time.

This case was perhaps the first time that administration of DTPA by inhalation was employed for a contaminated wound. It appeared to be less effective per gram than by intravenous administration, but is more acceptable to the patient. The inhalation route has been primarily used on the first and second day after inhalation exposures when it may be more effective than intravenous administration of DTPA.

This technician was restricted from future plutonium work and was assigned to nonradiation work. He continues to work without other limitations. His main complaint since the accident has been an ongoing anxiety about possible future health effects. The wound area is well healed. His ability to separate his index and middle finger is reduced. Certain impacts on his palm, such as catching a ball, are momentarily more painful than usual. This sensitivity is apparently due to the loss of some subcutaneous tissue in the wound area.

REFERENCES

1. Hall, R.M., Poda, G.A., Fleming, R.R., and Smith, J.A., A mathematical model for estimation of plutonium in the human body from urine data influenced by DTPA therapy, *Health Phys.*, 34, 419, 1978.
2. Lagerquist, C.R., Putzier, E.A., and Piltingsrud, C.W., Bio-assay and body counter results for the first 2 years following an acute plutonium exposure, *Health Phys.*, 13, 965, 1967.
3. Schofield, G.B., Howells, H., Ward, F., Lynn, J.C., and Dolphin, G.W., Assessment and management of a plutonium contaminated wound case, *Health Phys.*, 26, 541, 1974.
4. National Council on Radiation Protection and Measurements, Management of Persons Accidentally Contaminated with Radionuclides, NCRP Rep. 65, NCRP Publications, Washington, D.C., 1980.

26 Internal Contamination in the Goiânia Accident, Brazil, 1987

Carlos Nogueira de Oliveira, Dunstana R. Melo, and Joyce L. Liptzstein

CONTENTS

Description of the Accident 355
Internal Contamination 357
Efficacy of the Prussian Blue Therapy 357
References 360

DESCRIPTION OF THE ACCIDENT

This accident involved significant whole-body exposure, local radiation injuries, and major internal contamination; however, this chapter will focus predominantly on the treatment of the internal contamination. On September 13, 1987, in the city of Goiânia (Brazil), two individuals found a source of ionizing radiation used for medical teletherapy that contained 50.9 TBq (1375 Ci) of cesium-137, which had been abandoned in the interior of an empty building where a radiotherapy clinic had been functioning. They removed the rotating assembly of the shielding head of the medical teletherapy unit containing the radioactive source and brought it to the house of one them. There, they violated the shielding and ruptured the source canister, thus originating the radiological accident known as the "Radiological Accident in Goiânia."[1]

Part of the rotating shielding assembly containing the damaged source was sold to a scrap yard owner, who brought it home because he admired the blue glow that appeared in the dark. Small fragments of the source were distributed among relatives and friends. Some of them rubbed the material on their skin to appreciate its brightness.[2]

The accident was aggravated during the 16 days that elapsed between the rupture of the source and notification of competent authority. The source, in the form of cesium chloride salt (a highly soluble chemical compound), and its inappropriate handling contributed to the dissemination of the cesium and, as a consequence, the contamination of many people and the urban environment. The passing of contaminated materials from one individual to another, social and professional contacts among people, the movements of animals, wind and rain were the major pathways for the dispersion of the cesium.

The preliminary radiometric surveys and reports from individuals identified as having been in contact with the cesium necessitated the implementation of intervention measurements for the public and the urban environment. In the environment, seven areas were identified, isolated, and designated as the major foci of contamination. Of 159 houses monitored, 42 were evacuated and decontaminated, six were demolished and 53 were repaired. In all, 58 different public places were decontaminated, including pavement, squares, shops, and bars, along with 64 vehicles. The emergency response, which lasted 6 months, involved significant resources as, for example, the

730 emergency workers assigned to decontamination tasks, which generated some 3500 m³ of radioactive waste. The accident had a major economic impact on the region and depressed trade with other regions.

A soccer stadium known as the Olympic Stadium was chosen by the authorities as a triage and sorting center. There, an emergency monitoring program was implemented. This program consisted mainly of external skin contamination measurements. Portable gamma radiation detectors were used. Those persons who presented positive results were referred for repeated showers with water and neutral soap.

The measurements performed at the stadium lasted from September 30 to December 21, 1987. A total of 112,800 persons from the general public, out of approximately 1 million inhabitants of the Goiânia population, were registered and surveyed during this period. Of this total, 249 persons showed some signs of contamination. These individuals had clinical laboratory evaluation, monitoring, and screening of internal contamination by urine analysis. Of the 249, 120 people had contamination only on their clothing and shoes, and the other 129 showed internal contamination. After this period, 22 additional individuals were also found to be internally contaminated.

The medical-radiological triage was based on the level of effect on the hematological system, the seriousness of the radiation-induced lesions, and the intensity of the external skin contamination. In all, 49 individuals needed some type of medical treatment, 28 of whom presented with localized radiation-induced lesions (Figure 26.1); 20 individuals were hospitalized and 14 were transferred to the Marcilio Dias Navy Hospital (HNMD), located in the city of Rio de Janeiro (1348 km from Goiânia). Six patients, who were classified as needing secondary care since they did not require special isolation measures or replacement therapy but had moderate to severe internal contamination, remained at the Goiânia General Hospital (HGG). At the HNMD, 8 of its 14 patients developed a severe degree of bone marrow impairment, presenting with nausea, vomiting, and severe diarrhea, characterizing the acute radiation syndrome. Four of them died of bleeding disorders and sepsis within 4 weeks of admission to the hospital, having received total-body radiation doses of 2.9 to 4.4 Gy, as estimated by cytogenetic technique. The 29 individuals who did not require hospitalization, presenting with external skin and/or slight internal contamination, were interned at the State Children's Welfare Foundation (FEBEM), located in the city of Goiânia, in a facility adapted to function as a treatment unit.

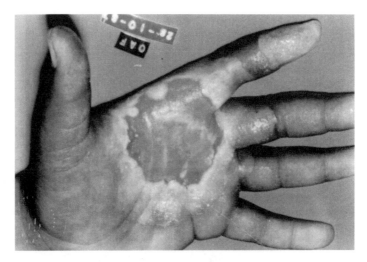

FIGURE 26.1 About 36 days postexposure, a bulla of palm has ruptured and moist desquamation can be seen over the proximal digits and distal second digit.

INTERNAL CONTAMINATION

Whole-body counting, excreta analysis, and the combination of both techniques were used to assess the internal contamination of the individuals. In the first 2 months of the Goiânia accident, the internal cesium contamination was evaluated through excreta analysis (feces and urine). During this period, 90 contaminated individuals were monitored using this technique. These measurements were used to ascertain the effectiveness of the cesium decorporation therapies, mainly the administration of Prussian Blue (PB), as well as other medical treatments including the administration of diuretics.

In November 1987, a whole-body counter was installed at HGG. As the body burdens of some of the patients were very high, they were placed on a fiberglass chair, approximately 2 m from the detector. This system, which has been described elsewhere,[3] was very useful in this situation. The minimum detectable activity (MDA) was 9 kBq for a 2-min count and the dead time was lower than 8% for the highest internal contamination. The system was relocated in January 1988, with shielding improvements, to a laboratory built inside a house on the street where the source had been breached. In July 1991, a multiple geometry system with electrical mechanical movement in the vertical and horizontal directions was installed in the laboratory. New detector shielding was installed (10-cm of lead wrapped around the crystal). For a whole-body measurement geometry at 70 cm from the subject, for example, the MDA was 218 Bq for a 30 min counting time.[4] A total of 616 individuals were subjected to whole-body counting in Goiânia from 1987 to 1994. Of these, 151 (64 females and 87 males) presented results above the minimum detectable activity for the systems. The highest measured activity was 79 MBq (2.1 mCi).

During a short period of time, both *in vivo* and *in vitro* monitoring techniques were simultaneously applied and showed similar results in terms of body burdens and biological half-lives.

The data from people internally contaminated in the Goiânia accident have shown that cesium-137 retention in the body consists of the sum of three exponential terms. The first term, with a short biological half-life, represents mainly the elimination of cesium-137 filtered by the kidneys within a few hours of its entry into blood. The second term, with a long biological half-life, represents the progressive loss in urine and feces of cesium retained in tissues. The second term biological half-life is a function of body weight until adulthood is reached. Skeletal muscle dominates the second retention term due to the predominance of active transport in the cells of that tissue and the fact that muscle is a slowly exchanging tissue. The third exponential term, with a very long biological half-life, may reflect retention in a subcellular fraction of skeletal muscle.[5]

Among the individuals who did not use PB, the second term biological half-life varied from 39 to 90 days for the adult females (average = 63 days) and from 66 to 141 days for the adult males (average = 89 days). For children between 1 and 16 years old, the second term cesium-137 retention was characterized by a stepwise function of body weight. Based on these data, a cesium retention model for children was derived, predicting half-times of 13 days for a body weight of 3 to 6 kg, 19 days for 7 to 10 kg, 25 days for 11 to 15 kg, 37 days for 16 to 30 kg, 49 days for 31 to 40 kg, 57 days for 41 to 50 kg, and 65 days for a body weight of 51 to 60 kg.

By 4 years after the accident, four individuals still had measurable activities in their bodies, suggesting a third biological half-time of about 500 days and corresponding to 0.1% of the initial body burden. Although insignificant in terms of dose, it is important in retrospective dosimetry to monitor an accident for several years after it has occurred.

EFFICACY OF THE PRUSSIAN BLUE THERAPY

Radiogardase, or Prussian Blue (PB), a "ferric ferrocyanide," was used to enhance the cesium elimination from the body. This drug, when administered orally, acts in the lumen of the intestine, decreasing the enterohepatic circulation and increasing the cesium amount excreted in the feces.

Other therapeutic measures, such as increasing the ingestion of liquids, the use of diuretics, sessions in the sauna, and exercising were also used on a case-by-case basis. No significant effect on the decorporation of cesium-137 was observed due to the administration of a diuretic or to the increase in the ingestion of liquids.[6] Melo et al.[7] have reported that a high consumption of water did not alter the whole-body clearance of cesium-137 in beagle dogs.

Of the 151 internally contaminated individuals in the Goiânia accident, 46 were treated with Radiogardase. Although the manufacturer recommended 3 g/day, 0.5 g every 2 h, the prescriptions of the medical team changed according to the ages of the patients and their internal contamination levels. The dosages administered for adults and adolescents were 3, 6, and 10 g/day, and 1 and 3 g/day for children. The drug was given orally two, three, or six times a day, depending on the total dosage, with a minimum of 2 h between consecutive administrations. The same individual sometimes received different dosages of the drug at different time intervals. In four cases, 20 g were administered during a 24-h period, but prior dosage was promptly reestablished, due to gastric distress to the patients and the number of PB pills taken — 40 in a single day. PB proved to be nontoxic, well tolerated, and refractory to absorption from the gastrointestinal tract, as described in the literature.[8] The only side effect observed was related to a complaint of constipation.

Because the accident was communicated to the authorities some days after it had happened, PB treatment started at the earliest 10 days after the cesium intake and, thus, did not have a significant influence on the fast clearance of cesium from the plasma (2 to 3 days half-life). The elimination of the nuclide from the body, with or without the PB treatment, followed a first-order biokinetic model. After ceasing the PB treatment, the cesium biological half-lives increased to values similar to those observed in the individuals of the same age and weight range who did not receive treatment.[9] It is worth mentioning that a 6-year-old girl had an intake on the order of 1.9×10^9 Bq (5.2 mCi), the highest internal contamination in Goiânia. She died 29 after days after exposure, despite the administration of PB.

Figure 26.2 shows the biological half-lives of cesium for seven children, five adolescents, and 13 adults during treatment with different dosages of PB and after treatment was ended. The average values of the biological half-lives for the adults were 25 ± 9 days for 3 g/day, 25 ± 16 days for 6 g/day, and 26 ± 6 days for 10 g/day of PB administered. There were no statistically significant differences in the half-lives among the different dosages of PB that were given ($P < 0.05$). The five adolescents under PB treatment whose biological half-lives could be estimated received 10 g/day, and showed average results of 30 ± 12 days. The average biological half-life of cesium for the seven children who received 3 g/day of PB was 24 ± 3 days. There were no statistical differences between the biological half-lives for the children, adolescents, and adults ($P < 0.05$). When PB is administered with a delay of several days after the intake of cesium (10 days for Goiânia), the biological half-life of cesium-137 is reduced to about 26 ± 10 days, independent of the PB dosage administered and of the age of the individuals. The average reductions of the biological half-life while PB treatment was under way in comparison with the values after the end of the treatment were 69% for the adults, 46% for the adolescents, and 43% for the children.[10]

After PB administration, as expected, feces became the prevalent pathways for cesium excretion. The feces-to-urine ratios increased with drug dosage, giving a false indication of an increased efficacy of the decorporation treatment. Further studies have shown that increased PB dosages enhanced the fraction excreted in feces and decreased the amount of cesium in urine. Overall, it did not change the total quantity of cesium that was excreted. For the adult individuals treated with different dosages of PB, a significant correlation between the feces-to-urine ratios with the dosage was observed. However, there was no significant statistical difference for the cesium-137 half-times under PB dosages of feces-to-urine ratios were 0.2, 1.5, 2.0, and 4.7 for 0, 3, 6, and 10 g/day.

In an experiment using male dogs of three different ages, Melo et al.[7] showed that PB caused an increase in the early clearance fraction, although the biological half-lives related to the first term — about 2.0 ± 0.7 days for all dogs — remained unchanged. The fraction of initial activity that is eliminated rapidly nearly doubled under the influence of PB. The results observed in the people

Internal Contamination in the Goiânia Accident, Brazil, 1987

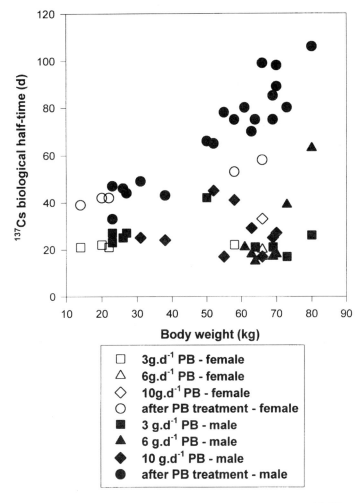

FIGURE 26.2 Cesium biological half-lives and treatment with PB.

affected by cesium-137 in Goiânia followed the same pattern as the biological half-life related to the long-term retention in dogs.

The data gathered from the individuals treated with PB in Goiânia in the dosage range of 1 to 3 g/day for children and 3 to 10 g/day for adolescents and adults, and from the experiment with dogs, were used to derive a mathematical equation for the retention of cesium in the body, $R(t)p$, under the influence of PB, namely,

$$R(t)p = a1pe^{-0.693/T1p} + a2pe^{-0.693/T2p} \qquad (26.1)$$

where the first term refers to the fast clearance of cesium from the body and the second term to the long-term clearance. The fraction related to the fast elimination from the body $a1p$ is equal to 0.5 for children and adolescents while the fast clearance half-life, $T1_p$, remains unchanged and equal to about 3 days. The long-term half-life, $T2_p$, is reduced to 26 days for all ages, and $a2_p = 1 - a1_p$. It was then concluded that the effectiveness of PB is dependent on the time treatment is started.[10] When PB treatment starts before or immediately after cesium intake, its effectiveness is increased since it acts by doubling the short-term elimination fraction, as demonstrated in the experiment with the dogs.

For the Goiânia patients, the rate of elimination of cesium from the body, under PB administration, was shown to be independent of the dosage, sex, age, body weight, and height. A minimum dosage (g/kg of body weight) of PB probably should be given to patients to make it effective. In the dosage range used in Goiânia, PB action overwhelmed the influence of the biological parameters on the clearance of cesium from the body.

Although the start of treatment was late, there was a significant reduction on the committed absorbed dose, e.g., an average reduction of 59% on the committed absorbed dose, with a range of between 84 and 41%.[5] Although the committed absorbed dose decreased, the higher concentration of cesium in the feces and the constipation induced by the PB may have increased the irradiation of the cells of the intestine wall. This increased concentration of cesium and transit time of the fecal content in the intestine were not considered in the standard dose calculations. The evaluation of the intestinal wall absorbed dose and the associated risks should be taken into account when deciding on PB dosage to be given to patients and the duration of administration of the drug.

REFERENCES

1. International Atomic Energy Agency, The Radiological Accident in Goiânia, IAEA, Vienna, 1988.
2. International Atomic Energy Agency, Dosimetric and medical aspects of the radiological accident in Goiânia in 1987, IAEA-TECDOC 1009, IAEA, Vienna, 1988.
3. Oliveira, C.A.N., Lourengo, M.C., Dantas, B.M. and Lucena, E.A., Design and operation of a whole-body monitoring system for the Goiânia radiation accident, *Health Phys.*, 60, 51–55, 1991.
4. Oliveira, C.A.N., Contribuição para a avaliação da contaminação interna atravis de medidas in vivo realizadas em decorrência do acidente radiológico de Goiânia, Doctoral dissertation, Institute of Biophysics, Rio de Janeiro Federal University, 1994.
5. Melo, D.R., Lipsztein, J.L., Oliveira, C.A.N., Lundgren, D.L., Muggenburg, B.A., and Guilmette, R.A., A biokinetic model for ^{137}Cs, *Health Phys.*, 73(2), 320–332, 1997.
6. Farina, R., Brandao-Melo, C.E., and Oliveira, A R., Medical aspects of ^{137}Cs decorporation: the Goiânia radiological accident, *Health Phys.*, 60, 63–66, 1991.
7. Melo, D.R., Lundgren, D.L., Muggenburg, B.A., and Guilmette, R.A., Prussian Blue decorporation of ^{137}Cs in beagles of different ages, *Health Phys.*, 71(2), 190–197, 1996.
8. Richmond, C.R., Acceleration of the turnover of internally deposited radiocesium, in, *Diagnoses and Treatment of Deposited Radionuclides: Proceedings of a Symposium*, Richland, WA, Komberg, H.A. and Norwood, W.D., Eds., Excerpta Medica Foundation, New York, 1968, 315–328.
9. Melo, D.R., Lipsztein, J.L., Oliveira, C.A.N., and Bertelli, L., ^{137}Cs internal contamination involving a Brazilian accident, and the efficacy of Prussian Blue treatment, *Health Phys.*, 66, 245–252, 1994.
10. Melo, D.R., Lipsztein, J.L., Oliveira, C.A.N., Lundgren, D.L., Muggenburg, B.A., and Guilmette, R.A., Prussian Blue decorporation of ^{137}Cs in humans and beagle dogs, *Radiat. Prot. Dosimetry*, 79(1-4), 473–476, 1998.

27 Fatal Accidental Overdose with Radioactive Gold in Wisconsin, U.S.A.

Fred A. Mettler, Jr.

The accident occurred in August 1968. A 73-year-old female, who had erythemic myelosis, was scheduled for a diagnostic nuclear medicine liver/spleen scan. The radiopharmaceutical being used was intravenously administered radioactive colloidal gold-198. The intended dose was 7.4 MBq (200 µCi), but the patient received 1000 times this, or 7.4 GBq (200 mCi). The estimated dose ultimately received by the bone marrow was 4 to 5 Gy, and the dose to the liver was estimated to be 70 to 90 Gy. Initially, there were no symptoms of acute radiation exposure. The patient was admitted to the hospital 30 h after the injection.

Unfortunately for this patient, there was and still is no known mechanism for mobilizing colloidal particles from the liver, spleen, or bone marrow following such misadministrations. A typical radiocolloid of this size will predominantly localize in the liver, but in patients such as this who have preexisting liver disease, a disproportionate amount may be displaced to the spleen and bone marrow. At admission, the patient had an enlarged liver, which had been present for several years. Available patient data are presented in Table 27.1.

It became clear that the major problems would be supporting the hematopoietic system and radiation damage to the liver. The patient was placed in protective isolation. Clothing, food, water, utensils, and all other items were presterilized. The air was filtered through laminar airflow hoods. Oral neomycin sulfate and Nystatin were started at admission in an effort to reduce the possibility of infection from intestinal flora. Vitamin K-1 pyridoxine and folic acid were given throughout the course of hospitalization. Allopurinol was started soon after admission and the serum uric acid returned to normal by day 10. The patient was given intermittent transfusions of fresh blood, white cells, and platelets. The lymphocyte count fell quite rapidly, and platelets decreased to their lowest levels at the end of the third week and could never be raised above 8000/mm^3 despite infusions of platelets.

Intermittent injections of androgen and corticosteroids were given with the hope of stimulating marrow function and reducing capillary fragility and possibly prolonging platelet life span. Despite these injections, the patient developed intermittent hematuria and subconjunctival hemorrhage. No significant deterioration of liver function tests was identified. This would have been expected if the calculated doses to the liver were correct. The patient remained alert and ambulatory until day 68, when she suddenly became dizzy and fell. She also complained of headache and then became comatose. She expired on day 69.

Autopsy revealed hypocellular marrow. Hepatocytes were seen to be hyperchromic. Lymph nodes were slightly atrophied. The patient had intracerebral, subdural, and subarachnoid hemorrhage as a result of the thrombocytopenia.

TABLE 27.1
Wisconsin Patient — Estimated Dose 4 to 5 Gy[a]

Findings	Postexposure	Value/mm³
Initial incapacitation	No	
Initial hypotension	No	
Nausea	No	
Vomiting	No	
Diarrhea	No	
Headache	No	
Weakness	No	
Fever	NR	
Edema	No	
Blistering	No	
WBC	1 day	6,600
	2 days	4,500
	4 days	3,500
	8 days	900
	16 days	200
	24 days	200
	32 days	150
	50 days	400
Lymphocytes	1 day	NR
	2 days	1,500
	4 days	300
	8 days	100
	16 days	100
	24 days	600
	32 days	600
	50 days	300
Thrombocytes	1 day	220,000
	4 days	150,000
	16 days	10,000
	24 days	8,000
	32 days	5,000
Epilation	No	
Death	Yes	69 days

Note: NR - not reported.

[a] Estimated liver dose 70 to 80 Gy.

REFERENCE

1. Baron, J.M., Yachnin, S., Polcyn, R. et al., Accidental Radiogold [198]Au liver scan overdose with fatal outcome, in *Handling of Radiation Accidents: Proceedings of a Symposium*, Vienna, May 19–23, International Atomic Energy Agency, Vienna, 1969.

28 Skin Wounds and Burns Contaminated by Radioactive Substances (Metabolism, Decontamination, Tactics, and Techniques of Medical Care)

Leonid A. Ilyin

CONTENTS

Introduction 364
General Characteristics of Radioactive Contamination of Wounds and Burns 365
Unique Aspects of Radionuclide Metabolism in Contaminated Skin Wounds and Burns 368
    Wounds 369
    Burns 379
    Radionuclide Metabolism in contaminated Wounds and Burns 384
Methods and Techniques of Control of Radioactive Contamination of Wounds and Burns 385
    Background 385
    Prevention of Radionuclide Body Absorption and Removal of Radionuclides from
        the Injured Area 385
    Decontamination of Burns Contaminated by Radioactive Substances 393
    Acceleration of Body Excretion of Radioactive Substances Resorbed in Wounds 394
    Experience with Human Wounds and Burns Contaminated by
        Radioactive Substances 399
    Summary: Control of Radioactive Contamination of Wounds and Burns 406
The Practice and Procedures of Medical Care of Skin Wounds and Burns Contaminated
        by Radioactive Substances 407
    Background 407
    Care at the Accident Site 408
    Medical Care at the Local Medical Facility 409
    Specialized Hospital Care 410
    Radioactivity Monitoring of Contaminated Wounds and Burns 412
References 414

INTRODUCTION

The measure of radiation exposure in an organism is the absorbed dose of radiation, which is determined by the quantity of energy absorbed in the unit of the exposed volume. For radioactive substances, the absorbed (tissue) dose is the product of multiplying three values: the quantity (concentration) of radionuclide in tissues, the kind and energy of the radiation emitted, and the time of contact of the emitter with the exposed biosubstrate. The kind and energy of radiation emitted by radioactive substances are constant, so it is necessary to find techniques to decrease the concentrations of the substances in tissues and to lower the duration of emitter exposure in biological structures, and in the whole body, to decrease the absorbed dose and, therefore, to mitigate radiation effects.

This obvious statement leads to the conclusion that medical measures should be based upon active (aim-directed) influence on the metabolism of radioactive substances at all phases of this in the body. This principle of control of radioactive exposure of the organism has been called "causal prophylaxis and therapy."[1] Three modes of intake of radionuclides in the body are known: inhalation, ingestion, and contact through intact and traumatized skin surfaces or mucosa membranes of the eye. Three major phases of the radionuclide metabolism can be schematically specified as follows: (1) the primary compartment (intact and traumatized skin surfaces, gastrointestinal tract, pulmonary organs), (2) transfer systems and radionuclide transportation (blood system and lymphatic system), and (3) incorporation in organs and tissues (including excretion organs).

To systematize general considerations of human body protection against radioactive substance exposure Table 28.1 provides a classification of causal protection and a list of medical interventions to modify radionuclide metabolism at different phases.

Table 28.1 demonstrates that techniques of the control of radioactive substances are based on prevention of their intake at the entry sites into the body, elimination of the nonresorbed portion from the primary entry compartment, binding of radionuclides that have penetrated into the blood and lymph into soluble, nondissociable complexes, decontamination of organs and tissues of the radionuclide, and, finally, on stimulation of radionuclide excretion from the body through excretion organs. Radionuclides of interest represent a large number of chemical elements; therefore, their metabolism in the body is predominantly determined by the chemical individuality of the corresponding stable element and by the radiochemical properties of the radionuclide.

In the framework of this scheme, it is obvious that the control of radioactive contamination of wounds and burns should presume the elimination of radionuclide from the injured area, prevention (limitation) of its resorption in the blood and surrounding tissues, and stimulation of the excretion of the resorbed portion from the body. At the same time, one should take into account that there is not a single pattern for tactics and techniques in medical care in such situations, due to the vast variety of skin injuries and the wide spectrum of radioactive contaminants, as well as the varied circumstances of contamination for a single-person and for wide-scale radiation accidents involving many people.

One of the postulates of radiation protection and radiation hygiene control is formulated as follows: when work or contact with radioactive materials is present in routine operations or after accidents, any injury to skin surfaces has to be considered potentially contaminated with radionuclides. Radiological precautions for such cases are always justified. Studies have shown that even small skin injuries such as excoriation and abrasions, which are negligible to the victims or the medical staff examining the patient, are dangerous intake routes for the uptake of radionuclides into the body. The radionuclide resorption rate through such injuries can be hundreds of times higher than that for intact skin.[2] Generally, any event related to contaminated wounds and burns must be considered a radiation incident with all consequences.

TABLE 28.1
Classification of Principles and Techniques of Causal Protection

No.	Metabolism Phase	Principal Influence in Radionuclide Metabolism	Technique of Protection
1	Intact skin surface	Cleaning (decontamination)	Mechanical, chemical, combined techniques and decontaminating agents
1	Injured skin surface	Prevention of the resorption in the blood and lymph; Elimination from the injured area	Limitation (cessation) of the blood flow from the injured area; nonspecific or selective absorption of radionuclide from the site of application; moist processing of the injured area; tissue dissection
2	Pulmonary organs	Prevention of the resorption and elimination of the radionuclide (including the digestive tract decontamination of ingested radionuclide)	Vasoconstrictive agents and substances amplifying the secretion processes, expectorants; washing of visible mucosa and upper pulmonary pathways and large bronchi; lung lavage; chelate agent inhalation; gastric lavage and absorbers
3	Digestive tract	Prevention of the resorption, elimination of radionuclides from upper parts, acceleration of the intestinal excretion, decrease of reabsorption	Absorbers and other agents binding radionuclides into the poorly soluble compounds; application of emetics, gastric lavage; salt purgatives
4	Blood, lymph, incorporation organs	Binding of radionuclides into soluble complexed compounds to enhance excretion; excretion stimulation through excretion organs	Chelating agents; soluble ion exchange compounds; isotope dissolution; competition of bioelements and antagonist elements; influence in the radionuclide metabolism through physiological and biochemical mechanisms using pharmacological agents and biologically active compounds

Source: Adapted from Ilyin, L.A., *Basics of the Human Protection against Radioactive Substances*, Atomizdat Publisher, Moscow, 1977.

GENERAL CHARACTERISTICS OF RADIOACTIVE CONTAMINATION OF WOUNDS AND BURNS

Skin wounds and inhalation are the major intake pathways for radionuclides in the occupational laboratory environment. As a rule, contamination of the wound results from contaminated objects. For example, according to the data of Reference 3, among 18 total cases of injuries accompanied by plutonium contamination, 6 cases resulted from glass splinters, 4 cases from slipped instruments, 1 case from the breakdown of a device operated at high velocity, and 3 injury cases from other causes. Acid and alkaline burns occur more frequently from spilled liquids or from explosions of vessel containers; thermal burns occur in cases of contact with flame or hot metal.[4,10]

Literature references contain detailed information on the rates and types of injuries, their localization, and dissemination, especially for radiation workers in plutonium (radiochemical) facilities and laboratories.[4-8] Hammond and Putzier[5] have elaborated on the radiological monitoring of 900 cases of hand skin injuries in plutonium industry workers and found that more than one third of these cases had plutonium wound contamination. Schofield[6] has reported on 1250 cases of radioactive contamination of wounds and microtraumas among personnel of the Windscale facility, while Johnson and Lawrence[7] have provided data on 137 injuries contaminated by transuranium elements at the Los Alamos National Laboratory from 1960 to 1972. Ohlenschläger[8] has reported that 148 cases of alpha emitter wound contamination have occurred in Karlsruhe Research Center (Germany).

According to data of Bazhin et al.[4] who examined 3968 radiation workers at the "Mayak" Association (Russia), 286 persons (7.2%) were recorded to have various skin injuries contaminated by alpha-emitting radionuclides. Of the workers examined, 10% had contact with poorly transportable compounds of americium and plutonium only, 25% had contact with relatively transportable compounds, but the majority of workers (more than 50%) worked with both classes of actinide compounds.

Table 28.2 lists the type, quantity, and localization of skin surface trauma. The most frequent injuries (wounds) of skin resulted from mechanical damage (86.7%), 10.4% of cases resulted from chemical (usually acid) burns, and about 3% of injuries were from thermal burns. The total number of injured skin sites was 415 in 286 victims. More than 90% of wounds were localized in arms and hands (fingers, predominantly). This general observation is found in other papers.[7,9] Table 28.3 presents the anatomical localization of wounds in the Los Alamos National Laboratory workers.

TABLE 28.2
Type, Quantity, and Localization of Skin Injuries Contaminated by Alpha-Emitting Radionuclides in Mayak Radiochemical Association Workers

Injury Type	No. of Victims	No. of Injured Sites	Localization			
			Hands and Arms	Feet and Legs	Head and Neck	Trunk
Wounds	248	349	332	7	9	1
Chemical burns	30	55	21	16	11	7
Thermal burns	3	11	7	2	2	—
Total	286	415	360	25	22	8

Source: Adapted from Bazhin, A.G. et al., Hyg. Sanit., 9, 27, 1994.

TABLE 28.3
Anatomical Localization of Contaminated Injuries

Localization	Quantity	Localization	Quantity
Fingers	96	Head	10
Hands	18	Hairy area	2
Palm surface	9	Face	8
Dorsal surface	9	Trunk	1
Forearm	12	Total number	137

Source: Adapted from Johnson, L.J., Lawrence, J.N.P., Health Phys., 27(1), 55, 1974.

The rate and types of injuries are strongly related to the working environment and the victim's occupation. Thus, at the Mayak facility mechanical injuries have been received by workers in foundries (28%), by turners (22%) employed at the mechanical shop, as well as by mechanical device operators in the chemical shop (13%). Among the mechanical device and lathe operators, the chemical burn factors consisted of nitric acid solutions (28 people), hydrochloric acid (1 person), and alkalines (1 person). Thermal skin burns were observed in foundry workers and lathe operators contacting hot metal.

When analyzing the character of mechanical damage of skin, it was shown that about 30% of injuries were epidermal with disturbance of the epidermis and the upper part of the papillary dermal layer (microtraumas), 65% of injuries were judged to be dermal injuries, and 4–5% were transdermal wounds.*

The last two kinds of injuries were conditionally combined into a "wound" group with damage depth of >1 mm.

Table 28.4 demonstrates that almost two thirds of all wounds were puncture wounds, less than one third of all wounds were incised, and 13% of all wounds were lacerated.

TABLE 28.4
Depth and Character of Mechanical Skin Injuries

Injury Depth	Injury Character					Total
	Puncture Wound	Incised Wound	Lacerated Wound	Slash Wound	Others	
<1 mm (microtrauma)	34	22	31	—	16[a]	103
>1 mm (wounds)	168	55	15	3	5[b]	246
Microtrauma and wounds	202	77	46	3	21	349

[a] Cases recorded as superficial skin injuries.
[b] Including three crushed wounds and two contusions.

Source: Adapted from Bazhin, A.G. et al., *Hyg. Sanit.*, 9, 27, 1994.

From the total number of recorded mechanical injuries (349), 119 wounds (34.1%) were contaminated by radionuclide burdens of the minimum detectable activity of the dosimetry equipment, when measurements were done following primary decontamination at the workplace and the medical facility. The minimum detectable activities equalled 14 Bq (plutonium-239) and 3 Bq (americium-241). Finally, the residual burden of alpha-emitting nuclides in 163 wounds (i.e., in almost half of all the cases) was below 74 Bq, which is the intervention level recommended in Russia (10% of the permissible plutonium-239 skeleton burden for occupational exposure[12]). This excess level found in 164 wounds (47%) was substantiation for the application of specialized care including, particularly, wound dissection or electric coagulation of wound surfaces and chelation therapy. The plutonium burden found in these wounds was wide ranging, 75 to 7400 Bq. In 22 cases that occurred in the 1940s and 1950s, the plutonium burdens were not measured because of the lack of adequate radiometry equipment; only the presence of wound contamination was stated.

From the total number of burn victims (38 people), 35 patients were hospitalized. In 3 people, burns contaminated with plutonium were revealed at routine medical examinations. The severity

---

* At facilities and laboratories, where the sanitary education of personnel and regular examinations of skin status and integrity are not well developed, the actual percentage of microtrauma can be significantly higher.

grades of 95% of the burns were diagnosed to be grade I to II (without damage of papillary layer and net layer of dermis), and only two victims were established to have grade III burns. This fact can be explained by timely and carefully applied therapy at the site of the accident, where special attention was paid to preservation of the integrity of blisters (detached epidermis). Major factors specifying the severity grade of burn injury are the concentration and exposure time of the chemical agent applied. Concentrated acids applied to the skin cause the coagulation (destruction) of albumins and create the acidic albuminates, which explains the low rates of the radiation emitter resorption through the burn surfaces. With such burns, a dense scab with a sharply limited demarcation borderline (dry necrosis) occurs. Concentrated alkaline dissolves albumin and creates alkaline albuminates, resulting in colliquative necrosis. Thus, for all other similar conditions, rates of the body resorption of radioactive substances are significantly lower for burn injury compared with wound surfaces (see below). At the same time, to absorb and resorb radionuclides the depth of the injury is of high importance, as is the integrity of the epidermal skin layer and dermal status. Dancer et al.[13] have described a case of intensive radioactive skin contamination resulting from spilled hot chlorine vinegar-like acid labeled by carbon-14. The radioactivity of the vessel content was about 2500 MBq. Despite immediate decontamination of the burn site, the body intake was 23.3 MBq of carbon-14, whose activity was evaluated using radiometry of the exhaled air; this activity was about 1% of the applied amount of the radionuclide.

In 1997, Kelsey et al.[10] described a case of radioactive contamination of the face and hair of the worker, who was contaminated by a chemical explosion of a container of 7-l volume with 740 MBq of iridium-192. The initial contamination was about 37 MBq. After immediate washing of the injured areas at the site of the accident, and consequent processing with sponges bathed with distilled water and a haircut in the hospital (where the patient was admitted 30 min after the accident), the local radioactivity in the application site was decreased five times. Within 24 h, about 1% of iridium-192 activity was excreted in urine. The authors evaluated the resorption rate of this radionuclide through the acidic burn to equal 0.1 to 3%. The described case is of specific interest because of the well-organized and adequate scope of radiological examinations.

UNIQUE ASPECTS OF RADIONUCLIDE METABOLISM IN CONTAMINATED SKIN WOUNDS AND BURNS

Knowledge of radionuclide metabolism peculiarities in cases of contaminated skin wounds and burns significantly determines the tactics and techniques of therapy for the victim. The multiplicity of possible types of injuries and the variable spectrum of radioactive contaminants, as well as the different aggregative states and chemical properties of radionuclide wound, together with the different conditions and events of radioactive contamination incidents make for significant experimental and clinical radiometric complications in the comprehensive examination of such problems. The scientific literature contains hundreds of references devoted to different aspects of this branch of radiation medicine. Apparently, the first attempt to systematize knowledge in this area was the attempt of Russian researchers, who generalized many years of experimental studies and literature references in the monograph *Radioactive Substances and Wounds (Metabolism and Decontamination)*,[2] in which the metabolism of radionuclides is represented in different groups of the periodic table of chemical elements together with evaluation of the efficiency of different measures taken in incidents of this kind. According to standardized protocol, the behavioral peculiarities of different biologically important radionuclides were examined for different groups of the periodic table, particularly those for group I (cesium-137), group II (strontium-85,89), group III (cerium-144), group VI (polonium-210), group VII (iodine-131) and the actinide group (plutonium-239, americium-241), to assess their metabolic parameters in the injured site, their resorption and behavior in the body in case of skin injuries of different kinds (abrasions, scratches, stab wounds, lacerations extending into skeletal muscle, incised wounds, thermal and chemical burns). Animal experiments were undertaken to investigate radioactive injury contamination control, and techniques and methods of decontamination.

Again, it is necessary to stress that world experience demonstrates that occupational radioactive wound contamination is most frequently related to plutonium and americium contaminants. These transuranium elements are a major issue for large contingents of atomic industry professionals in developed countries. The predominant importance of these radionuclides as possible sources of radioactive wound contamination in this category of radiation workers is likely to persist. At the same time, the wide application of different radioactive isotopes in medicine and in many other branches of science and technology, and the practical impossibility of avoiding radioactive material incidents completely must be considered.

One of the important parameters of radioactive substance behavior in contamination of wounds and burn surface trauma is the rate of their intake (resorption) into the blood and into the lymphatic system.*

It was previously remarked that radionuclide resorption throughout injured skin sites and skin burns depends on many factors and conditions, including which specific group or subgroup of the periodic table the radionuclide belongs, its aggregate state, whether it is an isotopic or nonisotopic carrier, and most significantly on the chemical form (solubility) of the applied contaminant compound, as well as the kind and character of skin injury and the duration of the emitter contact with the injured tissues.

Wounds

Generally, radioactive isotope resorption from wounds to the internal body medium can be specified for different chemical elements of the periodic table as follows.

The greatest level and rate of the resorption is found for radionuclides of the alkalines, alkaline-earth metals, and halogens dissolved into ion form and having poor ability to hydrolyze. The absorption of radionuclides of alkalines, alkaline-earth metals, and halogens from stab wounds (muscular tissue, subcutaneous cellular tissue) can reach nearly 100% of the applied contaminant.[1,2,14–16,18] Figures 28.1 and 28.2 illustrate this process using experimental data obtained in standardized experiments done in white rats for $^{137}CsCl$ and $Na^{131}I$ and different kinds of wounds.[2]

Table 28.5 shows differences of the resorption rates for stab wounds vs. cutaneous and muscle wounds as well as for skin abrasions in case of a number of radionuclide contaminants representing different groups of the periodic table at different times after the radionuclide application.[1,2,51] The data analysis shows a clear dependence of the resorption rate increase vs. the kind of skin injury independently from the radionuclide as follows: abrasions < cutaneous and muscle wounds < stab wounds. At the same time, the resorption rate depends upon the position of the radionuclide in a specific group of elements of the periodic table and the chemical compound of the radionuclide (note americium-241). The largest resorption ability was found for strontium chloride (alkaline-earth metal) among all tested elements.

High resorption rates of radiostrontium were certified by data obtained by Ducousso et al.[16] from experiments conducted in monkeys (macaques) who had a solution of strontium chloride ($^{85}SrCl_2$) injected intramuscularly or topically applied to the lacerated femoral wound. Just 40 min after the administration, 100% of radionuclide had been resorbed from the stab wound and the maximum blood concentration of strontium-85 was observed at minute 20. When radionuclide was applied to the lacerated wound, 22 and 37% of the administered amount was resorbed in the body

---

* The terms of *resorption* and *absorption* applied hereafter reflect the active physiology process of the penetration of substances throughout the cellular membranes into cells and then into the body including the penetration through intact and injured skin. The frequently used term absorption is common in physical chemistry and reflects the absorption of gases or dissolution of a substance in a liquid or solid medium. The terms *absorption*, *resorption*, and *penetration* hereafter are used synonymously to specify the radionuclide body intake throughout the injuries to cutaneous surfaces.

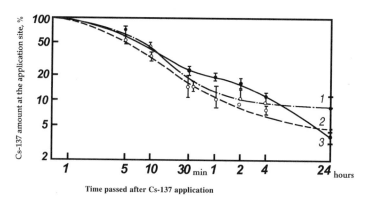

FIGURE 28.1 Cesium-137 wound resorption (related to the applied amount): abrasion (1), cutaneous and muscle incised wound (2), and subcutaneous compartment (3).

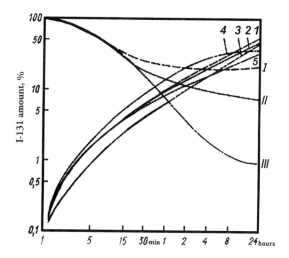

FIGURE 28.2 Resorption from abrasion (I), cutaneous and muscle wounds (II), and incised wounds (III) and iodine-131 thyroid accumulation for application to abrasion (1), cutaneous and muscle wound (2), peroral administration (3), and subcutaneous (4) and intraperitoneal (5) injection (related to administered amount).

at minutes 15 and 100, respectively, which is predetermined by the morphological peculiarities of lacerated wounds.

Actually, studies elaborated for different radioactive substances have shown that resorption (as well as the rate of absorption) of radionuclides is significantly dependent on the kind of wounds, especially for radionuclides that hydrolyze. Certainly, stab wounds (modeled by intramuscular injection) show higher absorption as compared with cutaneous and muscle wounds and to lacerated wounds.

For the last case, if massives tissue injury occurs, it is accompanied by blood vessel and lymphatic vessel damage, which may result in uptake comparable to stab wounds. Massive injury also causes vascular thrombosis and stasis phenomena. Obviously, these factors create conditions promoting a relative decrease of the rate of radionuclide resorption into the internal medium of the body.

Observations in 12 volunteers have provided data on radiostrontium resorption rates ($^{85}SrCl_2$, pH 7.0) in cases of skin abrasion intake and intact skin intake.[1,2,17,22] Table 28.6 presents the results:

TABLE 28.5
^{89}Sr, ^{144}Ce, ^{241}Am, ^{210}Po Resorption from Abrasions, Cutaneous and Muscle Wounds, and Stab Wounds (white rats; in % from applied amount of the radionuclide)[1,2,51]

Kind of Injury	Time Passed, h	% Intake of Radionuclide, Compound, pH of the Solution				
		^{98}SrCl$_2$, pH-2	^{144}CeCl$_3$, pH-3	^{210}Po(NO$_3$)$_4$, pH-1.5	^{241}Am(OH)$_3$, pH-3	^{241}AmCl$_3$, pH-3
Abrasions	1	—	—	0.13 ± 0.07	—	—
	4	—	—	0.21 ± 0.08	—	—
	24	29.6 ± 3.4	1.0 ± 0.19	0.56 ± 0.25	0.40 ± 0.08	2.1 ± 0.1
Cutaneous and muscle wounds	1	27.6 ± 3.9	—	0.31 ± 0.06	—	—
	4	36.2 ± 3.7	—	2.45 ± 1.1	—	—
	24	48.6 ± 4.5[a]	2.0 ± 0.7	9.90 ± 2.5	—	—
Stab wounds	1	70	—	5.21 ± 2.1	—	—
	4	100	—	8.1 ± 1.1	—	—
	24	100[b]	8.8[c]	25.9 ± 3.7[b]	5.0[c]	19.0[c]

[a] Direct radiometry data.
[b] Balance experiment data.
[c] Data on integral burden in internal organs and tissues.

TABLE 28.6
^{85}Sr Body Resorption through Abrasions and Intact Skin of Human (related to the applied activity, %)

Application Site	^{85}Sr Contact Duration	Range[a]	Average Value
Abrasions	30 min	45.3–25.5	38.0
	6 h	65.3–45.3	57.4
Intact skin	6 h	0.14–0.37	0.26

[a] For six methods of assessment.

Source: Adapted from Ilyin, L.A., *Chernobyl: Myth and Reality*, Nasasaki Association for Hibakusha's Medical Care, Moscow, 1998.

at minute 30 after the application of strontium chloride solution on the abrasion surface, 38% of strontium-85 has penetrated into the body; and 57.4% has been resorbed at hour 6. If compared with the resorption of ^{85}SrCl$_2$ from the intact skin surface (0.26% at hour 6 after application), the body isotope absorption throughout such small cutaneous injuries, like abrasions, is increased more than 200 times. Obviously, this phenomenon results from the elimination of the epidermis which is the major barrier for the penetration of different chemicals and metal ions.[19,20]

If compared with radionuclides of alkalines and alkaline-earth metals, the wound metabolism of elements of extra subgroups of groups I and II of the periodic table (i.e., silver-111, gold-198, zinc-65, copper-64, etc.) is significantly determined by the chemical form of their compounds. There are indications that ^{111}AgNO$_3$ absorption from cutaneous and muscle wounds is specified by the rate of <0.5% (within 1 h), whereas ^{111}AgCl (pH 7 to 8) absorption from the subcutaneous cellular layer can reach 30%.[21] The low penetration of ^{111}AgNO$_3$ and ^{65}ZnCl$_2$ (4.8%) as well seems to be related to their burn and astringent action in surrounding tissues. Interest in the investigation of muscular tissue metabolism of colloidal gold (gold-198) is related to the development of the agent for oncology practice.[24,25] It was shown that at day 3 to 4 the percentage of gold-198 absorbed from the muscular tissue is 30% (with the lymphatic system the predominant pathway and selective accumulation in regional lymph nodes). Some compounds of the major subgroup of group V of the periodic table can be judged as rather well-metabolized agents, including phosphorus-32, in which resorption of $NaH_2{}^{32}PO_4$ from cutaneous muscular incised wounds of mice and rats can reach 51 to 56%,[2,21] cobalt-60, which represents the transient group of the periodic table (Co, Ni, Fe), and, probably, some compounds of elements of extra subgroups of group VI (Cr, Mo, W)* and group VII (Mn).

The importance of the kind of chemical compound of these group radionuclides applied topically is demonstrated by the information on cobalt-60. The detailed work of Japanese researchers[23] has established large differences in resorption rates of different compounds of cobalt-60 applied topically in superficial/deep wounds of white rats and guinea pigs. Thus, the absorption of cobalt chloride ($CoCl_2$) has reached ~60% at day 2, whereas that for cobalt acetate was 27% and that for cobalt hydroxide 0.4%. In contrast, according to data of Reference 21, $^{59}FeCl_2$ compound, representing elements of the transient group, is resorbed from cutaneous muscular wounds at the rate of <6% of the applied amount. The different absorption rates of chlorides of cobalt and iron can be explained by different inclinations of their salts to hydrolyze: Co^{2+} is hydrolyzed at pH 7, while Fe^{2+} is hydrolyzed at pH 2.

Detailed studies were elaborated for wound metabolism peculiarities of one of the most radiotoxic radioactive substances (polonium-210) representing group VI of the periodic table.[1,2,26] Table 28.7 provides data on resorption of polonium-210 from the intact skin, abrasions, cutaneous muscular wounds, and stab wounds of white rats.[51] The table shows that if the integrity of skin is disturbed, the polonium-210 ($Po(NO_3)_4$) body penetration is greatly increased. Thus, according to the criterion of daily resorption, polonium-210 abrasion absorption is increased to more than 40 times and that for stab wounds is increased to 2000 times if compared with intact skin. The most rapid resorption of polonium-210 was found for muscular tissue (stab wounds), where 5.2% of the applied activity has penetrated into the body within hour 1; i.e., 20% of incorporated polonium was accumulated within 24 h. The experiments (including histoautoradiography test) have revealed that nitrogen-acidic polonium-210 (pH 1.5) will penetrate deeply in the cutaneous muscular tissues surrounding the wound.

Apparently, this phenomenon is explained by the active interaction of polonium-210 with bioligands, particularly by the known affinity of this element for albumin sulfhydryl groups as well as by the developing edema and inflammation, which occurs in the connective tissue interlayers

TABLE 28.7
^{210}Po Resorption Rates for Intact and Injured Skin of Rats (relating to the applied amount, %)

Kind of Injury	Time Passed after ^{210}Po Application, h		
	1	4	24
Abrasions	0.13 ± 0.07	0.21 ± 0.08	0.56 ± 0.25
Cutaneous muscular wounds	0.31 ± 0.06	2.45 ± 1.1	9.9 ± 2.5
Stab wounds	5.21 ± 2.05	8.1 ± 1.1	25.9 ± 3.70
Intact skin	—	—	0.013 ± 0.004

Source: Adapted from Ilyin, L.A. et al., Health Phys., 32(2), 107, 1977.

---

* Experimental data on the wound/burn metabolism of these radionuclides are lacking.

(straight to the vascular pathways, essentially) around the wound. This process in turn promotes radionuclide penetration into tissues surrounding the wound. Therefore, wound dissection cannot guarantee the complete removal of such pure alpha emitters as polonium-210 from the injured area, if careful radiometry monitoring is not applied. Studies of the distribution of polonium resorbed from wounds to the body have not shown a principal metabolism difference if compared with other intake pathways. Generally, this result is also specific to other radioactive substances, including such easily metabolized elements as alkalines, alkaline-earth metals, and halogens.[1] Some nuances are possible here. Where radionuclides are able to hydrolyze, to create radiocolloids, and to be polymerized at pH close to neutral are of concern, the relationship of the blood resorbed high-dispersion fraction to the partially or completely hydrolyzed fraction transported throughout the lymphatic pathways is important. For example, nitrogen-acidic plutonium ($Pu(NO_3)_4$) at tissue pH creates large radiocolloids; complex compounds of this element (such as plutonium citrate) persist to maintain a high dispersion condition even if the interaction with bioligands occurs. According to this explanation, the first-mentioned compound can basically distribute inside the internal body medium, like liver seekers, and the last-mentioned compound would basically be the skeleton seeker.[27]

Information on the wound metabolism of such biologically important fission products as zirconium-95, niobium-95, ruthenium-103 and 106 is virtually absent in the literature. One can suppose that their wound resorption would be relatively low; taking into account the specific inclination of zirconium compounds to hydrolysis and polymerization, the absorption rates for stab wounds would not exceed less than one to several percent within the first 24 h after administration. Generally, the inclination for hydrolysis and creation of radiocolloids and poorly solvable hydroxides is specific to rare earth elements (REE), elements of extra groups IV (zirconium) and V (niobium), platinum group elements (ruthenium), and transuranium and transplutonium elements.

At the same time, it is necessary to stress again that even within a single group of elements the rate and level of wound resorption of specific radionuclides can be significantly different, because of the chemistry and solubility of the compound of the radiation emitter. For example, these metabolism parameters for REE and transuranium radionuclides can be ranged as follows: oxides << nitrates < chlorides < complex compounds (citrates, oxalates).

Tables 28.8 and 28.9 summarize the data given in two publications,[27,28] which provide the reader with a general impression of the range of values of different plutonium-239 chemical forms, including metal plutonium. Table 28.8 shows the most intensive resorption of soluble complex

TABLE 28.8
Rates of Plutonium Resorption from Skin, Subcutaneous Cellular Tissue, and Muscular Tissue (related to the applied amount, %)

Animal Species	Pu Compound Form	Administration Technique	Time Passed after Administration, h	^{239}Pu Resorption Rate, %
Pig	Nitrate (IV)	Intracutaneous	24	25
Suckling pig	Pentacarbonate (IV)	Subcutaneous	6	30
	Citrate	Subcutaneous	6	64
Rabbit	Metal	Subcutaneous	260–1048 days	0.16–1.2
Rat	Metal	Subcutaneous	356–580 days	0.09–0.28
	Chloride (III)	Intramuscular	4	19
	Nitrate (IV)	Intramuscular	4	7
	Plutonile (VI)	Intramuscular	4	35–40

Source: Adapted from Buldakov, L.A. et al., *Plutonium Toxicology Problems*, Atomizdat Publisher, Moscow, 1969.

TABLE 28.9
^{239}Pu Resorption and Distribution after the Intramuscular Injection[28]

Chemical Formula	Animal Species	Time after Administration, days	Amount of Plutonium Remaining at Administration Site Related to the Administered Amount, %	Skeleton	Liver	Spleen	Lungs	Kidneys
PuO$_2$Cl$_2$	Rat	4	70	65	14.0	0.4	0.3	1.9
		16	30	64	2.8	0.3	0.1	0.7
		64	34	56	4.2	0.5	0.2	1.7
		256	13	47	1.5	0.3	0.1	0.3
PuO$_2$(NO$_3$)$_2$	Rat	4	70	—	10.0	—	—	1.6
		10	51	52	2.4	0.2	—	0.7
		64	40	51	2.0	0.2	—	0.2
		406	20	38	1.1	0.2	—	0.2
Pu(VI)-citrate	Rat	7	29	80	9.6	0.3	—	1.2
		62	23	56	1.4	0.2	—	0.3
		420	12	34	1.1	0.1	—	0.2
	Dog	14	14	—	6.8	—	—	—
		103	0.001	58	8.3	0.1	0.06	—
		234	0.001	41	13.0	0.3	0.1	0.1
Pu(NO$_3$)$_4$	Rat	4	96	79	4.4	0.3	0.2	1.7
		16	88	69	6.0	0.3	0.2	2.5
		64	68	63	2.7	0.1	0.1	0.5
		256	67	50	1.8	0.2	0.1	0.3
		4	84	—	13.0	—	—	0.6
		6	56	71	9.0	0.3	—	—
		7	72	86	3.4	—	—	—
Pu(NO$_3$)$_4$	Rabbit	1	98	80	12.0	0.2	0.8	0.6
		8	90	85	13.0	0.05	0.2	0.9
		35	75	85	13.2	0.02	0.1	0.7
		56	52	54	21.2	0.06	0.1	0.7
		112	55	44	18.9	0.02	0.1	0.6

		280	33	27	23.1	0.0	0.04	0.1
		365	51	33	22.4	0.03	0.4	0.1
Pu(IV)-citrate	Rat	4	97	30	26.0	—	—	—
		7	19	96	2.7	0.1	0.4	1.9
PuCl$_3$	Rat	4	77	68	7.1	0.5	0.3	0.4
		16	68	83	3.8	0.4	0.3	0.5
		64	40	52	2.9	0.4	0.1	0.5
		256	24	46	1.4	0.3	0.1	0.5

Note: Roman numbers are the chemical valences of plutonium of complex compounds.

Source: Adapted from Vaughan, J.C., in *Uranium, Plutonium, Transplutonium Elements*, Hodge, H.C. et al., Springer-Verlag, Berlin, 1973.

plutonium compounds; the resorption intensity decreases for acidic solutions and plutonium implanted as fine dispersive metal is retained in the wound site for a long time. In the last case less than 1% is transported into the body within a period of years.

Data provided by Reference 27 gives the resorption of different plutonium compounds within the framework of nearest hour intervals after the administration. Thus, for example, 7% of nitrogen-acidic plutonium (IV) was resorbed from the muscular tissue inside the rat body at hour 4; 19% of the chlorine plutonium (III) and 35 to 40% of plutonile (VI) were resorbed at this time, as well. The plutonium pentacarbonate resorption from subcutaneous cellular tissue of suckling pigs reached 30% and that for citrate complex 64% at 6 h after administration.

The analysis of data on resorption and body distribution of soluble plutonium compounds given in Table 28.9 for intramuscular injection (stab wounds) reflects this nuclide behavior for a wide spectrum of chemical compounds. Actually, the most intensive absorption was found for complex (citrate) compounds of Pu^{+4} and Pu^{+6}. Their resorption found in rats at day 7 reached 70 to 80%. At a latter period the penetration had moderated and plutonium-239 was retained for a long time at the administration site (12% at day 420); this retention is obviously related to the compound translocation and fast linkage to bioligands in the injection site. In contrast, dog experiments have shown more complete absorption of citrate from muscular tissue; at day 103 only traces of plutonium were detected in the injection site. The resorption of chlorine plutonium, Pu^{+4}, and plutonium (VI) within 4 days has been found to be similar and equal to ~30%. Unfortunately, this unique summary of data,[28] which was basically compiled to analyze the distribution of soluble plutonium compounds in organs and tissues, did not examine the assessment of its resorption rates at shorter periods of time after the administration; such assessment is of great practical interest in the context of this chapter.

The rate of resorption of plutonium nitrate of valence IV was slower when compared with other soluble compounds. This finding was confirmed by other researchers.[30] The author's experiments in rabbits have revealed 51% of the nitrogen-acidic plutonium retained in the site 1 year after intramuscular injection. Norwood and Fuqua[31] have indicated the following plutonium absorption rates found at day 5 after intramuscular injection in rats: 23% (plutonium chloride) and 4% (plutonium nitrate of valence IV). According to data of Volf,[32,33] 7 to 16% of plutonium nitrate was resorbed within 1 day from muscular tissue of rats.

Experimental data on the behavior of different plutonium compounds applied topically to lacerated wounds of white rats are of interest.[35] According to the results obtained, the residual wound activity was 82 ± 3.5% ($Pu(NO_3)_4$), 33 ± 1.2% (Pu citrate), and 41 ± 5.7% (PuO_2) at day 7 after the contamination. These results confirm facts referred to above on the high wound mobility of complex plutonium compounds and relatively lower resorption of radioactive substances from lacerated wounds if compared, for example, with stab wounds. However, the unusually high wound mobility of PuO_2 is questionable if compared with that of $Pu(NO_3)_4$. It is known that combusted plutonium oxide of particle size <0.7 μm has relatively higher mobility than dispersive plutonium oxide.[36] However, the referred to paper has reliably demonstrated that relatively insoluble plutonium oxide (PuO_2) has much lower wound mobility than nitrogen-acidic plutonium.

Models of intramuscular radionuclide administration can estimate resorption rates from shallow stab wounds inflicted by sharp articles (for example, glass splinters, etc.) with specific reservations. It is important to assess the behavior of soluble, relatively soluble, and insoluble plutonium compound contaminants of skin abrasions. White rat experiments done by Bazhin[52] have shown that after 2 days the absorption rates of plutonium were 16, 0.18, and 0.046% of the administered amount applied to skin abrasions for plutonium monomer citrate, plutonium nitrate, and plutonium nitropolymer, respectively. Bazhin suggests that the body intake of soluble plutonium monomer citrate through abrasions is 65 times higher than that for intact skin.

The studies done by Bazhin and colleagues[37,38] are of significant practical interest, because they investigate the biokinetic behavior of industrial plutonium, which has poor transportability in wounds of different kinds. The compounds were sampled as fine dispersible powders at different technological phases of the plutonium production. These powders had plutonium oxide content as high as 96 to 97% in some samples. The alpha activity concentration of these materials was in the range of 0.48 ± 0.10 MBq/mg to 1.4 ± 0.2 MBq/mg of the sample. The solubility of aerosols in these powders was determined using a dialysis technique (fast soluble fraction) and assessed to equal 0.12 to 0.62%.[39]

The goal of these studies done in more than 800 rats was to investigate wound and body metabolism of industrial plutonium oxides of poor transportability, the efficiency of emergency aid measures, and late radiation effects. To investigate plutonium metabolism, animals were sacrificed at different times commencing at hour 3 until 128 days after the application. Table 28.10 provides the resulting data on the plutonium resorption rates throughout abrasions, cutaneous muscular incised wounds, and stab wounds within 4 days after the topical application of industrial plutonium oxides. One can see that absorption rates of the radiation emitter are in the range of 0.06 to 0.8% of the applied amount and correlate with the character and depth of the skin injury. The highest wound resorption intensity was observed within day 1 and then declined. Nevertheless, the level of the integral resorption of plutonium oxides has been found to be 1.6 times higher if compared with the first 4 days of the experiment. The studies found that 0.08, 2.4, and 2.85% of the activity were resorbed within 128 days from abrasions, cutaneous muscular wounds, and stab wounds, respectively. Within the same period of time, 86% of plutonium nitrate was resorbed from stab wound sites.[40]

TABLE 28.10
Technological Plutonium Oxide Resorption for Skin Injuries of White Rats

Kind of Injury	Resorption at Day 4, %
Abrasions	0.063 ± 1.4
Incised cutaneous muscular wounds of the depth of 3.5–4.5 mm	0.23 ± 0.02
Stab wounds of the depth of 5–6 mm	0.78 ± 0.25

Source: Adapted from Lubchansky, E.R. et al.[38]

The investigation of the body distribution and accumulation levels of the wound resorbed plutonium has demonstrated that the plutonium oxide used in these experiments has been distributed to bone and liver with ratio of 1:1.2.[38] The authors explained this finding by apparent blood vessel transportation of the radionuclide portion as insoluble complexes (large aggregates), which accumulated in organs of the reticular endothelial system, particularly, in liver. This idea is shared by other researchers.[41] One of early plutonium toxicology experiments found uptake of alpha activity in the body from the subcutaneous implantation of the metal plutonium.[42] According to the data of these authors, the plutonium resorption (due to the oxidized plutonium-239) was found to equal 0.16 to 1.2% within 260 to 1048 days (rabbits) and 0.09 to 0.28% within 356 to 580 days (rats), where percentages are related to the activity of the metal implanted.

The specific investigation of the wound behavior of exotic radionuclides, such as curium and einsteinium, was not elaborated. Nevertheless, there are experimental studies devoted to the investigation of the body distribution and metabolism of these actinides in cases of parenteral (basically, intramuscular) administration and to the evaluation of the efficiency of diethylene-trimethyl-pentacetate (DTPA) chelates to stimulate their excretion from the body. Durbin[53,54] has shown the similarity of body distribution and metabolism of actinides to that of rare earth elements (lanthanide series), which has been explained by the close values of their ion radii.[54] The resorption of actinides of valence III (including americium-241) from muscular tissue was highest for citrate complexes with consequent decrease of the resorption for chlorine salts and nitrogen-acidic salts, which was predicted.[2] According to Parker et al.,[55,56] Smith,[57] and Williams et al.,[58] the absorption of citrate complexes of americium-241, californium-252, curium-242, and einsteinium-253 from muscular tissue of mice and rats reached 95 to 98% within the first 4 days.

Obviously, information on dosimetry and kinetics of resorption of human wounds contaminated with radioactive substances, particularly, plutonium, is of great interest (Figure 28.3). It should be noted that significant difficulties might arise depending on the adequacy of the plutonium dosimetry and by the effects of therapy, especially chelation, on the natural course of the radionuclide metabolism processes in the wound and in the body.

According to assessments of Schofield[44] based upon accidental finger injuries resulting from plutonium-contaminated subjects (metal plutonium, plutonium oxide, and plutonium nitrate), the plutonium nitrate resorption does not exceed 3% of the wound contaminant activity for stab and lacerated wounds without damage of large blood vessels. The plutonium-239 absorption from the subcutaneous cellular tissue of humans is about 3.5% at hour 4.[45] Coinciding estimates are given by Hesp and Ledgerwood[46] for the example of stab wounds contaminated by plutonium-239 (oxide and nitrate) and by americium-241. According to estimates, the total blood uptake was about 2.3% of the wound contaminant alpha activity (before the wound dissection); the effective half-times (T_{eff}) of the wound excretion were 565 ± 42 days and 400 ± 100 days for plutonium-239 and americium-241, respectively (for 700 days of observation).

In the case of plutonium-239 oxalate contamination (with admixtures of plutonium-238 and 240 and americium-241) of the deep stab wound (total alpha activity of the contaminant was 525.4 kBq) the residual plutonium body burden was assessed in the range of 3.7 to 55.5 kBq after two wound surgeries, performed at minute 15 and at day 15 after the contamination, and DTPA chelate therapy.[47] Thus, the maximum body burden of the residual plutonium oxalate has reached 10.5% of the initial contaminant activity. This leads to the clear conclusion that actual resorption level of the soluble plutonium compound from the stab wound could be much higher, had the surgery and therapy not been applied.

Norwood and Fuqua[31] suppose that plutonium metal penetrated into the skin or subcutaneously through stab wounds and lacerated wounds is retained topically for a long time because of rapid oxidation (PuO_2). Actually, according to published data,[48] the wound plutonium burden persisted to be constant within the whole period of observation (from day 90 to day 400 after the incident) of a patient who had undergone many wound surgeries.

When discussing results of dosimetry examinations of protactinium-231 and actinium-227 contamination cases (stab palm wound), Newton et al.[49] also state the long-term retention of poorly solvable compounds of these radionuclides.

An illustration of the multiple processes specifying the wound behavior of plutonium and, obviously, other multichargeable cations can be provided by the plutonium metabolism scheme proposed by Schofield.[44] The author supposes that the major portion of the activity resorbed into the blood is then transported to organs and tissues as the complex compounds of different bioligands or in the form linked to proteins. Colloid plutonium fraction (including insoluble plutonium particles) moves from the wound into the body through the intermediate compartment (reticular endothelial system, RES) after the "partial dissolution." Actually, the lymphatic system is directly involved in the transportation of hydrolyzed plutonium compounds from wounds.[1,41,50,52,53] Therefore, it is possible that the regional lymphatic nodes providing the lymph outflow from the injured area also accumulate other radioactive substances inclined to the hydrolysis and creation of colloid forms (for example, rare earth and transuranium elements, polonium, etc.), as well as the radionuclide wound contaminants of insoluble oxides or fine dispersible particles of metal.[1,2] This circumstance has to be taken into account when planning dosimetry and medical care of victims. For example, according to experiments done by Cable et al.[50] in suckling pigs using intracutaneous administration of nitrogen-acidic plutonium of valence IV, 4.5 and 12% of the administered contaminant were found in regional lymph nodes at days 1 and 7, respectively.

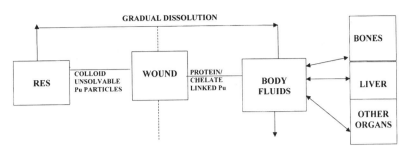

FIGURE 28.3 Scheme of plutonium wound dissemination.

Burns

In industrial facilities and research laboratories, the radioactive contamination of burns occurs less frequently than in skin wounds. At the same time, chemical burns are more frequent than thermal burns. Thus, according to Reference 4, of 286 skin injuries recorded to be contaminated by plutonium-239 and americium-241 only 8 cases (about 3%) were found to be thermal burns, whereas 30 people had chemical burns (10.5%). Several publications exist on clinical dosimetric aspects of specific cases of acidic applications (burns) of carbon-14, iridium-192, and plutonium-239.[10,13,60]

Information on the metabolism of radioactive contaminants in chemical and thermal skin burns has been obtained by a number of experimental studies. The first publications on these subjects, by Bock and Ivanov,[61,62] noted that radionuclide resorption rates from burns in white rats are not significantly different from that through intact skin, if all other conditions are similar. The authors have shown that application of weakly acidic solutions of cobalt-60, thallium-204, strontium-89, and barium-140 on the surface of grade II thermal burns in rats was found to result in an accumulation of these radionuclides of about 1% of the applied contaminant activity after 24 h. Cerium-144 absorption has reached several parts of a percent and that for iodine-131 was about 1.5 to 3% (see also Reference 2).

These first estimates were confirmed later by more-detailed studies done by the same group of researchers.[2,63,64,72] Table 28.11 provides summary results of experiments, where the standard thermal burns of different grades of severity* were inflicted by a special electric lamp generating filtered heat rays of 1.5 to 3.0 µm wavelength.[2]

Radionuclides of cesium, strontium, polonium, and americium in solutions of pH 1.5 to 2.0 were applied topically to the burn surface immediately after thermal exposure; from the analysis of results given in Table 28.11, one can conclude that the radionuclide uptakes rates from thermal burn are comparable to those through intact skin (within the experimental error range) and are independent of the physical and chemical properties of these radionuclides, which represent different groups of elements of the periodic table. For example, at hour 24 after the application of radionuclide contaminants, the differences of uptakes were limited to a factor of 2 for burns of severity grade II.

This phenomenon is best explained by the histological and morphological characteristics of cutaneous thermal burns of different grades of severity (see Reference 65, for example). It is known that burns of grade I do not induce large changes in the epidermis that could increase the penetrability of the corneous and basal layers that are crucial to the skin barrier function.[2,66] Histological changes of human skin in the case of grade I burns demonstrate pyknosis only of the external epidermal layer cell nuclei; the superficial vessels dilate, and edema of the net dermal layer develops. Apparently, the hyperemia itself does not increase the penetrability of superficial skin layers; moreover, the vascular network is situated under the epidermal layers that serve as the barrier.

---

* According to the adopted classification, four severity grades of skin burns are selected as follows: grade I (skin hyperemia), grade II (blistering), grade III (death of all derma layers), grade IV (death of tissues situated under the derma).

TABLE 28.11
Radionuclide Body Burdens (in % of applied contaminant activity) at Different Periods of Time after the Application of ^{137}Cs, ^{89}Sr, ^{131}I, ^{210}Po, and ^{241}Am to the Surface of Thermal Burns of Severity Grades of I–III (Balance Tests)[2,63,64]

Experiment Conditions	Time of Examination	^{137}Cs	^{89}Sr	^{131}I	^{210}Po	^{241}Am
Intact skin	1 h	0.4 ± 0.1	—	—	—	—
	3 h	—	—	—	0.008 ± 0.0006	0.007 ± 0.002
	6 h	2.6 ± 0.8	—	1.4 ± 0.2	0.012 ± 0.003	—
	1 day	2.0 ± 1.0	4.0 ± 0.9	2.4 ± 1.0	0.013 ± 0.004	0.03 ± 0.01
	5 days	1.3 ± 0.4	—	—	—	—
Grade I burn	1 h	—	—	—	0.004 ± 0.001	—
	3 h	—	—	—	0.011 ± 0.003	—
	1 day	1.8 ± 0.6	2.1 ± 0.8	2.2 ± 0.4	0.013 ± 0.003	0.06 ± 0.02
Grade II burn	1 h	0.3 ± 0.06	0.8 ± 0.3	0.8 ± 0.2	0.003 ± 0.0006	0.008 ± 0.002
	6 h	2.2 ± 0.8	2.1 ± 0.1	3.2 ± 0.7	0.014 ± 0.003	0.03 ± 0.003
	1 day	2.0 ± 1.0	2.5 ± 0.6	3.0 ± 0.5	0.025 ± 0.007	0.07 ± 0.04
	3 days	—	1.4 ± 0.5	3.3 ± 0.9	—	—
	5 days	1.8 ± 0.5	—	—	—	—
Grade III burn	1 h	—	2.0 ± 0.3	—	0.0004 ± 0.0002	—
	1 day	0.8 ± 0.2	1.8 ± 0.8	1.6 ± 0.3	0.0015 ± 0.0002	0.03 ± 0.077

However, the hyperemia can accelerate and partially amplify the radionuclide absorption throughout the corium (at the initial phase) or, alternatively, it can delay this process, when hemostasis (blood congestion) and edema develop. In the case of burns of severity grade II, epidermal necrosis begins. Cytoplasm becomes partially cellular and strongly oxyphilic through the whole depth of epidermal layer. The edema occurs in dermis, as well as infiltration of leukocytes and lymphocytes in the papillary layer and net layer of the skin; blisters occur with detachment of the part of epidermal layer. Experimental data in white rats (see Table 28.1) demonstrate that radionuclide resorption (iodine-131, polonium-210, americium-241, for example) throughout the surface of the thermal burn grade II is increased about twofold compared with intact skin, which indicates a relatively weak disturbance of the epidermal barrier function. Histoautoradiography tests have established that the character of the microdistribution of plutonium-210 applied to the intact skin of white rats is practically the same as the application to a skin burn grade I.[2] The major number of tracks were detected in epidermal corneal layers and in outlet ducts of hair follicles. In grade II burns, a lesser aggregation of polonium-210 in the epidermal surface was detected but with the same dominance of the alpha activity in corneum. The alpha activity is distributed as diffuse tracks and usually does not create dense accumulations ("stars"). Apparently, this phenomenon is related to the detachment of corneum filaments, which influences the stability of polonium-210 linkage to the superficial cutaneous structures. Thermal burns inflicted in white rats and guinea pigs do not induce blistering and, therefore, the detachment (rejection) of epidermis from skin does not occur. This raises the question of the validity of extrapolating data to humans. Apparently, such extrapolation is possible, if the integrity of blisters is not disturbed in grade II burns. Data published by Klyachkin and Filatov[67] have confirmed this conclusion in clinical studies, where they have shown that radioiodine absorption throughout burns of grades I and II (if blisters were intact) is not changed significantly. A much different picture was observed when the epidermal detachment has occurred and the dermis is uncovered. Radionuclide contamination of the skin, if not covered by epidermis, is practically the same as for wound contamination.

An experimental study elaborated in guinea pigs[68] has shown that strontium-89 contamination of skin burns, when the epidermis was removed (papillary and stem layers were naked), results in much larger resorption of the radionuclide (up to 76% of the applied contaminant activity at hour 1). Benes[14] describes the cauterization of thermal burns of grades II to III in white rats (600°C), when clear damage was inflicted both to corneous and lower epidermal layers and to deeper cutaneous structures. In such conditions the strong amplification of cesium-137 (pH 1) body resorption was observed to reach 21% of the applied contaminant activity at minute 30.

Thermal burns of grades III and IV are accompanied by induction of scabs; some publications[69] suppose that this barrier is practically nonpenetrable for radionuclide resorption. The experimental data provided by Table 28.11 and results of other works[70,71] indicate at least delay (decrease) of the absorption of radionuclides and some other substances (strychnine, methionine) from the inflammatory processes after the infliction of a grade III burn.

Thus, the data provided demonstrate that radionuclide resorption with thermal burns of grades I and II (if the epidermal integrity is not disturbed) and the more severe thermal burns of grades III and IV is not significantly different from that for intact skin. At the same time, thermal skin burns accompanied by blistering require specific attention, because rupture or destruction of blisters exposes underlying layers of epidermis and dermis, which in turn can increase radionuclide resorption from the injured site into the body. Therefore, when providing primary care of burns at the site of an incident, if intact blisters are present, the injured area should only be bandaged with a sterile bandage. Initial surgery (including decontamination) and, moreover, opening of blisters must be provided at a medical facility where appropriate precautions can be taken.

In cases in which the initial examination of a burn reveals the loss of epidermal integrity and dermis, primary care at the site of the incident must include careful antiseptic washing (primary decontamination) of the wound before application of the sterile bandage.

A number of publications on the experimental investigation of the metabolism of radionuclide skin contamination accompanied by concentrated acids, alkalines, or organic solvents exist in the literature. One of the first works of this kind[73] indicates that the body resorption rate of plutonium-239 applied to the skin with 10 N HNO_3 was 1 to 2% within 5 days and 0.1 to 0.3% if the radionuclide was applied with 0.1 N HNO_3 solution.* When plutonium-239 (10 µg) was applied to the palm of the hand together with 0.4 N HNO_3, the resorption rate (within 8 h) was 0.0002%[2] and total activity intake in the body was ~0.005% (within 24 h) of the total activity topically applied in the skin.[2]

Studies by Ilyin et al.[72,74] were devoted to intracutaneous distribution, absorption rates, and body metabolism of plutonium and americium applied to the intact skin of rats together with nitric acid solutions of different concentrations. Simultaneously, the pathomorphology and histoautoradiography pictures of plutonium-239 and americium-241 distributions in different cutaneous structures were investigated. Table 28.12 lists the body accumulation of plutonium-239 in rats at different times after application to the rat skin of 0.1 N 2.5 N, and 10 N HNO_3 solutions and plutonium polymer nitrate of pH 1 (0.1 N). Results of plutonium-239 experiments have shown that levels of percutaneous radionuclide intake are predominantly determined by destructive and necrotic changes of skin resulting from acidic burns.

A significant change (strong amplification) of emitter body intake was not found for acidic solutions of different concentrations. At important early time intervals, for example, 1 h after the application, plutonium accumulation body levels did not show significant differences. The levels were equal to thousandths of a percent of topically applied activity, excluding cases of 1 N HNO_3 plutonium solutions. By 24 h after the application, the plutonium body burdens were in the range of 0.017 to 0.058% of the activity applied in the rat skin. When 0.1 N HNO_3 plutonium-239 solution was applied, the histological structure of skin did not show significant changes and only mild epidermal changes such as thickening and enlargement of cells were observed 1 h after the

---

* Studies have shown that the barrier skin function already disturbed when 0.1 N concentration of strong acids is applied.

TABLE 28.12
^{239}Pu Body Burden in Rats (% of topically applied activity) after the Intact Skin Application of HNO$_3$ Solutions of Different Concentrations

HNO$_3$ Concentrations, N	Time Passed after Application, h			
	1	3	6	24
0.1	0.004 ± 0.001	0.0067 ± 0.0014	0.010 ± 0.002	0.017 ± 0.004
1.0	0.012 ± 0.004	0.020 ± 0.005	0.033 ± 0.01	0.058 ± 0.010
2.5	0.0068 ± 0.001	—	0.026 ± 0.006	0.038 ± 0.011
10	0.0045 ± 0.0017	0.008 ± 0.0015	0.015 ± 0.004	0.030 ± 0.005
Polymer nitrate, pH-1.0	0.0044 ± 0.0010	0.006 ± 0.001	0.009 ± 0.001	0.012 ± 0.002

Source: Adapted from Ilyin, L.A. et al., *Hyg. Sanit.*, 1, 26, 1982.

radionuclide application. At hour 24, focal intercellular edema and vacuolization of epidermal cells were found. A different picture was found in case of the application of 1 N HNO$_3$: morphological changes of cutaneous layer structures were already expressed at minute 5 after the application. Within 1 h, the skin damage and related plutonium microdistribution had significantly changed: the epidermis was thinning to single layer, nuclei were lysed, and enlargement of collagen fibers of the upper third of the dermis was observed. Histoautoradiography pictures show diffuse distribution of alpha particles within the skin itself and within the subcutaneous cellular tissue. Conglomeration of alpha particles was observed in the hair follicles and subcutaneous muscles as well as in the epidermis. An interesting finding was that consequent increase of acid concentration (up to 2.5 to 10 N) was not accompanied by increased plutonium body uptake. This finding is related to the rapid development of necrotic processes in tissues generating some extra barrier against radionuclide body penetration. Actually, within several minutes to 1 h after the application of 2.5 N HNO$_3$ or 10 N HNO$_3$, the necrotic zone has involved the whole skin, subcutaneous cellular tissue, and subcutaneous muscle layer.

Using the technique of consecutive horizontal skin slices of 20 μm thickness, it was established that the radionuclide has basically concentrated in the subcutaneous layers of the necrotic skin within 1 to 24 h after plutonium-239 application together with 2.5 N and 10 N HNO$_3$. The major portion (90%) of isotope found at depths between 20 and 900 μm below the surface was in the layer of 20 to 400 μm, a finding that certifies the low mobility of the radionuclide in the necrotic zone.

Similar associations of body resorption and accumulation were found in experiments with americium-241,[2] where the isotope was applied topically in white rat skin together with 0.5 N, 1 N, 2.5 N, 4 N, and 8 N HNO$_3$ solutions. Americium-241 body burden found at hour 24 did not have significant variation and was several tenths of a percent (0.14 to 0.32%).

Despite the fact that body intake of isotope with more concentrated solutions of nitrate acid is increased by a factor of 7 (see Table 28.13) if compared to the resorption of americium-241 applied with 0.05 N HNO$_3$ solution, the absolute levels of absorption can be interpreted as relatively low.

Nevertheless, one fact is clear: if skin contamination of radionuclide in concentrated acid solutions occurs, then the immediate careful (without brushes) decontamination of skin with neutralizing soap solutions of low alkalescence is strongly indicated. The paper referred to above[10] has proved that, in case of 37 MBq of ^{192}IrCl contamination of face and hair of the radiation worker, the immediate use of distilled water flushing provided at least a fivefold decrease in the topical contamination level. According to cautious assessments of the authors of this paper, the radionuclide body resorption did not exceed 0.1 to 3%.

TABLE 28.13
^{241}Am Skin Resorption and Body Accumulation in Case of the Application to the Intact Skin Together with Nitric Acid Solutions of Different Concentrations (in % of topically applied activity)[1,2]

HNO$_3$ Concentration, N	Time of Contact, h	Liver	Kidneys	Skeleton	All Soft Tissues[a]	Whole Body[a]
0.05	24	0.02 ± 0.008	0.001 ± 0.0007	0.01 ± 0.005	—	0.031
0.5	24	0.08 ± 0.02	0.01 ± 0.003	0.09 ± 0.002	—	0.18
1.0	24	0.08 ± 0.02	0.01 ± 0.001	0.08 ± 0.009	0.04 ± 0.004	0.22
	5 days	0.34 ± 0.04	0.03 ± 0.006	0.33 ± 0.06	0.45 ± 0.008	1.15
2.5	24	0.06 ± 0.003	0.01 ± 0.001	0.05 ± 0.006	0.02 ± 0.006	0.14
4.0	24	0.05 ± 0.005	0.009 ± 0.0008	0.04 ± 0.006	0.035 ± 0.006	0.14
8.0	24	0.04 ± 0.006	0.009 ± 0.008	0.04 ± 0.008	0.23 ± 0.07	0.32
	5 days	0.5 ± 0.06	0.05 ± 0.006	0.5 ± 0.05	1.0 ± 0.2	2.0

[a] Excluding ^{241}Am content in skin and subcutaneous tissues.

The analysis of experimental data on the dynamics of radionuclide distribution in organs and tissues as well as the body metabolism indicates that, in the presence of thermal and chemical burns of skin, the behavior of the resorbed portion of radionuclides maintains the general behavior specific to other body intake pathways (through the intact skin, for example). Some differences were found here for rates and levels of the radionuclide intake within the body. For example, low levels of plutonium and americium resorption in applications with low acidic solutions (0.1 N) are obviously explained by the influence of buffer skin systems and weak alkaline medium of deeper layers of skin, which promotes the neutralization of the contaminant. In this case, because of the hydrolysis and polymerization inclination of Pu^{+4} (where inclination is higher than that for Am^{+3} of valence III), polymer forms of plutonium hydroxide are created, which naturally decreases the radionuclide intake into the blood. If plutonium-239 skin contamination occurs together with concentrated acid solutions, then the neutralizing ability of skin becomes inconsistent and the acid damages the skin to deeper levels with increased plutonium infiltration (see above). In such case, plutonium is actually transformed into an ion-dispersible state and it is relatively more absorbable into the internal body medium. However, when the necrotic skin changes are growing, the resorption rate decreases with larger concentrations of acidic solution. One should suppose that such associations are also specific to the radionuclide behavior after radionuclide skin contamination with concentrated alkalies, as well. This general conclusion was confirmed by Japanese researchers, who have investigated the resorption of ^{58}CoCl$_2$ and ^{54}MnCl$_2$ applied to the bare skin of white mice together with 1 N, 5 N, and 10 N HCl or NaOH.[77] These experiments have assessed the dynamics of radionuclide resorption at minutes 15, 30, and 60 after application. Cobalt-58 experiments have shown that the concentration of acid or alkaline does not make a significant influence in radionuclide absorption if compared with intact skin resorption; the numerical range of these uptakes are 0.1 to 0.15% of the applied activity within 60-min contact. Manganese-54 experiments were devoted to acidic burns only, where similar conclusions were found (absorption rate below 0.1%), excluding 10 N HCl, in which case manganese resorption was increased by a factor of 5, i.e., 0.5% within 60 min.

It is clear that the resorption mechanism of intact skin for burns inflicted by chemicals (especially by relatively dilute acidic and alkaline solutions) is significantly determined by the character of the radioactive isotope interaction with specific biochemical components of the skin. For example, when investigating the skin distribution and resorption levels of plutonium applied to the intact skin together with 0.1 N HNO$_3$ or an organic solvent solution (tributylphosphate, TBP), where the nuclide is linked into a complex state; this complex penetrates into deeper skin layers and its body resorption rate is increased by a factor of 2.5 within 24 h.[75,76] The explanation for this phenomenon should be found in the dissolution of the water–lipid membrane that covers the skin surfaces by the organic solvent and in the change in character of the interaction of the plutonium–TBP complex with biocomponents of skin.

Investigation of the interaction peculiarities of radioactive substances with skin biocomponents was originally elaborated by Ilyin et al.[20] It was established that all examined fission product radionuclides and transuranium elements interact with albumin skin structures immediately after their penetration in the skin (up to 80 to 90% of the penetrated activity) but less with lipids (6 to 14% of the penetrated activity) and poorly soluble nonorganic compounds without any dependence on the radionuclide chemical individuality. The rather stable complex radionuclide compounds generated by functional groups of cutaneous albumin structures, apparently, determine low levels of the radionuclide resorption throughout the skin, including burns of severity grades I to II.

Radionuclide Metabolism in Contaminated Wounds and Burns

It is clearly demonstrated that mechanical damage of skin integrity strongly amplifies the intake of radioactive substances into the body. Taking the rate of the radioactive substance wound resorption within 24 h as the basis, one can consider that the highest body intake level is specific to radionuclides of alkaline and alkaline-earth elements, halogens, and, apparently, to other more easily metabolized elements (molybdenum, tellurium, cobalt, chromium, phosphorus, for example).

Where cutaneous muscular wounds are concerned, the resorption rate comprises several tens of percent of the radionuclide activity applied topically, and this index can reach 100% for stab wounds. The high absorption rate of soluble compounds of radioactive substances is a specific feature of their wound behavior; one can expect that about two thirds of soluble radionuclide contaminants in wounds will be absorbed within the first hour.

The resorption rate of soluble compounds of rare earth radionuclides from cutaneous muscular and stab wounds varies in the range of several percent; this index for polonium, plutonium, americium, and, obviously, other transplutonium elements is in the range of 10 to 25%. For some complex compounds (citrates, oxalates) higher uptakes are possible.

Within the first day after the occurrence of the wound contamination of poorly soluble/insoluble compounds of radioactive substances, the absorption rate is apparently below 1%. However, it is important to remember that wound resorption of easily hydrolyzed radionuclides continues for a long time, which is different from elements specific to ion dispersive state at body pH. Therefore, the importance of the initial compartment as the source of the prolonged internal body intake of radioactive substances seems to be very significant.

When generalizing results of experimental studies and clinical biophysical observations, one can prove that the elevation of rates of the radionuclide resorption throughout skin injuries can be ranged for all other similar conditions as follows: thermal burns < chemical burns < abrasions and excoriations of skin (microtraumas) < lacerated wounds < incised cutaneous muscular wounds < stab wounds.

It is possible to accept that radionuclide resorption rates through skin burns and particularly from thermal burn surfaces are in the range of their penetration rates throughout the intact skin with the elevation to complete absorption in case of stab or incised wounds contaminated by radionuclides dissolved to ion-dispersible state.

It is necessary to pay specific attention to the status and integrity of skin in radiation workers. It has been proven that radionuclide resorption through fresh skin microtraumas (abrasions, excoriations) can exceed the intact skin absorption for factors of tens to hundreds.

METHODS AND TECHNIQUES OF CONTROL OF RADIOACTIVE CONTAMINATION OF WOUNDS AND BURNS

BACKGROUND

Based upon the above metabolic considerations, one can expect that measures to control radioactive contamination of the injured skin are complex and designed (1) to prevent uptake and internal transport of radionuclides from the injured area and (2) to stimulate of the body excretion of radionuclides resorbed. Certainly, applied measures and means should not cause negative influence in consequent wound management and results of routine therapy of the contamination.

Apparently, the realization of the task should entail limitation of the blood outflow from the injured area to the systemic circulation (for example, use of a tourniquet or vasoconstrictive agent administration), application of absorption agent inhibition of radionuclides (sterile bandages or specific ion-exchange fabrics and absorbing compositions applied topically, etc.), and conversion of easily metabolized radionuclide compound into nonsoluble forms with consequent removal. Wound and burn decontamination can be done by washing the injured area with soap, detergent, or relevant solvents and/or by excision of contaminated tissues under radiometric monitoring.

The list of these measures is rather schematic because their sequence and application depend upon the kind and peculiarities of the injury, the radioactive contamination character, and upon other factors. For example, the solid binding of radioactive substances in the case of stab wounds is apparently not acceptable, and the surgical processing of the wound with wide dissection of its edges is not always convenient for cosmetic reasons (in the case of face trauma, for example, or risk of functional impairment).

In case of radioactive wound contamination, the application of agents that limit the body incorporation and that stimulate radionuclide excretion from the body is the obvious prophylactic measure. At the same time, this consideration can be limited in specific cases. It was found by experimental studies that the oral administration of modern agents stimulating the body excretion of polonium strongly increases its resorption from the injured area into the body.[1,2]

To obtain an impression of the experimental capabilities and clinical experience of the control of radioactive contamination of skin wounds and burns, the results of the prophylaxis measures applied at different phases of radionuclide metabolism are considered below.

PREVENTION OF RADIONUCLIDE BODY ABSORPTION AND REMOVAL OF RADIONUCLIDES FROM THE INJURED AREA

Information on the effectiveness of topical application of vasoconstrictive agents is very limited for the cases considered here. One publication[78] addressed the diagnostic aspects of radioactive indicators, particularly the possibility of delaying iodine-131 resorption after topical application of adrenaline and mezatone in the forearm where the radionuclide was injected intramuscularly in volunteers. The increase of the resorption time was found to be 50% of the administered amount of iodine-131 within 6 to 14 min. The same paper also stated the possibility of complete termination of iodine-131 blood absorption, if venous stagnation was arranged for 8 min using a blood pressure cuff. A number of indications in the literature refer to the convenience of using a tourniquet to prevent radionuclide resorption in cases of wounds accompanied by radionuclide contamination. Particularly, Ohlenschläger[79] recommends a tourniquet application in cases of arm and hand wounds as part of the first aid provided at the emergency site. To obtain quantitative assessment of the result of this technique on radionuclide intake, including the intake of various radionuclides with different metabolic behavior, corresponding studies were elaborated.[2] White rat experiments were done using iodine-131, cesium-137, polonium-210, and americium-241. Nuclide solutions were administered subcutaneously in the metatarsal area. A rubber tourniquet 1 mm wide with a cloth cover was applied above the tarsal–metatarsal joint at minute 1 or 5 after injection of radioactive solution. The duration of tourniquet application was 30 min. With this application, a significant decrease of the radionuclide blood resorption and organ accumulation was observed. The highest effectiveness was found after administrations of iodine-131 and cesium-137, if the tourniquet was applied at minute 1 after the administration. When the tourniquet was removed the iodine-131 thyroid burden did not exceed 0.1% of the administered amount and was almost 100 times lower than in control rats. Cesium-137 burdens in organs and tissues were equal to 0.6% of the administered amount and were 60 times less than in controls. Delaying the tourniquet application for 5 min strongly reduced its effectiveness; iodine-131 and cesium-137 burdens in organs and tissues of the experimental animals were found to be only two times lower than those in the control. At the same time, tourniquet application in cases of the administration of polonium-210 and americium-241, which are radionuclides of relatively low metabolic activity, has provided more modest results. If the tourniquet is applied 1 min after americium-241 injection, the total decrease of the radionuclide accumulation in skeleton, liver, and kidneys was only 18% compared with the control; i.e., this accumulation was several times less compared with the decrease of 60- to 100-fold found for iodine-131 and cesium-137. The tourniquet application deferred for 5 min decreased americium-241 and polonium-210 burdens in organs and tissues by only approximately threefold compared with that in controls. Therefore, the effectiveness of this technique significantly depends on the time of application and the type of radionuclide wound contaminant. If rapidly metabolized radionuclides contaminate the wound before the immediate tourniquet application, their incorporation is strongly decreased in organs and tissues and the effectiveness is reduced if the first aid is delayed even for only several minutes. If slowly metabolized radionuclides contaminate a wound in the same condition, the therapeutic effect is decreased and the absolute values are significantly lower.

The experiments have also demonstrated that the body resorption of different radionuclides after removal of the tourniquet is immediately restored, and the levels of deposition of iodine-131, cesium-137, americium-241, and polonium-210 in organs and tissues are similar to those found in controls at hour 24 after radionuclide administration.

The results of the investigation provide several general considerations concerning the effectiveness of tourniquets and their importance in the whole complex of first aid measures for radioactively contaminated wounds. The immediate application of a tourniquet should be obligatory for any kind of wound in a radioactive environment (obviously, if one can be applied to the specific wound localization). This measure is especially important when rapidly metabolized radioactive wound contaminants are present (for example, radionuclides of chemical elements of groups I, II, and VII). Wound decontamination, including initial surgery, should be accomplished within the time permitted for tourniquet application; one should remember that removal of the tourniquet results in resumption of radionuclide uptake into the blood.

Surgical excision is a very effective measure for radionuclide removal from the injured area. Its effectiveness is particularly high when poorly transported radionuclide contaminants of slow uptake are present. At the same time, wound tissue surgery deferred for 1 h or more is of little effect when rapidly metabolized radionuclides are present because of the massive uptake to the blood flow immediately following the injury. Thus, timely application of a tourniquet and implementation of surgery as soon as possible after the incident are obviously important. Aseptic wet and dry bandages, cotton-gauze tampons, or specialized adhesive bandage applied to cutaneous muscular wounds as a first-aid measure within first 5 min can absorb up to 20 to 50% of radionuclide wound contaminants.[2,14,80]

A general rule is that the effectiveness of first aid decreases proportionately with the time passed since the radionuclide wound contamination. For example, experiments with strontium-89, polonium-210, cerium-144, and americium-241 done by Ivannikov, Popov and Bajin[2,43,51] have shown that treating wounds or abrasions with two sequential tampons (wet and dry) 5 min after the contamination results in removal of 20 to 40% of radionuclide solutions applied to the wound, but the same procedure results in up to 50 to 60% removal if done after only 1 min.

Data on topical application of adsorbing materials, sorbents, and some compounds to bind radionuclides into soluble complexes have been published.[1,2,16,81,82] Cutaneous muscular wounds in rabbits were contaminated by phosphorus-32 (Na_2HPO_4) and immediately sprinkled with Jitnouk powder containing xeroformium, boric acid, streptocidium, and sugar. Phosphorus-32 body resorption was decreased 1.5 to 2 times as compared with control.[82]

Experiments in monkeys by Ducousso et al.[16,81] focused on treatment of radioactive strontium (strontium-85) in lacerated wounds using potassium rhodizonate, saturated $MgSO_4$ solution, calcium alginate, and aluminum phosphate gel.* All reagents were applied 5 min after the contamination and the strontium-85 blood concentration decreased by 35 to 45%. Delaying administration of agents 15 min after the contamination significantly decreased their effect; only potassium rhodizonate was found to have a moderate effect (strontium-85 blood concentration was decreased approximately 25 to 30% as compared with control). It was concluded that potassium rhodizonate is the best reagent to bind radioactive strontium within lacerated wounds, which decreases blood resorption. Such a conclusion could be reliable, if the authors had compared the effect of topical application of rhodizonate vs. the effect of common cotton-gauze tampon.

To absorb radioactive strontium within cutaneous muscular wounds and skin abrasions of white rats, highly oxidized cellulose (vocacite)[1] and sodium alginate were applied, as well as specialized cationic exchange gauze.[2] The results showed that early (at minute 5) application of sorbents and specialized gauze provided an effect essentially the same as that observed in experiments with wet cotton-gauze tampons. Applications deferred for 30 min result in a better effect if highly oxidized cellulose is applied.[1,2]

The effect of binding and removal of radioactive strontium from human cutaneous microtraumas was examined in six volunteers. These studies[1] were a part of the tests described above. To clean abrasions contaminated with strontium-85, 5% highly oxidized cellulose solution ($NaHCO_3$ solvent, pH = 7.2) was applied with subsequent flushing of the contaminated area with physiological solution and 2% hydrogen peroxide solution (Table 28.14). Skin abrasions were treated at minute 30 (first group) and at hour 6 (second group) after the application of radioactive solution. The cleaning technique included 3 min of processing of the strontium-85-contaminated area with sterile tampons moistened with highly oxidized cellulose and 30 s of physiological solution washing; thereafter, repeated processing with highly oxidized cellulose was done together with washing of the residual of this agent using physiological solution and 2% hydrogen peroxide solution.

TABLE 28.14
Decontamination Effectiveness of Human Cutaneous Abrasions Contaminated by ^{85}Sr[1,2]

		Residual activity ratio (to the initial value), %				
Moment of Process Start	Volunteer Code	First Processing with High-Oxidized Cellulose	Physiological Solution Washing	Second Processing with High-Oxidized Cellulose	Physiological Solution and H_2O_2 Washing	Total ^{85}Sr Removed, %
Minute 30	04	37.3	26.9	21.1	17.7	82.3
	05	35.0	27.4	23.8	21.8	78.2
	06	43.0	33.1	28.8	24.1	75.9
	Average	38.4	29.1	24.6	21.2	78.8
Hour 6	07	20.3	15.9	14.6	13.6	86.4
	08	23.5	15.3	13.6	12.7	87.8
	09	16.9	15.5	14.6	15.5	84.5
	Average	20.2	15.6	14.3	13.9	86.1

* These substances (calcium alginate and aluminum phosphate gel, especially) have been well investigated as agents able to bind radioactive strontium inside the gastrointestinal tract.[1]

Table 28.14 demonstrates that about 80% of strontium-85 is removed by the above procedure. This result certifies the real possibility of effective radioactive decontamination of superficial cutaneous injuries (those contaminated with radioactive strontium, particularly). The first application of highly oxidized cellulose was most effective and it has provided decontamination of 80 to 90% of the strontium-85. Each subsequent application was less effective than the previous one. This result was observed in all tests. Looking at the data, one obtains an impression that late processing of abrasions (at hour 6 after contamination) is more effective than at 30 min. This peculiar phenomenon results from the specificity of the direct radiometry of the injured area. One should remember that strontium-85 resorption is poor at hour 6 after skin contamination. The retained portion of strontium-85, which is incorporated in the skin, is also strongly decreased at this hour. Alternatively, at the period of early processing (at minute 30), a large amount of beta emitter is present in this area because of the intensive uptake of strontium-85 into the skin. This activity adds to the integral radioactivity at the contaminated site, which is measured by direct radiometry techniques. This circumstance can cause underestimation of the actual effect of the cleaning of the abrasion at the early period of decontamination.

The decontamination mechanism is obviously determined by the highly oxidized cellulose sorption of the available strontium-85. Removal of the strontium-85 results from both the action of this agent and the additional mechanical removal of the radionuclide by tampons moistened with physiological solution. Hydrogen peroxide washing did not significantly influence cleaning of strontium-85-contaminated abrasions.

Because of the small number of tests, limited by the small number of volunteers, investigation of other abrasion decontamination schemes was not done. For example, one can suppose that the application of physiological solution at the first washing could be less effective than highly oxidized cellulose sorption.

Several publications are devoted to the investigation of wound and burn decontamination including substances and solutions of different chemical compounds able to create complexes with different radioactive contaminants. Most detailed experiments on this subject were done by Benes.[14] The experiments were elaborated in white rats with cutaneous muscular wounds contaminated by strontium-89, phosphorus-32, iodine-131, cesium-137, and a uranium fission product mixture; the effectiveness of the application of solutions of EDTA, hexametaphosphate (HMP), sodium citrate, DTPA, and surgical dissection of wounds (as the comparative technique) was assessed. Wound processing was done at hour 6 after radioactive contamination using cotton-gauze tampons moistened with the various solutions.

Comparative analysis of the effect of the examined compounds for the specific radionuclide has revealed mild differences. For example, radionuclide amounts removed from wounds by water, EDTA, citrate, HMP, and DTPA have varied in the range of 50 to 67% (strontium-89), 50 to 79% (phosphorus-32), and 48 to 68% (uranium fission products). At the same time, there is an impression of higher effect for DTPA, although the high effect of this compound for iodine-131 and phosphorus-32 (which are not able to create chelates with DTPA) is doubtful. Based upon the results obtained, all data were integrated and the conclusion was reached that the fluid decontamination wound techniques provide about 45% removal of radioactive substances on average (it should be remembered that this result is related to late wound processing). At the same time, the comparison of data obtained by Benes for different radioactive substances reveals the significant difference of their "decontamination ability." For example, cesium-137 and iodine-131 were removed from wounds less well, as compared to strontium-89, phosphorus-32, and uranium fission products. This circumstance can be explained by the metabolic peculiarities of these radionuclides and by differences of the stability of their liaisons with wound biosubstrates.[1,2]

Studies done by Ilyin et al.[2,26] on the decontamination of cutaneous muscular wounds and abrasions of white rats have applied chelating compounds including EDTA, 2,2-diamino-diethyl ether of *N,N,N,N*-tetracetic acid (DEETA) (strontium-89), DTPA (cerium-144, americium-241), and sodium-2,3-dimercaptopropaneoxyethanesulfate (oxathyol) (polonium-210). Cotton-gauze tampons moistened with 5% solutions of these complexing compounds were tested. Early processing of cutaneous muscular wounds (at minute 5) with solutions of the various compounds has promoted the removal of 40 to 63% of radioactive contaminants. The abrasion cleaning efficiency was higher in all cases if compared with that for cutaneous muscular wounds. Apparently, this finding reflects the lower stability of binding of radioactive substances in the superficial structure of cutaneous abrasions and the larger "availability" of radionuclides for chelation. When treating cutaneous muscular wounds and abrasions at minute 30 after contamination, the decontamination effect was lowered. When comparing the effectiveness of various washing techniques of contaminated cutaneous injuries, the influence of chemical properties on the increase of the wound decontamination efficiency occurs for strontium, cerium, and americium as well as a purely mechanical decontamination effect.

It is necessary pay attention to whether the use of chelating agents for decontamination of injured skin may increase absorption of the radioactive substance in the body. Results of polonium-210 experiments for contamination of cutaneous muscular wounds and abrasions are informative for this subject. For example, moistened cotton-gauze tampons applied at minute 5 after contamination to cutaneous muscular wounds removed 25% of polonium-210, while 40% of this radionuclide was removed if the wound was processed with oxathyol. However, the latter case was also accompanied by a twofold increase in polonium-210 body intake. In abrasions, 44% of polonium-210 was removed by tampon mechanical processing and oxathyol has provided 59% removal. At the same time, the animal body radionuclide accumulation was elevated 4.5 times compared with the control, because of the strong uptake of the polonium–oxathyol complex and its consequent disintegration in kidneys.[1]

The topical application of DTPA at minute 5 after americium-241 contamination of wounds and abrasions has resulted in 63 and 68% of the radionuclide being removed from wounds and abrasions, respectively. Americium-241 body resorption has also been strongly elevated, which is verified by urine radioactivity measurements in the animals under study. However, americium-241 organ burdens (including kidneys) were lower than those in the controls, which differs from the results of the oxathyol tests with polonium-210.[1,2]

Thus, the results of these studies demonstrate that the application of complexing compounds for the decontamination of cutaneous muscular wounds and abrasions is an effective measure, but it is accompanied by increased radioactive substance uptake from the contaminated site. Obviously, the mechanism of this phenomenon follows from the creation of soluble radionuclide complexes that lead to easy resorption. When this complex disintegrates in the body, accumulation of radioactive substances in organs and tissues is increased. Alternatively, the complexing agent provides a soluble complex with the radionuclide, and it is nearly completely excreted from the body. The result is decreased incorporation of radionuclide in organs and tissues and decreased radiation doses. It follows *a priori* that the topical application of complex-creating agents is justified for the only those cases, in which it is known that this agent creates a highly stable complex compound with the specific radionuclide without disintegrating the body.* Because wounds contaminated with plutonium occur most frequently, experimental evaluation of the influence of topical application of complexing agent solutions and other agents able to remove plutonium from the contaminated site is of specific interest, as is the consequent behavior of this radionuclide in the body. Experiments done on white mice in Japan[86] have shown that the topical DTPA application to wounds contaminated by plutonium-239 monomer compounds provides significant topical cleaning of this radionuclide without increases in organ doses.

---

* The set of the effective agents of selective binding of polonium in the body is limited to the complex-creating dithyolic compounds of oxathyol, unithyol (sodium 2,3-dimercaptopropane sulfate), BAL (3,4-dimercaptopropanol). These agents are successfully applied for decorporation of polonium, cadmium, and mercury.[1,2,84,85] Nevertheless, these agents are not applicable for decontamination of wounds and burns, which is shown by data provided.

White rat experiments have focused on the efficiency of DTPA vs. physiological solution washing of lacerated wounds contaminated by different plutonium compounds.[35] Half of the experimental animals were also given DTPA intravenously in each series of the experiment. The lacerated wound was contaminated by solutions of plutonium nitrate, plutonium citrate, or plutonium dioxide suspension. At minute 30, the wound was washed by 500 ml of 0.8% NaCl solution or mild (0.2%) DTPA solution with 0.9% NaCl solution. The radioactivity in the first 40 ml of washing fluid was measured separately (which amount was considered as the plutonium-239 fraction was mechanically removed from the wound) and another 460 ml was measured thereafter. After the processing, the wound was bandaged and half of the animals were given DTPA (14 mg/kg of body mass) by repeated injections at days 1, 2, 3, and 4.

The analysis of data obtained (Table 28.15) demonstrates some disharmony in the comparison of data on washing fluid radioactivity vs. the residual plutonium in the wound. For example, tests of plutonium nitrate and plutonium citrate have shown the amount of plutonium-239 removed by physiological solution to be higher than that removed by DTPA, which leads to the conclusion that the processing of lacerated wounds with DTPA or physiological solution did not reveal any advantage of one compound over the other as concerns their decontamination effect.

Data analysis of the activity in organs and tissues of animals, which were not given additional intravenous DTPA injections, indicate that plutonium citrate-contaminated wounds washed with physiological solution have shown skeleton burdens of confidently lower levels than those found for wounds decontaminated with DTPA solution. Authors have objected to interpreting the results obtained for plutonium dioxide because of the uncertainty of the data obtained.

A general conclusion is drawn from the apparent predominance of the mechanical decontamination effect vs. the chemical abilities of DTPA when fluid washing is done. This conclusion agrees with other data.[14,66]

At the same time, alternative considerations exist for the importance of DPTA to the decontamination effect. Volf,[89] Schofield,[6,44] Schofield and Junn,[45] and other researchers[9,34] consider DTPA application for topical processing of plutonium-contaminated wounds preferable. Experimental data given above for other radionuclides that are able to bind stable DTPA complexes make it possible to expand the application of this recommendation; moreover, such processing decreases radionuclide body incorporation simultaneously with wound cleaning.[1,2]

One more possible technique for wound treatment must be discussed, namely, the injection of complexing agents, such as DTPA, in tissues surrounding deep puncture wounds contaminated by radionuclides because such cases show low effect from the wound washing technique in applying the decontamination solution. "Surrounding injection" of tissues is directed to create contact of the medicating agent with the radioactive substance for consequent removal of the contaminant by increasing its excretion from the body.[2,32,86]

Experiments in white rats with puncture wounds of intramuscular injection of ^{144}CeCl$_3$ or ^{241}AmCl$_3$ involve administering 5% DTPA solution into tissues surrounding the wound by four injections of a total amount of 1.0 ml 1 h after radioactive contamination.[1,2] Table 28.16 shows that DTPA injections at americium-241 and cerium-144 wound sites were very effective. The radioactivity of tissues dissected at the americium-241 injection site at hour 24 was twofold lower than that in control; the radionuclide burdens in skeleton and liver were decreased by more than 90%. Therefore, it can be concluded that this method of chelate application can provide direct interaction of the chelate and the radionuclide in the contaminated site. However, if deep wounds are contaminated by insoluble radionuclide compounds (including plutonium compounds), the efficiency of DTPA infiltration within the tissues surrounding the wound will be apparently insignificant. This consideration is confirmed by data obtained by clinical observations of injection of DTPA into surrounding tissues for PuO$_2$ contamination of a stab wound in a human finger.[91]

The removal of radioactive substances from wounds using surgical dissection of contaminated tissues has been examined by a number of experiments and clinical studies.[7,9,31,34,44,46] The high effectiveness of this technique of radioactive wound contamination control is mentioned for

TABLE 28.15
Lacerated Wound Decontamination Experiment Results for Different Plutonium Compound Contaminants

^{239}Pu Compound	Processing Scheme	Washing Fluid Activity Ratio to the ^{239}Pu Wound Applied Activity, %		Organ and Tissue Activities at Day 7 (related to ^{239}Pu amount applied), %				
		Total Fluid Amount	Last 460 ml of Fluid	Wound Area	Femur	Liver	Kidneys	Body
Nitrate	Physiological solution washing	4.7 ± 0.84	4.1 ± 1.9					
	Control			82 ± 3.5	0.088 ± 0.008	0.57 ± 0.024	0.029 ± 0.003	2.7 ± 0.18
	DTPA i.v.			73 ± 7.5	0.080 ± 0.005	0.28 ± 0.037	0.022 ± 0.002	3.0 ± 0.57
	DTPA washing	3.1 ± 0.44						
	Control			76 ± 5.8	0.12 ± 0.01	0.59 ± 0.04	0.031 ± 0.002	3.0 ± 0.18
	DTPA i.v.			60 ± 7.5	0.08 ± 0.01	0.31 ± 0.02	0.028 ± 0.003	2.8 ± 0.48
Citrate	Physiological solution washing	46 ± 2.9						
	Control			33 ± 1.2	2.8 ± 0.23	9.1 ± 1.8	0.54 ± 0.04	38 ± 1.8
	DTPA i.v.			30 ± 1.9	1.3 ± 0.28	2.5 ± 0.18	0.241 ± 0.028	22 ± 1.9
	DTPA washing	37 ± 4.3						
	Control			31 ± 1.7	17 ± 0.24	7.4 ± 0.69	0.50 ± 0.054	32 ± 3.9
	DTPA i.v.			36 ± 4.0	0.8 ± 0.017	8.4 ± 0.83	0.29 ± 0.041	19 ± 2.4
Dioxide	Physiological solution washing	3.4 ± 0.7						
	Control			41 ± 5.7	0.006 ± 0.005	0.018 ± 0.008	0.0032 ± 0.0008	0.64 ± 0.20
	DTPA i.v.			90 – 28	0.001 ± 0.0003	0.03–0.013	0.0017–0.0005	1.3 ± 0.38
	DTPA washing	5.5 ± 0.99						
	Control			88 ± 16	0.0010 ± 0.0001	0.016 ± 0.006	0.0012 ± 0.0004	2.0 ± 0.75
	DTPA i.v.			70 ± 17	0.0062 ± 0.004	0.012 ± 0.006	0.0012 ± 0.0005	2.3 ± .81

Source: Adapted from McClanahan, B.J., Kornberg, H.A., in *Diagnosis and Treatment of Deposited Radionuclides, Proc. Symp.*, Richland, WA, 1967.

TABLE 28.16
The Effect of Na$_3$CaDTPA Surrounding Injection of ^{144}Ce and ^{241}Am Injection Site in the Organ Radionuclide Incorporation and Radionuclide Wound Burden Found in Wound at Hour 24 (related to the administered radionuclide amount, %)

Radionuclide Compound	Liver	Ratio to the Control Value	Skeleton	Ratio to the Control Value	Kidneys	Ratio to the Control Value	Wound Surrounding Tissues	Ratio to the Control Value
^{241}AmCl$_3$	0.06 ± 0.1	2.4	0.9 ± 0.1	5.3	0.2 ± 0.2	40.0	22.9 ± 4.7	51.0
^{144}CeCl$_3$	2.3 ± 0.2	4.4	1.7 ± 0.1	5.8	0.5 ± 0.5	67.6	42.1 ± 11.8	52.3

Source: Adapted from Ilyin, L.A., *Basics of the Human Protection against Radioactive Substances*, Atomizdat Publisher, Moscow, 1977.

insoluble and low-solubility radionuclide compounds, especially. It is found that 70 to 90% and more of wound radioactivity can be removed. These evaluations should be accepted as general indications, because each specific case shows the effect of surgical dissection of contaminated wounds is dependent on many factors (kind and physiochemical condition of the radionuclide, injury character, time of the surgery, etc.). It is obvious that the time factor is especially important for surgical aid in cases of radionuclide contaminants of rapid blood uptake (iodine, strontium, cesium, etc.). If tourniquet application is possible in such situations, depending on location and character of the injury, to prevent the blood outflow from the injured area, then surgery (dissection) of the contaminated wound done as a first-aid measure can be quite effective. When comparing effects of surgical treatment of wound (tissue dissection) vs. wound decontamination therapy using different solutions, the higher effectiveness of surgery was recognized by the majority of researchers. Some researchers[14] consider this technique to be approximately 20% more effective than the others. However, possible immediate washing (decontamination) of the wound just after the injury was not taken into account, which is quite different from the surgical technique. Analysis of the original data and available references indicates that both techniques are additive. However, there are some exceptions to this rule. Polonium-210 investigation results have demonstrated an increase in body deposition of radionuclide after application of decontamination-washing techniques using the complex agents unithyol and oxathyol. At the same time, if early surgery (at hour 1) was tried, polonium-210 burdens were strongly decreased in the body (95%) and kidneys (82%) when compared with control animals.

Some remarks should be made concerning the influence of anesthetics in radioactively contaminated wound metabolism. Chromov[80] has mentioned that Novocain does not have any influence on the rate and character of iodine-131 resorption from subcutaneous cellular tissue and muscles and has recommended the local anesthesia of Novocain with the addition of antibiotics as the method of choice for initial wound surgery. Antibiotics are considered to promote radioactive substance removal from wounds as well as to decrease the danger of wound infection.[83] Information exists on a twofold delay of radionuclide substance resorption from the injured site if ether anesthesia is applied.[83,87] Nevertheless, one can suppose that the choice of the technique and the specific means of anesthesia for surgery of wounds and burns contaminated by radioactive substances should not concern the surgeon when analyzing possible influences in radionuclide wound and body metabolism.

DECONTAMINATION OF BURNS CONTAMINATED BY RADIOACTIVE SUBSTANCES

It was mentioned above that radionuclide resorption rate throughout the surface of thermal and chemical burns is similar to that for the radionuclide penetration through intact skin. It follows that major efforts should be directed to decontamination of injured skin when such kinds of trauma are present. Benes[14,105] has applied water, 2% solution of $Na_3CaDTPA$, 3% solution of $Na_2CaEDTA$, and 2% solution of HMP for initial washing of grade III thermal burns contaminated by fission products from a ground nuclear explosion. The early application of chelates has promoted the removal of about 60% of radionuclides from the burn area.

To decontaminate thermal burns of grades II and III from iodine-131 and polonium-210, solutions of soap (3%) and $KMnO_4$ (1.5%) were applied, respectively, as well as 3% soap solution together with subsequent use of 5% unithyol/oxathyol solutions.[2] It was shown that the most effective technique was the application of 3% soap solution: about 80 to 85% of radionuclides were removed at hour 1. Polonium-210 tests have combined complexing agents and the previously mentioned technique, which promoted greater cleaning of the burn area (up to 95%) but increased polonium-210 body deposition (approximately fivefold). Similar to experiments of wound decontamination using oxathyol/unithyol, the creation of soluble complexes in the polonium-210 contact sites, their uptake in the systemic circulation, and subsequent partial deposition in kidneys are the explanations.[1] The investigation[62] established that the application of bandages with Vishnevsky ointment to a grade II thermal burn surface contaminated with a uranium fission product mixture increased the body uptake by two- to threefold.

A few publications[2,64] have focused on the experimental investigation of decontamination of acid burns. White rat skin burns from 1 N and 8 N HNO$_3$ and contaminated by americium-241 have been tested with water, 2% NaHCO$_3$ solution, 3% soap solution, and 5% Na$_3$CaDTPA solution.[2] The control group comprised rats topically exposed to americium-241 in a 0.05 N HNO$_3$ solution. Table 28.17 provides the major results of these studies.

Table 28.17 demonstrates that application of 3% soap solution was very effective in cleaning the chemical area of americium-241 and preventing its incorporation in the body. Loss of cleaning efficiency is related to increases of treatment start time and acid concentration.

Experimental data, including acid burns contaminated by polonium-210, have confirmed the necessity of washing the injured area with alkaline agents, particularly soap solutions.[2] The application of chelating agents, which are able to create stable radionuclide complexes that are not dissociated in the body, is not contraindicated for decontamination of thermal and chemical burns, excluding the cases referred to above.

A number of experimental studies[14,98,99] have found high efficiency (up to 90 to 100%) for traditional surgery of burns of grades II and III, when the burns are dissected. In such cases, the removal of necrotic tissue (blisters, particularly) is strongly indicated, if appropriate precautions are taken.[80,83] However, a number of surgeons have a different attitude concerning the tactics of handling "common" burns noncontaminated by radionuclides. For example, Ariev,[106] in a basic monograph on thermal injuries, presents several pieces of evidence for the advantages of sparing washing of burns and for the inconvenience of opening blisters in cases of grade II burns. One piece of evidence indicates that "most frequent adhesion of grade II burns will occur when blisters persist intact; if they were removed the epithelization of viable tissue is decreased by 40%." It should be stated that in cases of radionuclide-contaminated burns physicians should give primary surgical consideration to treatment of the burn; if it is necessary to open and remove blisters, as well as necrotomy of damaged tissues, specific precautions should be taken to exclude radionuclide contamination of naked surfaces of viable tissues.

ACCELERATION OF BODY EXCRETION OF RADIOACTIVE SUBSTANCES RESORBED IN WOUNDS

When considering the metabolism of radionuclides transferred from blood to the initial compartment, the need to use excretion stimulators is obvious. However, in cases of the "wound" intake pathway, the question of the possible influence of the excretion stimulators, usually applied parenterally, on the behavior of radionuclides situated in the wound should be asked. The tactics of parenteral application of complexing agents in cases of radioactive contamination of wounds have been widely discussed. The subject of this discussion involves possible amplification of radionuclide resorption from the injured area and an increase of the radionuclide accumulation in critical organs, if the complexing agent is prescribed early. Based upon the literature data and specific studies rather than the necessity of the administration of chelates (DTPA, particularly), is justified independently of the initial cleaning of the contaminated wound (tissue dissection or cleaning).

Detailed information summed from many experimental studies devoted to this subject is given in a monograph.[2] The majority of the studies have dealt with the application of chelate polyaminocarbonates (DTPA, particularly) to stimulate body excretion of plutonium, transplutonium elements, and rare earth radionuclides. Recently, results of studies devoted to experimental tests of new ligands — 3,4,3-LI (1,2-HOPO), TREN-(ME-3,2-HOPO), and other hydroxypyridinone derivatives — were published in cases of intramuscular administration of plutonium, americium, thorium, and neptunium.[100–102] These studies, establishing higher effectiveness of these new chelates compared with DTPA, have not yet reached the clinical test phase. Nevertheless, if clinical tests resolve

TABLE 28.17
Skin Decontamination Efficiency after the Topical Application of ^{241}Am HNO$_3$ Solutions of Different Concentrations (% of the applied amount; data at hour 24)

HNO$_3$ Concentration, N	Processing Start Time after ^{241}Am Application	Processing Agents and Schemes	% of ^{241}Am Activity Removed	% of ^{241}Am Activity Resided	^{241}Am Organ Burdens		
					Liver	Kidneys	Skeleton
0.05	5 min	3% soap solution	98.2	1.8 ± 0.5	0.002 ± 0.003	0.000 ± 0.0001	0.004 ± 0.001
0.05	24 h	3% soap solution	91.3	8.7 ± 3.2	0.02 ± 0.008	0.001 ± 0.0007	0.01 ± 0.005
1	5 min	3% soap solution	98.7	1.3 ± 1.3	0.009 ± 0.002	0.002 ± 0.0001	0.009 ± 0.002
1	5 min	Water + 2% NaHCO$_3$ solution, 3% soap solution (at hour 1)	98.3	1.7 ± 0.5	0.04 ± 0.02	0.006 ± 0.002	0.04 ± 0.02
1	5 min	Water + 3% soap solution (at hour 1)	97.6	2.4 ± 0.4	0.05 ± 0.01	0.008 ± 0.01	0.04 ± 0.009
1	5 min	Water + 3% soap solution (at hour 1)[a]	97.6	2.4 ± 0.4	0.03 ± 0.006	0.004 ± 0.001	0.045 ± 0.01
1	24 h	3% soap solution[a]	76.0	24.0 ± 3.6	0.34 ± 0.04	0.03 ± 0.006	0.33 ± 0.06
1	1 h	3% soap solution[a]	87.9	12.1 ± 1.0	0.09 ± 0.02	0.01 ± 0.002	0.09 ± 0.02
1	1 h	3% soap solution + DTPA	82.5	17.5 ± 2.9	0.1 ± 0.03	0.02 ± 0.005	0.1 ± 0.04
1	24 h	3% soap solution	72.1	27.9 ± 4.7	0.09 ± 0.02	0.01 ± 0.001	0.08 ± 0.009
8	5 min	Water + 3% soap solution[a]	85.8	14.2 ± 2.5	0.1 ± 0.03	0.02 ± 0.002	0.2 ± 0.03
8	24 h	3% soap solution[a]	34.7	65.3 ± 8.1	0.5 ± 0.05	0.05 ± 0.006	0.5 ± 0.05

[a] ^{241}Am organ burdens were measured in rats of this group at day 5.

Source: Adapted from Ilyin, L.A. and Ivannikov, A.T., *Radioactive Substances and Wounds (Metabolism and Decorporation,* Atomizdat, Moscow, 1979.

problems of toxicity and sustainability, the practical application of this class of chemical compounds is very promising.

Experimental data verify the dependence of the effectiveness of complexing agents on the scheme and dosage of the agent, the kind of radionuclide, its compound, and the physiochemical state of this compound within the wound and from the character of the injury. An example of DTPA application in a case of a cutaneous muscular wound contaminated by radiocerium shows that a single administration of this ligand at minute 30 after ^{144}CeCl$_3$ application results in a decrease of liver incorporation (up to 80%), but it did not influence radionuclide deposition in the skeleton of white rats. At the same time, multiple DTPA administrations started at hour 4 and continued for 9 days provided a highly protective effect in organs of major deposition[1] (Table 28.18).

TABLE 28.18
^{144}Ce Burdens in Liver and Skeleton of White Rats after Parenteral DTPA Administration in Case of Cutaneous Muscular Wound Radionuclide Contamination (percents of applied amount of radionuclide)

DTPA Administration Scheme	Time of Examination, day	Liver	Ratio to the Control Value	Skeleton	Ratio to the Control Value
Single administration at minute 30	1	0.04 ± 0.007	19	0.42 ± 0.07	—
Control		0.21 ± 0.12	—	0.45 ± 0.09	—
Single administration at hour 4 after contamination and daily administration within 9 days	14	0.09 ± 0.05	2.7	1.19 ± 0.50	22.2
Control		3.26 ± 0.47	—	5.35 ± 0.72	—

Note: Na$_3$CaDTPA was administered intraperitoneally at a dose of 500 μmol. Wound decontamination was not applied.

The multivariant study of DTPA treatment efficiency after intramuscular administration of different compounds of curium-242, americium-241, californium-252, and einsteinium-253 in white rats has given results demonstrating the importance of factors of time, agent dosage, frequency of administration, and site and method of chelate administration.[28] Similar to the previous work,[1] DTPA has been administered to rats for continuous radionuclide resorption from the initial compartment (muscular tissue) (Table 28.19). In all cases, DTPA administration promoted a decrease in actinide incorporation in the skeleton, which is one of the major organs of transplutonium element deposition. Obviously, early chelate topical injection at the site of intramuscular radionuclide administration was most effective; DTPA inhalation administration was less effective than parenteral administration (predominantly due to the lower dosage of the agent). Naturally, addition of surgical excision of a puncture wound greatly reduces radiation doses in the skeleton and the whole body.

If one concludes that parenteral administration of DTPA and other chelates at any time after wound contamination by radioactive substances will cause these ligands to bind into stable soluble complexes, which are nondissociable in the body, that treatment is justified as well as clinically substantiated for the majority of cases (see below). There are other complexing agents and radionuclides whose action has not yet been finally judged. For example, Zotova[103] has referred to work of Izorgina,[104] where a single injection of unithyol resulted in almost complete uptake (86%) of polonium-210 from a subcutaneous injection site. This finding contraindicates administration of this complexing agent before surgical excision of contaminated tissues, but its administration is recommended after surgical treatment.

TABLE 28.19
DTPA Application Efficiency in Case of Intramuscular Actinide Administration in Rats

Compound	Observation Period, days	DTPA Therapy					Radionuclide Bone Burden (related to the control value), %
		Time of the Therapy Start (after the radionuclide administration)	Number of Treatments	DTPA Dosage per One Treatment, mmol/kg	Total DTPA Dosage, mmol/kg	DTPA Administration Pathway	
$^{242}Cm(NO_3)_3$	1	Minute 30	1	0.12	0.12	Intramuscular in the radionuclide administration site	3.6
$^{242}Cm(NO_3)_3$	20	Days 1, 5, 10, 15	4	0.12	0.48	Intramuscular but to the intact extremity	12
	42	Day 21, 2 times/week	6	0.12	0.72		45
	81	Day 21, 2 times/week	16	0.12	1.92		50
	111	Day 21, 2 times/week	24	0.12	2.88		35
$^{241}Am(NO_3)_3$	10	Days 1 and 7	2	0.12	0.24	Intramuscular but to the intact extremity	21
	90	Day 1, 1 time/week	13	0.12	0.565	Inhalation	24
	10	Days 1 and 7	2	0.0012	0.0024		84
$^{241}Am(SO_4)_3$	90	Day 1, 1 time/week	13	0.12	1.56	Intramuscular but to the intact extremity	13
$^{253}Es(NO_3)_3$	21	Hour 1, days 1–3, 5, 7, 9, 12, 15, 17	10	0.33	3.3	Intraperitoneal	42.3
^{241}Am citrate	4	Hour 2, days 1–3	4	0.11	0.44	Intraperitoneal	34
	14	2 h, days 1–4, 7–11	10	0.11	1.10		34
^{252}Cf citrate	4	Hour 2, days 1–3	4	0.11	0.44	Intraperitoneal	46
	14	Hour 2, days 1–4, 7–11	10	0.11	1.10		38.5
^{252}Es citrate	1	Hour 2	1	0.11	0.11	Intraperitoneal	76.5
	4	Hour 2, days 1–3	4	0.11	0.44		68.5
	14	Hour 2, days 1–4, 7–11	10	0.11	1.10		50

Source: Adapted from Scott, K.G. et al., *J. Biol. Chem.*, 176, 283, 1948.

Reference 2 evaluates different variants of oxathyol application in puncture and cutaneous muscular wounds of white rats contaminated by polonium-210. In particular, it states that the duration of the application of this complexing agent is of major importance in obtaining effective treatment for puncture wounds contaminated by polonium-210. If the agent is applied for a short term (3 to 7 days), the kidney burden of polonium-210 was 1.6 to 5 times higher than that in the control, while the burdens in whole body, liver, and spleen were decreased. However, if the term of administration was prolonged to 2 weeks (two injections of 100 mg/kg each per day), a 50% decrease in polonium-210 kidney burden was achieved compared with the control value. It is necessary to stress that this experimental model was not "aggravated" by surgical wound treatment.

Table 28.20 provides the results of applying topical oxathyol and surgical treatment to cutaneous muscular wounds contaminated by polonium-210 in rats. Comparison of these data leads to the conclusion that the combination of surgical wound treatment and parenteral oxathyol renders significantly poorer results than surgical dissection of contaminated tissues alone. For example, polonium-210 kidney burden found at hour 24 after the wound dissection was 5.7 times lower than that in the control, and this burden was ten times less than that when oxathyol was also applied.

The available experimental data are not sufficient to form straightforward recommendations as yet. However, one can conclude an absence of benefits of short-term application of oxathyol (and, apparently, other chelates) combined with early surgical treatment of cutaneous muscular wounds, as is clear for the prophylaxis of polonium-210 incorporation, if the combined treatment is compared with results using surgical treatment alone. At the same time, one can also conclude that long-term parenteral oxathyol application with thorough clinical and dosimetric monitoring is indicated, if the surgical dissection of a polonium-210-contaminated wound is impossible or if surgery is delayed for a long time.

TABLE 28.20
Radioactivity Burdens in Organs and Tissues of White Rats after the Surgical Treatment and Oxathyol Administration in ^{210}Po-Contaminated Cutaneous Muscular Wounds (related to the applied radionuclide amount, %)

Test Scheme	Trunk M ± m	Trunk Related to Control Value (%)	Kidneys M ± m	Kidneys Related to Control Value (%)	Whole-Body Burden M ± m	Whole-Body Burden Related to Control Value (%)
Cutaneous muscular wound dissection	0.38 ± 0.08	5.2	0.3 ± 0.05	17.6	0.71 ± 0.06	7.7
Dissection + parenteral oxathyol	0.72 ± 0.20	9.9	4.3 ± 0.4	253	5.0 ± 1.5	54
Oxathyol topical application, dissection, oxathyol injections	0.77 ± 0.18	10.5	3.6 ± 0.8	212	4.4 ± 0.8	48
Control	7.3 ± 1.8	—	1.7 ± 0.1	—	9.2 ± 1.9	—

Notes: 1. Tissue dissection at hour 1 after the wound application of ^{210}Po nitrate; subcutaneous oxathyol injection immediately after the dissection and at hour 3; oxathyol wound treatment was done just before the dissection. 2. Data are given for hour 24 after ^{210}Po wound contamination.

Source: Adapted from Ilyin, L.A. and Ivannikov, A.T., *Radioactive Substances and Wounds (Metabolism and Decorporation,* Atomizdat Publisher, Moscow, 1979.

Finally, one can conclude that peroral, inhalation, topical, or parenteral administration of medications to prevent radionuclide incorporation and to increase excretion of radionuclides is necessary. This conclusion is applicable for any type of prophylactic measures applied topically to the injured area at any time after radionuclide wound contamination. Availability of treatment by chelation should be included in planning for first-aid and emergency medical care. For example, after radioiodine contamination of a cutaneous muscular wound in rats, the peroral administration of stable iodine agent (KI) at minutes 5 and 30 reduces the uptake of iodine-131 in the thyroid gland to 0.8 to 1.6% at hour 24. In comparison, 46 to 48% of iodine-131 activity was found in the thyroid of control animals at the same time. Topical application of 5% iodine tincture in skin abrasions contaminated by this radionuclide was similarly effective, so this simple treatment can be recommended for microtraumas and small traumas of skin contaminated by iodine radionuclides.[2,97]

At present, no effective decorporation agents have been tested clinically for radionuclides of groups I and II of the periodic table (cesium, rubidium, thallium, strontium, barium, lanthanium, radium[1]); therefore, oral administration of selective sorbents is indicated to limit the resorption of these radionuclides in the intestinal tract in cases where wound intake is combined with inhalation of radionuclides. Compounds of the ferric/ferrocyanide class (Prussian Blue, Ferrocyne) are the proper agents for radioactive isotopes of cesium and rubidium, while alginic acid preparations, highly oxidized cellulose, or polyantimonyl are applicable for radiostrontium, barium, or lanthanum wound contamination.[1] Obviously, all such cases need to be considered for such factors as start time, dosages, and duration of agent application. Detailed procedures for application of such agents to contaminated wounds are given in the literature.[2,3,79,92–97]

EXPERIENCE WITH HUMAN WOUNDS AND BURNS CONTAMINATED BY RADIOACTIVE SUBSTANCES

Radiation medicine has had some experience with human wounds and burns contaminated by radioactive substances. The majority of observations relate to plutonium-contaminated wounds. More than 90% of known cases are finger wounds inflicted by sharp articles while the victim is handling radioactive materials. These wounds are predominantly punctures or cuts; in some cases, they are rather deep (with tendon and periosteum involvement). Analysis of literature data indicates that medical care for such injuries consists of surgical treatment (excision) of the wound and administration of complexing agents to prevent resorption of the radionuclide into the systemic blood circulation and deposition into other organs. For a general impression of the efficiency of these measures, see Table 28.21, which sums up the basic results of observations available in the medical literature. It should be noted that some cases were published several times in different versions as a result of corrections in the radiometric data and extension of the observation period of the patient.

Table 28.21 illustrates that wound surgery to excise tissues contaminated by radioactive substances is the one of most effective ways of contamination removal and prophylaxis of body intake. According to data of different authors this procedure (repeated in some cases) provides a strong reduction of wound contamination of plutonium and americium.

Data given in Reference 44 illustrate this aspect and generally compare wound excision and chelate (DTPA) effect on the increasing the excretion of plutonium in wounds (Table 28.22). Three cases of wound contamination of different plutonium compounds show the effectiveness as follows: 91% (PuO_2), 99.8% ($Pu(NO_3)_4$), and 99.96% (metal plutonium). Analysis of other cases shown in Table 28.21 also demonstrates the effect of decontamination by wound excision. However, to provide high radionuclide removal with the procedure, the authors were forced to make repeated excisions in some cases. For example, the case described in Reference 48 had four sequential excisions, which removed 99% of the radioactivity in the wound. In some cases (particularly deep stab wounds) the surgery was less effective. For example, References 45 and 46 report that surgical

TABLE 28.21
Summary Data on Victim Treatment (wounds contaminated by radioactive substances)

Radionuclide	Compound	Agent	Application Time	Administration Route	Administration Schedule	Single Dosage, g	Integral Dosage, g	Treatment Results: Urine Excretion Acceleration, Times	Additional Information	Ref.
^{239}Pu	Nitrate	EDTA	Day 3	i.v.	Two daily injections (days 1–4 and 7–18)	2.5	80	100	Wound tissue excision was done before EDTA therapy. Radionuclide excretion acceleration for 100 times was found at the end of therapy day 1. EDTA administration termination caused the strong delay of radionuclide excretion. Pathological symptoms were found at day 11: albumins, parenchymal cells, erythrocytes and leukocytes were found in urine. Headache and nausea complains. Radionuclide body burden was 0.5 MPa.	108
^{239}Pu	Nitrate	DTPA	Hour 9	i.v.	Daily injections within 5 days	1.0	—	50—100	First dissection of finger wound was done at hour 2 after the incident. After the second dissection 222 Bq (0.006 µCi) remained. Initial ^{239}Pu body burden was assessed to be 1.3 kBq (0.035 µCi). Excretion efficiency (~37%) is given by author with relation to initial deposition. Maximum radionuclide urine excretion amplification was found at DTPA therapy day 1.	9
			Day 51	i.v.	Daily injections within 5 days	3.0	12	—		
			Days 52–55	i.v.	Daily injections within 5 days	1.0	—	—		
^{239}Pu	Nitrate	DTPA	Hour 9	i.v.	Once per day	1.0	28	70	After two dissections 237 Bq (0.0064 µCi) remained. During the therapy 70 times excretion was found for days 51–54, 79, 81, 83 if related to the previous level.	109
			Days 3-6	i.v.	Twice per day	1.0				
			Day 15	i.v.	Twice per day	3.0				
			Days 51–54	i.v.	Twice per day	1.0				
			Days 79, 81, 83	i.v.	Twice per day	1.0				
			Days 98–105	i.v.	Twice per day	1.0				

Radionuclide	Form	Chelator	Time	Route	Injection	Dose 1	Dose 2	Dose 3	Comments	Ref.
239Pu	Metal	DTPA	Hour 1.2	i.v.	Single injection	1.0	—	—	After the removal of metal plutonium debris of 3.1 MBq (83 μCi) from the index finger wound 126 kBq (3.4 μCi) were found in the wound before dissection and 0.5 kBq (0.014 μCi) after the dissection. Within day 1 after the accident 137 Bq (3690 pCi) of 239Pu was excreted, which was equal to 75% of radionuclide eliminated by DTPA within 40 days.	45
			Hour 24	i.v.	Single injection	1.0	—	—		
			Days 4–14	i.v.	Single injection	0.25	4.25	—		
239Pu, 241Am	Mixture of oxide and nitrate	DTPA	Days 1–4	i.v.	Single injection	0.25	—	—	Deep stab wound of finger. 28.6 kBq (0.773 μCi) of 239Pu was found in wound before the dissection and 5.4 kBq (0.147 μCi) of 239Pu after dissection (~19%). Analysis of 239Pu urine excretion curve has concluded to the absence of any significant influence of DTPA in 239Pu body excretion.	45
						0.1	0.55	—		
						0.1	—	—		
						0.1	—	—		
239Pu	Oxide	DTPA	Hour 11	i.v.	Single injection	0.25	0.55	—	Stab wound of fourth finger of the right hand. After washing with water and soap the surgery was tried at hour 11 and DTPA therapy was started immediately thereafter. Initial 239Pu wound burden was 37 kBq (1 μCi) and 3.3 kBq (90 nCi) was found after the dissection. ~740 Bq (20 nCi) was removed from the body and 1.1 kBq (30 nCi) remained.	44
			Days 1–3	i.v.	Single injection	0.1	—	—		
239Pu	Nitrate	DTPA	Minute 30	i.v.	Single injection	1.0	—	—	Incised wound of soft tissue of the distal phalanx of the third finger of left hand. After water and soap washing, the intravenous droplet DTPA injection was done at minute 30. Wound surgery was tried at hour 9. 37 kBq (~1 μCi) of 239Pu was found in wound before processing and 74 Bq (2.0 nCi) was found after dissection. Residual body burden is 1.1 kBq (30 nCi). 239Pu total amount excreted by DTPA is 148 Bq (4 nCi).	44
			Hour 9	i.v.	Single injection	0.4	—	—		
			Days 1–10	i.v.	Six injections	0.25	3.9	30–40 at days 10–15		
			Day 14	i.v.	Single injection	1.0	—	—		

TABLE 28.21 (CONTINUED)
Summary Data on Victim Treatment (wounds contaminated by radioactive substances)

Radionuclide	Compound	Agent	Application Time	Administration Route	Administration Schedule	Single Dosage, g	Integral Dosage, g	Treatment Results: Urine Excretion Acceleration, Times	Additional Information	Ref.
^{239}Pu and ^{241}Am traces	Chloride, dioxide	DTPA	Hour 1	i.v.	Single injection	1.0	—	—	Wound was treated surgically. 274 kBq (7.4 µCi) of ^{239}Pu was excreted at first 60 days and 22.2 kBq (0.6 µCi) was excreted at next 66 days. Authors refer to high efficiency of DTPA. Quantitative characteristics of the agent effect are not provided.	111
			Hour 3.5	i.v.	Single injection	1.0	—	—		
			Days 3–5	i.v.	Twice per day	1.0	62	—		
			Days 6–18	i.v.	Once per day	1.0	—	—		
			Days 22–50	i.v.	Once per day	1.0	—	—		
			Days 51–78	i.v.	Once per week	1.0	—	—		
			Days 79–113	i.v.	3 times per week	1.0	—	—		
			Days 114–148	i.v.	3 times per week	0.33	—	—		
^{239}Pu	Monoxide					—	—	—	Incised wound of finger. Initial contamination of 3.9 kBq (106 nCi). After the wound washing 2.4 kBq (65 nCi) was found at minute 55. Surgery has decreased the burden to 259 Bq (7 nCi). ^{239}Pu excretion stimulation was not tried.	112
^{239}Pu and ^{241}Am	Mixture of oxide and nitrate	DTPA (see [45])	—	—	—	—	—	—	Deep stab wound of finger (bone surface involved). 29.2 kBq (0.79 µCi) and 5.6 kBq (0.15 µCi) of alpha activity were found before and after the wound dissection (80% decrease). ^{239}Pu and ^{241}Am body burden was 0.44 kBq (0.012 µCi). The initial amount of radioactivity blood uptake was 67 Bq (0.0018 µCi). 3.3–3.7 kBq (0.09–0.10 µCi) of ^{39}Pu and 148–370 Bq (0.004–0.01 µCi) of ^{241}Am have been resorbed to the blood and deposited in the body at day 695. The total wound resorption of ^{239}Pu and ^{241}Am intake is 2.3%.	46, 45

Nuclide	Form	Agent	Dose	Timing	Route			Notes	Ref.
^{241}Am		EDTA, zirconium citrate	4 g per day	Zirconium citrate was tried twice		—	—	EDTA amplified ^{241}Am excretion 2 times if compared to periods when the agent was not administered. Zirconium citrate had no effect.	Referred from 57
^{241}Am ^{239}Pu	Mixture of oxide and nitrate	DTPA	Dosage and administration rhythm are not given.			—	—	DTPA administration resulted in the increase of radionuclide excretion.	Referred from 57
^{239}Pu	Monoxide	DTPA		Day 1	i.v.	1.0	81	Shoulder wound. Initial wound contamination was 1.3 MBq (36 μCi) (+ 263 MBq, 7100 μCi, as the piece of metal plutonium). After four sequential dissections 11.8 kBq (0.32 μCi) remained in wound. Thereafter, the wound was washed by 4 l of 0.1% solution of Na$_4$DTPA (the remained activity was ~5.9 kBq (~0.16 μCi, 50% of initial one). At day 4 the wound activity has decreased to 2.6 kBq (0.07 μCi). ^{239}Pu body burden was assessed to be 8.1 kBq (0.22 μCi). Authors^{12} suppose that DTPA has resulted in the removal of 60% of the initial activity of ^{239}Pu.	48, 31
				3 times per week within 50 weeks with intervals					
^{241}Am	Perchlorate	DTPA		Day 1	i.v.	0.5		Stabbed incised wound of finger. The wound was covered by bandage of adhesive bactericidical plaster. ^{241}Am initial wound contamination was ~ 9.3 kBq (~250 nCi) and it was 1.65 kBq (44.5 nCi) after the surgery. Second dissection has decreased the wound radioactivity to 0.14 kBq (3.8 nCi) (~1.5% of the initial level). Wound washing with water and DTPA was ineffective. After the third dissection the wound activity was 28 Bq (0.75 nCi). The paper does not provide the quantitative evaluation of DTPA efficiency for stimulation of ^{241}Am body excretion.	66
								At day 1 the strong amplification of ^{241}Am excretion was found; at days 13–15 ten times amplification was found.	
				Day 12	i.v.	0.5			
^{239}Pu O$_2$	Ceramics	DTPA		Minute 90	i.v.	1.0	1.0	Finger wound processed with DTPA. Initial contamination was 4.4 kBq (120 nCi) and 7 Bq (0.2 nCi) remained after the surgery. Whole-body burden was 19 Bq (0.5 nCi). Authors considered DTPA ineffective for enhancing excretion of insoluble nuclide compound.	113

TABLE 28.21 (CONTINUED)
Summary Data on Victim Treatment (wounds contaminated by radioactive substances)

Radionuclide	Compound	Agent	Treatment Scheme					Treatment Results: Urine Excretion Acceleration, Times	Additional Information	Ref.
			Application Time	Administration Route	Administration Schedule	Single Dosage, g	Integral Dosage, g			
238Pu	Nitrate	DTPA	Day 1	i.v.	Single injection	1.0	—	—	Stab wound of hand. 0.0055 µCi of ^{239}Pu was found in the wound after the surgery. 0.031 µCi body burden was assessed. DTPA and EDTA efficiency data are indirect; 35-fold increase in the nuclide excretion has been observed at the first period of therapy. Patient did not complain about the length of DTPA therapy, with 943 days of therapy (intervals existed).	110
			Day 2	i.v.	Single injection	1.0	—	35		
			Days 4–19	i.v.	4 times/week	1.0	—	—		
		EDTA	Days 20–30	i.v.	4 times/day	0.335	13.4	—		
		DTPA	Days 31–47	i.v.	4 times/week	—	—	—		
			Days 61–82	i.v.	4 times/week	1.0	—	—		
			Days 312–597	i.v.	4 times/week	1.0	56.35	—		
			Days 4–82	i.v.	4 times/week	—	—	—		
			Days 452–597	Inhalation	4 times/week	1.0	—	—		
			Days 598–943	Inhalation	Two days in a row per month		—	—		

TABLE 28.22
Wound Surgery and DTPA Body Elimination of ^{239}Pu

Pu Compound	Initial Wound Burden, kBq	Time Passed Before the Wound Dissection, min	Pu amount in Wound after Surgery, kBq	DTPA Therapy Start Time, min	Pu amount Excreted by DTPA, Bq	Residual Amount of Pu in the Body, kBq
PuO$_2$	37	690	3.3	690	0.74	1.1
Pu(NO$_3$)$_4$	37	540	0.074	30	148	1.1
Pu metal	185	140	0.074	75	185	0.74

Source: Adapted from Schofield, G.B., in *Handling of Radiation Accidents, Proc. Symp.*, Vienna, 1969.

removal of plutonium-239 and americium-241 from a deep stab wound reduced the radionuclide burden by only 20% of the initial value.

In the majority of cases described, wound excision was preceded by cleaning of surrounding healthy tissues with water and soap or with other neutral means. In one case,[60] the wound was covered with a waterproof bandage of bactericidical plaster and intact skin was decontaminated with NaEDTA solution. Sodium hypochlorite solution is also reported to be applied for cleaning plutonium from tissues surrounding wounds.[114]

Adsorbents were not used in any of the cases described, which is apparently related to both the trauma peculiarities and to the presence of insoluble compounds of plutonium and americium. Unfortunately, in those cases where a cotton-gauze bandage was applied, the quantitative data showing the sorbing effect of the bandage is not given (for example, see Reference 47). Reference 115 evaluates the amount of plutonium-239 in the bandage material. After the first surgery, 381.5 kBq of plutonium-239 oxalate remained in the wound. The wound activity measured before the second surgery had decreased to 285 kBq; at the same time 16.7 kBq of plutonium-239 was found in the bandage. The radioactivity retained on the plutonium-239-absorbed bandage was about 17% in this case.

The subject of wound cleaning using specific decontamination agents or conventional sterile preparations for routine surgery and wound cleansing is insufficiently described in the available literature; the existing data are discordant. In case of plutonium oxide contamination, washing the wound with water and soap (including mechanical cleaning with a brush) has little effect.[44,108,112] After an excision of a wound contaminated by americium-241 the subsequent washing with antiseptics and 10% DTPA solution did not significantly reduce wound activity.[31]

Norwood and Fuqua[31] propose the immediate washing of contaminated wounds with DTPA solution, dilute hydrochloric acid and water, if the condition of the wound permits this procedure.

According to Reference 48, the application of 4 l of a 0.1% Na$_4$DTPA solution after four surgeries on a shoulder wound contaminated with plutonium metal was relatively effective. Wound activity decreased by 50% of the initial value recorded after the fourth surgery.

Analysis of the literature devoted to the treatment of wounds contaminated by plutonium and americium show that DTPA is almost always given to control body incorporation of these nuclides. Materials provided by Table 28.21 lead to the conclusion that this complexing agent has promoted the elimination of significant amounts of nuclide; a number of observations indicate moderate DTPA efficiency and a few cases have not demonstrated an effective response to DTPA. Apparently, the causes for different DTPA experiences in chelation of plutonium and americium are explained by two factors: (1) the physiochemical state of the nuclide within the wound and (2) the extent of injury, including its character and the scope of vascular damage.[6,9] The latter circumstance determines the quantity, rate, and duration of blood uptake of the radioactive substance and, therefore, its "availability" for chelation. Thus, the opinion[116] expressed that effective DTPA therapy depends on the quantity of plutonium in the blood rather than on the quantity of the nuclide found in the wound is valid.

Analysis of available clinical data does not lead to a straightforward conclusion regarding the DTPA therapy effectiveness vs. peculiarities of the physiochemical state of the plutonium in wounds. One significant impression is that DTPA effectiveness is higher in wounds contaminated with soluble plutonium compounds (nitrates and oxalates). It was also demonstrated that, in some cases of wound contamination with mixed forms (nitrates and oxides) of plutonium-239, DTPA therapy was ineffective. At the same time (see Table 28.21), in cases of wounds contaminated with plutonium-239, a clear amplification of nuclide excretion induced by DTPA was observed. Reference 7 suggests that an insignificant portion of plutonium metal in wounds is transferred to an ionic form, which becomes available for chelation after the blood uptake. In this case the duration of the blood uptake of the ionic form of metal (and, therefore, the time of its "dissolution" in wound) was longer than that for plutonium nitrate.

SUMMARY: CONTROL OF RADIOACTIVE CONTAMINATION OF WOUNDS AND BURNS

Medical measures applied for radioactive wound contamination should be multiple and should assure removal of radioactive substances from the injured area while increasing their excretion from the body.

Because of the relatively low rates of radioactive substance resorption from thermal and chemical burns, medical care should focus on prophylaxis of local radiation exposure by removal of radioactive substances from the injured area.[10,60]

To decontaminate wounds, the following techniques can be applied: surgical excision of contaminated tissues, processing (washing) of the injured area with neutral and specific solutions, and sequential tampon and bandage applications including bandages moistened with soluble ion-exchange compounds. In all other similar conditions, the most effective technique of wound decontamination consists of surgical dissection of tissues, which removes more than 90% of radioactive wound contaminant in some cases. The other techniques listed above provide about a twofold decrease in the local radioactivity.

These quantitative assessments are approximate and depend upon (1) the character and kind of radioactive contamination, (2) the kind of injury, and (3) the time elapsed since the wound occurred. Obviously, the wide range of combinations of these three basic factors excludes formulation of a template of tactics and specific methods for medical care.

In the framework of these considerations, it seems necessary to draw specific attention to how the factor of time influences the effectiveness of first-aid and emergency care measures. If the wound is contaminated by radioactive substances with a high resorption rate, first aid (including tourniquet application) given in first few minutes will be more effective in preventing uptake of the contaminant than excision of tissues, which can be done later. Along with this consideration, if the wound is contaminated by slowly resorbed radionuclides, then surgical excision of tissues done several hours after the incident can provide effective removal of wound contaminants.

The application of washing techniques to clean contaminated wounds may also promote increase in radionuclide uptake. One might suppose that solutions of compounds able to provide better decontamination may also promote an increase in the systemic uptake of the radionuclides. These compounds, which bind radionuclides into stable, nondissociable, soluble complexes within the body, are unconditionally indicated for wound decontamination. In such cases, the elevation of radiation dose rates in the short term during the transportation of radionuclides throughout the internal media of the organism will be completely compensated for by the decrease in the levels of their eventual cumulative incorporation in organs and tissues; therefore, the absorbed dose will be greatly decreased.

Parenteral administration of such compounds to prevent radionuclide incorporation in the body should be done at the earliest time possible after radioactive contamination and are independent of other wound decontamination efforts.

A number of problems for radiation medicine in the area of wound contamination remain unsolved. There are insufficient data on the metabolism of radionuclides of both individual chemical elements and groups of chemical elements of the periodic table. The metabolism of radioactively contaminated burns has been poorly investigated, especially chemical burns from concentrated acids. The existing state of the art reflects a dearth of experimental evaluations of the effectiveness of different techniques and means of decontaminating wounds and burns, as well as prophylaxis of the incorporation of corresponding radionuclides in the body.

A need exists for experimental investigation of the best means to manage radionuclides incorporated in regional lymph nodes. One possibility is performing a lymphadenectomy to remove insoluble plutonium compounds in nodes as proposed in Reference 117. Information on the biological effects from radiation due to wound intakes is insufficient.[2,40] Together with the investigation of the pathophysiological aspects of the influence of radiation on wound healing, the data on follow-up health effects of the incorporated radionuclides are of special future interest. The discussion of this problem is beyond the scope of this chapter, but this information is integral to understanding of the consequences and the need for treatment of radionuclide incorporation in the body.

THE PRACTICE AND PROCEDURES OF MEDICAL CARE OF SKIN WOUNDS AND BURNS CONTAMINATED BY RADIOACTIVE SUBSTANCES

BACKGROUND

The control of radioactive contamination of skin wounds and burns is an important medical aspect of protecting humans from ionizing radiation exposure.

A number of monographs, manuals, and recommendations have been published on the subjects of decontamination and therapy of personnel in cases of internal radionuclide contamination, including radioactive contamination of skin injuries (see References 1, 2, 79, 92–97, for example). The report, "Recommendations on Medical Care of Traumas Contaminated by Radioactive Substances," was published in Russia specifically for local medical facilities located near atomic industry facilities and other institutions that have contact with radioactive material.[97]

These recommendations particularly emphasize that "the wound surfaces of soft tissues, burns and other skin injuries are one of most hazardous pathways of intake of radioactive substance into the body. Any skin injury occurring in persons working with radioactive materials is suspected to be potentially contaminated by radioactive substances."

The organization and tactics of the care of each specific case are determined by many circumstances. For example, to make a decision on the scope of care at the time of rescue of victims, one should take the following into account:

1. The accident (incident) peculiarities, the number of victims, the general characteristics of the radiation accident, and its specific location;
2. The status of victim(s), kind and localization of injury, the availability of means of emergency care and individual protection at the site;
3. The possibility of rapid assessment of the character and level of radiation exposure, the radionuclide content, and the amount and physicochemical state of radioactive material contaminating the wound and body surface;

4. The availability of a specialized decontamination room and a local dispensary equipped with necessary devices and dosimetric instruments;
5. The distance from this room to the accident location, as well the distance to a specialized medical facility.

Transportation time is one factor that determines the time delay before specific treatment.

Three major phases of medical care can be specified as follows: (1) care at the accident site (first aid), (2) medical care at the local medical facility of the nuclear facility (paramedical care and physician assistance), and (3) in-patient medical care (qualified medical assistance).

CARE AT THE ACCIDENT SITE

Proper and timely first aid at or near in the accident site (including self-assistance and colleague assistance provided before the arrival of medical staff and safety service personnel) significantly determines the effectiveness of medical care provided at later periods. The considerations explained previously show the obvious great importance of a fast response time in such cases when the wound contaminants include rapidly resorbed or slowly metabolized radionuclides suitable for chelating into soluble compounds.

It is clear that the radiometry of wounds and burns and the dosimetry of the incorporated radionuclides are the obligatory elements of measures to be taken in accidents like this. However, the actual accident situation dictates the application of these measures according to specific circumstances of the accident. Actually, experience indicates that the emergency measures by self-assistance and colleague assistance to treat wounds and burns should not be postponed while collecting data on the character and levels of contamination. This is especially important for alpha-emitting radionuclides. The organization and elaboration of such measurements takes some time even if adequate dosimetric equipment is available; if treatment is delayed, the major portion of radionuclides can be transferred into blood and lymph systems.*

All radiation workers should be trained on the behavior (immediate termination of work, reporting on the accident, etc.) and skills necessary for first aid of wounds and burns. The importance of education concerning the danger of radioactive contamination of wounds and burns, which are frequently ignored by workers, should be stressed.**

Generally, the goal of self-assistance and colleague assistance consists of the application of simple measures to remove radioactive material and to limit its uptake from wounds and burn surfaces. This goal can be fulfilled by (1) mechanical removal of contaminants from the injury site (for example, using intensive water washing if a decontaminating solution is not available), (2) nonspecific absorption of radionuclide using gauze tampon or any other bandaging material, and (3) applying a tourniquet to create venous stagnation around the wound, if wound localization permits (a tourniquet should not be applied for skin burns).

Simple and available means to provide first aid should be in each workplace, at the site where radiation work is done. First-aid equipment should include a rubber tourniquet with a surgical

---

* Generally, there is no single template for the medical emergency care of radiation accidents. For example, for a radiation accident resulting in intensive beta/gamma exposure to victims and to radioactive contamination of injured and intact skin, the priorities and sequence of medical staff actions should be predominantly determined by the severity and prognosis of the major factor of the combined radiation injury (total-body beta/gamma dose). One practical example is the hospital admission of personnel and firefighters from the Chernobyl accident, who had high levels of radioactive contamination of the intact skin. All standards of medical care require radioactive decontamination before hospital admission. However, the severe status of the majority of victims and the expressed symptoms of the initial reaction to the intensive total-body exposure forced the clinicians of the radiation medicine department of the Institute of Biophysics (Moscow, Russia) to object to time delays for decontamination procedures at the emergency room and to apply these procedures later, when the basic medical activities for the major disease were finished.[123]
** Personnel at radiation operations should be provided with regular monitoring of radioactivity and integrity of skin (especially hands and forearms).

clamp, sterile bandaging packages, and containers with solutions for decontamination and neutralization. These containers should be placed near a source of tap water.

The application of a venous tourniquet is one first-aid measure that is applicable during the first 30 minutes even if subsequent dosimetric measurements and assessments show that it, in fact, was not necessary.

If the character of the accident and the victim status permit, the initial decontamination of a wound should be done after tourniquet application and a 3- to 5-min washing of the injury using tap water or a decontaminating solution. A 2 to 5% solution of $Na_3CaDTPA$ chelate should be used for contamination by radionuclides of alkaline elements, rare earth elements, and actinides. The application of bandages and tampons after a 5 min washing does not prevent wound uptake of the radionuclide, but it decreases its magnitude due to nonspecific adsorption.

In cases of skin contaminated by concentrated acid or alkali solutions, the major task is to prevent or mitigate the chemical effects of the acid or alkali on skin. Initial treatment consists of abundant flushing of the contaminated area with water and washing with a 3% soap solution, a 2 to 3% $NaHCO_3$ solution for acids, or a 3% boric acid or 10% sodium hexametaphosphate solution. Obviously, these procedures are predominantly directed mitigation of the damaging effects of acids and alkalis. Thermal burns should not be decontaminated at the incident site, but simply covered with sterile bandage.

After first-aid measures are completed, the victim should be transported to the decontamination room, where the clothes are removed and the injured area is covered by a waterproof material; depending upon the victim's condition, partial or complete decontamination should be continued with radiological monitoring.

MEDICAL CARE AT THE LOCAL MEDICAL FACILITY

In a number of cases the local medical facilities are not able to implement the full scheme of medical care, including surgery, for radiation injury. As a rule, only conservative therapy can be provided at this primary medical care facility. Surgery can be performed in some cases only if general revision of the wound needs be done or necrotic tissue and foreign bodies can be removed. Apart from this, stabilization of the patient's vital signs should be done here according to normal medical practice. The status of tetanus immunization should be checked and tetanus vaccine administered, if necessary.

In the framework of conservative therapy, the intravenous injection of 10.0 ml of 5% $Na_3CaDTPA$ solution should be given, if indicated (for example, if plutonium or transplutonium wound contaminants are present). If the wound is contaminated by radioactive iodine, one tablet of sodium iodide (0.25 g) should be administered orally to prevent iodine deposition in the thyroid gland and 3 to 4 g of Ferrocyne or other preparations of ferricoferrocyanides should be administered orally in case of radioactive cesium contamination.

The decontamination of skin surrounding the wound area should be done before medical manipulations in a specially equipped room of the local medical facility. The wound area should be isolated by waterproof film and the surrounding area should be processed with "Zaschita" agent[1,20] or other decontaminating agents.

It is known that bandaging material is able to absorb radionuclides from open wounds. Therefore, the sterile bandage applied at the accident site should be removed and additional wound cleansing by tampons moistened with decontaminating solution (5% $Na_3CaDTPA$ solution, for example) and with 3% hydrogen peroxide should be done at the local medical facility. Thereafter, a sterile bandage with adsorbing material should be applied. These procedures should be accompanied with radiological monitoring of the wound and surrounding tissues.

All washing waters, initial bandage material, tampons, and foreign bodies removed from the wound, as well as the victim excreta should be collected and placed in containers or packages for radiological measurements. This requirement is also applicable for in-patient treatment.

Some authors recommend taking a 50-ml blood sample before the administration of medications to have a control sample for subsequent radiological measurements. This recommendation should be obligatory because a reliable sum of the radiometric data can be obtained if excreta, decontaminating solutions, and bandages are collected properly.

SPECIALIZED HOSPITAL CARE

Specialized medical care and quantitative radiometric measurements should be done in a hospital with an emergency plan that includes the availability of dosimetric instruments and a qualified staff.

To provide the most effective therapy, the time between the incident and in-patient admission should be as brief as possible. The victim should be admitted to the decontamination room, where complete decontamination of the body (excluding the injured site) should be done if indicated. The decontamination room should adjoin rooms for radiometric monitoring and whole-body counting. Equipment for measurement of alpha, beta, and gamma radiation should be available. Measurements will be done here to obtain data on the character and magnitude of radioactive contamination of the wound and surrounding tissues, as well as a preliminary assessment of incorporated radionuclide(s) in the body. A thorough decontamination of the intact skin surrounding the wound should be done before any surgery procedure is undertaken.

It is extremely desirable that the surgery room be equipped with small wound counters of different designs to obtain information on the location of radioactive substances within the wound, i.e., to obtain the topography of radioactivity distribution in the injured area and, therefore, to measure the effectiveness of surgery during its course. If conventional wound decontamination activity was not able to decrease the radioactivity in the wound to background levels, then the question of the permissible wound burden will arise. Concerning plutonium and transplutonium elements, the maximum permissible wound burden is proposed to equal 0.1 of the maximum permissible burden calculated for the critical organ. This recommendation can be considered as the reference level by which the medical staff judges the course of wound tissue decontamination. Ohlenschläger[8,79] has noted that amputation (of finger or finger phalanx, for example) can be considered for lifesaving purposes. This extreme action might be taken when lesser surgical excisions are inadequate to decrease the radioactivity to a safe level. This is most likely in complex situations of transuranium element wound contamination. Actually, such cases are possible and have been described in Reference 114.

Agents for decorporation therapy (chelates, etc.) should be administered at the specialized hospital according to indications; the necessary radiological examinations (excreta radioactivity measurements, whole-body counting, radiometry of bandaging materials, instruments, etc.) should be continued as necessary. After the surgery, the victim should be admitted to the hospital or treated on an outpatient basis following radiometric tests.

The organization and tactics of the medical care considered above indicate only general considerations on the first aid transport and definitive management of victims. Obviously, the multiplicity of possible occurrences and characters of an accidental situation as well as a number of side circumstances can significantly alter the sequence and scope of medical care. It is interesting to consider one practical case that resulted from an accident involving intensive radioactive wound contamination.

During glove box operations to replace one of the elements of a pipeline system filled with plutonium solution, the operator injured the first finger of his right hand. According to procedure, the operator stopped his work and called his colleague, who was working at the same location. The victim put on a respirator, switched on the alarm signal, and left his injured hand inside the glove box to avoid dissemination of the contamination. In response to the alarm signal, the radiation protection officer arrived at the site of the incident. Using the portable alpha and beta survey meter, he measured the radioactivity on the forearm and hand of the victim, who slowly removed it from the glove box. Visual examination revealed a 1.5-cm-long wound on the flexor surface of the distal phalanx of the first finger. The bleeding was stopped with a cotton tampon. Significant contamination of this cotton tampon was found. The glove port was sealed to provide containment within the glove box. The injury was immediately reported to the local medical service. The nurse at the plant arrived 5 min after the incident and informed the physician. The victim was attended at an on-site decontamination room, where the wound was washed several times using warm water with soap. A monitoring survey showed that wound contamination remained. The wound was bandaged with a sterile dressing and the forearm was covered; the victim was moved to the decontamination facility at the plant.

The medical service started actions recommended for incidents of this kind. A questionnaire was completed. The victim's supervisor and radiation protection officer provided their information on the radionuclide contaminant. The contaminant was plutonium-239 with very probable admixture of americium-241. The health physicist provided quantitative information on the radioactivity of blood sampled from the injured area (9.7 Bq/sample). The nasal smear showed the insignificant radioactivity (~0.037 Bq). The wound was washed with warm water with soap, detergent, and, finally, with DTPA. The decontamination effect was negative. It was concluded that there was deep wound contamination. By using a proportional counter, it was confirmed that the wound was contaminated by plutonium-239 and americium-241. At minute 30 after the injury, quantitative evaluation of wound contamination was estimated to be 670 Bq. At 25 min after the injury, the intravenous injection of 20 ml of 5% $Na_3CaDTPA$ was given. Thereafter, a decision to surgically dissect the contaminated wound was made. The surgeon was called immediately and the surgery room prepared.

The surgery was started about 70 min after the incident. Under local anesthesia, an incision 2 cm long, 2 mm deep was made. To monitor the radioactive contamination in the surgical wound, a NaI(Tl) gamma probe connected to a multichannel analyzer situated in the adjoining room was used for measurement. The measurement results were provided by telephone to the surgeon. He had the measured intensity of gamma and X-ray readings posted on a board in the surgery room, which gave a visual record of the progress of radioactivity measurements. After the surgery, no elevated radioactivity was found in the wound area. The wound was sutured.

Excision of the wound had eliminated 1.33 kBq of plutonium-239 and 1.15 kBq of americium-241. The difference between the activity found in the tissue excised and the activity measured *in vivo* (670 Bq) was explained by the absorption of low-energy gamma radiation in the material of the sterile bandage applied to the finger.

The patient was monitored over the next 5 months. Feces and urine were periodically measured for the presence of radioactivity to evaluate possible internal contamination.

The described case demonstrates the general order of phase-by-phase medical care for radioactively contaminated wounds. The proper actions of the victim, the radiation protection service, and the medical service should be noted. These efforts assured a minimal time delay between the contamination event and medical care.

The decontamination of the plutonium-contaminated wound started 5 min after the injury and $Na_3CaDTPA$ solution was injected intravenously 20 min later. The surgery was started 70 min after the accident. All these activities were preceded by radiological measurements, which determined the extent of the radioactive contamination and the amount of radionuclides in the wound. These data justified the decision to excise the contaminated wound tissues.

The description given above clarifies the importance of the instrumental diagnosis of radioactive wound contamination at all phases of the victim's care. Therefore, some brief information on wound radiometry is given in the next section, but detailed description of these techniques should be obtained from the corresponding manuals.

Radioactivity Monitoring of Contaminated Wounds and Burns

The selection of the device applicable for wound monitoring depends upon the type of radiation emitter and its physiochemical properties.

Uranium fission product contamination is relatively easy to measure by beta or beta/gamma survey meters, which are able to provide quantitative evaluation of the radioactivity in the wound. Beta radiation has lower penetrative ability than gamma radiation and will be attenuated by tissue in case of deep wounds; the degree of this attenuation depends on the energy of the beta particles. In case of superficial injuries, beta measurements can provide sufficiently accurate evaluations of wound contamination by beta emitters.

The most difficult task consists in the detection of alpha emitters in wounds. Because of the absorption of alpha particles in blood, tissue fluid, or coagulated blood, direct alpha measurements do not provide objective information. In case of deep wounds, pure alpha emitters situated in the depth of a wound are completely hidden for detection applied at the wound surface. In such cases, the measurement will be an assessment of surface alpha contamination on the injured area and surrounding skin. Therefore, the detection of alpha emitters in wounds at a count rate above background is an indication for the application of decontamination measures. For example, in earlier cases all wounds suspected to be contaminated by plutonium in the Los Alamos National Laboratory (U.S.A.) were excised, if the surgery was possible without functional impairment.[7] This situation existed until the development of specialized devices that were able to detect the low-energy X rays emitted by plutonium.[6] After the invention of scintillator and semiconductor detectors, the quantitative assessment of wound burdens of plutonium and transplutonium elements became possible using their X-ray and low-energy gamma radiation.

Scintillation counters are the more common. According to Reference 7, a probe (1.27 cm diameter, 0.127 cm thickness) is able to detect 4 Bq of superficial wound plutonium above the background at a 95% confidence level.

Reference 79 provides the following order for the measurement of radionuclide contamination localized in wounds:

1. Measurement of alpha and beta activity of a wound using an ionization counter (~150 cm^2 area; the measurement field is limited by a plastic plate with a slit).
2. Measurement of alpha and beta activity of wound using a semiconductor detector.
3. Measurement of the area surrounding a wound to determine the total area and level of contamination.
4. Measurement of the radioactivity of plutonium or americium in a wound using a scintillation detector.

If the wound is contaminated by a uranium fission product mixture, a multichannel analyzer should be applied to visualize the radiation energy spectrum and to identify the specific radionuclides, including the presence of a plutonium and americium admixture.

To increase the accuracy of quantitative evaluation of wound plutonium in cases of minor injuries to fingers, the finger is placed into a specially designed individual plastic form to provide the exact distance between the wound and probe.

To check decontamination efficiency, measurements should be done before and after decontamination. Pieces of the dissected tissues, wound blood, washing fluid, and the initial bandage should also be measured.

To cleanse wounds contaminated by transuranium radionuclides of plutonium-239 and americium-241 rapidly and consistently, information on the localization of the radionuclide in the wound is necessary as is estimation of the depth of the radionuclide deposition. The deposition depth of plutonium-239 in a wound can be assessed using comparison of the relationships of emitted X-ray radiation of different energies.

To determine the depth of radioactive substance deposition, proportional counters are applied, which can measure the energies of X-ray and gamma radiation emitted from the wound. The magnitude of the plutonium penetration into tissues is very important in determining the scope of surgery, which can be illustrated by the following case of plutonium wound contamination.[7] While working in a glove box, an operator suffered two puncture wounds of the finger. With a NaI(Tl) detector, 1.67 kBq of plutonium was detected. A proportional counter determined the depth of the plutonium penetration to be 1.5 mm from the skin surface. The radioactive material was removed by surgical excision. Radiological measurements of the dissected tissue and autoradiography confirmed the localization and depth of plutonium deposition (1.5 mm).

The accumulated experience from treatment of wounds contaminated by radioactive substances has formulated some basic requirements for measurement devices, as follows:

1. High sensitivity to determine the radionuclide burden in the wound in an amount of 0.1 of maximum permissible body burden;
2. High spatial resolution to provide the measurements of radioactivity of the volume of < 30 mm^3 near the probe;
3. Brief time requirements for measurement;
4. Easy handling when making measurements and the ability to fix the probe above the contaminated area (this feature will provide the surgeon with real-time information on changes in the radioactivity level during the surgery);
5. Possibility of the probe sterilization.

Taking into account the requirements given above, measurement systems were designed and improved to determine the localization and burden of the wound activity of transuranium elements both within wounds and on their surface.[92,119,120] For example, one measurement system[119] contains a set of probes including two NaI(Tl) scintillation detectors to determine and localize the amounts of low-energy gamma or X-ray emitters and one NaI(Tl) scintillation detector to measure the gamma radiation with energies up to 1 MeV. This system also contains a multichannel analyzer. The detectors are designed as a lightweight wound probe.

Wound probes of small scintillation detectors (3 and 6 mm diameters and 1 mm thickness) are able to measure activity inside the wound. A NaI(Tl) scintillation detector of 12 mm diameter and 1 mm thickness is used for application to the wound surface. It can be replaced by a detector of 12 mm thickness, which expands the measurement range of gamma radiation up to 1 MeV. The sensitivity of all detectors equals 37 Bq of plutonium-239 and the measurement time is 100 s. Sterilization is provided using aseptic solution processing and a sterile colorless lacquer coating on the probe. The probe can be fixed in any spatial position within several tens of millimeters from the wound. The energy resolution of the wound probe equals 25%, with a spatial resolution of 30 mm^3 from the probe. The authors recommend a preliminary "sound" survey of the wound using headphones connected to the counter. This measurement system, successfully applied, recognized a plutonium-239 deposition at month 4 after a puncture wound and determined the radionuclide quantity and localization.[120] The description of this case is given below.

During the removal of radioactive waste, a worker punctured the soft tissue of the distal phalanx of the third finger of his left hand. The occurrence of this injury was not reported, and the wound healed. During a routine examination 2 months after the incident, the victim's urine contained radioactivity. The worker remembered this injury. Radioactivity measurement of the distal phalanx indicated a deposition of about 104 Bq of plutonium-239.

Medical examination of the distal phalanx of the third finger did not show any sign of the wound. Another radiological measurement, of the left hand, using a large-area proportional counter, including the former wound area, did not detect alpha radiation. Nevertheless, another scintillation detector measurement of low-energy gamma and X rays confirmed the previous results obtained by the same device. After local anesthesia, the end point of the finger was incised at the edge of the measured activity site. The plutonium deposition was mapped using a wound probe. To confirm the detected magnitude of wound plutonium, a test plutonium source of known activity was measured. After excision of contaminated tissues, the wound probe measurement confirmed the removal of the activity. The radiation source found in the dissected tissue was a 2-mm piece of glass pipette debris.

REFERENCES

1. Ilyin, L.A., *Basics of the Human Protection against Radioactive Substances*, Atomizdat Publisher, Moscow, 1977, 256 (in Russian).
2. Ilyin, L.A. and Ivannikov, A.T., *Radioactive Substances and Wounds (Metabolism and Decorporation)*, Atomizdat Publisher, Moscow, 1979, 256 (in Russian).
3. Kiy, M.K. and Schneider, V.M., Erfahrungen mit Wundkontamination: Erste Hilfe an Arbeitsplatz, presented at Seminar uber Strahlen Schutzprobleme deim Umgang mit transsuz Anelementen, Karlszuhe, 21–25 Sept. 1970, No. 29.
4. Bazhin, A.G., Khokhriakov, V.F., and Shevkunov, V.A., Skin wounds and burns contaminated by alpha-emitters in radiochemical facility personnel, *Hyg. Sanit.*, 9, 27–29, 1994 (in Russian).
5. Hammond, S.E., and Putzier, E.A., Observed effects of plutonium in wounds over a long period of time, *Health Phys.*, 10(6), 399–406, 1964.
6. Schofield, G.B., Absorption and measurement of radionuclides in wound and abrasions, *Clin. Radiol. Rad.*, 15(1), 50–54, 1963.
7. Johnson, L.J. and Lawrence, J.N.P., Plutonium contaminated wound experience and assay techniques at the Los Alamos Scientific Laboratory, *Health Phys.*, 27(1), 55–59, 1974.
8. Ohlenschläger, L., Chirurgische Versogung der mit alpha-aktivitot kontaminierten Verletzung, presented at Seminar on Radiation Problems Relating to Transuranium Elements, Karlsruhe, Sept. 1970, No. 28.
9. Norwood, W.D., Removal of plutonium and other transuranic elements from man, in *Diagnosis and Treatment of Radioactive Poisoning*, IAEA, Vienna, 1963, 307–318.
10. Kelsey, C.A., Mettler, F.A. et al., ^{192}IrCl acid skin burn: case report and review of the literature, *Health Phys.*, 74(5), 610–612, 1998.
11. Ilyin, L.A., Ed., *Manual on Organization of Medical Examination of Persons Exposed to Ionizing Radiation*, Atomizdat Publisher, Moscow, 1986 (in Russian).
12. NRB 76/87 Standards of Radiation Protection, OSP-72/87 Basic Sanitary Rules, Atomizdat Publisher, Moscow, 1988 (in Russian).
13. Dancer, G.H., Morgan, A., and Hutchinson, W.P., A case of skin contamination with carbon-15 labelled chloroacetic acid, *Health Phys.*, 11(10), 1055–1058, 1965.
14. Benes, A., Radioactive zamorene rana popalemia, in *Sbornik Vedeckych Praci Vejenskeho Lekarskeho Vyzkumniho a Doskolovaciho Ustavu*. JEP, Avazek 23, Hradec Kralove, VZDu, 1967 (in Czech).
15. Stojanovic, D.B. and Milivojevic, K.S., Effect des rajonnements ionisants sur la penetration du radiocesium par des lesions de la pean et possibilite de decontamination, in *Diagnosis and Treatment of Incorporated Radionuclides, Proc. of the International Seminar on Diagnosis and Treatment of Incorporated Radionuclides*, 8–12 December 1975, IAEA, Vienna, 1976, 99–106 (in French).
16. Ducousso, R., Causst, A., and Pasquer, C., A study of the translocation of radioactive substances from wounds and therapy by local instabilization, presented at 3rd Internat. Congress of the IRPA, Washington, D.C., 1973, 90.
17. Ilyin, L.A., Ivannikov, A.T., Parfenov, V.D., and Stolyarov, V.P., Strontium absorption through damaged and intact human skin, *Health Phys.*, 29(1), 75–80, 1975.
18. Ilyin, L.A., Ivannikov, A.T. et al., Radiation hygiene assessment of the hazard and protection efficiency in case of ^{85}Sr contamination of abrasions and intact skin of humans, *Med. Radiol.*, 11, 44–49, 1975 (in Russian).
19. Kolpakov, F.I., *Skin Penetrability*, Medicina Publisher, Moscow, 1973 (in Russian).
20. Ilyin L.A., Noretz, T.A., Schvydko, N.S., and Ivanov, E.V., *Radioactive Substances and Skin (Metabolism and Decontamination)*, Ilyin, L.A., Ed., Atomizdat Publisher, Moscow, 1972, 301 pp. (in Russian).

21. Tcylourik, I.T., *The Penetration of Radioactive Substances through Skin and Wound Surface*, Ph.D. thesis, Kharkov, 1959 (in Russian).
22. Ilyin, L.A., *Chernobyl: Myth and Reality*, Nagasaki Association for Hibakusha's Medical Care (NASHIM), 1998, 497 (Japanese edition; in Japanese).
23. Suzuki-Yasumoto, M. and Inaba, J., Absorption and metabolism of radioactive cobalt compounds through normal and wounded skin, in *Diagnosis and Treatment of Incorporated Radionuclides, Proc. of Int. Seminar on Diagnosis and Treatment of Incorporated Radionuclides*, Vienna, 8–12 December 1975, IAEA, Vienna, 1976, 119–136.
24. Sedov, V.V., Serebryanov, N.G., and Tarasov, N.F., Perspectives of the radioactive isotope application for the therapy of malignant neoplasms of the lymphatic nodes, *Med. Radiol.*, 3, pp. 3–12, 1964 (in Russian).
25. Levin, J.M., *Problems of Interstitial and Lymphatic Vascular Therapy in Oncology*, Medicina Publisher, Moscow, 1976 (in Russian).
26. Borisov, N.B., Ilyin, L.A., Margulis, U.Ya., Parkhomenko, G.M., and Krusch, V.T., *Radiation Protection of Polomium-210 Operations*, Petrianov, I.V. and Ilyin, L.A., Eds., Atomizdat Publisher, Moscow, 1980, 262 pp. (in Russian).
27. Buldakov, L.A., Lubchansky, E.R., Moskalev, J.I., and Nifatov, A.P., *Plutonium Toxicology Problems*, Atomizdat Publisher, Moscow, 1969 (in Russian).
28. Vaughan J.C., ^{239}Pu metabolism with special reference to the skeleton, in *Uranium, Plutonium, Transplutonium Elements*, Hodge, H.C., Stannard, J.N., and Huroh, J.B., Eds., Springer-Verlag, Berlin, 1973, 351–391.
29. Scott, K.G., Axelrod, D., Fisher, H. et al., The metabolism of plutonium in rats following intramuscular injection, *J. Biol. Chem.*, 176, 283–293, 1948.
30. Taylor, D.M., The metabolism of plutonium in adult rabbits, *Br., J. Radiol.*, 42, 44–50, 1969.
31. Norwood, W.D. and Fuqua, P.A., Medical care for accident deposition of plutonium (^{239}Pu) within body, in *Handling of Radiation Accidents*, IAEA, Vienna, 1969, 151–157.
32. Volf, V., Combined effect of DTPA and citric acid on a intramuscular deposit in rats, *Health Phys.*, 27(1), 152–153, 1974.
33. Volf, V., The effect of combinations of chelating agents on the translocation of intramuscularly deposited ^{239}Pu nitrate in the rat, *Health Phys.*, 29(1), 61–68, 1975.
34. Foreman, H., Medical management of radioactively contaminated wounds, in *Diagnosis and Treatment of Radioactive Poisoning*, IAEA, Vienna, 1963, 387–411.
35. McClanahan, B.J. and Kornberg, H.A., Treatment of contaminated wounds with DTPA in rats, in *Diagnosis and Treatment of Deposited Radionuclides, Proc. of Symposium*, Richland, WA, 15–17 May 1967, 390–402.
36. Bistline, R.W., Watters, K.L., and Lebel, J.L., A study of plutonium and americium from simulated puncture wounds in beagle dogs, *Health Phys.*, 22(6), 829–831, 1972.
37. Lubchansky, E.R., Bazhin, A.G. et al., The improvement of measures of specialized medical care in case of the accidental ^{239}Pu intake through pulmonary organs and injured skin, Report of the Affiliated Branch No. 1 of the Institute of Biophysics, 1992, IBP Library (in Russian).
38. Lubchansky, E.R., Bazhin, A.G. et al., Experimental justification of plutonium-239 exposure levels in combination with physical and chemical factors of industry and the assessment of resorption coefficients of poorly transportable plutonium compounds through injured skin, Report of the Affiliated Branch No. 1 of the Institute of Biophysics, 1991, IBP Library (in Russian).
39. Khokhriakov, V.F. and Suslova, K.G., Modified model of lung clearance, in *Actual Subjects of the Internal Exposure Dosimetry, Abstracts of All-Union Conference*, Gomel, 20–22 September 1989, Moscow, 1989, 14–15.
40. Bazhin, A.G., Lubchansky, E.R. et al., Behavior and biological effect of ^{239}Pu in case of intramuscular administration and chelate therapy application, *Radiobiology*, 1, 129, 1984 (in Russian).
41. Buldakov, L.A. et al., Plutonium-239 uptake through skin and subcutaneous cellular tissue of sucklingpigs, *Radiobiology*, 7(4), 591–601, 1967 (in Russian).
42. Lisco, H. and Kisileski, W.E., The fate and pathological effects of plutonium metal implanted into rabbits and rats, *Am. J. Pathol.*, 29, 305–321, 1953.
43. Ilyin, L.A., Ivannikov, A.T., Popov, B.A., Konstantinova, T.P., Altukhova, G.A., and Bazhin, A.G., Radioisotope resorption through injured skin, *Hyg. Sanit.*, 8, 48–54, 1976 (in Russian).

44. Schofield, G.B., Comparison of the medical management of three cases of plutonium contaminated wounds, in *Handling of Radiation Accidents, Proc. Symposium*, Vienna, 19–23 May 1969, pp. 163–172.
45. Schofield, G.B. and Junn, C.A., A measure of the effectiveness of DTPA chelation therapy in cases of plutonium inhalation and plutonium wounds, *Health Phys.*, 24(3), 317–321, 1973.
46. Hesp, R. and Ledgerwood, R.M., The study of case which involved a wound contamination with plutonium-239 and americium-241, presented at Seminar on Radiation Protection Problems Relating to Transuranium Elements, Karlsruhe, 21–25 Sept., 1970, No. 13.
47. Schofield, G.B., Howells, H. et al., Assessment and management of a plutonium contaminated wound case, *Health Phys.*, 26(6), 541–554, 1974.
48. Larson, H.V., Newton, C.E., and Baumgarten, W.V., The management of an extensive plutonium wound and the evaluation of the residual internal deposition of plutonium, *Phys. Med. Biol.*, 13(1), 45–53, 1968.
49. Newton, D., Rundo, J., and Sandals, F.J., A case of internal contamination with ^{213}Pa and ^{227}Ac via a puncture wound, in *Diagnosis and Treatment of Deposited Radionuclides, Proc. Symposium*, Richmond, WA, 15–17 May 1967, 521–533.
50. Cable, J.W., et al., Effects of intradermal injections of plutonium in swine, *Health Phys.*, 8(7), 629–634, 1962.
51. Ilyin, L.A., Ivannikov, A.T., Bazhin, A.G. et al., Intake of Po-210 into the body through the damaged skin and efficiency of some methods in preventing its absorption, *Health Phys.*, 32(2), 107–111, 1977.
52. Bazhin, A.G., Assessment of ^{239}Pu resorption rate in case of skin injury and the efficiency of decontamination, *Hyg. Sanit.*, 6, 43–46, 1983 (in Russian).
53. Durbin, P.W., Metabolism and biological effects of transplutonium elements, in *Uranium, Plutonium, Transplutonic Elements*, Hodge, H.C., Stannard, J.N., and Huroh, J.B., Eds., Springer-Verlag, Berlin, 1973, 739–896.
54. Durbin, P.W., Distribution of transuranic elements in mammals, *Health Phys.*, 8(7), 665–671, 1962.
55. Parker, H.G. et al., The metabolism of ^{253}Es in mice, *Health Phys.*, 22(6), 647–651, 1972.
56. Parker, H.G., Low-Beer, A., and Isaac, E.L., Comparison of retention and organ distribution of ^{241}Am and ^{252}Cf in mice: the effect of in vivo DTPA chelation, *Health Phys.*, 8(7), 679–684, 1962.
57. Smith, V.H., Therapeutic removal of internally deposited transuranium elements, *Health Phys.*, 22(6), 765–778, 1972.
58. Williams, M.H., Jeung, N., and Durbin, P.W., Effect of complexing agent and mode of administration on distribution of curium-242 in the rat, UCRL-9617, 1961, 35–38.
59. Lebel, J.L. and Watters, R.J., Study of the translocation of plutonium and americium from puncture wounds, *Nucl. Sci. Abstr.*, 26(24), 59–136, 1972.
60. Lagerquist, C.R., Allen, J.B., and Holman, K.L., Plutonium excretion following contaminated acid burns and prompt DTPA treatments, *Health Phys.*, 13(1), 1–4, 1967.
61. Bock, M.I. and Ivanov, E.V., Resorption of radioactive substances through burned skin, in *5th Scientific Conference on Burn Problem*, 6–8 June 1967, Part 1, VMOLA Publisher, Leningrad, 1967, 45–46 (in Russian).
62. Ivanov, E.V. and Bock, M.I., Radiation evaluation of some methods of the initial processing of burns contaminated by radioactive substances, in *5th Scientific Conference on Burn Problems*, 6–8 June 1967, Part 1, VMOLA Publisher, Leningrad, 1967, 143–144 (in Russian).
63. Ilyin, L.A., Ivannikov, A.T., Popov, B.A., and Parfenova, I.M., Radionuclide resorption through the thermal burn surface and decontamination problem, *Hyg. Sanit.*, 4, 6–9, 1981 (in Russian).
64. Bazhin, A.G. and Parfenova, I.M., ^{210}Po resorption through intact skin and burn wounds, *Hyg. Sanit.*, 10, 36–39, 1976 (in Russian).
65. Berlin, L.B., *Skin Morphology after Burns and Free Grafting*, Medicina Publisher, Leningrad, 1966 (in Russian).
66. Ohlenschläger, L. Bericht über eine mit Americium-241 Kontaminierte stichschmittverletzung am linken Leigefinger. *Strahlentherapie*, 142(1), 73–79, 1971.
67. Klyachkin, L.M., Filatov, V.I., Results of 131 application to evaluate the capillary blood flow and penetrability of vascular degree in human burns, *VMOLA Proc.*, 114, 38–40, 1960 (in Russian).

68. Kazimirko, N.Z., Burn Penetrability and Novocaine Blockade Influence in Resorption Properties of Combusted Wounds, Ph.D. thesis proffered paper, Ivanovo-Frankovsk Medical Institute, Ivanovo-Frankovsk, 1965 (in Russian).
69. Gukasian, A.A. and Jijin, V.N., Principles of therapy of wounds and burns contaminated by radioactive substances, *Mil. Med. J.*, 3, 14–18, 1964 (in Russian).
70. Zolotarevsky, V.Y. and Pereverzeva, R.A., On the resorption ability of burn, *Mil. Med. J.*, 5, 57–59, 1959 (in Russian).
71. Troynikova, A.D., On the uptake of combusted tissues, in *Etiology and Pathogenesis of Burn Shock, Proc. of Leningrad Institute of Blood Transfusion*, Vol. 9, Leningrad, 1950, 103–107 (in Russian).
72. Ilyin, L.A., Ivannikov, A.T., Beliayev, I.K., Bazhin, A.T., and Altukhova, G.A., Percutaneous intake of ^{239}Pu in rats in case of nitric acid burn, *Hyg. Sanit.*, 1, 26–29, 1982 (in Russian).
73. Weeks, M.H. and Oakley, W.D., Influence of plutonium concentration on effectiveness of therapeutic agents, in *Biology Research Annual Report*, 1953, USAEC Rep., H.W. 30437, Hanford Atomic Products Operation, General Electric Co., 1954, 109–110.
74. Beliayev, I.K., Ivannikov, A.T., and Ilyin, L.A., Intracutaneous distribution of ^{239}Pu in case of chemical burn inflicted by nitric acid, *Hyg. Sanit.*, 5, 78–79, 1979 (in Russian).
75. Beliayev, I.K., Ivannikov, A.T., Parfenov, I.M., and Bazhin, A.G., Effectiveness of the sanitary processing in case of ^{239}Pu skin contamination of organic solvents, *Hyg. Sanit.*, 2, 87, 1984 (in Russian).
76. Ilyin, L.A., Beliayev, I.K., Bazhin, A.G., and Ivannikov, A.T., Investigation of percutaneous ^{239}Pu body intake, *Hyg. Sanit.*, 11, 32–35, 1981 (in Russian).
77. Kusama, T., Hon, S., and Voshizawa, V., Absorption of radionuclides through wounded skin, *Health Phys.*, 51(1), 138–141, 1986.
78. Protyakov, K.M. and Kondratyeva, A.P., Change of ^{131}I resorption time from the intracutaneous compartment under the influence of some physical and pharmacological factor, *Med. Radiol.*, 6, 29–32, 1966 (in Russian).
79. Ohlenschläger, L., *First Medical Aid in Case of Injuries Complicated by Radioactive Contamination*, Merle, G., Ed., (translated from German into Russian), Medicina Publisher, Moscow, 1975, 121–135 (in Russian).
80. Chromov, B.M., Wounds contaminated by radioactive substances, *Vestn. Chir.*, 3, 110–120, 1957 (in Russian).
81. Pasquier, C., Ducousso, R., and Regnauld, M., Emergency treatment of wound contaminated by a mixture of fission products, *Nucl. Sci. Abst.*, 26(1), 23–78, 1972.
82. Sheiko, V.Z., Application of powder mixture to control the radioactive substance uptake from soft tissues, in *Abstracts of 2nd Municipal Conference of Young Surgeons*, SPG-Medgiz Publisher, Leningrad, 1956, 10–11 (in Russian).
83. Berkutov, A.N., Surgical processing of wounds in case of combined injuries, *Mil. Med. J.*, 1, 17–22, 1956 (in Russian).
84. Nigrovic, V., Einfluß von Chelatbildem auf Verhalten Quecksilber in Organism, *Arzneimittel-Forschung*, 13(7), 787–789, 1963.
85. Niemmejer, B., Der Einfluß von Chelatbildem auf Verteiung und Toxicitat von Codmium, *Int. Arch. Gevebepathol. Gevebehyg.*, 24(1), 160–163, 1967.
86. Jishima, H., Kashima, M., and Matsuoka, O., Decontamination of internally deposited ^{239}Pu — treatment of plutonium contaminated wounds with CaDTPA in mice, NIRS, Chiba, *Abstr. Radiat. Res.*, 13(1), 214, 1972.
87. Mayzelis, M.H., On the influence of medication dream in rabbit skin penetrability, *Vestn. Dermatol. Venerol.*, 1, 19–20, 1954 (in Russian).
88. Volf, V., Actual state and problems of chelation therapy, presented at Seminar on Radiation Protection Problems Relating to Transuranium Elements, Karlsruhe, 1970, No. 10.
89. Volf, V., Experimental background for prompt treatment with DTPA of Pu-239 contaminated wound, *Health Phys.*, 27(3), 273–277, 1974.
90. Harrison, J.D. and David, A.J., A comparison of different chemical forms of plutonium from simulated wound sites in the rat and hamster and effect of DTPA on clearance, in *Annual Research and Development Report*, 1976, NRPB, Harweel, Didcot, March 1977, 68–70.

91. Schulte, H.E. and Whippe, H.O., Chelating agents in plutonium deposition: a minority view, in *Diagnosis and Treatment of Deposited Radionuclides, Proc. Symposium*, Richland, WA, 1968, 587–590.
92. Gerber, G.B. and Thomas, R.G., Eds., Guidebook for the treatment of accidental radionuclide contamination of workers, *Radiat. Prot. Dosimetry*, 41(1), 27–36, 1992.
93. Management of persons accidentally contaminated with radionuclides: recommendations of the NCRP, NCRP Rep. 65, Washington, D.C., 1980, 205 pp.
94. Schulte, B., Wissenwerttes für den Arzt zur Behandlung Strahlenexponierter/Institut für Strahlen Hygiene. 1989 – h. 132 – 67 S.
95. Ilyin, L.A., Ed., *Emergency Care of Acute Radiation Exposure*, 2nd rev. ed., Atomizdat Publisher, Moscow, 1976, 100 (in Russian).
96. Ilyin, L.A., Ed., *Manual for Organization of Medical Assistance of Persons Exposed to Ionizing Radiation*, Energoatomizdat Publisher, Moscow, 1986, 190 (in Russian).
97. Recommendations on Medical Care of Traumas Contaminated by Radioactive Substances, 1st and 2nd eds., Ministry of Health of the USSR, Moscow, 1981; 1984, 22 pp. (in Russian).
98. Moiseev, V.M., ^{32}P uptake from burn surface, in *Proceedings of Military Medicine Faculty of Kuybishev Medical Institute*, No. 3, Kuybishev, 1957, 43–47 (in Russian).
99. Izmukhanov, A.K., On Therapy of Thermal Burns Contaminated by Radioactive Substances in the Experimental Conditions, Ph.D. thesis, Alma-Ata Medical Institute, Alma-Ata, 1967 (in Russian).
100. Stradling, G.N., Gray, S.A. et al., Efficacy of TREN (Me-3,2–HOPO), 5L-(Me-3,2–HOPO) and DTPA for removing plutonium and americium from rat after inhalation and wound contamination as nitrates: comparison with 3,4,3–Li(1, 2 HOPO), *EULEP Newsl.*, 79, 17, 1995.
101. Stradling, G.N., Gray, S.A. et al., Comparative efficacies of TREN-(Me-3,2–HOPO), 5–Li-(Me-3,2–HOPO) and 3,4,30Li(1,2–HOPO) from removing thorium from the rat after inhalation and wound contamination, *EULEP Newsl.*, 79, 18, 1995.
102. Metivier, H., French strategy in decorporation research, *EULEP Newsl.*, 79, 20–22, 1995.
103. Zotova, M.G., ^{210}Po body intake through wounds, in *Distribution and Biological Effect of Radioactive Isotopes*, Moskalev, Ju., Ed., Atomizdat Publisher, Moscow, 1966, 83–88 (in Russian).
104. Izorgina, A.G., Some peculiarities of polonium body excretion in case of unithyol administration subcutaneously and perorally, in *Complexing Agents: Synthesis, Properties, Application in Biology and Medicine*, Sverdlovsk, 1958, 119–131 (in Russian).
105. Benes, A., Vstrebavani modelone smesi jaderneno vybuchu kuzi popaleninou a ranou, *Vojen. Zdrav.*, 37(2), 52–55, 1968 (in Czech).
106. Aryev, T.Y., *Thermal Injuries*, Medicina Publisher, St. Petersburg, 1966.
107. Bazhin, A.G., Evaluation of body intake and efficiency of decontamination of wounds and abrasions contaminated by ^{239}Pu, *Hyg. Sanit.*, 12, 74–76, 1985 (in Russian).
108. Foreman, H., Experimental administration of ethylenediaminetetraacetic acid in plutonium poisoning, *Arch. Ind. Hyg. Occupat. Med.*, 10(3), 226–233, 1954.
109. Swanberg, F. and Henle, R.C., Excetion of ^{239}Pu in a patient with plutonium contaminated injury, *J. Occupat. Med.*, 6(4), 175–178, 1964.
110. Jolly, L.J., Treatment and evaluation of a plutonium-238 nitrate contaminated puncture wound: two year case history, *Health Phys.*, 23, 331–341, 1972.
111. Putzier, E.A. et al., Evaluation and treatment of an acute internal exposure to plutonium, *Personal Dosimetry for Radiation Accidents, Proc. of Symposium*, 8–12 March, IAEA, Vienna, 1965, 549–566.
112. Laylee, D.M., Fraser, D.C., and Johns, T.L., *A Plutonium Contaminated Wound*, Med. Branch and Radiological Safety Division of AEE, Winfrith, 1966, 1–15.
113. Testa, C. and Delle Site, A., The study of a case which involved a wound contaminated with insoluble ^{239}Pu and ^{241}Am, in *Health Physics Problems of Internal Contamination, Proc. of the IRPA Second European Congress on Radiation Protection*, Bujdoso, E., Ed., Academiai Kiaido, Budapest, 1973, 573–600.
114. Lagerquist, C.R., Putzier, E.A., Pietingrud, G.W., Bioassay and body counter results for the first 2 years following an acute plutonium exposure, *Health Phys.*, 13(9), 965–972, 1967.

115. Howells, H., Schofield, G.B., Lynn, J.C., and Ward, F.A., Assessment and management of a plutonium contaminated wound case, in *Health Physics Problems of Internal Contamination, Proc. of the IRPA Second European Congress on Radiation Protection*, Bujdoso, E., Ed., Academiai Kiaido, Budapest, 1973, 601–604.
116. Freke, A.M. and Dolphin, G.W., Rationale for the use DTPA in the treatment of plutonium contamination in humans, in *Second Int. Congress of the IRPA*, 3–8 May, Brighton, England, 1970, 226.
117. Gomez, L.S., Lebel, J.L., and Watters, R.L., The effect of lymph node removal of PuO_2 translocation, *Health Phys.*, 22,(6), 833–836, 1972.
118. Laalu, P., Controle d'un accident de boite a gants: traitment chirurgical d'une blessure contaminee par un melange de plutonium-239 et americium, in *Handling of Radiation Accidents, Proc. of a Symposium*, Vienna, 28 February–4 March, IAEA, Vienna, 1977.
119. Fromhein, O., Ohlenschläger, L., and Rapp, W., A new approach for an improved short-time procedure for localization and measurement of low activity, low energy transuranium deposits in wound, in *Diagnosis and Treatment of Incorporated Radionuclides, Proc. of Int. Seminar on Diagnosis and Treatment of Incorporated Radionuclides*, Vienna, 8–12 December 1975, IAEA, Vienna, 1976, 223–230.
120. Ohlenschläger, L., Removal of a four-month-old ^{239}Pu deposit in a puncture wound at the tip of left middle finger, in *Diagnosis and Treatment of Incorporated Radionuclides, Proc. of Int. Seminar on Diagnosis and Treatment of Incorporated Radionuclides*, Vienna, 8–12 December 1975, IAEA, Vienna, 1976, 491–496.
121. Deveataykin, E.B., Technique of ^{239}Pu activity measurement in hands, *Med. Radiol.*, 12, 61–64, 1973 (in Russian).
122. Yuan, Z.Q. et al., Medical treatment for plutonium contaminated wounds in three cases, *Chin. J. Radiol. Med. Prot.*, 2(6), 23–26 (Abstr. of original articles, p. 78), 1982.
123. Ilyin, L.A., *Chernobyl: Myth and Reality*, Megapolis Publisher, Moscow, 1995, 398 (English edition).

29 Iridium-192 Acid Skin Burn in Albuquerque, New Mexico, U.S.A.

Charles A. Kelsey and Fred A. Mettler, Jr.

Management of contaminated wounds has been thoroughly discussed in the previous chapter. This chapter presents a case example of a contaminated acid burn. At approximately 3:00 P.M. on March 25, 1997, a worker was mixing approximately 740 MBq (20 mCi) iridium-192 chloride in a 0.75 N nitric acid solution with toluene. The reaction was designed to label the toluene with the radioactive iridium-192. There may have been up to 30% of iridium-194 present as a contaminant. The volume in the container was approximately 7 ml. This reaction had been processed many times previously with no problems.

The reaction suddenly and unexpectedly exploded, ejecting approximately half the solution out of the mixing container. Some of the solution splashed on the worker. He was wearing eyeglasses, gloves, and protective clothing but was not wearing a head cover or a full face shield. The radioactive acid solution was deposited on his left cheek and the hair above his left ear (Figure 29.1). After immediately rinsing his face with water and removing his protective apparel, the worker was driven to the hospital where he arrived within 30 min of the accident.

Upon arrival, the exposure rate at the skin surface was 1.3×10^{-5} C/kg/h (50 mR/h) with the beta shield in place. After about 30 min of gentle cleaning with 4×4 sponges soaked in distilled water, the exposure rate was reduced to 2.6×10^{-6} C/kg/h (10 mR/h). Gamma camera scintillation images of the left side of the worker's face demonstrated the remaining contamination to be localized to the cheek and hair above the left ear. Subsequent removal of the contaminated hair reduced the surface exposure rate to 1.29×10^{-7} C/kg/h (0.5 mR/h). The worker was released to return to his home after treatment of his superficial acid burns. The surface exposure rate was 5.2×10^{-1} C/kg/h (0.2 mR/h) over a single localized spot 16 days after the accident.

An estimate of remaining contamination was made using the exposure rates when he was seen initially and when he was sent home and the iridium-192 gamma factor of 3.3×10^{-11} C/kg · cm^2/Bq/h (4.8 R · cm^2/mCi-h). The amount of isotope trapped in the skin was initially about 37 MBq (1000 µCi) and about 7 MBq (200 µCi) when he was sent home.

Urine samples were taken at 2, 3.5, 6.5, 14, and 23 h after the accident. Table 29.1 presents the results of the urine sample measurements. Integration of the values in Table 29.1 yields an estimated total 1.3×10^5 Bq (3.6 µCi) excreted during the first 24 h after the accident. Figure 29.1 shows the worker's face 2.5 days after the accident.

Iridium-192 decays primarily by beta minus emission to platinum-192 with a 74-day half-life. It has a complicated decay scheme with platinum characteristic X rays. The majority of the X rays have energies of approximately 300 keV with the maximum energy of 612 keV (Radiological Health Handbook, 1990). The 18-h half-life of the possible contaminant iridium-194 might have contributed to the apparent rapid decay of the residual contamination. No spectroscopic analysis was performed. The initial concern was whether the iridium-192 chloride had entered the bloodstream. The annual limit on intake (ALI) is 33 MBq (900 µCi). The critical organ receiving the

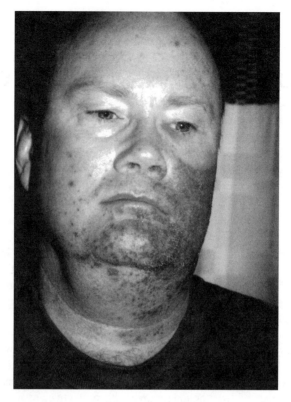

FIGURE 29.1 Acid burns on the left side of the face 2.5 days postexposure. The acid contained iridium-192 chloride.

TABLE 29.1
Results of Urine Sample Measurements

Time after Accident (h)	Activity Bq/ml
2	115
3.5	425
6.5	103
14.0	27.4
23	8.5

highest dose is the kidney. The urine sample results indicate that the amount absorbed through the skin was less than 1.8×10^5 Bq (5 µCi).

Calculations using the LUDEP program from NRPB (National Radiation Protection Board, Chilton, U.K.) based on the absorption of 1% of the material on the skin surface give an effective dose of 5.1×10^{-4} Sv and a dose to the kidneys of 2.6×10^{-3} Sv.

Literature sources indicated that penetration of these radioactive solutions through the intact skin is low and only twofold to threefold higher through acid or alkali burned skin.[1-12] One should begin decontamination efforts as early as possible, but it is important to protect the integrity of the skin. NCRP Rep. 65[13] states that acidic solutions fix the contamination to proteins. This would explain why only about 1% of these solutions is found systemically following an acid burn. The same report gives apparently conflicting comments regarding absorption of radionuclides through acid-burned skin, indicating that acid burns decrease absorption. However, it also states that dilute acid burns tend to facilitate absorption, at least in the case of plutonium.

The authors' experience confirms that usually only a small fraction (0.1 to 3%) of contamination passes through acid-burned skin. Decontamination efforts are most effective using mild soap solutions within the first hour of contamination. Vigorous scrubbing or any efforts that break the skin are to be strictly avoided. Decontamination efforts delayed beyond 3 h are ineffective and abrading the skin may increase uptake 100-fold or more. Simply waiting allows the skin to normally exfoliate over 1 to 2 weeks, removing the remaining surface contamination.

REFERENCES

1. Beliaev, I.K. and Altukhova, AG., Intracutaneous ^{239}Pu distribution after its application in nitric acid solutions, *Gig. Sanit.*, 11:80–83, 1981 (in Russian).
2. Beliaev, I.K., Ivannikov, A.T., and Ilyin, L.A., Intracutaneous distribution of ^{239}Pu in chemical skin burns with nitric acid, *Gig. Sanit.*, 5:78–79, 1980 (in Russian).
3. Blank, I.H. and Scheuplein, R.J., The epidermal barrier, in *Progress in the Biological Sciences in Relation to Dermatology*, Ilyin, L.A., Ed., Cambridge University Press, New York, 1964, 245.
4. Ivannikov, A.T., Beliaev, I.K., Bazhin, A.G., and Altukhova, G.A., Percutaneous ^{239}Pu uptake in rats with skin burns from nitric acid, *Gig. Sanit.*, 1:26–9, 1982 (in Russian).
5. Ilyin, L.A., Ivannikov, A.T., Parfenov, I.D., Konstantinova, T.P., and Popov, B.A., Hygienic evaluation of the radiation hazard and the effectiveness of protection during contact of ^{85}Sr with excoriations and intact integument of man, *Med. Radiol.*, 20:44–49, 1975 (in Russian).
6. Ilyin, L.A., Ivannikov, A.T., Parfenov, I.D., and Stolyarov, V.P., Strontium absorption through damaged and undamaged human skin, *Health Phys.*, 29:75–80, 1975.
7. Ilyin, L.A., Ivannikov, A.T., Popov, B.A., Altukhova, G.A., and Parfenova, I.M., ^{241}Am resorption and microdistribution in the skin of rats with a nitric acid burn, *Gig. Sanit.*, 4:23–26, 1980 (in Russian).
8. Ilyin, L.A., Ivannikov, A.T., Popov, B.A., Konstantinova, T.P., and Alukhova, G.A., Radioisotope resorption through injured human skin, *Gig. Sanit.*, 8:48–54, 1976 (in Russian).
9. Ilyin, L.A., Ivannikov, A.T., Popov, B.A., and Parfenova, I.M., Percutaneous resorption of ^{137}Cs and ^{89}Sr in acid solutions and deactivation of the burn surface, *Gig. Sanit.*, 10:38–41, 1981 (in Russian).
10. Ilyin, L.A., Ivannikov, A.T., Popov, B.A., and Parfenova, I.M., Radionuclide resorption through the surface of thermal burns and problems of deactivation, *Gig. Sanit.*, 4:6–9, 1981 (in Russian).
11. Kusama, T., Itoh, S., and Yoshizawa, Y., Absorption of radionuclides through wounded skin, *Health Phys.*, 51:138–141, 1986.
12. Oakley, W.D. and Thompson, R.C., Further studies of percutaneous absorption and decontamination of plutonium in rats, in Biology Research Annual Report 1955, Hanford Laboratories, Richland, WA, Rep. HW 41500, 1956, 106. Radiological Health Handbook, U.S. Department of Health, Education, and Welfare, Richland, WA, 1990.
13. NCRP, Management of Persons Accidentally Contaminated with Radionuclides, Rep. 65, National Council on Radiation Protection and Measurements, Bethesda, MD, 1980.

30 Hospital Preparation for Radiation Accidents

Fred A. Mettler, Jr.

CONTENTS

Introduction 425
Communications 426
Area Designation 427
Supplies 428
Area Setup 429
Floor Covering 430
Ventilation 431
Patient Decontamination 431
Shielding 431
Protective Clothing 432
Instrumentation 432
Procedures 433
Security 434
Drills 434
Summary 434
References 434

INTRODUCTION

Historically, major hospitals located near nuclear facilities, whether commercial reactors, other industrial sites, or universities, have a reasonably predictable chance of seeing a patient involved in a radiation accident. On the average, such hospitals will treat at least one seriously injured and radioactively contaminated patient every 2 to 4 years. The reason for presentation of most patients is a medical or surgical emergency such as myocardial infarction, hypotension, thermal steam burns, or trauma with resultant fracture, etc. As might be expected, many of the patients come to the hospital during the evening or night shift. Whatever preparations have been made, there needs to be certainty that the designated procedures can be carried out with limited staffing.

Depending on the severity of the accident, the level of medical aid to persons irradiated or contaminated will include the following:[1]

1. First aid provided at the place of the accident (without a physician or nurse necessarily in attendance);
2. Initial medical examination (triage will be required if large numbers of persons are exposed), detailed clinical and laboratory investigations and medical treatment in a general hospital;
3. Complete examination and treatment in a specialized radiation medical center, when there is evidence of serious irradiation or internal contamination.

In the 1970s as nuclear reactors were becoming more common, it was suggested that regional centers should be set up to handle radiation accidents. Currently, there are 16 World Health Organization (WHO)-designated radiation accident centers that can provide advice on management of difficult cases. These are listed with their telephone numbers in Appendix 2. Experience during the decade has indicated that immediate local medical and surgical support is critical and except for major accidents (such as Chernobyl) regional support is less important.

Many of the early designs of hospital facilities for radiation accidents had a permanently installed decontamination tabletop in a dedicated room. There was often rigid plumbing with drainage to a specific holding tank for radioactive materials. Now patients are initially treated in the emergency room using specific precautions.[2-7]

Another major change in immediate medical care of radiation accidents has been that the radiation aspects of the case have become secondary, and associated trauma, thermal burns, and myocardial infarctions have become the primary medical concern. Thus, patients must be able to be treated in the area of the emergency room where life-support equipment exists and appropriate supplies are nearby. This has the added advantage that emergency personnel are familiar with where their supplies are located. Now most hospitals maintain equipment that is not fixed and therefore can be readily moved, not only to the emergency room but to other parts of the hospital (in case a radioactive spill occurs within the hospital).

Most hospital plans regarding radiation accidents have assumed the possibility of one to five severely injured and contaminated patients from some industrial or research facility. It is now known from the experience at Three Mile Island and Chernobyl that hospitals also need to be prepared to be able to evaluate large numbers of the public for radioactive contamination. In spite of local emergency plans to evaluate these persons elsewhere, many people living near a nuclear facility that has had release of radioactivity will come to the hospital even though they are not injured just to check whether they have become contaminated with radioactive materials. Unless specific arrangements are made, these people usually will come to the emergency room and possibly in very large numbers. Any plan therefore must include several personnel with monitoring equipment who can make such evaluations, keep appropriate records, and still leave the emergency room capable of handling severely traumatized patients. A classification of the treatment of radiation accident patients at general hospitals is outlined in Chapter 2, Table 2.3.

COMMUNICATIONS

Communication undoubtedly is one of the most important aspects of preparation for a radiation accident. Early in the plan-writing process, the hospital should develop some idea of the various facilities in its area that handle radiation sources and radioactive material. Once this has been done, one can roughly predict the type of accident that may come from each facility. The facilities and ambulance personnel should be aware that, in the case of a suspected or actual radiation accident, the hospital will need advance notice to prepare for the patient's arrival. This information should be directed to the charge nurse in the emergency room. Directing such information to the hospital switchboard has not proved satisfactory in many experiences. The emergency room charge nurse should have a specific procedure manual immediately available. This manual should include a call sheet (see Appendix 1) that prompts certain questions to be asked of the caller, including number of patients, type of injuries, and if the accident is simply a case of overexposure (external irradiation) or if contamination is involved or suspected. A telephone in the room where the patient is to be treated is necessary. This will allow the physician in the room to communicate directly with the industrial facility and consultants as may be necessary.

AREA DESIGNATION

If there is a possibility of radioactive contamination, then a *Radiation Emergency Area* (REA) should be set up. The purpose of this area is to control the spread of radioactive materials (Figure 30.1). Choice of a radiation emergency area is made on the basis of several factors: (1) the area chosen must be suitable to appropriate life support and medical stabilization, (2) the area should be located close to an entrance or have an entrance directly into the treatment room from the outside (this will minimize the possibility of tracking contamination throughout the emergency room), and (3) the area should also be easily accessible to the ambulance so that an ambulance can back up close to the entrance to be utilized. Procedures should designate that the ambulance is to be roped off and watched by security or other personnel. The reason for this is that the ambulance may be contaminated.

The REA is usually set up to have a *contaminated room*, i.e., a room that may become contaminated while treating the patient, and a second area outside the contaminated area referred to as the *buffer zone*. This buffer zone is an area with access controlled by means of doors or ropes. Figure 30.1 shows a buffer zone. The object is to try to keep this area clean of contamination but with the realization that there may be breaks in technique that allow radioactive materials to escape the contaminated room into the buffer room. Beyond the designated buffer zone is the clean (radiation-free) area of the hospital.

The entrance to the contaminated room, optimally, is directly from the outside of the hospital directly into the room. Thus, portions of the emergency room that have a fire exit are ideally suited to become an REA (Figure 30.2). If such an entrance is not available, it usually is not practical or economical to install an entrance specifically for radiation accidents. In the situation in which no such entrance already exists, there are two acceptable alternatives. The one most commonly utilized is to have a floor covering material rolled out from the REA down the hall and out the emergency room entrance. The patient is then taken from the ambulance (on the ambulance stretcher) into the

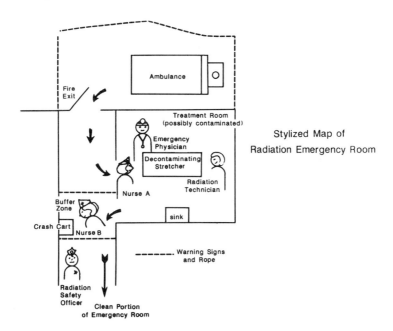

FIGURE 30.1 Schematic design of an area to treat radiation accident victims in an emergency room.

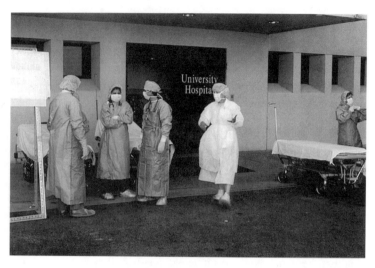

FIGURE 30.2 Hospital staff awaiting multiple radiation accident patients outside the main emergency room entrance.

treatment room. It is important to keep the ambulance personnel and the stretcher on the floor covering. This method is only practical if the hospital has had advance notice, time to put down the floor covering, and if the area chosen for the REA is not too far from the emergency room entrance.

If there has been no advance call of patient arrival or if the REA is located at a fair distance from the emergency room entrance, the simplest alternative is to take a clean hospital stretcher (with a sheet opened on it) out to meet the ambulance (Figure 30.3). The patient can be transferred from the ambulance stretcher onto the hospital stretcher, wrapped up in the cloth sheet, and brought into the hospital (Figure 30.4). A cloth sheet is almost always sufficient to contain the radioactive contamination. In addition, under circumstances in which the patient needs to proceed immediately to the operating room, this method can also be utilized very effectively. The only requirement for this latter technique is that the ambulance personnel must know not to bring a potentially contaminated patient to the emergency room itself but rather to ask the emergency room staff to come out to the ambulance. The use of plastic sheets to wrap the patient is generally inadvisable.

SUPPLIES

One of the first considerations is how to store the necessary supplies. Three possibilities that are often utilized: a closet, locker, and part or all of a large lockable box, i.e., a steamer trunk. Whichever one is utilized, however, it must be lockable. The keys to these supplies normally are kept with the narcotics key by the emergency room charge nurse. The author's particular preference is for storage of the supplies in a manner that they can be easily moved, for example, a locker or cart on wheels, or a steamer trunk. The reason is that, if there is an accidental spill in the hospital, the supplies can easily be moved to the site for appropriate cleanup. These supplies should be organized with an inventory list, to be checked every 6 months, and brief, explicit directions for the use of the items. This will make handling of an accident much easier if persons unfamiliar with radiation accident drills actually have to handle a contaminated and injured patient. The general category of supplies that are included are protective clothing, instrumentation and dosimeters, material for securing the area and controlling contamination, i.e., rope and signs, materials for bioassay and labeling, decontamination supplies, and a long pair of forceps to handle potentially radioactive metallic fragments.

Hospital Preparation for Radiation Accidents

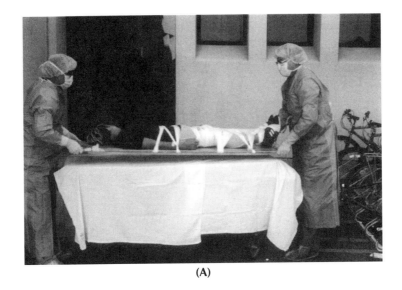

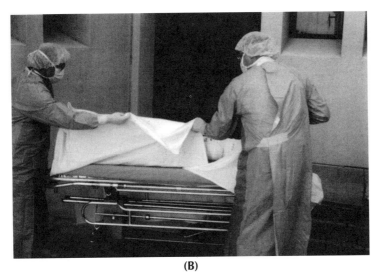

FIGURE 30.3 (A) Placement of a contaminated patient with a traumatic back injury on a stretcher. (B) Folding a cloth sheet over the patient will contain contamination and allow transport to most portions of the hospital.

AREA SETUP

The REA can be set up in many different ways. The critical factor is the amount of time between notification to expect a patient exposed to radiation and the actual arrival of the patient. Most areas need to be able to be set up within 15 to 20 min, although on a historical basis one out of three or four patients will arrive at the emergency room without any prior notification. Under these circumstances, if the patient is seriously injured, the area may have to be set up while the patient is being treated. The setup may be accomplished by emergency room personnel, radiology and nuclear medicine personnel, radiation safety personnel, or the housekeeping and engineering department. The difficulty with having either the radiation safety officer or nuclear medicine personnel in charge of this is that they are not immediately available on evening or night shifts. Most hospitals rely

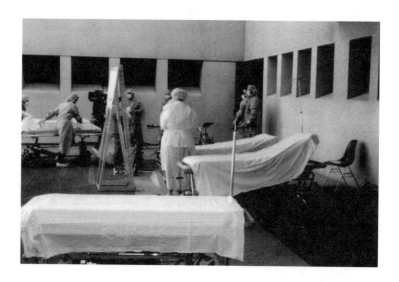

FIGURE 30.4 Patient being taken in a side entrance to a trauma treatment room.

upon either housekeeping or the emergency room personnel themselves to set up the area. The placement of the rope, signs, etc. can be very confusing to someone who has never been through a training session and who is reading the procedure manual for the first time. In this regard, it is extremely valuable to take photographs of the setup in various stages during the course of a drill. These photographs are placed in the procedure manual so that they can be looked at to facilitate REA setup. A map of the floor space and traffic flow also is valuable.

FLOOR COVERING

Special floor covering is not necessary for treatment of a radioactively contaminated patient. The sole purpose of placing floor covering down is to make cleanup of contamination easier after the patient has been treated and has left the area. There is no excuse for delaying medical treatment of a patient because there is no floor covering in place. There are a number of large hospitals that have elected not to use special floor covering for radiation accidents, since it is cumbersome and can delay patient treatment. Most of these hospitals have treatment areas with permanent one-piece floor covering. These have become more commonplace in hospital construction since they allow easy cleanup of blood and pathogens (not to mention radioactive materials).

If one elects to lay floor covering, the following considerations apply. Prior to patient arrival, most hospitals try to cover the floor in the contaminated room and the buffer zone. Several materials have been utilized for floor covering. Paper products are unacceptable since they tear easily when they become wet. Clear or black plastic has been utilized but extreme care should be taken with these materials because they become very slippery when wet. Some heavy duty and nonskid plastic materials have been successfully utilized. The cheapest and most available material for floor covering is probably barbecue cloth. This is most commonly use for tablecloths at picnics and has a nonskid back with a plastic top. It comes in 4-ft-wide rolls and can be purchased at most fabric stores. In the interests of saving time for area preparation, many hospitals have taken the floor covering material and taped it together so that it fits the floor plan of a certain room and can simply be unfolded. If floor covering is used, all of the materials mentioned need to be taped down at the edges to avoid tripping.

VENTILATION

Ventilation in an area where a radioactively contaminated patient is being treated is always a matter of concern. Some institutions have installed high-speed exhaust fans with respirable particle filters. In fact, most residual radioactive contamination usually is not in the form of easily respirable particles, but rather heavy and large particles similar to dirt. The primary reason that surgical masks are worn during treatment of radioactively contaminated patients is not to prevent inhalation of the contamination but rather to keep the hands of doctors and nurses away from their faces (thus preventing oral internal contamination). In spite of the fact that such residual radioactive contamination on patients is not easily airborne, it is still wise to cover the exhaust duct of the hospital ventilation system from the REA with a piece of plastic and masking or duct tape. While this has little effect from a scientific viewpoint, it provides a great amount of reassurance to patients and staff in other portions of the hospital who do not understand that X rays, gamma rays, etc. are not carried along by air currents. A particular caveat to be kept in mind is the special instance in which contamination involves transuranic elements such as plutonium or americium. Under these circumstances, if there is a lot of contamination, respiratory protection may be necessary. Respirators usually are only necessary in hospitals near weapons or very large research facilities. Since hospitals usually do not keep these type of respirators, arrangements to bring appropriate respiratory protection along with the patient should be made prior to an accident.

PATIENT DECONTAMINATION

Decontamination of the patient may pose a problem in terms of disposing of the water utilized. Certainly, if the patient only has a minor traumatic injury, the patient probably should have been kept at the facility where the contamination occurred, decontaminated there, and then brought to the emergency room as a "clean" patient. A patient who has been brought to the emergency room and is severely traumatized obviously will be unable to stand up in a shower.

Perhaps the simplest way to decontaminate a patient who is lying down is to remove the clothing and place it in a plastic bag. This usually will remove about 70 to 90% of the contamination. The residual contamination is typically on the hands, face, neck, and hair. The simplest thing to do is to use a series of washcloths with lukewarm water and mild soap to wash these areas. The washcloths, once used, are placed in a plastic bag.

Decontamination tabletops for supine patients have been developed and are available from several manufacturers. These are lightweight tables that have straps supporting the patient in the supine position and allow the patient to be washed off and the water collected from a drain in the table. A showerhead is sometimes used but there should be a mixing valve to assure that the water may be adjusted to lukewarm rather than being simply hot or cold. If a decontamination tabletop is available, there must be a mechanism for water drainage and collection. Decontamination tabletops should have seatbelt-type straps so that they can be firmly affixed to a standard stretcher. Specific consideration must be given to contaminated patients who present to emergency rooms and have suspected myocardial infarctions. In such circumstances, it is not wise to place such patients on metallic tables (such as a morgue table) or even on a metallic decontamination table, since the patient may need electrical defibrillation.

SHIELDING

Shielding may provide some protection from radiation. This may be in the form of lead bricks, lead aprons, or leaded glass. Unfortunately, experience has demonstrated that shielding is only of limited value in most radiation accidents. Lead aprons of the type available in radiology departments are predominantly useful for low-energy X rays; radiologists and emergency room physicians sometimes feel these are necessary. However, lead aprons of this type provide good shielding only for X and gamma rays in the low energy range (about 30 keV). Most radionuclides involved in accidents have energies that range from 100 keV to over 1000 keV. Thus, in most of the circumstances, one or even two lead aprons do not provide a significant shielding.

Previously, many REAs were designed to include heavy lead shielding that could be placed about the patient. Often these lead shields weighed hundreds of pounds and were not only cumbersome but also top-heavy, so that sometimes they presented more of a danger to the patient than protection to the medical staff. Under most accident circumstances in management of a patient at a hospital, radiation protection for medical staff is best obtained by (1) increasing the distance from the radiation source and (2) spending less time near the radiation source. There is one circumstance in which shielding is important. If a radioactive metallic fragment has been removed from the patient, a lead container (such as may be found in nuclear medicine departments) should be used for placement of the item. Most nuclear medicine departments also have lead bricks that can be obtained as necessary for special shielding purposes. Another item that is useful for radiation protection purposes is a clock. This should be clearly visible in the REA. With this, the radiation safety officer or radiation technician can keep track of the amount of time various individuals have spent in the radiation area.

PROTECTIVE CLOTHING

Protective clothing should be utilized in handling contaminated patients. Typical garb for handling a radioactively contaminated patient is the same as used for "universal precautions" in handling patients with infectious diseases (Figure 30.5). "Protective" clothing is somewhat of a misnomer, since it does not actually protect the wearer from penetrating radiation. Protective clothing usually consists of plastic or water-repellent gowns, jumpsuits, etc., which do not provide significant attenuation of either gamma rays or beta rays. The reason the clothing is termed *protective* is that it prevents radioactive contamination present on the patient from getting onto the skin of the attendants. If contamination gets on the protective clothing, it can be removed by removing the clothing. Full anticontamination gear of the type used in nuclear power plants is not useful in hospitals, especially when working with a seriously injured patient.

A surgical mask is always used to reduce the possibility of hand–oral contamination. A surgical cap is also recommended, particularly for women who have long hair. Gloves are also necessary. The best gloves to utilize are surgical gloves, since it is often necessary to handle wounds, begin intravenous lines, etc. While heavier gloves may not rip as easily, they are often more cumbersome. Some authors have recommended initially wearing two pairs of surgical gloves so that, if the outer pair becomes contaminated, it can simply be removed. This is not absolutely necessary since, if only one pair of gloves is worn and it becomes contaminated, it simply can be changed.

Plastic shoe covers are always utilized. Paper booties (as can be found in operating rooms) are insufficient since they often become wet and disintegrate. If the plastic shoe covers have a relatively high ankle portion, this should be secured with tape.

INSTRUMENTATION

Radiation instrumentation and dosimeters are also necessary. The instrumentation should include as a minimum a Geiger counter. This should preferably be able to operate on batteries as well as on standard electrical current. A Geiger counter really is only utilized to determine whether contamination is present and, if so, where. If very high levels of contamination are present, such that there might be a medical hazard to attendants, the radiation exposure may exceed the capability

Hospital Preparation for Radiation Accidents

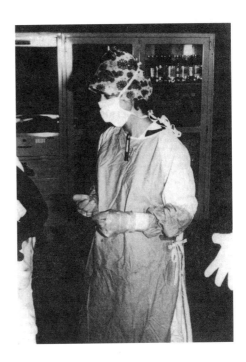

FIGURE 30.5 Universal precaution dress to prevent contamination of the medical staff. Note personal dosimeter on collar.

of the meter and thus a higher-range exposure meter is also useful. Many Geiger counters have a maximum exposure capability of about 50 to 200 µSv/h.

Personnel dosimeters are necessary to determine the dose of radiation received by an individual attendant during the course of accident management. Three forms of dosimeters are utilized. The first is a pen dosimeter, which is basically a small ionization chamber. This is set to zero or has had a baseline reading taken prior to being worn, and it is placed on the outside of the collar of the individual. These dosimeters have the advantage of being instantaneously readable. At any time during the accident, the pen dosimeter may be held up to the light and the radiation exposure read. While very convenient, these do not provide a permanent record and are not as accurate as film badges or thermoluminescent dosimeters (TLDs). These latter two items are familiar to most radiologists and often to nurses as well. They are worn underneath the protective clothing and provide a very accurate record of the dose actually received. Unfortunately, they cannot be read immediately and must be processed. It is important not to let them get contaminated prior to their processing or the dose indicated will be erroneously high.

PROCEDURES

Despite all the planning that is done and the procedures that are written, the management of the patient needs to be able to proceed even with a physician and/or nurses who have never participated in a drill or read the procedure manual. In this regard, it is often helpful to create a poster and include it with the supplies.

The procedure for handling a radiation accident should be written, with copies kept in the emergency room and radiation safety office, as well as in the radiology and nuclear medicine departments. The procedures should be kept on floppy disks so they can be easily and quickly updated. The procedure manual should include a distribution list as well as table of contents. Sample procedures for a hospital that can be easily adapted are found in Appendix 1.

SECURITY

An often-overlooked area in management of these accidents is the need for security as well as the news media aspects. The security personnel should be intimately involved, not only to direct the ambulance to the appropriate entrance, but to be able to secure the entire area in the event of a contaminated patient. A radiation accident of any size merits intense news media coverage. News media continuously scan and monitor ambulance transmissions and, in some accidents, the reporters have actually arrived at the hospital ahead of the patients. Reporters will often cross REA boundaries to be able to talk to the patient and get a story. Under these circumstances, there is potential spread of radioactive materials by the reporters. To circumvent this, hospital administration should be notified when there is a radiation accident. This should allow an area to be set up where information can be given to reporters as it becomes available. At the same time, security should focus on keeping reporters out of the radiation emergency area.

DRILLS

Drills are essential to prepare adequately for handling radiation accidents. The purpose of the drill is twofold: first, to assure that the written procedures are in fact functional, and also to provide training for the personnel. Radiation accidents, as has been mentioned in earlier chapters, are very uncommon and, therefore, unless drills are held it is unlikely that management of such patients will be optimal or even acceptable. These drills should be held on at least an annual basis, and the drill may be included as part of the annual radiation disaster drill for the hospital. It is useful to inject as much realism as possible in the drill by going through the entire procedure with protective clothing and a simulated patient. It is often useful to videotape drills and then edit them down to a 12- to 15-min tape with audio dubbing to explain each of the steps involved. These tapes can be made available to the emergency room for training during the course of the year. As new emergency room physicians and their nursing staff are hired during the course of the year, these tapes can be used to provide a relatively short but efficient training experience. At the end of each drill, a critique should be held, at which time each of the deficiencies or questions can be addressed. Reports derived from the critiques and suggestions are normally forwarded to the radiation safety office and the disaster control committee.

SUMMARY

Effective management of radiation accidents requires a large amount of preparation and thought. In addition, training of the staff is absolutely essential. This is best accomplished through annual drills, but also may be accomplished through the use of videotapes. The critical points to be remembered in the handling of such accidents and in writing the procedures are that treatment of nonradiation-related injuries and medical stabilization are paramount. The second point is that it is important to be able to distinguish between a patient who has been irradiated from an external radiation source and one who is contaminated with radioactive materials. The handling of these two types of accidents is entirely different and this distinction needs to be made early. All of the items outlined in this chapter concern the care of individuals who have been severely injured and radioactively contaminated.

REFERENCES

1. International Atomic Energy Agency, Planning the Medical Response to Radiological Accidents, Safety Rep. Series No. 4, IAEA, Vienna, 1998.

2. National Council for Radiation Protection and Measurements, Developing Radiation Emergency Plans for Academic, Medical or Industrial Facilities, NCRP Rep. 111, National Council for Radiation Protection and Measurements, Bethesda, MD, 1991.
3. International Atomic Energy Agency, What the General Practitioner (MD) Should Know about Medical Handling of Overexposed Individuals, IAEA-TECDOC366, Vienna, 1986.
4. International Atomic Energy Agency, Medical Handling of Accidentally Exposed Individuals, Safety Series No. 88, LAEA, Vienna, 1988.
5. International Atomic Energy Agency, Assessment and Treatment of External and Internal Radionuclide Contamination, IAEA-TECDOC-869, Vienna, 1996.
6. International Atomic Energy Agency, World Health Organization, Diagnosis and Treatment of Radiation Injuries, Safety Rep. Series No. 2, IAEA, Vienna, 1998.
7. International Atomic Energy Agency, Emergency Planning and Preparedness for Accidents Involving Radioactive Materials Used in Medicine, Industry, Research and Teaching, Safety Series No. 91, IAEA, Vienna, 1989.

31 Emergency Room Management of Radiation Accidents

Fred A. Mettler, Jr.

CONTENTS

Introduction 437
Decontamination 438
Radiation Emergency Team Duties 439
Radiation Accident Management Example 440
Specific Problems 445
      Psychological 445
      Blood and Other Laboratory Studies 445
      Electrocardiograms 445
      Radiographs 445
      Surgical Emergencies 446
      High-Activity Source or Metal Fragments in a Patient 446
Summary 446
References 447

INTRODUCTION

The treatment of radioactively contaminated patients is a rare occurrence. The techniques for management of radioactive contamination are also applicable to handling contamination with other toxic substances and, with appropriate modifications, may therefore be used in those circumstances. This chapter is concerned with emergency room management of accidents involving a limited number of radioactively contaminated and medically injured patients. Such circumstances may happen in transportation accidents of radioactive materials, accidents in a medical or research laboratory, or small accidents at nuclear power stations. There are four different kinds of radiation accident patients (see Chapters 1 and 2).

    External Irradiation Only — These persons are not radioactive; however, they may have received very large doses of radiation from an external source. External whole-body or local radiation overexposure is primarily a medical disease and the patient is managed symptomatically in a regular hospital or emergency room without modification. Accidents of this sort occur from irradiation by radioactive industrial sources or accelerators. The pathogenesis, recognition, and definitive treatment of whole-body irradiation has been extensively discussed in Chapters 4 and 5. Evaluation and definitive management of external local overexposure is discussed in detail in Chapter 14.

Internal Contamination Only — Internal contamination could be secondary to inhalation ingestion or wounds involving radioactive materials. This may be from an industrial accident, a very severe misadministration of nuclear medicine materials, or even bizarre circumstances such as attempted suicides. If there is no concurrent external contamination, these patients, again, may be treated in routine medical or emergency rooms; however, vomitus, urine, or feces may be contaminated and must be handled with care. More detail on specific management of internal contamination is presented in Chapter 23.

A Highly Radioactive Metallic Source Embedded within a Patient — Such accidents are exceedingly rare and are typically associated with an explosion. By their nature, therefore, such accidents are almost always associated with physical trauma. Since activated pieces of metal can have very high specific activity, there may be a significant exposure hazard to treatment personnel. Dose rates from such fragments may be as high as 0.5 Sv/h very close to the object. Such accidents could occur from an explosion in the reactor of a nuclear power plant.

External Contamination with or without Internal Contamination — This type of accident may occur as the result of a transportation accident, a nuclear power plant accident, or a spill in a nuclear medicine facility. When serious injury accompanies the contamination, this group requires special precautions to avoid spread of the radioactive contamination to the environment and to medical personnel, and to minimize or prevent internal contamination of the patient.

These patients may need emergency treatment of their injuries concurrently with radiation monitoring and decontamination. It must be emphatically noted that radioactive contamination (whether internal or external) is never immediately life-threatening and, therefore, decontamination should never take precedence over significant medical or surgical injuries. It is, however, important to minimize the internal contamination if at all possible.

One can then give general objectives in approximate order of importance for the emergency room management of seriously injured and contaminated patients.

1. First aid and resuscitation;
2. Medical stabilization;
3. Definitive treatment, if possible, of serious injuries;
4. Prevention/minimization of internal contamination;
5. Assessment of external contamination and decontamination;
6. Treatment of other minor injuries;
7. Containment of the contamination to the treatment area and prevention of contamination of other personnel;
8. Assessment of internal contamination;
9. Treatment of internal contamination (this could be concurrent with many of the above);
10. Assessment of local radiation injuries/radiation burns;
11. Careful long-term follow-up of patient with significant whole-body irradiation or internal contamination;
12. Careful counseling of patient about expected long-term effects and risks.

DECONTAMINATION

The theory of decontamination is relatively simple. Most radioactive contamination on intact skin behaves like loose dirt and may be removed by routine washing. Chapter 28 has a very detailed discussion of contaminated skin wounds and burns. The effectiveness of decontamination procedures of most radionuclides is easily monitored by a Geiger counter. Radionuclides on the *intact skin* surface rarely, if ever, cause a high enough gamma radiation dose to be a hazard to the patient or to medical staff. Even large amounts of fresh fission contamination on a patient are unlikely to cause dose rates of more than 10 mSv/h. To date, the highest recorded absorbed dose in the

United States to a medical person treating patients from a commercial reactor has been 140 μSv. Medical staff treating the Chernobyl victims and spending a lot of time in contact with them received doses in the range of 10 mSv. The intact skin is a very effective barrier to internal contamination. Internal contamination may be a hazard depending upon activity and residence time within parts of the body. Since the main hazard of external contamination is the possibility of internal contamination, external contamination procedures are designed to (1) minimize or prevent internal contamination and (2) decrease the external contamination that is present.

All efforts are made to clean the contamination from the skin, which usually is in the form of loose radioactive dirt, but occasionally may be fixed or embedded in the skin. The skin barrier must be preserved so that procedures such as shaving or harsh scrubbing are not done. If hair needs to be removed, clipping is effective. Warm water, not hot, is used for washing so that a hyperemia is not induced, which may increase absorption of any contaminants through the skin. Cold water is not used since it would tend to close skin pores and trap radioactive contamination. Decontamination is done by progressive cleansing, starting with mild agents such as soap and water and working up to somewhat more involved procedures. The decontamination end point is reached when:

1. No further decrease occurs as determined by monitoring.
2. The contamination is considered low enough to no longer be a significant hazard, i.e., twice background levels.
3. When further decontamination would be more harmful than helpful. This is particularly important in contaminated wounds where debridement might result in permanent or potential deficits in areas such as hands or face.

RADIATION EMERGENCY TEAM DUTIES

The duties of the members of a radiation emergency team are as follows.

Maintenance — It is essential to have the necessary equipment such as gowns, gloves, monitoring devices, and protective floor covering transported to the appropriate area and assembled. The team should also consider closing off the ventilation of the area, as well as placing appropriate warning ropes and signs.

Security Personnel — The radiation area may well be contaminated and must be isolated and protected from visitors. Security may be necessary to direct the ambulance to a designated site or special entrance to the treatment area.

Physician — At least one emergency physician should be present in the decontamination room to deal with the acute medical emergencies. Other medical specialists may be needed as dictated by the other injuries in the case. A medical checklist of useful information to be obtained is given in Table 31.1.

Technical Personnel — A radiation technician, nuclear medicine technologist, or health physicist must ensure that monitoring instruments are operating properly and must assign, collect, and distribute the personnel dosimeters. This individual should perform surveys to determine the extent and magnitude of radioactive contamination.

Nursing Personnel — At least two nurses will be needed inside the decontamination room, one for direct patient care and decontamination, and the other assisting with transfer of equipment in and out of the room, labeling the specimens, etc. Additionally, a third nurse who controls the buffer zone of the decontamination suite is required. This is usually the busiest and one of the most important positions. One other person is required to bring equipment as needed to and from the radiation emergency area (REA) from the rest of the hospital. If possible, another person generally in or near the buffer zone, whose job is solely to monitor everything leaving the room for possible contamination, should be available.

TABLE 31.1
Medical Information Checklist

These can be used by the attending physician at the hospital for obtaining historical information to assist in the early management of radioactively contaminated persons.

Circumstances of the Accident

When did the accident occur and what are the circumstances of the accident? What are the most likely pathways for exposure?
How much radioactive material is potentially involved?
What injuries have occurred?
What potential medical problems may be present besides the radionuclide contamination?
What radioactivity measurements have been made at the site of the accident, e.g., air monitors, smears, fixed radiation monitors, nasal smear counts, and skin contamination levels?
Are toxic or corrosive chemicals involved in addition to the radionuclides?
Have any treatments been given for these?

Present Status of the Patient

What radionuclides now contaminate the patient?
Where and what are the radiation measurements at the surface?
Was the patient also exposed to penetrating radiation? If so, what has been learned from processing personal dosimeters, e.g., film badge, TLD, or pocket ionization chamber? If not yet known, when is the information expected?
What information is available about the chemistry of the compounds containing the radionuclides? Soluble or insoluble? Any information about probable particle size?
What decontamination efforts, if any, have already been attempted? With what success?
Have any therapeutic measures, such as blocking agents or isotopic dilution, been given?

Follow-Up of Patient

Has clothing removed at the site of accident been saved in case the contamination still present on it is needed for radiation energy spectrum analysis and particle size studies?
What excreta have been collected? Who has the samples? What analyses are planned? When will they be done?

Public Relations/Administrator — Since radiation accidents are of intense public and media interest, one can expect reporters and photographers to arrive in droves. The hospital administration needs to be prepared to deal with such individuals, as well as to maintain liaison with the facility where the accident occurred.

An optimum radiation accident management team for one or two patients would therefore include the following:

1. One physician
2. One buffer zone nurse
3. Two nurses in the decontamination room
4. One "go-for" person outside the decontamination room
5. Two survey personnel; one inside the room, one outside
6. Administrator and security staff

RADIATION ACCIDENT MANAGEMENT EXAMPLE

To give a clear understanding of the workings of an emergency room during a radiation accident, a scenario and the handling of such an accident will be given. The scenario involves a small chemical explosion at a nearby nuclear power plant, causing a serious physical trauma and radioactive contamination to worker A. Another (B) is contaminated and has minor injuries and other workers (C and D) have skin contamination only.

The initial response in any accident would be emergency personnel arriving at the scene. In any industrial scene, this would be the first aid team and/or security personnel at the plant. Notification would be made to the control room of the power plant (or, outside of the power plant, to police personnel). Immediately, first aid should be given to the two injured as required and the area cordoned off. An ambulance is called as soon as significant injuries are identified. If the site of the accident is in a high enough radiation field, greater than 0.3 to 0.5 Gy/h, the patients should be carefully moved to a nearby lower radiation field area. The hospital should also be notified to begin preparation of the REA. It is essential that the ambulance be given specific instructions regarding where to enter the plant and where to park. Ambulance personnel should be given dosimeters, be accompanied by security guards from the main plant gate, and be instructed on how they are to dress. Gowns, surgical gloves, and boot covers are usually adequate. It is particularly critical to avoid contamination of the ambulance by parking upwind if there are fumes or a fire. The ambulance personnel will perform the usual medical stabilization, make an assessment of the injuries, and again notify the hospital. Specifically, notification should be given to the emergency room of the number of victims, the nature of the injuries, and whether or not patients are or are suspected to be contaminated.

At this point, triage is important. Workers C and D, who only have skin contamination, should probably be kept at the plant and decontaminated. There are several reasons for this. First, plant personnel usually are much more familiar with decontamination procedures than are emergency room personnel. Second, if all four workers are taken to the hospital, the ambulance will be needlessly crowded and the activities at the hospital REA may be more confused than necessary. Worker B, who has minor injuries and surface contamination, can be taken to the plant's first aid room and have decontamination done as well. If some wound contamination persists, this worker can have the wound covered and be driven to the hospital in a private automobile. Only worker A, who is seriously injured, needs to be transported to the hospital while still contaminated. If time permits, initial decontamination may be done in the ambulance. This involves careful removal of outer clothes and washing contaminated areas (usually face and hands). The ambulance then transports the patient to the emergency treatment area. Since the entrance to the REA may not be the usual emergency room entrance, the ambulance personnel must be so informed. It is useful for security personnel to be stationed at appropriate locations to direct the ambulance.

When the hospital emergency room receives notification of the accident, it puts its radiation accident plan into action. This requires coordination of several different groups as already outlined. It takes approximately 20 to 30 min to set up an average decontamination suite for one or two patients. When the ambulance arrives, the patients are conducted into the treatment area. If there is no outside door to the treatment room, there are several ways to move the patients without spreading contamination. One way is to lay nonskid plastic sheeting down the hallways over which the ambulance stretcher may be wheeled. It is also possible, if the victim's injuries are not too serious, to transfer the patient from the possibly contaminated stretcher in the ambulance onto a clean stretcher with the patient wrapped in clean blankets or sheets. The patient can then be transported down the usual hallways with the contamination contained inside the sheet (Figure 31.1).

Upon arrival, the usual medical assessment should be performed to ensure that the patient is, in fact, medically stable. This is likely to include routine blood work, physical examination, and history. If intravenous lines are needed, they should be started, preferably in skin areas that are uncontaminated; however, intravenous or central lines, if necessary, could be started through regions that are possibly or known to be contaminated if the area is routinely cleansed. Again, external contamination is not immediately life-threatening and should not be allowed to interfere seriously with emergency or resuscitative medical procedures. If, by chance, a patient is routinely admitted

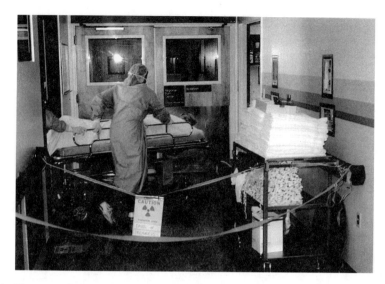

FIGURE 31.1 Entrance of a radioactively contaminated and injured patient to a trauma treatment room. The patient has been wrapped in a sheet and the nearby area has been roped off.

to the emergency room and radioactive contamination is subsequently discovered, the following steps should be taken:

1. Continue attending to the patient's medical needs;
2. Secure entire area where victim and attending staff have been;
3. Do not allow anyone or anything to leave area until cleared by the radiation safety officer;
4. Establish control lines and prevent the spread of contamination;
5. Completely assess patient's radiological status;
6. Personnel should remove contaminated clothing before exiting area, they should be surveyed, shower, dress in clean clothing, and be resurveyed before leaving area.

With appropriate notification, and the patient medically stabilized, initial decontamination of the patient should be started. The most effective step, which may be done in the ambulance on the way to the hospital, involves the removal of all clothing. This is likely to remove over 90% of the contamination with the exception of the hands, face, and other exposed skin areas. Clothing should be carefully removed to avoid contamination of clean skin from the dirty clothing, and to keep the contamination contained. This procedure is most easily accomplished by carefully and correctly cutting off the clothes. The cuts of the clothes are best made in the midline along the leg, the arms, in the middle of the chest, and abdomen. The clothes are then carefully folded back away from the skin so that any dislodged contamination will not fall on the patient, but will tend to fall away from the patient. The clothes can then be folded outside and removed from the patient. Shoes and/or boots should also be removed if possible as this will also remove a large amount of contamination. If the clothes are heavily contaminated, they should be placed in a plastic bag and removed to a far corner of the decontamination suite so as not to affect the radiation measurement of the patient.

Following removal of the clothing, the patient should again be carefully monitored from head to toe (including the back, if possible) and the locations and readings of any contamination remaining on the patient's skin should be carefully recorded. Swabs should be made of these contaminated areas, and the site and time recorded. The distance of the probe to the patient should be a standard distance of approximately 2–3 cm. This is essential for comparison with subsequent readings, which will be made to determine the effectiveness of decontamination. If there are sufficient personnel, decontamination and removal of clothing could be done concurrently with medical assessment and stabilization. If contamination on skin persists, there are several items that should be considered prior to the use of more aggressive scrubbing or the use of stronger decontaminating agents. Often the persistent counts may come from contamination that is in skin folds of the ears, about the nose, etc. It also may be the result of radioactive material under or next to the fingernails. Thus, before more aggressive tactics are employed, a careful washing of these areas should be performed. A second point to remember is that not all counts on an instrument may be coming from skin contamination. They may in fact be coming from internal contamination, such as inhaled or ingested materials, radioiodine in the thyroid, or even contamination of the Geiger counter probe. Internal contamination should be assessed at a minimum by swabs of the nares and mouth. Internal contamination should be suspected if nasal or oral swabs show contamination although, since oral and nasal contamination may be rapidly cleared, negative swab readings should not be construed as an indication that internal contamination is not present. All swabs should be placed in a bag and labeled (Figure 31.2). The swabs can be counted either on a Geiger counter or in nuclear medicine. Nasogastric suction should be considered if there is the serious possibility of recently swallowed radioactive materials. All excreta, such as urine, feces, etc., should be collected, labeled by site and time, and examined for contamination. Contamination found in any of these documents internal contamination, and the samples may be analyzed for the isotopes and compounds involved.

If there are open wounds and they are free of contamination, they should be covered with a waterproof dressing such as Op-cite[R] to prevent cross-contamination. Contaminated wounds may be cleaned by gentle scrubbing with a surgical sponge and irrigation (Figure 31.3). Debridement for removal of contamination should be carefully considered before it is performed. Emergency management of thermal burns that are radioactively contaminated is a difficult problem. The immediate instinct of emergency staff is to wash such burns thoroughly to remove the contamination. This should not be done for several reasons. If the thermal burn is extensive, any washing will place the patient in grave danger of hypothermia and hypotension. Even if the thermal burn is localized, scrubbing may remove marginally viable skin and make the burn treatment much more difficult. Usually, gentle rinsing of local burns is all that is necessary initially. The burn is then

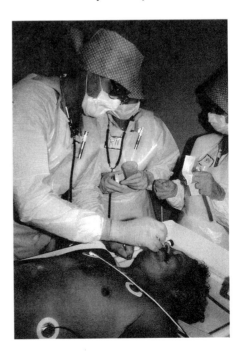

FIGURE 31.2 After the patient has been medically stabilized, an assessment of possible internal contamination via inhalation is done by checking for radioactivity on nasal swabs.

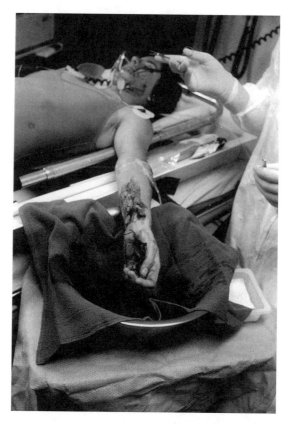

FIGURE 31.3 A contaminated wound should be irrigated and the washings collected in a container.

covered and over the next few days the exudate will lift out a lot of the contamination into the dressings. When the patient is stable and clean, he can be moved from the room. "Clean" would suggest a contamination level at or below twice background level although, depending upon the region of contamination, more or less may be tolerated. When the patient is clean, he or she should be transported carefully to a clean table or stretcher for removal from the room. When this is done the personnel should have on clean gloves. The appropriate procedure for removal is to roll in a new stretcher over a clean plastic sheet parallel to the patient's decontamination table. The patient is then transferred to the clean stretcher; and the clean patient is wheeled out of the room. The patient, stretcher, all supplies, the intravenous bags, and everything leaving the room must be monitored to prevent the spread of contamination outside the REA.

At this point, it is only the personnel who will have to deglove and degown carefully as they exit the room. This involves a progressive removal of the outer toward the inner garments, leaving all possibly contaminated articles in the REA. The personnel are then monitored, particularly the feet, as they exit the room to be sure that they are not contaminated. The usual approach is removal of the outer pair of gloves, followed by the mask and/or hat. Aprons are removed, followed by the external surgical gown, which is carefully removed from the outside keeping the contamination off the personnel. Finally, the booties or shoe covers are removed one at a time with the person then stepping from the room toward the outside one foot at a time and, while leaning back in the room, the gloves are then removed one at a time. The pen-reading dosimeter and film badge thermoluminescent dosimeter (TLD) should be given to the radiation safety officer for recording and processing, if necessary. Be sure that the proper name is affixed to the dosimeter or film badge. Once all the personnel have left, one now has simply a contaminated room. This is usually cleaned up by the persons responsible for the contamination, such as the power plant or regulatory authorities. It is essential that the contaminated waste is disposed of properly.

SPECIFIC PROBLEMS

PSYCHOLOGICAL

The psychological aspects of the patient are all too often forgotten in the emergency management of such patients. Specific pyschological issues are covered in more detail in Chapter 41. Certainly, the emergency room is a strange environment for most patients. This feeling, coupled with the appearance of frightened medical staff all suited up in gowns, etc. is even more unsettling for the patient. If one now adds the patient's own fears about radiation effects, there are the makings of a genuine psychiatric consult. A calm and reassuring attitude of all concerned is essential not only in management of the patient, but of the family, news media, and hospital administration. Careful discussion with the patient about the short- and long-term effects of the radiation are almost as essential as the decontamination. This should include the reassurance that the patient is not a hazard to friends and families.

BLOOD AND OTHER LABORATORY STUDIES

Questions often arise regarding how to perform certain medical procedures in a decontamination suite. This list is not exhaustive, and neither are the explanations; however, they do give a good indication as to how these procedures may be easily and efficiently performed.

Blood can and should be taken for the usual routine diagnostic tests. If possible, venipunctures, including intravenous lines, should be performed outside the areas of known contamination. If this in not feasible, then the selected area should be cleansed in the usual fashion and the venipuncture performed. The puncture does not usually introduce significant contamination into the patient. The blood products should then be monitored before leaving the suite. If contamination is identified on the blood sample tubes, it is most likely to be contamination on the outer tube surface and significant contamination of the blood is unlikely. This surface contamination may then be cleaned off.

Certain laboratory studies should be obtained in the initial evaluation of radiation accident patients. These include:

- Full blood count
- Cytogenetic analysis (usually best done 24 h postexposure)
- Blood sample for later analysis of radionuclide content
- Serum amylase
- Urine and stool samples for later evaluation of radionuclide content

ELECTROCARDIOGRAMS

The easiest method of performing an electrocardiogram (ECG) if necessary is to leave the ECG cart outside the room in a clean or buffer area and only introduce into the room one set of ECG leads. The leads are attached to the patient and a clean end is left attached to the ECG machine. The procedure is performed and the ECG leads can then be left in the room for decontamination or disposal, leaving the machine available for use elsewhere in the hospital.

RADIOGRAPHS

Routine portable radiographs can be performed. The X-ray machine can be left outside the decontamination room and only the head of the machine projected into the room (Figure 31.4). The patient can be wheeled on the stretcher toward the door and then the chest, abdomen, or extremities

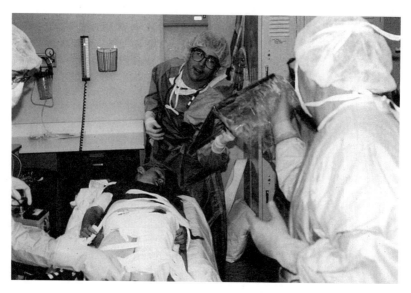

FIGURE 31.4 An X-ray cassette has been covered with plastic prior to being used in the contaminated room to keep the cassette from becoming contaminated.

can be radiographed as needed. The film, of course, must be moved into and then out of the room. This can be done most easily by placing the clean cassette inside a plastic bag, which is then placed under the patient as required. The cassette with the bag is then handed toward the outside of the room, the clean cassette inside the bag is removed, and the contaminated bag left within the decontamination suite. The X-ray machine, not being contaminated, may now be removed.

SURGICAL EMERGENCIES

In the worst case, a patient with a surgical emergency could be moved to the operating room while still contaminated and have the emergency surgery performed. During surgery, minimization of internal contamination should be attempted; however, any life-threatening emergency requiring immediate surgery should not be deterred or deferred by the presence of external contamination. In this case, the operating room would be contaminated and would need to be decontaminated prior to use by other patients. One could assess the presence and level of contamination in this room with a careful survey using a Geiger counter.

HIGH-ACTIVITY SOURCE OR METAL FRAGMENTS IN A PATIENT

It is possible for small, highly radioactive metal fragments to be embedded in the patient. Because they may have a very high dose rate at their surface, it is essential that they be handled with forceps or pick-ups to avoid possible radiation burns to personnel. A lead container or "pig" from nuclear medicine is useful to shield personnel from these fragments once they are removed.

SUMMARY

Emergency room management of radioactively contaminated patients who have an associated medical injury requiring immediate attention must be handled with care. Radioactive contamination of the skin of a worker is not a medical emergency and is usually dealt with at the site of the accident. Effective preplanning and on-the-scene triage will allow the seriously injured and contaminated patients to get to the medical care they need with a minimum of confusion and interference. Immediate medical and surgical priorities always take precedence over radiation injuries and radioactice contamination.

Probably the most difficult aspect of emergency management is the rarity of such accidents, and hence the unfamiliarity of the medical staff with the appropriate procedures. The simplest answer to these problems is preplanning, having a simple and workable procedure, and finally having 24-h access to experts. The World Health Organization Coordinating Centers and their telephone numbers are listed in Appendix 2.

REFERENCES

1. Leonard, R.B. and Ricks, R.C., Emergency department radiation accident protocol, *Ann. Emerg. Med.,* 9, 462, 1980.
2. NCRP, Management of Persons Accidentally Contaminated with Radionuclides, NCRP Rep. 65, National Council on Radiation Protection and Measurements, Washington, D.C., 1980.
3. Jankowski, C.B., Radiation emergency, *Am. J. Nurs.,* 82, 90, 1982.

32 Application of Radiation Protection Principles to Accident Management

Fred A. Mettler, Jr.

CONTENTS

Introduction 449
Accidental Exposure 449
Intervention 450
Limitation of Occupational Exposure in Emergencies 450
Dose Limits and Overexposure 450
References 452

INTRODUCTION

Radiological protection is primarily concerned with procedures and practices to control exposures to ionizing radiation in a way that provides an appropriate standard of protection without unduly limiting benefits of the uses of radiation.[1]

The radiation from a source or practice needs to be justified. This means that no practice involving radiation exposure should be adopted unless it produces sufficient benefit to the exposed individuals or to society to offset the radiation detriment. In addition, doses should be kept as low as reasonably achievable (ALARA), taking economic and social factors into account.

Control of occupational exposure is done at the source (by fixing its characteristics in the environment, e.g., ventilation or shielding) and at the individual (requiring working practices). Public exposure is only controlled at the source.

Finally, individuals should be subject to dose limits or some control of risk (in the case of accidents). This is done to assure that individuals are not exposed to radiation risks that are judged to be unacceptable from these practices in normal circumstances. Dose limits do not apply to accidental exposures but rather to control of existing practices..

ACCIDENTAL EXPOSURE

Even with radiation protection programs in place, accidents will occur. Accidents are sometimes referred to as "potential exposures." In the application of radiation protection, the probability and magnitude of accidents should be considered as part of the original justification process.[2] In general, design of equipment and facilities should have less than a one in a million chance per year of a sequence of events that may cause death and a 1 in 100,000 to 1,000,000 chance of a sequence of events that results in doses to persons that will cause deterministic injury.

INTERVENTION

Accidents, once they have occurred, give rise to situations in which the only available action is intervention.[3] Intervention is intended to reduce radiation dose from a source that is already present in the environment. Examples of intervention would include removal of radioactive contamination, administration of potassium iodide, sheltering, evacuation, and interdiction of contaminated foods (Table 32.1).

TABLE 32.1
Examples of Protective Actions (Interventions) for Averting Exposures via Various Pathways

Route of Exposure	Protective Action
External irradiation from a source	Control of access, shielding
Radionuclides in air or on ground	Control of access, sheltering, evacuation
External contamination	Protective clothing, decontamination
Inhalation of radioiodine	Stable iodine administration
Ingestion of radionuclides	Restriction of contaminated food and water supply, decreasing incorporation into food chain, decontamination

Three general principles form the basis for taking decisions on intervention.[4] The first of these is that all possible efforts should be made to prevent serious deterministic health effects. There is no specific dose level at which intervention should be undertaken, although at levels of dose that would cause serious deterministic effects, some kind of intervention would be almost mandatory. The second principle is that the invention should be justified in the sense that the protective measure should do more good than harm. While this may seem obvious, inappropriate actions have been taken in accidental situations to reduce dose at an extremely high social and monetary cost.

The third principle is that the levels at which intervention is introduced and at which it is later withdrawn should be optimized. After an intervention action is applied (e.g., administration of DTPA chelating agents after a plutonium inhalation), there still needs to be optimization of the action to determine the scale and duration of the intervention. Obviously, the costs and benefits of such actions will change over time. If people have been relocated and the radioactivity decays sufficiently, they may be allowed to go back home. A summary of the International Commission on Radiological Protection (ICRP) and International Atomic Energy Agency (IAEA) recommended intervention levels is shown in Table 32.2.

LIMITATION OF OCCUPATIONAL EXPOSURE IN EMERGENCIES

When it is clear that an accident has occurred, it may be necessary knowingly to allow individuals to be exposed to relatively high levels of radiation. This may be necessary to perform an urgent intervention or even to save lives. The ICRP has recommended that effective doses that exceed about 0.5 Sv and skin doses that exceed about 5 Sv should not be permitted except for life-saving actions. Very similar guidance comes from the U.S. National Council on Radiation Protection and Measurements (NCRP) (Table 32.3). Most organizations are silent regarding how much whole-body dose above 0.5 Sv should be permitted for life-saving actions. Given the uncertainties in dosimetry during an accident, as well as the sharp rise in serious deterministic effects above 1 Sv, this should be regarded as a practical upper limit.

TABLE 32.2
Summary of ICRP and IAEA Recommended Intervention Levels[a]

ICRP

Type of Intervention	Intervention Level of Averted Dose (mSv)	
	Almost Always Justified	Range of Optimized Values
Sheltering	50	Not more than a factor of 10 lower than the justified value
Administration of stable iodine-equivalent dose to thyroid	500	
Evacuation (<1 week)		
Whole-body dose	500	
Equivalent dose to skin	5000	
Relocation	1000	5–15 mSv per month for prolonged exposure
Restriction to a single foodstuff	10 (in 1 year)	1,000–10,000 Bq/kg (beta/gamma emitters) 10–100 Bq/kg alpha emitters

IAEA

Type of Action	Dose Avertable by Protective Action	
Sheltering (up to 2 days)	10 mSv	
Evacuation (up to 1 week)	50 mSv	
Temporary relocation	30 mSv in first month, 10 mSv in a subsequent month	
Permanent resettlement	1 Sv in a lifetime	
Iodine prophylaxis	100 mGy	

Restricting Foods Containing	General Consumption	Milk, Infant Foods, Water
^{134}Cs, ^{137}Cs, ^{103}Ru, ^{106}Ru, ^{89}Sr	1000 Bq/kg	1000 Bq/kg
^{131}I	—	100 Bq/kg
^{90}Sr	100 Bq/kg	—
^{241}Am, ^{238}Pu, ^{239}Pu, ^{240}Pu, ^{242}Pu	10 Bq/kg	1 Bq/kg

[a] These are generic guidelines and specific accident circumstances that need to be taken into account. For example, food and water restriction depends upon alternative supplies being readily available.

TABLE 32.3
Guidance for Emergency Occupational Exposure

Type of Action	Organ	Level (mSv)
Life-saving		
ICRP	Whole body	May exceed 0.5 Sv effective dose
	Skin	May exceed 5 Sv equivalent dose
NCRP	Whole body (or large part)	May approach or exceed 0.5 Sv
Urgent		
ICRP	Whole body	0.5 Sv or less effective dose
	Skin	5 Sv or less equivalent dose
NCRP	Whole body	Occupational limits up to 0.5 Sv effective dose
	Skin	5 Sv equivalent dose

DOSE LIMITS AND OVEREXPOSURE

Despite source control and intervention, in accidental situations an individual or the public can exceed the annual recommended dose limits. As noted in earlier chapters, dose assessment during the early phases of accident management is, at best, difficult. Individual dose assessment is ultimately based upon physical dosimetry, accident reconstruction, or biological markers and clinical examination.

Ultimately, a decision needs to be made whether the individual can be permitted to go back to work. Workers or employers may be hesitant to allow more occupational exposure knowing that the individual received more than the annual recommended dose limit. A number of misconceptions exist about the use of dose limits. They are widely and erroneously thought of as the demarcation between "safe" and "dangerous." The annual dose limit is an amount that a worker could receive each and every year of his work life. Thus, slightly exceeding an annual effective dose limit has little biological significance. The major factor is the total cumulative dose and the risk that the individual has incurred. Risk from exceeding the dose limit in 1 year can be offset by being below the dose limit in other years.

The ICRP has no specific guidance relative to allowing a person to return to work after exceeding a dose limit; however, the NCRP has discussed the issue of occupational radiation exposure in excess of the dose limits.[5] The NCRP recommends that individuals whose cumulative effective dose exceeds the age-related limit (10 mSv × age in years) should be restricted in their exposures to no more than 10 mSv/year until the age-related lifetime limit is met. If additional flexibility is warranted, particularly for older workers, in a dialogue between the employer and worker, an exposure of up to 100 mSv in 5 years and 50 mSv in any year may be considered.

Intake of long-lived radionuclides poses additional problems. Doses are often calculated in terms of "committed dose." This usually refers to the dose an individual would be expected to receive from that intake over the next 50 years. Although this may make sense for a young worker, it has little relevance to a 60-year-old worker. Nonetheless, a number of governments have chosen to remove workers from a radiation environment if their committed dose exceeds the lifetime dose limit. An additional issue is that doses from intakes of radionuclides are often calculated on the basis of models and the ICRP reference manual. There may be significant individual deviations from these estimates and, with significant exposures, individual information should be used. This is particularly important if there has been an intervention (such as administration of potassium iodide) that substantially affects the clearance and biological half-life of the radionuclide.

REFERENCES

1. ICRP, 1990 Recommendations of the International Commission on Radiological Protection, ICRP Publ. 60, *Ann. ICRP*, 21(1–3), Pergamon Press, Oxford, U.K., 1991.
2. ICRP, Protection from Potential Exposure: A Conceptual Framework, Publ. 64, International Commission on Radiological Protection, *Ann. ICRP*, 23(1), Pergamon Press, Oxford, U.K., 1993.
3. ICRP, Principles for Intervention for Protection of the Public in a Radiological Emergency, International Commission on Radiological Protection, ICRP Publ. 63, Pergamon Press, Oxford, U.K., 1993.
4. IAEA, Intervention Criteria in a Nuclear or Radiation Emergency, Safety Series No.109, International Atomic Energy Agency, Vienna, 1994.
5. NCRP, Limitation of Exposure to Ionizing Radiation, National Council on Radiation Protection and Measurements, NCRP Rep. 116, Bethesda, MD, 1993.

33 Monitoring and Epidemiological Follow-Up of People Accidentally Exposed

Shirley A. Fry and Fred A. Mettler, Jr.

CONTENTS

Introduction 453
Medical Monitoring 454
    Effects of Accuracy of Monitoring and Disease Prevalence 455
    Assessment of the Benefit of Medical Monitoring 456
    Costs of Medical Monitoring...456
    Monitoring Sensitive Populations 456
    Screening for Specific Cancers...457
    Summary of Medical Monitoring Considerations..457
Epidemiological Follow-Up..457
    Issues of Study Design 458
    Choice of Population and Outcome to Be Studied 458
    Data Sources and Quality 458
    Summary 459
References 460

INTRODUCTION

After the acute effects of accidental high-dose radiation exposure are dealt with, there is often a discussion about the utility of long-term medical monitoring, creation of an accident registry, or epidemiological evaluation. This chapter will not deal with early clinical care or follow-up for specific deterministic injuries since these are covered in other chapters. A wide range of issues related to follow-up of potentially exposed soldiers has been recently published in a report of the U.S. Institute of Medicine.[1] This chapter draws heavily upon that report.

Some issues clearly affect the identification of long-term health effects. Major issues include the need for good dosimetry and availability of records. A number of additional issues must also be recognized as important. A bias may well occur when an accidentally exposed worker does not report a potential radiation-induced illness for fear of losing his or her employment. This will result in assuming that there may not be a problem (or that it is small) when the problem is actually significant. On the other hand, if there is a chance for economic gain, there may be a tendency to overreport and overestimate potential problems.

After high doses of radiation there may be long-term health effects such as bowel obstruction, skin ulceration, and thyroid hypofunction. These issues will be specific to a given accident and to a given patient. The best approach to these potential problems is to relate the patient's estimated organ doses to the organ effects listed in Chapters 5 and 6 and then to design an individual program. In accidental situations, the number of persons requiring this is likely to be in the range of several hundred or less. Some accidental situations have exposed very large numbers of people to doses of radiation less than 1 Sv. These people are the focus of this chapter and concern is primarily related to the development of malignant disease and psychological effects.

For purposes of this chapter, medical monitoring refers to the screening of asymptomatic populations to detect preclinical disease with the purpose of delaying or preventing the development of disease in those individuals. Epidemiological follow-up tracks a defined population with the purpose of identifying deviations from normal health parameters.

MEDICAL MONITORING

As early as 1922, the American Medical Association endorsed routine physical examinations for the general population to reveal current and prevent future illnesses. This approach, along with the use of multiphasic testing, yielded little new information or served to confirm already diagnosed illnesses. Therefore, in 1983, the American Medical Association issued a policy statement withdrawing its support for the standard adult physical examination. Canadian and Australian authorities have reached similar conclusions.

Similarly, medical monitoring after radiation exposure is not routinely suggested or practiced for individuals with known or suspected exposures to radiation. An exposure or a presumed exposure to radiation is not by itself sufficient to justify a medical monitoring program. The decision about whether a medical monitoring program is appropriate and necessary in a given situation should be based on consideration of a number of factors including a rigorous cost–benefit analysis. This analysis should take into account the following characteristics:

1. The exposure of concern (e.g., its certainty, dose, and temporal relationship of exposure to observation);
2. The disease of interest (e.g., its natural history and prevalence in the population);
3. The characteristics of the available screening tests (e.g., their effectiveness, sensitivity, and specificity);
4. The potential that the screening tests will actually cause harm;
5. The potential for action when test results are positive (e.g., the availability of and risks from follow-up evaluation); and
6. Whether there is evidence that an intervention can improve the clinical outcome.

Those malignant diseases that have been associated epidemiologically with prior radiation exposure are termed *radiogenic*; they include leukemia (all types except chronic lymphocytic leukemia); cancer of the female breast; cancers of the lung, stomach, thyroid, esophagus, small intestine, colon, liver, skeleton, central nervous system, and ovary; nonmelanoma skin cancer; and cancer of the salivary glands.[2,3] For some tumors (such non-Hodgkin's lymphoma) whether there is an increased risk is not clear. For a number of cancers such as cervix, uterus, pancreas, multiple myeloma, and prostate, there is little evidence of increased risk associated with radiation exposure.[4] Unfortunately, many times the approach to medical follow-up of potentially exposed individuals is based not on scientific knowledge but on sociopolitical considerations.

A number of investigators have discussed the principles for cancer screening in general. Taplin and Mandelson[5] suggest a series of steps beginning with evaluation of the existing epidemiology literature in terms of the normal incidence of the disease of interest. It is not reasonable scientifically to screen for a disease that is extremely unlikely to occur as a result of a given exposure. If, for example, 100,000 people were exposed to a radiation dose that was estimated to increase the risk of developing cancer by one in a million, less than one additional case of cancer would be expected to result from that exposure. Screening of that population would not yield useful results. Screening is done for cervical cancer, which is diagnosed in 6 of 100,000 U.S. women annually, and for breast cancer, which is diagnosed in 85 of 100,000 U.S. women annually.

The justification for a proposed screening or monitoring program can be assessed by considering the normal incidence rates and comparing these to the excess number of cases expected as a result of some exposure. Consider the case of a disease that spontaneously occurs at an annual incidence of about 25 cases/100,000 population at age 50 but whose incidence rises to 50/100,000 at age 55. Excess cases induced by some toxic exposure would justify monitoring only if monitoring was also justified (and performed) for the increase (25 cases/100,000 population) that occurred spontaneously.

The latent period between radiation exposure and the development of a clinically detectable tumor may have an effect on the design of a screening program. If a population is exposed between the age of 20 and 40 years, most radiation-induced tumors would be expected to become clinically evident at ages older than 40, and in most cases older than 50. Since most cancers occur spontaneously at older ages, Berg[6] has looked at cancer screening of a nonexposed general population over the age of 50. For such a population, he recommends periodic physical examination of the breast, mammography, a Pap test, physical examination of the skin, flexible sigmoidoscopy to 35 cm, and oral examination.

Recommended screening tests for cancer change with time as randomized clinical trials are completed and as technology develops. Probably the best comprehensive source of current information and guidance is the report of the U.S. Preventive Services Task Force.[7] It is of interest to note that most of the more than 50 screening interventions reviewed in the 1996 edition had insufficient evidence of effectiveness to warrant a U.S. Preventive Services Task Force recommendation.

EFFECTS OF ACCURACY OF MONITORING AND DISEASE PREVALENCE

Since actions are taken or are not taken on the basis of test results, that false-positive and false-negative results can and do occur must be considered when planning a test program. The U.S. Agency for Toxic Substances and Disease Registry (ATSDR), which is charged by statute with evaluating the need for medical monitoring programs at Superfund sites (sites subject to cleanup of hazardous materials, including radioactivity), has developed criteria for the establishment of medical monitoring. These are designed in recognition of the serious consequences that can result from both false-positive and false-negative test results. ATSDR has also addressed the psychological consequences of false-positive results.

The prevalence of the disease of interest in the population has an effect on screening test accuracy. When a test is performed on a symptomatic population, the prevalence of the expected disease is reasonably high. However, in the screening of an asymptomatic population, the probability that the disease is actually present is low. As an example, if the test is being used with a population of 10,000 persons with a disease prevalence of 1 in 10,000 and the test has a 5% false-positive rate, there will be 501 positive results, of which 1 will represent true disease and 500 will be false-positive results (a positive predictive value of 1/501, or 0.2%). The use of more than one test further reduces the positive predictive value. Even if the prevalence of disease in the screened population is quite high (e.g., 1%), the positive predictive value of a one-test screening program rises only to 16%.

ASSESSMENT OF THE BENEFIT OF MEDICAL MONITORING

Even with the availability of an accurate test, there must be a demonstration of the benefit of early detection. There must also be lead time during which a disease can be found as a result of monitoring before symptoms occur. If the patient presents with symptoms at the same time that the test becomes positive, then periodic testing will be of no benefit.

The availability of a sensitive and accurate test that detects a disease before symptoms occur still is not sufficient reason to justify the use of such a test to monitor the health of a population. There must also be an intervention or a therapy that is effective, available, and acceptable to the patient. A number of screening programs have found smaller tumors in high-risk populations (e.g., chest radiographs of smokers), but the mortality rate was unchanged, probably because the tumor had already spread to distant sites in the body. As a result, chest radiographs are not recommended for monitoring or screening even of smokers, who are at five to ten times higher risk for lung cancer than nonsmokers.

Randomized trials using the screening tests must show a benefit. The benefit can be measured in a number of ways. Commonly used parameters are the percentage of people who are cured or the percentage of fatalities that are averted. More difficult to measure — and therefore less desirable as study end points — are a decrease in years of life lost or an increase in quality of life remaining.

Finally, effective use of a test depends on the clinician's sufficient understanding of the test to know the appropriate interval for repeat testing, as well as the costs and risks of the test.

COSTS OF MEDICAL MONITORING

The International Agency for Research on Cancer (IARC)[8] has pointed out that screening costs to be considered should include not only the financial cost of the initial medical actions but also the

- Cost of intensive follow-up for false-positive results,
- Emotional cost for false-positive results,
- Cost of delayed diagnosis due to false-negative results,
- Extension of period of morbidity for those in whom early detection does not improve survival,
- Unpleasantness of screening test (e.g., colonoscopy), and
- Risk from screening (e.g., mammography).

An example of the major psychological costs[9] associated with screening programs involves mammography. Mammography has rates of false positivity of 70 to 80%, so three of every four women who test positive must have a biopsy or surgery — with the accompanying physical risk and psychological fear — before they learn that they do not have a malignancy.

MONITORING SENSITIVE POPULATIONS

There are situations when risk is low (and monitoring the general population is not warranted) but a monitoring program might be justified for selected subgroups.[10,11] Such subgroups might include those who are genetically susceptible to a particular disease such as cancer. Relative to radiation exposure, the predominant general factor that appears to affect radiation sensitivity to a number of cancers is age at the time of exposure (with more risk per unit dose at the younger ages). Gender is also related to the incidence of cancer following radiation exposure: females have a slightly higher risk per unit dose than men due to the occurrence of breast and thyroid cancers.

At present, genetic testing is only beginning to be used, and its ramifications are not clear.[12] The issues of efficacy of intervention, test cost and accuracy, and disease prevalence considered throughout this chapter also apply to genetic testing. At present, genetic testing is used only in the clinical management of families with well-defined inherited cancer syndromes.

SCREENING FOR SPECIFIC CANCERS

Although certain types of leukemia and some cancers are generally accepted as having a scientific basis for their designation as "radiogenic cancers," to date screening programs have been shown to reduce mortality effectively only for cancers of the female breast and colon among this group of potentially radiogenic tumors. Although the Pap smear for the early detection of cervical cancer has proved to be highly successful in reducing the rate of mortality due to this cancer among women, association of the cancer with exposure to radiation is equivocal. The Pap smear is therefore unlikely to be useful for the detection of potentially radiogenic cervical cancers. The same may be said for prostate cancer screening tests.

SUMMARY OF MEDICAL MONITORING CONSIDERATIONS

A medical monitoring program for asymptomatic persons exposed to radiation must take account of a wide variety of major factors before it is instituted. The major long-term effect that one might find after exposure to radiation in the dose range of 50 to 1000 mSv is cancer. The risk of cancer is high even in nonexposed populations, and few tests have been shown to be of benefit in terms of improving either survival or quality of life. Those that have been endorsed include the Pap smear and mammography. However, the incidence of radiation-induced tumors among those exposed to the dose range of interest would almost always be less than the normal spontaneous incidence. If a monitoring or screening test is developed and an effective therapy is available, it is the spontaneous cancer risk (not the radiogenic cancer risk) that should drive a decision to do monitoring. It is theoretically possible that a test may be developed that could assess radiation-induced genetic damage likely to lead to malignancy. If such a test were developed it could prove useful. None of the above should prevent symptomatic persons from receiving appropriate diagnostic tests.

EPIDEMIOLOGICAL FOLLOW-UP

All the medical follow-up processes described in the preceding sections involve direct contact with *individuals* who may have been exposed to radiation. Epidemiological follow-up is based primarily on the *records* for *groups* of those individuals. Epidemiological studies seek to identify the distribution and determinants of disease among human populations by comparing groups that have some experience or exposure, such as radiation, in common. Although such research may benefit the individuals studied, it contributes primarily by increasing scientific understanding of the relationships between exposure and subsequent health outcomes.

Epidemiological follow-up of a group of persons known or presumed to have been exposed to a potentially hazardous agent may be implemented to

- Identify adverse health effects in an *at-risk* group and to determine whether the risk of such effects is greater than that for a comparable but nonexposed group of individuals;
- Determine whether the increased risks that may be identified are associated statistically with the exposure;
- Determine whether the increased observed risk is related to or influenced by other factors associated with or independent of the exposure, such as tobacco smoking and radon; and
- Add to the scientific knowledge base, which can then be used to derive and refine risk estimates and to develop interventions.

Epidemiological follow-up studies may describe a disease situation in a defined group at a specific point in time (cross-sectional prevalence studies) or may collect information about group members over an extended time period (longitudinal studies). In prospective longitudinal studies, a defined population (or cohort) that has a common experience or exposure is followed forward in time to determine if there is an increased risk of disease among this cohort relative to that among a comparable nonexposed cohort. Alternatively, groups of individuals with and without a specific disease, condition, or cause of death can be compared retrospectively, using recorded data, to determine if the risk of exposure was greater in the diseased than in the nondiseased group.

Issues of Study Design

The planning and implementation of epidemiological research involve many practical concerns,[13] including the

- Availability of a clearly defined and appropriate study population with unique individual identifiers;
- Size and composition of the study population (as a general approximation, a population of 1000 persons is needed to evaluate the carcinogenic effects of a dose of 1 Gy, 100,000 people are needed to evaluate the effects of 0.1 Gy and 10,000,000 people are needed to evaluate the effects of a 10 mGy dose);
- Completeness (and lack of bias) with which study subjects can be enrolled;
- Magnitude and distribution of exposure to the hazard being studied; accuracy — including the unbiased collection of data and adherence to a defined time frame — with which the exposure can be measured (measurement of absorbed dose, as in the atomic bomb survivors, is extremely important since the most compelling evidence of causality is the demonstration of a dose–response relationship); disease identification (history of disease should be confirmed from hospital records, and causes of death should be determined by obtaining copies of death certificates);
- Background rate of the disease being studied;
- Expected increase in the incidence of disease among the exposed group;
- Availability of information on other factors that might determine disease;
- Procedures to ensure valid consent for those research settings in which it is appropriate.

Choice of Population and Outcome to Be Studied

An epidemiological follow-up study typically begins by identifying two groups of people — those exposed and those unexposed to the agent, treatment, or characteristic being studied — and then seeks to determine whether the groups experience different health outcomes. The choice of an outcome — the measure of health — affects study design, complexity, and feasibility.

Mortality is the outcome most conducive to an epidemiological study because the occurrence is clearly definable, happens at most once per person, and relatively complete records are available. Mortality is not, however, always the health outcome of interest. Many questions involve diseases and conditions that affect the quality of life but that do not kill the individual. Physical and emotional health are often grouped under morbidity, yet concomitant employment, economic, and social well-being outcomes are increasingly being used as measures of effect. Finally, although not a direct measure of an individual's health, health care use — and its cost to the individual and other government agencies — is a reasonable choice of outcome for some epidemiological follow-up studies. The study of each of these outcomes — death, illness, and cost — poses substantial challenges to the epidemiologist.

Data Sources and Quality

A robust study design includes a clearly defined and identified study population and assurances that adequate data (in terms of completeness and lack of bias) regarding those individuals can be acquired. All of the products of the exposure monitoring and record-keeping activities need to be available for use in epidemiological follow-up studies. Assessing whether and to what extent potentially hazardous exposures (e.g., ionizing radiation) are present is complicated by the demanding conditions arising from the hazard itself, as well as by limitations associated with the devices used to quantify the exposure. The quality of the exposure data tremendously influences the feasibility and usefulness of such studies.

In part because of the very limited existence of prospectively designed and funded epidemiological studies, researchers often turn to available databases. Administrative databases and registries are prime examples. They can be very useful in the consideration of some questions, but they have severe limitations in many epidemiological applications.

Because of the need for unbiased sample selection and exposure and outcome measurements, it is a great advantage for epidemiologists to choose the population to be studied and to measure prospectively the baseline characteristics (demographic, clinical, and risk factors) of the individuals in that population. Also, outcome information must be sought in ways that make all members of the population equally likely to be identified. Registry data are therefore not necessarily well suited for use in epidemiological analyses. The drawbacks of registry data include the following: (1) the individuals with adverse outcomes may be more likely to register; (2) even among those with adverse outcomes, only a subset will register; (3) the outcome is influenced by more than the putative exposure, and those confounding factors — such as access to medical care (diagnosis and treatment) or health-related behaviors such as tobacco use — are usually not recorded in registry databases; and (4) reports to registries are often associated with compensation claims.

Confounding factors, including disease-causing behaviors such as smoking and alcoholism, may obscure the relationship under study. This often is exacerbated when studies begin many years after the occurrence of an exposure and require many years to complete.

Measurement of exposures, outcomes, and possible confounding factors is further complicated by the availability and quality of event records (e.g., medical and dose records). Records may be poorly maintained, stored in decentralized locations, or discarded after a set time period. Record systems may also inconsistently document events in situations in which examiners, such as pathologists and physicians, do not use standardized diagnostic routines.

A major consideration in the design of a study and the analysis and interpretation of its data is statistical power. To determine whether there is a difference in outcome between an exposed and an unexposed population, each population must be large enough (sample size) so that normal variation does not dwarf any real differences. That sample size is determined by the prevalence of the outcome in the unexposed population and the level of uncertainty that the researcher is willing to take in terms of false-negative results (not finding an exposure–outcome relationship in the data when there actually is one).

SUMMARY

Attempts to study the late health effects of exposure to radiation — assuming that malignant disease is the major concern—include other specific difficulties:

- No unique disease: All malignancies are pathological and clinically the same regardless of cause.
- Population size and dose need to be large enough to be able to detect a statistically significant difference in risk between exposed and nonexposed populations.
- There is a long interval between time of exposure and occurrence of disease (latent period); dose uncertainties may overwhelm the true dose at low-dose levels.
- Confounding factors may mask a radiation effect if there is one.

Epidemiological studies necessitate consideration of the privacy and confidentiality concerns associated with the use of personal records. Privacy refers to keeping sensitive information about oneself secret. Confidentiality refers more generally to keeping personal data from being used by others without informed consent.[13]

REFERENCES

1. Committee on Battlefield Radiation Exposure Criteria, Potential Radiation Exposure in Military Operations: Protecting the Soldier Before, During, and After, Institute of Medicine National Academy Press, Washington, D.C., 1999.
2. National Research Council, Health Effects of Exposure to Low-Levels of Ionizing Radiation (BEIR V), National Academy Press, Washington, D.C., 1990.
3. International Agency for Research on Cancer (IARC), IARC Monographs of the Evaluation of Carcinogenic Risks to Humans, Vol. 75, Ionizing Radiation, Part 1: X- and Gamma Radiation and Neutrons, IARC, Lyon, France, 2000.
4. Sources and Effects of Ionizing Radiation, United Nations Scientific Committee on the Effects of Atomic Radiation, Report to the General Assembly, United Nations, New York, 2000.
5. Taplin, S. and Mandelson, M., Principles of cancer screening for clinicians, *Cancer Epidemiol. Prev. Screening Primary Care*, 19:513–532, 1992.
6. Berg, R., Cancer prevention and screening in the light of health promotion and prevention of disability for the second 50 years, *Cancer*, 68:2511–2513, 1991.
7. U.S. Preventative Services Task Force, *Guide to Clinical Preventive Services: Report of the U.S. Preventative Services Task Force*, 2nd ed., Williams & Wilkins, Baltimore, MD, 1996.
8. IARC (International Agency for Research on Cancer), Cancer: Causes, Occurrence and Control, Tomatis, L., Ed., Rep. 100, IARC Scientific Publications, Lyon, France, 1990.
9. Wardle, J. and Pope, R., The psychological costs of screening for cancer, *J. Psychometric Res.*, 36:609–624, 1992.
10. Fearon, E.R., Human cancer syndromes: clues to the origin and nature of cancer, *Science*, 278:1043–1050, 1997.
11. Perera, F.P., Environment and cancer: who is susceptible?, *Science*, 278:1068–1073, 1997.
12. Ponder, B., Genetic testing for cancer risk, *Science*, 278:1050–1058, 1997.
13. Institute of Medicine (IOM), Adverse Reproductive Outcomes in Families of Atomic Veterans, The Feasibility of Epidemiologic Studies, Medical Follow-up Agency, National Academy Press, Washington, D.C., 1995.

34 Issues Involved in Long-Term Follow-Up of People after Radiation Exposure

Shigenobu Nagataki and Kazuo Nerishi

CONTENTS

General Considerations 461
    Epidemiological Methods 461
    Biological Dosimetry 462
    Time and Human Factors 462
Tests for Cancers 464
    Hematology 464
    Tumor Markers 464
    Ultrasound Examination 464
    Molecular Biology 464
Tests for Noncancer Diseases 464
    Psychological Problems 464
    Ophthalmological Diseases 465
    Cardiovascular Disease 465
    Parathyroid Diseases 465
    Infectious Diseases 465
    Immunological Abnormality 466
    Subclinical Inflammation 466
Follow-Up over a Generation 466
    Storage of Biological Materials 466
    Examination of Second Generation 466
References 466
Appendix 468

GENERAL CONSIDERATIONS

EPIDEMIOLOGICAL METHODS

It is well known that people exposed to radiation may suffer from acute and/or late effects of radiation exposure, depending on dose received. The studies on A-bomb survivors in Hiroshima and Nagasaki have shown that late effects are still observed, more than 50 years after the atomic bombings. Therefore, to elucidate the as yet unknown late effects of radiation exposure, follow-up of the exposed will be necessary for many years. Because most of the radiation induced health disorders are not radiation pathognomonic, they cannot be differentiated from health disorders due to other causes. Thus, an epidemiological approach is the only way to associate specific health disorders with radiation exposure; that is, incidence of a particular health disorder needs to be compared between a radiation-exposed group and a matched nonradiation-exposed group. If the incidence in the former is significantly higher statistically than that in the latter, the health disorder in question is judged to be associated with radiation exposure. However, a causal association should not be concluded hastily. Rather in epidemiology, the determination of causal associations requires that the following five items be satisfied: consistency, strength, specificity, temporality, and coherence.

Thus, the epidemiological method for assaying the health risks of radiation exposure is to identify a numerator of those with health abnormalities among a denominator population defined by exposure dose. In Hiroshima and Nagasaki, the identification of the denominator population was delayed because of confusion after the war. A greater delay has occurred in Chernobyl, and only the numerator has been emphasized. This is regrettable, and every effort should be made to provide an appropriate denominator as soon as possible to pursue long-term follow-up studies of persons after radiation exposure.

Hematological and immunological laboratory tests are necessary for long-term follow-up because it is those organs that are radiosensitive. It is also important to employ cancer detection tests, especially for thyroid, breast, and liver, organs in which a significant radiation association has been observed.

From the point of view of laboratory test accuracy, sensitivity, and specificity in human cohort studies, a variety of confounding factors, such as lifestyle and socioeconomic factors, must be considered. Inter- and/or intraobserver variation are also great problems, especially in morphological observation. Tumor and/or tissue registries are useful for repeated diagnostic procedures among observers and should be established.

Table 34.1 presents a summary of test items used in Japan for long-term follow-up of radiation-exposed individuals.

BIOLOGICAL DOSIMETRY

Although an approximate radiation dose can be determined by acute symptoms, such as erythema, epilation, and bleeding, and by blood cell count, this is not necessarily an accurate means for estimation. For repetitive reevaluation of radiation effects, biological dosimetry is required. Stable chromosome aberrations, such as translocation and inversion, are effective markers for estimating dose long after radiation exposure.[1] G banding has been used to detect chromosome aberration, and the fluorescence *in situ* hybridization (FISH) method has become available for easy translocation detection. Glycophorin A (GPA) assay for MN allele mutation, which shows significant radiation dose response,[2] is limited to MN heterozygous persons (see Chapter 40).

Electric spin resonance (ESR) is useful to detect stable radicals in the teeth enamel of radiation-exposed persons, including those chronically exposed, and ESR correlates well with chromosome aberration.[3] However, one must keep in mind that ESR is affected by sunlight and medical X-ray exposure.

TIME AND HUMAN FACTORS

During long-term follow-up, as new technology is developed a conversion of old methods to new must be periodically considered. A proportion of the study population could also be skewed for a variety of reasons, including migration, cooperation rate, diseases, dropout, and others.

In those exposed *in utero* and as infants, who tend to be retarded in height, head growth, and mental function,[4,5] long-term observation is required.

In a systemic physical examination, organs in which association with radiation has been observed, such as the lens, thyroid, and breast, should be carefully examined. At examination, physicians should also pay attention to the psychology of the radiation-exposed and instruct patients

TABLE 34.1
Test Items for Long-Term Follow-Up of Atomic Bomb Survivors

Category	Test Items	Radiation Association	Radiation Specificity
Biological dosimetry	Acute symptoms	+	+
	Blood cell count		
	Chromosome aberration, such as translocation and inversion		
	G banding		
	Fluorescence *in situ* hybridization		
	Glycophorin A		
	ESR in tooth enamel		
Physical examination	Height, head growth, and mental function in those exposed *in utero* and as infants	+	−
Laboratory tests	Hematological and immunological laboratory tests	+	−
	Cancer detection tests, especially for thyroid, breast, and liver		
Ultrasound examination	Thyroid cancer, thyroid nodules, breast cancer, liver cancer, and uterine myoma	+	−
Hematology	Hematological tests	+	−
	Protein electrophoresis		
	Serum iron and unsaturated iron-binding capacity		
Molecular biology	Genetic polymorphism	?	?
Psychological problems	Cornell Medical Index	+	−
	General Health Questionnaire		
	Composite International Diagnostic Interview		
Ophthalmological diseases	Slit-lamp examination	+	−
	Lens photographs		
Cardiovascular disease	Electrocardiogram	+	−
	Funduscopy		
	Computed tomography		
	Aortic pulse wave velocity		
	Radiography for aortic calcification		
Parathyroid diseases	Serum calcium	+	−
	Phosphorus		
	Alkaline phosphatase		
	Ultrasound		
	Parathyroid hormone		
	Bone radiography		
	Bone mineral densitometer		
Infectious diseases	Hepatitis B virus antigen	+	−
	EB virus antibody		
Immunological abnormality	T-cell surface markers	+	−
	Cytokines		
	Antibodies		
Subclinical inflammation	Erythrocyte sedimentation rate		+
	Leukocyte count		
	Acute–phase proteins		
	Sialic acid		
	C-reactive protein		
Examination of second generation	Chromosome aberrations	−	−
	Anomaly		
	Sex ratio imbalance		
	Cancer		
	Protein variants		

concerning radiation effects, explaining diseases associated with exposure, early signs of those diseases, screening tests for them, and preventive measures.

TESTS FOR CANCERS

HEMATOLOGY

Leukemia is a typical radiation-related cancer,[6] and is usually detected by hematological tests. The peak incidence for leukemia is 6 to 7 years after exposure. For multiple myeloma, protein electrophoresis is useful in detecting the monoclonal spike of monoclonal gammopathy.[7] Myelodysplastic syndrome is suspected to be responsible for the increased risk of hematological death other than from leukemia.[8] Serum iron and unsaturated iron-binding capacity are useful routine tests to differentiate iron deficiency anemia from other anemia, including myelodysplastic syndrome. Malignant lymphoma is not increased in radiation-exposed persons.[9] Since the normal range of hemoglobin in each person is narrower than that of the normal population, close longitudinal observation enables detection of malignancies by subtle changes in hemoglobin levels.

TUMOR MARKERS

There are several markers for specific cancers, and some are radiation associated. However, since most tumor markers are expensive, their introduction into the follow-up of radiation-exposed persons as a method for cancer screening may not be practical. C-reactive protein and stool occult blood tests are more practical. Family information is important to find one's predisposition to radiation-induced malignancies, such as ataxia-telangiectasia, xeroderma pigmentosum, Fanconi's anemia, Bloom syndrome, and Cockayne's syndrome.

ULTRASOUND EXAMINATION

Ultrasound examination is noninvasive, inexpensive, and the most effective screening method for solid tumors, such as thyroid cancer, thyroid nodules,[9] breast cancer, liver cancer, and uterine myoma.[10] Although there is no specific finding unique to radiation, following leukemia,[7] thyroid disease is second highest in radiation-exposed persons. Papillary carcinoma is relatively predominant among pathological types of thyroid cancer in radiation-exposed persons.

MOLECULAR BIOLOGY

While genomic instability, apoptosis, adaptive response, and hormesis are common concentrations for study in experimental animals, in humans they prove difficult because it is difficult to obtain materials before cancer development. By accumulating data on genomic polymorphism in certain cancers, one can predict preferential occurrence of radiation-induced cancers, such as *RET* oncogene of papillary thyroid carcinoma.

TESTS FOR NONCANCER DISEASES

PSYCHOLOGICAL PROBLEMS

During physical examinations, physicians should pay attention to the psychology of people who have been exposed to radiation, although lack of an assessment instrument makes it difficult to evaluate the psychological effects of radiation. Several trials use the Cornell Medical Index (CMI),[11] General Health Questionnaire (GHQ),[12] and Composite International Diagnostic Interview (CIDI),[13] and, overall, those instruments show significant associations with radiation dose. However, it is not likely that radiation causes this radiophobia. Rather, socioeconomic, familial, and psychotraumatic reasons underlie the psychological disturbances of the exposed. Although there is no significant increase of somatic diseases in Chernobyl cleanup workers in Estonia, their suicide rate is reportedly double that of controls.

Psychological and hygienic rehabilitation are highly recommended. In addition to instruction regarding radiation effects, as mentioned before, physicians should instruct patients concerning hygienic rehabilitation and/or lifestyle improvement, such as cessation of smoking, diet modification to include increased intake of fresh vegetables and fruits and decreased consumption of fat and salt, and proper exercise; such instruction alone lowers cancer risk.

OPHTHALMOLOGICAL DISEASES

Subcapsular axial opacity and polychronal changes of the lens are relatively radiation specific in radiation-exposed persons,[14] and changes are relatively stable after development up to 6 months after exposure. Therefore, patients do not develop a visual disturbance. However, recent reports indicated the possibility of the development of late-onset subcapsular axial opacity as well as early-onset peripheral opacity in those exposed in infancy.[15,16] Such long-term observation has never been conducted and is required to confirm the evidence in another population. Slit-lamp examination is noninvasive, inexpensive, and the most effective method for screening for subcapsular axial opacity and polychronal changes of the lens. For objective observation, use of photographs and/or a grading system may be useful. One problem is that the opportunity to assess the association between late-onset cataract and radiation dose may be lost when affected individuals undergo a recently developed resection surgery for treatment.

CARDIOVASCULAR DISEASE

In one study, cardiovascular disease has been associated with radiation dose in radiation-exposed persons.[8] Since disease risk is not large as compared with cancers among the radiation-exposed, careful investigation that incorporates a variety of confounding factors and diagnostic precision factors is required. Confounding factors, such as smoking, cholesterol, obesity, diabetes mellitus, diet, and exercise habits, are important to estimate disease risk precisely. Objective tests, such as an electrocardiogram (ECG) for ischemic heart disease, computed tomography for cerebrovascular disease, funduscopy, aortic pulse wave velocity measurements, others for arteriosclerosis, and radiographs for aortic calcification, are useful to evaluate disease risk. For those unable to undergo these tests at the clinic, health monitoring, such as periodic mail and/or telephone survey, may be effective to ascertain health problems in radiation-exposed persons in a timely manner.

PARATHYROID DISEASES

Hyperparathyroidism has been reported to increase in radiation-exposed people.[17] Serum calcium, phosphorus, and alkaline phosphatase are recommended as screening tests. For those with high levels of the mentioned serum factors, ultrasound examination of the parathyroid organ and measurement of parathyroid hormone levels are to be followed to identify parathyroid tumors. Bone radiography is useful to detect pathological fracture, as is bone mineral densitometry to detect osteoporosis. Past history of radiotherapy for thymoma and tinea capitis is important because of these patients risk developing hyperparathyroidism.

INFECTIOUS DISEASES

The prevalence of antigens for type B hepatitis virus[18] and Epstein–Barr (EB) virus antibody titration[19] has been reported to be associated with radiation. This suggests that continuous infection with such viruses in radiation-exposed people may be due to immune deficiency. There may be other infectious diseases not yet tested.

Immunological Abnormality

Radiation-exposed people reportedly have immunological changes. Two characteristic changes are a decrease in T cells and an increase in B cells.[20]

The immunological tests for detecting changes may include T-cell surface markers,[21] serum cytokines, and autoantibodies. They have specific and/or common functions in the immune system, including autoimmunity, infection, and tumor development. Decrease in CD4 T cell is reported to be significantly associated with increased inflammation.[22] Although autoimmune disease is not increased in radiation-exposed persons, inflammation is enhanced by radiation.

Subclinical Inflammation

Increased erythrocyte sedimentation rate and leukocyte count have been reported in A-bomb survivors.[23] Consistent with previous studies, recent analysis shows significant association with radiation dose in several other inflammatory tests, such as acute-phase proteins and sialic acid.[22] As a routine test, C-reactive protein is useful as a specific indicator for inflammation.

FOLLOW-UP OVER A GENERATION

Storage of Biological Materials

It may be useful to store biological materials for long-term follow-up of radiation-exposed people because new evidence may be obtained with technology not currently available. Tissues, lymphocytes, sera, and plasma are possible storage materials. Tumor and/or tissue registries enable diagnostic procedures to be repeatedly conducted among observers to avoid inter- and/or intraobserver variation in epidemiological study. Establishment of tumor and tissue registries is important.

Examination of Second Generation

Several tests have been conducted to identify the possible radiation effects in offspring of A-bomb survivors, but none of the findings has proved significant. There is no increase of anomaly,[24] sex ratio imbalances,[25] chromosome aberration,[26] cancer,[27] or protein variants[28] in offspring born to A-bomb survivors. However, since it is possible that some radiation effects in DNA-level mutation exist, it is necessary to store the DNA of offspring born to radiation-exposed people as immortalized lymphocytes until radiation-specific DNA probes become available. The Radiation Effects Research Foundation (RERF) has just started examining the second generation with the same methods used in first-generation studies.

REFERENCES

1. Awa, A.A., Honda, T., Sofuni, T., Neriishi, S., Yoshida, M.C., and Matsui, T., Chromosome-aberration frequency in cultured blood cells in relation to radiation dose of A-bomb survivors, *Lancet*, 2(7730):903–905, 1971.
2. Kyoizumi, S., Akiyama, M., Cologne, J.B., Tanabe, K., Nakamura, N., Awa, A.A., Hirai, Y., Kusunoki, Y., and Umeki, S., Somatic cell mutations at the glycophorin A locus in erythrocytes of atomic bomb survivors: implications for radiation carcinogenesis, *Radiat. Res.*, 146(1):43–52, 1996.
3. Nakamura, N., Miyazawa, C., Sawada, S., Akiyama, M., and Awa, A.A., A close correlation between electron spin resonance (ESR) dosimetry from tooth enamel and cytogenetic dosimetry from lymphocytes of Hiroshima atomic-bomb survivors, *Int. J. Radiat. Biol.*, 73(6):619–627, 1998.
4. Otake, M. and Schull, W.J., Radiation-related brain damage and growth retardation among the prenatally exposed atomic bomb survivors, *Int. J. Radiat. Biol.*, 74(2):159–171, 1998.

5. Otake, M., Schull, W.J., and Lee, S.. Threshold for radiation-related severe mental retardation in prenatally exposed A-bomb survivors: a reanalysis, *Int. J. Radiat. Biol.*, 70(6):755–763, 1996.
6. Preston, D.L., Kusumi, S., Tomonaga, M., Izumi, S., Ron, E., Kuramoto, A., Kamada, N., Dohy, H., and Matsuo, T., Cancer incidence in atomic bomb survivors. Part III. Leukemia, lymphoma and multiple myeloma, 1950–1987, *Radiat. Res.*, 137(2 Suppl):S68–97, 1994.
7. Neriishi, K., Yoshimoto, Y., Carter, R.L., Matsuo, T., Ichimaru, M., Mikami, M., Abe, T., Fujimura, K., and Kuramoto, A., Monoclonal gammopathy in atomic bomb survivors, *Radiat. Res.*, 133:351–359, 1993.
8. Shimizu, Y., Kato, H., Schull, W.J., and Hoel, D.G., Studies of the mortality of A-bomb survivors, Vol. 9, *Mortality*, 1950–1985: Part 3. Noncancer mortality based on the revised doses (DS86), *Radiat. Res.*, 130:249–266, 1992.
9. Nagataki, S., Shibata, Y., Inoue, S., Yokoyama, N., Izumi, M., and Shimaoka, K., Thyroid diseases among A-bomb survivors in Nagasaki, *J. Am. Med. Assoc.*, 272:364–370, 1994.
10. Kawamura, S., Kasagi,, F., Kodama, K., Fujiwaa, S., Yamada, M, Ohama, K., and Ito, K., Prevalence of uterine myoma detected by ultrasound examination in the atomic bomb survivors, *Radiat. Res.*, 147(6):753–758, 1997.
11. Yamada, M., Kodama, K. et al., The long-term psychological sequel of atomic bomb survivors in Hiroshima and Nagasaki, in *The Medical Basis for Radiation-Accident Preparedness, III*, Elsevier Science, New York, 1991, 155–163.
12. Goldberg, P., *The Detection of Psychiatric Illness by Questionnaire*, Oxford University Press, London, 1972.
13. World Health Organization, *Composite International Diagnostic Interview (CIDI)*, Core version 1.1, American Psychiatric Press, Washington, D.C., 1993.
14. Choshi, K., Takaku, I., Mishima, H., Takase, T., Neriishi, S., Finch, S.C., and Otake, M., Ophthalmologic changes related to radiation exposure and age in the Adult Health Study sample, Hiroshima and Nagasaki, *Radiat. Res.*, 96:560–579, 1983.
15. Wilde, G. and Sjostrand, J., A clinical study of radiation cataract formation in adult life following gamma irradiation of the lens in early childhood, *Br. J. Ophthalmol.*, 81:261–266, 1997.
16. Hall, P., Granath, F., Lundell, M., Olsson, K., and Holm, L.E., Lenticular opacities in individuals exposed to ionizing radiation in infancy, *Radiat. Res.*, 152(2):190–195, 1999.
17. Fujiwara, S., Sposto, R., Ezaki, H., Akiba, S., Neriishi, K., Kodama, K., Hosoda, Y., and Shimaoka, K., Hyperparathyroidism among atomic bomb survivors in Hiroshima, *Radiat. Res.*, 130(3):372–378, 1992.
18. Neriishi, K., Akiba, S., Amano, T., Ogino, T., and Kodama, K., Prevalence of HBs antigen, HBe antigen, HBe antibody and HBs antigen subtypes among atomic bomb survivors, *Radiat. Res.*, 114:215–221, 1995.
19. Kusunoki, Y., Kyoizumi, S., Fukuda, Y., Huang, H., Saito, M., Ozaki, K., Hirai, Y., and Akiyama, M., Immune responses to Epstein-Barr virus in atomic bomb survivors: study of precursor frequency of cytotoxic lymphocytes and titer levels of anti-Epstein-Barr virus-related antibodies, *Radiat. Res.*, 138(1):127–132, 1994.
20. Akiyama, M., Kusunoki, Y., and Kyoizumi, S., Overview of immunological studies on A-bomb survivors, *J. Radiat. Res.*, 32(Suppl.):301–309, 1991.
21. Kusunoki, Y., Kyoizumi, S., Hirai, Y., Suzuki, T., Nakashima, E., Kodama, K., and Seyama, T., Flow cytometry measurements of subsets of T, B and NK cells in peripheral blood lymphocytes of atomic bomb survivors, *Radiat. Res.*, 151:227–236, 1998.
22. Neriishi, K., Nakashima, E., and Delongchamp, R.R., Laboratory indicators of inflammation among atomic-bomb survivors, RERF MS 9-99.
23. Sawada, H., Kodama, K., Shimizu, Y., and Kato, H., Adult Health Study Report 6. Results of six examination cycles, 1968–1980, Hiroshima and Nagasaki, RERF TR 3-86.
24. Otake, M., Schull, W.J., and Neel, J.V., Congenital malformations, stillbirths, and early mortality among the children of atomic bomb survivors: a reanalysis, *Radiat. Res.*, 122(1):1–11, 1990.
25. Schull, W.J., Neel, J.V., and Hashizume, A., Some further observations on the sex ratio among infants born to survivors of the atomic bombings of Hiroshima and Nagasaki, *Am. J. Hum. Genet.*, 18(4):328–338, 1966.

26. Awa, A.A., Bloom, A.D., Yoshida, M.C., Neriishi, S., and Archer, P.G., Cytogenetic study of the offspring of atom bomb survivors, *Nature*, 218(139):367–368, 1968.
27. Yoshimoto, Y., Schull, W.J., Kato, H., and Neel, J.V., Mortality among the offspring (F_1) of atomic bomb survivors, 1946–85, *J. Radiat. Res.*, (Tokyo), 32(4):327–351, 1991.
28. Satoh, C., Awa, A.A., Neel, J.V., Schull, W.J., Kato, H., Hamilton, H.B., Otake, M., and Goriki, K., Genetic effects of atomic bombs, *Prog. Clin. Biol. Res.*, 103(A):267–276, 1982.

APPENDIX — LABORATORY TESTS CONDUCTED AT RADIATION EFFECTS RESEARCH FOUNDATION IN HIROSHIMA AND NAGASAKI

Physical examination
Anthropometry (weight, height, blood pressure)
Chest radiograph
Electrocardiogram
Ultrasonography
Urinalysis
Occult blood test in stool
Complete blood count
Erythrocyte sedimentation rate
C-reactive protein
Blood chemistry
Total protein
Albumin
Protein electrophoresis
Lactate dehydrogenase
Aspartate oxoglutarate aminotransferase
Alanine oxoglutarate aminotransferase
Alkaline phosphatase
Total bilirubin
Cholinesterase
Leucine aminopeptidase
Gamma-glutamyl transpeptidase
Thymol turbidity test
Zinc turbidity test
Glucose
Hemoglobin$_{A1C}$
High-density lipoprotein cholesterol
Triglyceride
Blood urea nitrogen
Calcium
Phosphorus
Uric acid
Iron
Unsaturated iron-binding capacity
Sodium
Potassium
Chloride

Questionnaire
Medication
Smoking
Alcohol
Nutrition
Health monitoring
Telephone and/or mail

35 Long-Term Follow-Up after Accidental Exposure to Radioactive Fallout in the Marshall Islands

Fred A. Mettler, Jr.

CONTENTS

Introduction 471
Study of U.S. Servicemen 471
Evaluation of the Marshall Island Population 473
References 476

INTRODUCTION

The United States conducted 66 nuclear tests in the Marshall Islands prior to a 1958 moratorium. These tests exposed both U.S. serviceman and the local populations to radiation of different types and to different degrees. The largest test in 1954 was 15,000 kilotons in yield, and was code-named "Bravo." It predominantly exposed Marshall Islanders and fisherman. Earlier tests exposed the U.S. military. These early tests included Operation Crossroads that involved approximately 40,000 military personnel who were in the Bikini Atoll of the Marshall Islands in 1946. The Marshall Islands as a testing site subsequently generated requests for retrospective evaluation of a large number of U.S. serviceman and a prospective medical study of a much smaller number of Marshall Islanders. It is instructive to examine both the study design and outcome in both cases. Some of the problems are similar to accidentally exposed populations at other test sites, such as in Russia (see Chapter 37).

STUDY OF U.S. SERVICEMEN

The purpose of the Crossroads test was to determine the effects of nuclear weapons on ship equipment and material. The first series of tests included nuclear detonation Able, which was detonated at an altitude of 520 ft, and Baker, which was detonated 90 ft under water. Each had a yield of 23 kilotons. There were 90 vessels positioned as a target fleet and 150 other ships accommodated technical service laboratory workshops, etc. The original air detonation sank five ships. Most surviving target ships were reboarded within 24 h. The underwater Baker explosion sprayed radioactive water and debris over most of the target fleet.

This epidemiological design was a retrospective cohort study. The study began in 1986 and was conducted by the U.S. Institute of Medicine, Medical Follow-up Agency.[1] As with most epidemiological studies, to design it appropriately, the question that has been posed needs to be articulated. In this case, the question was "Did Crossroads participants have more or earlier deaths from all causes than did similar military personnel who were not engaged in these activities?"

The first challenge was to ascertain the accuracy and completeness of the participant list. The second was to find an appropriate comparison group, and the third issue was to locate data and come to conclusions about the mortality experience of both groups. The study was solely a mortality study and did not consider the incidence of nonfatal or not yet fatal diseases. The mortality measures were (1) all-cause mortality, (2) all-cancer mortality, and (3) leukemia mortality. The reference groups that were utilized included a military nonparticipant cohort, the U.S. male population, and mortality rates from other relevant published studies. This epidemiological study was purely retrospective. Large numbers of people and doses were relatively low. Large comparison groups were also available.

This study is in sharp contrast to the medical follow-up study of the Marshall Islanders themselves. In that follow-up, there has been prospective analysis of the population with annual medical evaluation. The number of people involved, however, was very small, the doses were relatively high, and the background incidence of disease in the population was uncertain.

There are some interesting points relative to data collection in the Crossroads study. When looking at mortality, information can be obtained from records such as death certificates. However, under such circumstances it will not be clear, if a death certificate cannot be found, whether the person is, in fact, dead or alive. Conversely, if one attempts to get information from the subjects who are alive, if a person cannot be found, it will not be clear initially whether they are dead or alive either. Initially, data were obtained from each military service. Subsequent to that time, however, the U.S. Defense Nuclear Agency had consolidated the records of nuclear tests, personnel, and reviews and had identified the exact ships that participated in the Bikini Atoll during the operational period.

In any such retrospective evaluation, as always, the potential exists for personnel to self-identify themselves for any number of reasons, including potential future compensation. As a result, it is important to examine the validity of the participant group, and in this particular study, it was estimated that 2 to 4% of individuals had not participated. It also becomes important to identify whether the participants had engaged in only this set of nuclear tests or in additional ones, and it was determined that 90% of the participants had not engaged in any other military nuclear tests. For selection of a comparison cohort, Navy and shipboard Marines, both in the Atlantic and Pacific, who had not engaged in nuclear activities were matched. In addition, it was also important to match them, not only on job type but on military rank.

Exposure definition, measurement, and verification also is a major problem, particularly in a study involving thousands of subjects. Although the Defense Nuclear Agency's nuclear test personnel review program had attempted to assign individual doses, it was decided that these data were not appropriate for epidemiological studies. As a result, it was necessary to use other proxies, and exposure was categorized by adding data from individual radiation badges that had been issued to some participants, although this was not a common practice, and to examine the boarding records of the various ships with the assumption that those who are on board ship at the time of the detonations were more likely to be contaminated. Finally, a general ranking of exposure by listed occupational specialty category was also used.

Mortality ascertainment was done primarily by using Veterans' Affairs records, particularly the beneficiary identification and record locator system. In this system, there is a record of death benefit requests. In the cases in which this occurred, a death certificate was requested and sent to a certified nosologist to classify the causes of disease.

The results and comparison of the different groups showed that 31% of the Crossroads participants had died vs. 30% of the control group. Approximately 11 to 12% of each group was lost to follow-up. Date and cause of death was available in 85 to 90% of cases.

Results of this study indicate that among Navy personnel, who were the primary analysis group, there was a higher mortality for the participants than in the comparable group of nonparticipating military controls. The increase in all-cause mortality was 4.6%, with a relative risk of 1.046, with a 95% confidence interval of 1.020 to 1.074. This was statistically significant. For malignancies, there was a slight nonstatistical elevation in mortality with a relative risk of 1.014, with confidence interval of 0.96 to 1.068. Leukemia was elevated, but also in a nonsignificant fashion. The relative risk for leukemia was 1.020 (confidence interval 0.75 to 1.39).

The increase in all-cause mortality did not concentrate in any specific group studied. In addition, the mortality due to all malignancies and leukemia did not vary among those who boarded the ships after detonation vs. those who did not, or by occupation specialty. The conclusion was that the elevated risk of all-cause mortality in the Crossroads participants is probably the result of an unidentifiable factor, other than radiation, but associated with participation in or presence at the test, and the second is a self-selection bias within the participant roster.

EVALUATION OF THE MARSHALL ISLAND POPULATION

The Bravo test was detonated on a tower at Bikini Atoll in the early morning of March 1, 1954. Radioactive debris from the thermonuclear weapon test deviated from the predicted path and contaminated several atolls in the northern Marshall Islands (Figure 35.1). Marshallese inhabiting Rongelap, Alinginae, and Utirik atolls, as well as a group of servicemen on the Rongelap Atoll were caught within the downwind fallout field for 2 to 3 days before they could be evacuated. In addition, the Japanese fishing vessel, *Fukuryu Maru* (Lucky Dragon) was also exposed. Overall, 239 native inhabitants, 28 U.S. servicemen, and 23 Japanese fisherman received variably severe exposures. Fallout material largely consisted of mixed fission products with small amounts of neutron-induced radionuclides and minimal amounts of fissionable elements. The individuals were exposed to penetrating whole-body gamma radiation, surface beta radiation, and internal contamination by inhalation or ingestion.

Nausea occurred within 48 h in two thirds of those residing on Rongelap (the most heavily exposed group) with vomiting and diarrhea in 10%. By contrast, none of those on Utirik, who were the least-exposed group, had these findings, and only 5% of those on Ailingnae experienced nausea. One fourth of those on Rongelap and Alinginae complained of skin irritation and itching, and one fourth had eye irritation This was due to direct exposure by high-energy beta emitters; most of the individuals later developed epilation, and a few developed conjunctivitis. Some of these symptoms may have been aggravated by the alkaline calcium oxide produced by fireball vaporization of the coral island. Dermal effects were most pronounced on the scalp, neck, dorsum of the feet, axilla, and antecubital fossa (Figure 35.2). On Rongelap, the fallout was described as similar to snowfall

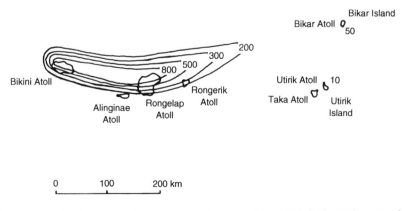

FIGURE 35.1 Approximate gamma dose rates (roentgens per hour) at 3 ft above the ground, 1 day after detonation.

and actually whitened the hair and adhered to the skin. Partial epilation began within 2 weeks in half of the group. A less dense, powdery mist fell on Alinginae and Rongerik, and dermal effects were less evident with epilation beginning at 3 weeks and affecting less than 20% of the population.

Hematological profiles were extensively studied, and in the Rongelap population, the absolute neutrophil counts in all groups fell 20 to 30% in the second postexposure week, and 50% by the fifth week, gradually returning to normal after 1 year. Peripheral lymphocyte counts dropped rapidly to about one half of normal by day 3; 2 years later, they were nearly normal. Lymphocyte depression was greater in the younger age groups with lymphocyte depression down to 25% of normal values. Platelet counts reached a low of about one third of normal during the fourth postexposure week and eventually required more than 2 years to return to normal. Similar but less severe hematological alterations were observed on Alinginae, and the low-exposure group on Utirik did not develop significant alterations, except for a slight transient depression of platelets.

Radiation doses, as well as the number of people affected, on each of the atolls are shown in Table 35.1. After resolution of the early radiation effects, a program for observation of the Marshallese was set up under the U.S. Atomic Energy Commission, and headquartered at Brookhaven National Laboratory. The program later came under aegis of the U.S. Energy Research and Development Administration, and subsequently of the Department of Energy. The program is a cooperative effort with support from the U.S. Department of Defense and Department of Interior (trust territory of the Pacific Islands). From its inception, the primary objective of the program was early detection and treatment of any medical conditions that might evolve as a consequence of radiation exposure. A longitudinal prospective follow-up study of the exposed individuals and a control population was organized.

It was clear from the beginning that the study had significant difficulties. The dose assessments were complex, the population size was very small, and data on the incidence of various diseases in Micronesia were meager, nonexistent, or unreliable. In the first decade following the accident, there were few clinical findings that could be reasonably related to radiation. Cutaneous scarring and depigmentation were the only residue of the beta burns, and no evidence of skin malignancy was identified. Some children exhibited growth retardation, and peripheral blood elements remained minimally below comparison with the control group for about 5 years. Some chromosomal defects were also identified.

In the second decade, the development of hypothyroidism and thyroid nodules in a significant number of individuals was identified, and there was a fatal case of acute myelogenous leukemia. Other than this, the general health of the population appeared to be no different from comparison populations. There was no clear evidence of accelerated aging or cataract formation, decreased longevity, or of increased incidence of malignancy other than in the thyroid gland.

During the third decade postexposure, chief among the responsibilities of the ongoing program was a cancer-related evaluation. In general, the guidelines used were those of the American Cancer Society, which include:

- A review of systems and complete medical examination
- Advice on decreasing risk factors and on the self-detection of lesions
- Pelvic examination with Pap smear
- Stool testing for occult blood
- Annual mammography

Rectal examination and stool testing for occult blood was done annually, starting at age 40. Routine flexible sigmoidoscopy was offered before age 50, and would be repeated every other year or more frequently if clinically indicated.

Overall, the program was generally aimed at attempts to identify malignant disease. The exposed Marshallese received additional attention for two reasons: first, because their type of radiation was quite unique and, second, because data collected by the Brookhaven team suggested that there

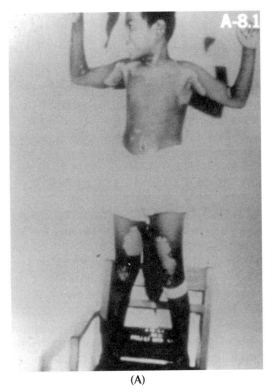

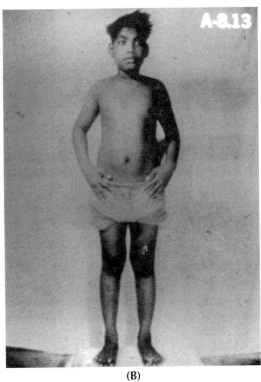

FIGURE 35.2 (A) Beta burns from the fallout. These are most pronounced on the thighs, axillary regions, and antecubital fossae. (B) After healing.

TABLE 35.1
Estimated Radiation Doses in Exposed Populations

Atoll	Number Affected[a]	Estimated Whole-Body Gamma Dose Sv	Estimated Thyroid Dose Sv by Age (Years) at Exposure		
			<10	10–18	>18
Rongelap	67	1.75	8–18	3.3–8.1	3.35
Alinginae	19	0.69	2.75–4.50	1.9	1.35
Utirik	163	0.14	0.60–0.95	0.3–0.6	0.3

[a] Includes *in utero* exposures (three on Rongelap, one on Alinginae, and six on Utirik).

might be previously undocumented late effects. There have been reports of an increased incidence of pituitary neoplasms (although this is not identified in other radiation literature of long-term survivors) and a trend toward lower blood cell counts. Hypothyroidism was documented in the earlier years of the program.

Relative to the thyroid, there were annual clinical thyroid examinations as well as thyroid function studies annually or biennially. In addition, thyroid suppression with Synthroid was offered for all exposed at Rongelap with the intent to decrease the likelihood of thyroid malignancy. As of 1984 in the exposed population, there had been at least 31 adenomatous nodules compared with 4 in the comparison population, at least 8 papillary carcinomas compared with 2 in the control population, and at least 4 occult papillary carcinomas compared with 2 in the control population. The latter lesions are felt to be of little clinical significance. One follicular carcinoma was identified in the exposed group.[2,3]

Antithyroid antibodies were found to be elevated in 4% of the exposed group vs. 2% in the comparison group. As of 1994, of the original 253 Marshallese exposed, 147 were still alive.

REFERENCES

1. Mortality of Veteran Participants in the Crossroads Nuclear Test, Report of the Medical Follow-Up Agency, Institute of Medicine, National Academy Press, Washington, D.C., 1996.
2. Conard, R.A. et al., Review of Medical Findings in the Marshallese Population 26 Years after Accidental Exposure to Radioactive Fallout; Brookhaven National Laboratory Rep. BNL51261, TID-4500, Brookhaven National Laboratory Associated Universities, Inc., U.S. Department of Energy, 1980.
3. Adams, W.H., Heotis, P.M., and Scott, W.A., Medical Status of Marshallese Accidentally Exposed to 1954 Bravo Fallout Radiation, January 1985 through December 1987.

36 Manhattan Project Plutonium Workers at Los Alamos

George L. Voelz

CONTENTS

Introduction 477
History of Manhattan Project Workers 477
Dosimetry 478
Mortality Data 480
Clinical Data 481
Summary 482
References 483

INTRODUCTION

Plutonium (^{239}Pu) was deposited internally in a group of 26 young males who worked in the Manhattan Engineer District's Project "Y" at Los Alamos, New Mexico in 1944 and 1945. They were engaged in processing plutonium that fueled the atomic bombs used in the Trinity test and the Nagasaki bombing.

HISTORY OF MANHATTAN PROJECT WORKERS

The working conditions for these young men have been described as being "extraordinarily crude."[1] Some procedures, such as centrifuging and weighing of plutonium, were done in open rooms. Ordinary open-faced chemical hoods offered the principal protection against air contamination during chemical and metallurgical procedures. Half-faced, filter paper respirators were what was available at Los Alamos at this time and were used during more hazardous operations. In the absence of air samplers for radioactive dusts (the first ones became available in the fall of 1944), nasal swipes were routinely taken at the end of the working day or if accidental inhalation exposures were suspected. After nose counts above 50 counts per minute (cpm), the person was questioned about possible accidental inhalation or breakage of safety regulations. Contamination of nasal swipes was common after workdays. For example, from June through August 1945, a total of 373 nose counts from 50 cpm to above 5000 cpm was measured among the 18 members of this cohort who worked in a plutonium area during this period. Swipes of benchtops, floors, and equipment were counted with laboratory alpha counters because semiportable alpha counters were not available until early 1945. They proved to be bulky and inconvenient, so the swipe technique was continued in some laboratory rooms until June 1945. Areas from which swipes exceeded 500 cpm were decontaminated. In June, July, and August 1945, the number of decontamination procedures carried out was 1980, 3489 (of which 760 exceeded 30,000 cpm), and 5347, respectively. Kilogram quantities of plutonium began arriving at Los Alamos for processing and fabrication by April 1945.

Fortunately, by this time semiportable alpha counters, continuous air samplers, and dry boxes (predecessors to glove boxes) were being developed to help with monitoring and controlling contamination in certain rooms. In July 1945, a special face mask, called the Kennedy–Hinch mask after its designers, was developed to give better protection against airborne radioactivity.

By March 1945, a plutonium urinary assay method had been developed at Los Alamos to the point where it could be applied to monitor worker exposures. Contamination during collection of urine samples for use with this procedure was a serious problem for several years. It resulted in false positives that indicated plutonium deposition many times acceptable levels. A system of urine collection under controlled conditions was designed to minimize contamination of urine samples, reducing precipitously the radioactivity measurements.

Inhalation of plutonium particles was the main exposure pathway for all these workers. No therapy was available for plutonium inhalation exposures at that time. Seven of eight potentially contaminated minor cuts or puncture wounds were excised. Four of the excised tissues were measured for plutonium activity. Of these, subject 20 had 55 Bq in his excised tissue; the other three had less than 1 Bq. Contaminated wounds do not appear to be a source of significant intake to these workers; nevertheless, subject 1 still has about 300 Bq (~ 8 nCi) of plutonium in his right index finger at a site of a contaminated wound received in July 1944. There have been no abnormal physical findings at his wound site. Three individuals have a history of a chemical burn on the skin from acidic plutonium solutions; no radioactivity measurements are recorded.

Of the 26 workers, 21 had left Los Alamos by 1946 or earlier. The other 5 of the 26 men worked in or around plutonium facilities after 1945, but additional plutonium exposures were minor compared with their wartime work. Wright Langham, a biochemist, and Louis Hempelmann, a physician, were on the laboratory staff during World War II and were concerned that these men might have long-term health effects from their plutonium exposures. They are to be credited and commended for having started this follow-up study as a long-term health surveillance program.

In 1951, this cohort of 26 men was selected by Wright Langham based on their individual job histories, work conditions, and urine plutonium bioassay results. Members of the cohort have been examined medically about every 5 years since 1952. From 1952 to 1972, the examinations were conducted by physicians at or near the place of residence of each person. Only one or two urine samples from each person were collected for plutonium measurements over these 20 years, except for four men who were still working at Los Alamos and contributed many samples. In 1971, it was decided that future examinations, including urinalyses for plutonium, *in vivo* chest counts, and sputum cytology sample collections, should be done at Los Alamos. Since then, medical and plutonium dosimetric studies were done in 1971,[1] 1977,[2] 1982,[3] 1987,[4] 1992,[5] and 1997.

DOSIMETRY

Cumulative effective whole-body doses, calculated from plutonium excretion values in urine samples from 1945 through 1997, are listed on Table 36.1. Most of the men have no recorded external radiation doses in their records because personal dosimeters (film badges) were not in use at Los Alamos until late 1945, shortly after the wartime plutonium work was done. Gamma radiation doses were probably minimal because the americium-141 (60 keV gamma) content was very low in the plutonium being processed in 1944 to 1945 (e.g., 2 to 5% of the americium-241 dose from a comparable amount of plutonium processed in the 1980s). Small but unknown neutron doses were likely for all of them during their work in 1944 to 1945. The effective doses from internally deposited plutonium-239 (sum of calculated annual effective doses from first exposure through 1996 or the year of death) range from 0.11 to 7.2 Sv with a median dose of 1.3 Sv (mean dose = 2.1 Sv). The doses to workers in this cohort, most of which occurred in a period of less than 6 months, are 5 to 360 times greater than the dose estimated to occur after exposure to the currently recommended annual limit of intake. Internal plutonium depositions as of 1996 range from 80 to 3080 Bq (2.4 to 83 nCi) with a median activity of 515 Bq (14 nCi). These depositions are what remains in their

TABLE 36.1
Estimated Plutonium Depositions and Effective Doses as of 1996 or Year of Death

ID No.	Pu Deposition[a] (Bq)	Effective Dose (Sv) Pu	External
1	1440	3.9	
2	300	0.62	
3[b]	3080	7.2	
4	2220	5.3	0.10
5	1330	3.0	
6	2180	3.7	
7	3220	5.1	
8	1850	2.5	
9	2440	5.8	
10[b]	740	1.4	<0.01
11	440	1.3	<0.01
12	440	1.6	
13	80	0.11	
15[b]	380	0.41	
16[b]	550	0.42	
17	1040	3.6	
18	920	3.0	
19	370	1.1	
20[b]	580	1.3	
21	440	1.0	
22	480	0.64	
23	220	0.89	
24	370	0.85	
25	130	0.30	0.04
26	110	0.23	
27	270	0.50	0.09

[a] Deposition estimated as of 1996 or the year of death based on urine excretion data using J.N.P. Lawrence's PUQFUA4 and PUIDE computer program.
[b] Deceased (see Table 36.3 for year of death).

bodies more than 50 years later or at death. Plutonium has an estimated half-time of 20 years in liver and 50 years in bone. Lung retention is variable depending on the solubility of the plutonium compound inhaled. It is likely that the original plutonium incorporation in these workers was two to three times the 1996 estimated depositions.

Direct *in vivo* measurements over the chest, using phoswich detectors and an array of hyperpure intrinsic germanium planar detectors, have not detected plutonium or americium (americium-241) in these men. An exception was one individual who had a measurement of 7 Bq (0.2 nCi) of americium-241. The absence of positive lung counts for plutonium-239 is attributable to the low transmission rate through the chest wall of the characteristic U-L X rays (17 keV average energy) being measured. The detection limit of these chest counters is of the order of 1000 to 2000 Bq for plutonium-239, depending on the chest wall thickness of the individual.

Measurements of plutonium in blood, urine, and feces from 17 of these men were made in 1976–1977, about 31 years after their exposure. Excretion of plutonium in their feces was widely variable, at least partly due to difficulty in determining the time span represented by a fecal sample. Fecal elimination compared with urinary excretion had a median ratio of 30%, but individual values

($n = 12$) range from 6 to 133%. The fecal-to-urinary excretion ratios on these occupationally exposed persons appear to be consistent with ratios (40%) observed in two patients 27 years after being injected with soluble plutonium compounds. The median value for blood/urine ratios in the workers is 17.5. The plasma clearance rates per day are 0.166 ± 0.034 l by urine excretion and 0.218 ± 0.032 l by urine plus fecal elimination.

MORTALITY DATA

Of the 26 men, 7 had died by the end of 1996. The mortality rate in this cohort is compared with those of white males in the U.S. general population, adjusted for age and calendar year of death. The results are listed in Table 36.2. The standardized mortality rate (SMR) for all causes of death is 0.37, which is significantly low. Another significant finding is the exceptionally low SMR of 0.22 for the category, all cardiovascular diseases. The SMR of 0.65 for all malignant neoplasms is not a statistically significant finding. Three of the seven deaths were due to malignancies; the underlying causes of death were from cancers of lung, prostate, and bone. The bone tumor, an osteogenic sarcoma, gives a significantly high SMR of 90 in this small cohort.

Mortality rates of an internal control group of 876 unexposed Los Alamos workers from the same period were used to determine a mortality risk ratio for the Manhattan plutonium worker cohort. For all causes of death, the risk ratio was 0.77; for all malignant neoplasms, it was 0.94. Neither result is statistically significant, but both values suggest the mortality rate of the plutonium-exposed persons is probably not greater than that of their fellow unexposed workers.

Plutonium deposition and the underlying cause of death for each of the deceased is listed in Table 36.3. Comparison of the plutonium depositions determined by radiochemical analysis of autopsy tissue and estimates by plutonium excretion in urine show reasonably good agreement between the two methods. The autopsy tissue samples for Subject 3 did not include lung so his autopsy data account only for systemic deposition. Thus, the difference between the two methods is undoubtedly greater than the numbers indicate. Subject 20 had extensive bone metastases and emaciation by the time of his death. This wasting process may have resulted in a lower value in the autopsy data than that calculated from the urinary excretion data. A urine sample from Subject 20 in 1989, less than a year before his death, did not show an elevated rate of plutonium excretion compared with previous samples.

TABLE 36.2
Standardized Mortality Ratios (SMR) of Manhattan Project Plutonium Workers Based on Mortality of U.S. White Males through 1996

Categories	Observed	Expected	SMR	95% C.I.	P Values
All causes of death	7	18.8	0.37	0.15–0.77	<0.001
All malignant neoplasms	3	4.6	0.65	0.13–1.9	0.33
Lung cancer	[1]	1.6	0.60	0.01–3.4	0.51
Prostate cancer	[1]	0.37	2.7	0.04–15	0.31
Bone	[1]	0.01	90	1.18–502	0.01
All cardiovascular	2	9.1	0.22	0.02–0.80	0.006
All respiratory	1	1.47	0.68	0.01–3.77	0.56
All external causes	1	1.33	0.75	0.01–4.19	0.63

Note: Person-years of survival = 1246. C.I. = confidence interval.

TABLE 36.3
Causes of Death in 7 of 26 Manhattan Project Workers Exposed to Plutonium from 1944 to 1945

ID No.	USTUR No.	Age at Death	Year of Death	Underlying Cause of Death	Total Plutonium Deposition (Bq) by	
					Autopsy[a]	Urine Data
15	—	36	1959	Myocaridial Infarction	—[b]	
16	0060	52	1975	Trauma (Accident)	620	550
27	0193	62	1982	Pneumonia	246	270
10	—	71	1985	Lung cancer	—[b]	740
25	0255	70	1988	Arteriosclerotic heart	98	130
3	0778	66	1989	Prostate cancer	3300[c]	3080
20	0769	66	1990	Osteogenic sarcoma	252[d]	580

[a] Autopsy data from the U.S. Transuranium and Uranium Registries, Washington State University, Richland, WA.
[b] No autopsy done.
[c] Systemic deposition only. No lung autopsy data available.
[d] Preliminary data.

CLINICAL DATA

Comprehensive medical examinations were made on 15 of the 19 living persons in 1997. Four individuals were not able to travel to Los Alamos, so medical data were obtained by telephone interview and from personal physicians near their places of residence. Ages at the end of 1996 of the 19 living persons range from 71 to 88 years; median and mean ages are 74 and 75.8 years, respectively. The median age for all 26 individuals in the original group is $72^{1}/_{2}$ years using the age of the living subjects in 1996 and age at death for the deceased.

Diseases, including past medical histories, recorded in the 19 living individuals in 1997 are those frequently seen in males above 70 years of age. The more common diagnoses are hearing loss (10), history of coronary atherosclerosis or abnormal electrocardiogram (9), hypertension (8), cancer (6) exclusive of 4 persons with a history of skin cancer, cataracts (6), glaucoma (4), circulatory system disease (4), pulmonary obstructive disease (4), and hypercholesterolemia or hypertriglyeridemia (4). Diagnoses with a frequency of three or less in this cohort are not identified here.

Cancer diagnoses within this cohort are the principal interest. Among the seven deceased persons as of 1997, the underlying causes of death by malignant neoplasms (see Table 36.3) are prostate cancer (subject 3), lung cancer (subject 10), and osteogenic sarcoma (subject 20). Additional cancer diagnoses listed on the death certificates, but not the underlying cause of death, are two lung cancers (subjects 3 and 25). Among the 19 living persons examined in 1997, there are 6 malignancies: papillary carcinoma of bladder (subject 9), 3 prostate cancers (subjects 12, 13, and 24), colon cancer (subject 11), and lung cancer (subject 6). In addition, subject 13 has a history of malignant melanoma of skin, which was successfully resected in 1971.

The most significant new finding from the 1997 examinations was a large asymptomatic lung cancer found by chest radiograph on subject 6. His sputum cytology was normal. The tumor, adenocarcinoma of the lung, was treated by surgical excision and chemotherapy. He died in 1998 at age 77. He was a heavy cigarette smoker for about 30 years, but had quit smoking in 1978.

Combining cancers diagnosed in both the living and deceased subjects, 10 of the 26 persons in this cohort have had a history of malignant neoplasm (not including basal and squamous cell carcinoma of the skin). The types and numbers of malignancies are cancers of the prostate (4), lung (4), bone, colon, bladder, and skin (malignant melanoma). Two individuals were diagnosed with two separate malignancies. The size of this cohort is so small that analysis of cancer incidence is not particularly meaningful for specific cancers. All four individuals with lung cancer were moderate to heavy cigarette smokers throughout much of their adulthood.

Sputum cytology has not been very helpful in this series of studies. The results have ranged from being normal to having mild or moderate atypia. Over the 25-year period that sputum cytology has been done on members of this cohort, no *in situ* cancer cells or malignant neoplasms were reported. A sample from each of two heavy cigarette smokers (Subjects 3 and 4) in 1972 was read as marked atypia. Bronchoscopy of subject 3 in 1975 showed no evidence of neoplasia. Changes in his exfoliated bronchial cells were attributed to bronchitis secondary to smoking. Subsequent samples were read as mild atypia for both individuals who had the marked atypia. The underlying cause of death for Subject 3 in 1989 was prostate cancer, but lung cancer was also diagnosed as a second malignancy.

The observation of one osteogenic sarcoma in this small cohort warrants special attention. Animal studies have clearly demonstrated an excess of osteogenic sarcomas associated with plutonium exposures, and osteogenic sarcoma was also the most frequent radiation-induced cancer observed in persons with high radium depositions. Subject 20 began having pain in his lower back in late 1988. X-ray examination identified a large bone tumor of the sacrum. A radiograph of his sacrum at his 1986 examination was normal. The latent period from exposure to clinical appearance of his malignancy is 43 years. The cumulative dose to the surfaces of bone is estimated to be 0.44 Gy and to the average skeletal (volume) is 0.016 Gy.[1] The presence of one case of osteogenic sarcoma in this small study group is statistically significant compared with mortality rates of U.S. white males (Table 36.2) and also with a group of 876 unexposed Los Alamos workers.[1] This same individual was also included in an independently selected cohort of all plutonium-exposed males ($n = 303$) who worked at Los Alamos from 1943 through 1977. In that study, the bone tumor death rate in the plutonium-exposed workers was not significantly elevated compared with unexposed workers. The cause and effect relationship between this man's relatively low plutonium deposition and induction of his osteogenic sarcoma remains speculative.

Two cytogenetic studies of peripheral blood from these men, 27 and 32 years after exposure, observed that the total aberration rates are relatively low and there is no apparent correlation between aberration rate and the plutonium body burden. Blood samples taken on 19 men of this cohort, 47 years after exposure, were also examined at the cytogenetic laboratory of the Oak Ridge Institute of Science and Education. Although the chromosome aberration rate was high in several men, the elevated rates did not correlate well with plutonium depositions. Estimated bone marrow doses range from 0.05 to 3.0 Sv with a median dose of 0.89 Sv.

Measurements of mononuclear cells in peripheral blood of 18 subjects of this cohort indicate a preferential reduction in suppressor T lymphocytes in some individuals.[7] The decrease in T_s cells is apparently due to altered radiosensitivity, which is demonstrated in cultured cells subjected to *in vitro* X-ray radiation. The increase in ratios correlates with the quantity of plutonium deposition in these subjects, but there are wide individual differences. Confirmatory studies are needed in other persons with long-term alpha or chronic gamma radiation exposure. If confirmed, the implications would include recognition of a potential mechanism for an enhanced immune system reactivity in some individuals exposed to chronic low-level radiation.

SUMMARY

Data on 26 workers exposed to plutonium-239 in 1944 to 1945 and observed for a period of more than 50 years have consistently shown that the mortality rates for all causes of deaths and for all cancers are not elevated compared with either U.S. white males or unexposed Los Alamos male workers with comparable hire dates. This finding differs from some popular misperceptions that large health risks occur after any exposure to plutonium. The median effective dose to these men is 1.3 Sv (mean dose = 2.1 Sv). The incidence of specific cancers, especially lung cancer (4) and osteogenic sarcoma (1), is interesting, but additional data are needed to draw conclusions about the relationship between plutonium doses comparable to those in this study and the induction of excess cancers.

REFERENCES

1. Hempelmann, L.H., Langham, W.H., Richmond, C.R., and Voelz, G.L., Manhattan Project plutonium workers: a twenty-seven year follow-up study of selected cases, *Health Phys.*, 25, 461, 1973.
2. Voelz, G.L., Hempelmann, L.H., Lawrence, J.N.P., and Moss, W.D., A 32-year medical follow-up of Manhattan Project plutonium workers, *Health Phys.*, 37, 445, 1979.
3. Voelz, G.L., Grier, R.S., and Hempelmann, L.H., A 37-year medical follow-up of Manhattan Project plutonium workers, *Health Phys.*, 48, 249, 1985.
4. Voelz, G.L. and Lawrence, J.N.P., A 42-year medical follow-up of Manhattan project plutonium workers, *Health Phys.*, 61, 181, 1991.
5. Voelz, G.L., Lawrence, J.N.P., and Johnson, E.R., Fifty years of plutonium exposure to the Manhattan Project plutonium workers: an update, *Health Phys.*, 73, 611, 1997.
6. Wiggs, L.D., Johnson, E.R., Cox-DeVore, C.A., and Voelz, G.L., Mortality through 1990 among white male workers at the Los Alamos National Laboratory: considering exposures to plutonium and external ionizing radiation, *Health Phys.*, 67, 577, 1994.
7. Voelz, G.L., Stevenson, A.P., and Stewart, C.C., Does plutonium intake in workers affect lymphocyte function? *Radiat. Prot. Dosimetry*, 26, 223, 1989.

37 Epidemiological Evaluation of Populations Accidentally Exposed Near the Techa River, Russia

Angelina K. Guskova

The brief survey of data given in this chapter deals with the health effects in a population living near a nuclear weapons facility and exposed to long-term irradiation. The activities of the "Mayak" industrial complex began in 1948. This facility is located 1848 km west of Moscow, about 100 km northwest of Chelyabinsk, and 220 km southeast of Yekaterinburg.

In the period between 1949–1956, there was continuous discharge of radiochemical industry waste into the Techa river. Approximately 95% of doses to the population were from radionuclides of strontium-90 and cesium-137. In addition, some short-lived radionuclides were released from March 1950 until November 1951. Maximum levels of water contamination in the upper stream were 2000 to 3000 times above the permissible level of ^{90}Sr and 100 times above permissible levels of ^{137}Cs and ^{89}Sr. Gamma dose rates reached 50 mGy/h on the river shore, 35 mGy/h near a village named "Metlino" and 0.10–0.15 mGy/h inside its dwellings. After 1952, the maximum outdoor dose rate in this village dropped to 0.006 mGy/h. Maximum individual annual doses of external gamma exposure in some of the population of Metlino and Techa-Brod villages were up to 2 Gy/year. Partial relocation of village residents started in the end of 1951 and during 1951–1957 practically all the people living in the upper stream area were relocated.

During the following years, there was a significant decrease of radionuclides into the lower river due to dam construction in the upper river system. As a result, the radionuclide concentration in the lower river system decreased 100-fold during the next 30 years and dose rates along the upper Techa river shore decreased threefold.

In 2000, four settlements (more than 8000 people) live in the Techa valley. In 1988 the maximum dose rates found around these villages were in the range of 1.4–0.8 µGy/h. Whole-body counting done 25–30 years after the major radiation impact has revealed that about 1% of the people living in the Techa river area have ^{90}Sr body burdens above 74 kBq (2 µCi) with the highest burdens in people who were exposed during the 1950s as children and adolescents. Calculated internal exposure doses have shown that about 87%, 10%, and 3% of red bone marrow doses resulted from ^{90}Sr, ^{137}Cs, and ^{89}Sr, respectively.

The effective equivalent dose distribution in the Techa river population (28,000 people) is as follows: <200 mSv (73%), 200–500 mSv (~7%), >500 mSv (12%), and >1 Sv (~8%). Single cases of 3–4 Sv of effective dose were found. The average effective equivalent dose was assessed to be 320 mSv in the affected area of the Chelyabinsk region and ~70 mSv in the Kurgan region.

Medical examinations of the upper Techa river village population began in 1951 and continue until the present time. It is interesting to note that a detailed analysis has shown that while some of the population of the Techa valley was exposed to different radiation sources (river discharge, 1957 atmospheric fallout, etc.), the majority of the people was not irradiated at all.

Early examinations suggested chronic radiation disease (ChRD) in 935 individuals. This estimate was later revised down to 66 people after more accurate dose assessment and evaluation of concurrent somatic diseases. The average dose in the initial group of 935 people was 130 mGy and the dose after revision was 0.7–1.2 Gy in the 66 substantiated ChRD patients. The hematological changes in these patients have confirmed the importance of external gamma exposure in ChRD induction.

Medical observation and data analysis have continued for three cohorts of the Techa river population (31,000 people) who were exposed to the 1957 accidental release resulting from a radioactive waste storage tank explosion. A cohort includes the progeny of parents exposed. Mortality analysis of these cohorts has demonstrated that the major difference is the elevation of mortality due to malignant neoplasms (Table 37.1).

TABLE 37.1
Mortality Structure of the Population Exposed in Techa River vs. Control Indices

	Mortality Rates per 100,000 Man Years			
Cause of Death (ICD-9 classes)	Exposed, Ethnic Group A; 360/700 mSv Average Dose[a]	Ethnic Group A Control	Exposed, Ethnic Group B; 130/250 mSv Average Dose[a]	Ethnic Group B Control
Infectious diseases	136.0[c]	88.4	69.1	712
Neoplasm	145.8[b]	114.9	197.0[c]	168.6
Endocrine system	12.5[c]	3.8	7.1	5.8
Blood	3.6	2.4	1.0	22
Mental disorders	3.6	4.3	3.5	2.5
Nervous system	16.9	10.2	11.9	12.5
Blood circulation system	417.9	401.5	615.0	592.2
Pulmonary organs	128.0	144.0	123.7[b]	105.3
Digestive organs	32.9	23.4	25.5	28.9
Urogenital system	6.2	5.6	6.8	9.1
Pregnancy complications	53	4.6	5.2	3.6
Skin	0.9	1.6	1.3	1.4
Bone-muscular system	1.8	0.8	1.3	1.4
Congenital abnormalities	2.7	0.3	4.2	1.2
Perinatal period states	7.1	4.3	5.2	3.1
Unclear	48.0	56.4	47.2	67.8
Traumas	102.2	115.5	145.7	162.9

[a] Doses are averaged in soft tissues/red bone marrow.
[b] 90% confidence difference vs. control.
[c] 95% confidence difference vs. control.

To assess radiation cancer induction, the population was grouped according to age, gender, ethnicity, age at exposure, and cause of death. The data was analyzed with EPICURE software, which was also used for A-bomb survivor mortality analysis. The predicted and excess cases of leukemia and solid cancers were assessed in relation to bone marrow and soft tissue doses (Table 37.2). The leukemia excess was >40%, and when red bone marrow doses were above 0.5 Gy, the excess was >60%. Excess solid cancer incidence was 3.1% (30 cases), and in the >0.5 Gy dose group the excess was 15%. Malignant neoplasm morbidity in the nonirradiated general public of the Chelyabinsk region increased from 244 cases per 100,000 man years in 1979, to 294

TABLE 37.2
Leukemia and Solid Cancer Mortality Rates in Techa River Population Exposed to Radiation

Dose Groups, Gy[a]	Leukemia			Solid Cancer		
	Man Years	Observed Cases	Excess	Man Years	Observed Cases	Excess
0.005–0.1	103031	3	−1	459576	716	5
0.1–0.2	194858	13	4	96297	126	1
0.2–0.5	200144	16	6	19582	34	10
0.5–1.0	93873	9	5	32204	52	6
1+	49398	9	7	33645	41	8
Total	641304	50	21	641304	969	30

[a] Doses in red bone marrow/soft tissues applied for analysis of leukemia/solid cancer, respectively.

in 1989. The cancer morbidity rates for all ages of irradiated and nonirradiated groups were similar and there was no decrease in risk with attained age. The most frequent sites of cancer were the lungs and the digestive system.

Ethnic differences in mortality can be noted in Table 37.3. It is clear that ethnic differences were more important in cancer risk than was radiation exposure. Environmental contaminants were also important; for instance, the population living in the area affected by Chelyabinsk metallurgical enterprise had increasing cancer incidence (per 10^5 people): 958 in 1985, 1097 in 1987, and 1114 in 1989. Some elevation of general mortality incidence in the irradiated population was also caused by an elevated childhood infectious mortality in the 1950s.

TABLE 37.3
Mortality Rates in the Techa River Ethnic Groups Exposed to Radiation vs. Ethnic Controls

Index	Kunashak Area (Bashkirs and Tatars)		Krasnoarmeisk Area (Russians)	
	Irradiated	Nonirradiated	Irradiated	Nonirradiated
General mortality (/10^3)	10.78	9.82	12.27	11.36
Malignant neoplasm mortality (/10^5)	144.9	114.1	215.4	177.2

The incidence of acute leukemia, chronic myeloleukemia, and total leukemia was generally found to be higher in irradiated population than in nonirradiated controls. As of 2000, the total number of myeloproliferative disease cases in the exposed population was 70. As a percentage, this was significantly higher than that in a control population (36.5% vs. 21.2% for acute leukemia and 23.1% vs. 11.9% for chronic myeloleukemia). The maximum leukemia excess was reached during the period of 5–20 years after the beginning of exposure. There was also an increased incidence of the combination of leukemia and tumors of other sites (lung, stomach, and thyroid) in irradiated people.

The cumulative baseline incidence rate of all congenital diseases was less than 3% for a nonirradiated population. The mental retardation incidences were very different even in villages of the same area without any clear radiation dose-effect. For instance, in two villages (Bolshoy Kuyash and Tatarskaya Karabolka) where the average effective doses were similar (47 mSv), the incidence of congenital mental retardation was 1.9% and 7.4%, respectively. In the Muslumovo village (average gonadal dose of 120 mSv), the mental retardation incidence was 5.3%, vs. the Khalitovo village (nonirradiated area) where this incidence was 5.9%. It should be noted that a 10% mental retardation incidence was recorded in villages that were located at long distances from the radioactively contaminated territories.

During 1950–1953, there were 1677 people born and exposed *in utero* in the Techa villages. They lived there until January 1, 1995. They were medically examined, and 27 mental retardation cases were found (1.6%). This rate is confidently below the control group in which there were 220 cases per 10,577 people (2.1%), and is also below the congenital mental retardation incidence among the irradiated parent progeny born in 1954–1983 (3.39%). An analysis of family history has indicated that more than 25% of all retarded children had close relatives who suffered from retardation. Nonradiation hereditary factors were believed to account for 55–76% of mental retardation cases, and other factors such as the age of the parents, twin or triplet delivery, parental addiction to alcohol, pregnancy and delivery complications, infectious diseases with brain damage during the first year of life, may account for another 30% of cases. The progeny of the irradiated population had an incidence rate for Down syndrome below that of the general public. The major risk factor for Down syndrome was maternal age during pregnancy.

In summary, many years of medical observation of the population irradiated in the Techa river valley have confirmed radiation effects in people with the highest radiation doses. There was an increase in the incidence of malignant neoplasms (particularly leukemia) as the major late radiation effect. A low number of documented chronic radiation disease cases were found and follow-up examinations demonstrated some recovery of disturbed functions. The health status and the background morbidity rate of hereditary diseases of first and second generation progeny was not found to be affected by parental irradiation. An increase of mental retardation incidence rate was not found for people exposed *in utero*.

REFERENCES

1. Akleev, A.V., Goloshapov, P.V., Kossenko, M.M., and Degteva, M.O., Radioactive environmental contamination in south Urals and population health impact, *TcniiAtomInform*, Moscow, 1991, p. 66. In Russian.
2. Seligman, P.J., The U.S.-Russian health effect research program in southern Urals, *Health Physics*, 79(1), 3–8, 2000.
3. Vorobieva, M.I., Degteva, M.O., Burmistrov, D.S. et al., Review of historical monitoring data on Techa river contamination, *Health Physics*, 76(6), 605–618, June 1999.
4. INFOR — 2000, Information Analytic Journal of Urals Region, pp. 58–61, 62–65, 45–44, 18–23. In Russian.

38 Instrumentation and Physical Dose Assessment in Radiation Accidents

Charles A. Kelsey and Fred A. Mettler, Jr.

CONTENTS

Introduction 489
Radiation Detection Instruments 490
    Ionization Chamber Survey Meters 490
    Geiger–Mueller Counters 490
    Scintillation Detectors 492
Personal Dosimeters 492
    Pencil or Pocket Dosimeters 492
    Thermoluminescent Dosimeters 494
    Film Badges 496
Physical Assessment of Absorbed Dose 497
    Personal Dosimeters 497
    History 497
    Accident Reconstruction 498
Radiation Accidents, Incidents, and Nonaccidents 498
Use of Personal Monitors to Estimate Effective Dose 499
Issues Related to Radiation Exposure Records 499
Summary 499
References 499

INTRODUCTION

In the management of a radiation accident patient, a hospital must have instrumentation available to locate and assess the amount of radioactive contamination as well as to assess absorbed radiation dose to both the patient and the medical staff. The purpose of this chapter is to describe (1) basic types and characteristics of radiation monitoring instruments, (2) methods for assessing personal absorbed dose, and (3) how to use physical methods to assess absorbed dose to the patient.

    One of the most important steps in coping with a radiation accident should be taken before any accident occurs. This step is the assembly and periodic testing of a radiation instrumentation kit. Such a kit should contain instrumentation for real-time detection of various types of radiation that might be expected, and be capable of assessing both high and low levels of radiation exposure. The kit should also contain devices such as film badges that can be used to estimate individual absorbed doses. It is important that any kit be tested and inventoried at least every 6 months. Calibration procedures should be in place.[1]

RADIATION DETECTION INSTRUMENTS

Radiation detection instruments generally measure either alpha particles or beta/gamma radiation.[2,3] Only a very sophisticated and expensive piece of equipment can measure alpha as well as more penetrating radiation types. The extremely short range of alpha particles usually requires a special alpha detector, and such meters are very delicate since the detector portion must have a window thin enough to permit passage of alpha particles. High-activity alpha emitters are found almost exclusively in defense facilities or in very large research facilities and, in general, it is not necessary for most hospitals to have an alpha detection capability. Some of the difficulties related to alpha detection equipment are related to the poor penetrating power in air or through other substances. Most weapons-grade plutonium contains sufficient other radionuclides such that one may choose to detect low-energy X rays rather than the alpha particles themselves.

Beta- and gamma-emitting radionuclides are in common use throughout industry and medicine, and accidental contamination with such radionuclides is a real possibility. Thus, a hospital should maintain an instrument for detection of these types of radiation. Various types of radiation detection instruments are shown in Table 38.1.

IONIZATION CHAMBER SURVEY METERS

Ionization survey meters contain an air-filled chamber for detection purposes. These ionization meters can operate over a wide range of radiation levels. Thus, if high exposure levels are suspected, an ionization chamber should be initially utilized. The range of such meters is on the order of 10^{-5} Gy to tens of Gy per hour. Unfortunately, such ionization chambers often have a relatively slow (several seconds) response time, and this means that the detector probe must be moved slowly over suspected areas. The ionization survey meter shown in Figure 38.1 has a thin mylar end window protected by a plastic end cap. The end cap must be removed only when searching for beta contamination. If the window is torn or punctured, the detector cannot be used and must be returned to the supplier for repair.

GEIGER–MUELLER COUNTERS

Geiger counters are the instruments of choice for radiation surveys when one is attempting to localize areas of contamination or detect very small amounts of radiation. The detector, or probe, on the Geiger counter contains a pressurized gas in a sealed tube. Geiger counters are relatively fast in responding and relatively inexpensive. Most Geiger survey probes have a protective cover over a thin entrance window so that the machine can be used to detect poorly penetrating radiation (such as beta) when the shield is moved into the open position. Figure 38.2 shows a Geiger counter with the probe having its protective shield partially rotated to expose the thin window underneath. Both the instruments shown in Figure 38.2 are civil defense-type instruments. The instrument shown in Figure 38.2 is low-range instrument with a maximum exposure range of 1.25×10^{-5} C/kg (50 mR/h). The instrument shown in Figure 38.3 has a maximum rate of 125 10^{-5} C/kg (5 R/h), but since it does not have a probe or thin window, it has no beta sensitivity.

The first application of such monitoring or survey instruments is to determine whether or not the patient is contaminated. This is accomplished by performing a radiation survey of the patient. The detector is slowly scanned over areas of suspected or possible contamination (Figure 38.4).

Prior to performing a survey, it is important to ascertain whether or not each instrument is functional. With instruments that operate on batteries, this is usually done by initially turning the selector switch to the "BAT" or "BATT" position. If the batteries are adequate, the indicator needle on the meter will go near the top end of the scale face. After this is done, one turns the selector switch to the x1 position. This will allow the survey instrument to begin detecting. If the instrument has an audible output or makes a clicking sound, background radiation should be identified. For many Geiger-type meters, background radiation is about 60 clicks/min. Often it is useful to have

TABLE 38.1
Radiation Survey and Monitoring Instruments

Instrument Type	Radiation Detected	Typical Use	Minimum Energy Detected (keV)	Typical Dose Rate or Dose Range	Advantages	Disadvantages
Ionization chamber survey meter	X, beta, gamma	Survey	20	5 μSv/h–5 Sv/h	Response independent of photon energy	Slow response, low sensitivity
Pencil dosimeter	X, gamma	Personal monitoring	50	2 mSv–2 Sv	Small, inexpensive, instant reading of integrated dose	May discharge if dropped
Film badge	X, beta, gamma	Personal monitoring	20	>10 μSv	Measured integrated dose, gives permanent record	Must be processed under controlled conditions; heat and vapor can produce falsely high readings
TLD	X, beta, gamma	Personal monitoring	20	>10 μSv	Measures integrated dose, gives permanent record	Must be processed before reading is available
Geiger–Mueller counter	X, beta, gamma	Survey	20	5–200 μSv/h	Rapid response, rugged instrument	Very energy-dependent response
Scintillation counter	X, beta, gamma	Survey	20	0.5–200 μSv/h	Very sensitive reading response	Fragile, expensive

a very tiny radioactive "check" source taped on the side of the instrument case. The probe should be placed next to this tiny source and the needle should show a response. Once this is done, one can begin surveying for contamination. Any indications of radiation levels higher than natural background radiation represent potential areas of contamination and, in general, areas that register more than twice the background level are considered contaminated.

Contamination usually refers to the presence of unsealed and unwanted radionuclides; however, survey meters are also capable of detecting continuous radiation emitted from other sources, such as an encapsulated radioactive source perhaps used for industrial radiography. If a radiation field is present, it is difficult to assess the possibility or presence of contamination on a patient until the patient is removed from the radiation field. This is because the survey meters are essentially unable to distinguish between radiation from a source and radiation emanating from radioactive contamination. Use of the audio portion of the meter has both advantages and disadvantages. If the audio portion is turned off, one must simultaneously watch both the position of the probe with respect to the patient and the meter. Under these circumstances, it is easy to touch the probe to a contaminated area and contaminate the probe itself. To avoid contaminating the probe, it may be covered with a plastic food storage bag or a surgical glove. The main disadvantage of the use of the audio portion is that in a situation in which the patient is already apprehensive about radiation, even a small amount of contamination will result in a significant audio output. This may significantly increase the patient's apprehension and concern out of proportion to the actual hazard.

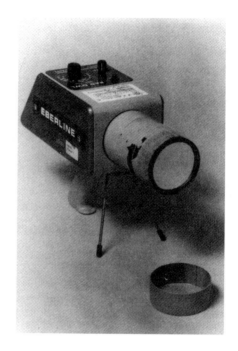

FIGURE 38.1 Ionization survey meter.

SCINTILLATION DETECTORS

Scintillation detectors are much more expensive than either ionization chambers or Geiger-type counters. They are also very sensitive to physical shock. However, these disadvantages are overcome by a considerably improved efficiency. These detectors utilize a dense crystal. Interaction of ionizing radiation with the crystal results in a scintillation, or light flash, which is recorded by a photomultiplier tube. The major advantage of such a detector over the other types of detectors is that it is possible to assess the energy of the incident radiation since the intensity of the light flash is proportional to the amount of energy. Another advantage of such a detector is that once the energies of the incident radiation are identified, one can identify the radionuclide involved.

PERSONAL DOSIMETERS

The purpose of personal dosimeters is to provide an estimate of individual absorbed dose. Hospital personnel are already familiar with at least one form of these devices, i.e., film badges. There are two basic types of personal dosimeters: (1) the pencil or pocket dosimeter and (2) the thermoluminescent dosimeter (TLD) or film badge.

PENCIL OR POCKET DOSIMETERS

These devices are approximately 1.5 cm in diameter, about 15 cm long (Figure 38.5), and have a clip to attach the dosimeter to the user's clothing. The dosimeter is basically an air-filled ionization chamber. The dosimeter must be charged prior to use (Figure 38.6A). Pushing down on the dosimeter while the distal end is inserted into a charging device performs this. When this is done, the scale at the end of the device is illuminated and, by turning a knob on the charger, the scale indicator can be positioned to the zero mark. This charges the unit and, as ionization occurs, the charge within the unit is reduced and the indicator line moves up the scale. Reading the dosimeter requires no special instrumentation and can be done immediately. Reading is accomplished by looking through the dosimeter at a bright light, as illustrated in Figure 38.6B. An example of the image that one might see at the end of a dosimeter is shown in Figure 38.7.

Instrumentation and Physical Dose Assessment in Radiation Accidents 493

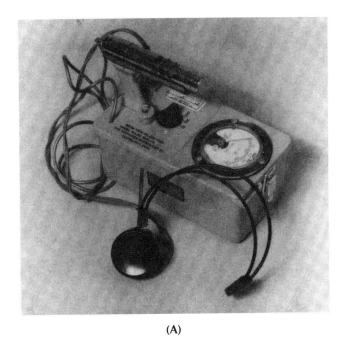

FIGURE 38.2 (A) Model CDV-700 low-range Geiger counter. (B) Geiger counter probe with thin window partially open.

Pencil ionization dosimeters are easy to use and provide an instant measure of the accumulated exposure to that portion of the individual. Thus, while caring for a patient who is contaminated, one is able to look occasionally at the dosimeter to obtain an estimate of one's own absorbed dose. Unfortunately, the pencil dosimeters do not provide a permanent record and, thus, it is important to record this information. Another disadvantage is that these dosimeters are very sensitive to shock and they may go off scale by being dropped on the floor or bumped against a hard surface. Pocket dosimeters can be purchased in a varied range of sensitivities, for example, from 0–2.5×10^{-5} C/kg (0 to 100 mR) or 2.5×10^{-3} C/kg (0 to 10 R). Overall, the accuracy of the devices is not as great as TLDs or film badges.

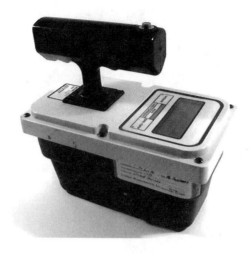

FIGURE 38.3 Pressurized ion chamber survey meter.

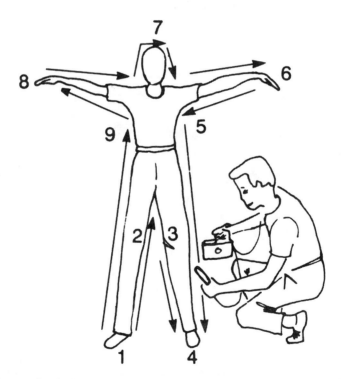

FIGURE 38.4 Survey of an individual. The same survey pattern is repeated on the back of the individual.

THERMOLUMINESCENT DOSIMETERS

These devices are very similar in appearance to a standard film badge. Both TLDs and film badges suffer from the disadvantage of not providing an instantaneous readout and the absorbed dose to an individual is only ascertained after the fact. TLDs contain crystalline or powdered material, which, when heated, gives off light in proportion to the amount of radiation absorbed. These

Instrumentation and Physical Dose Assessment in Radiation Accidents

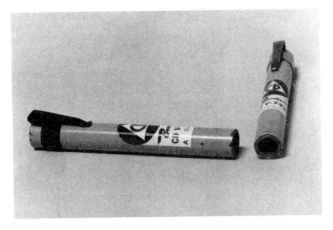

FIGURE 38.5 Personal or "pencil" dosimeters.

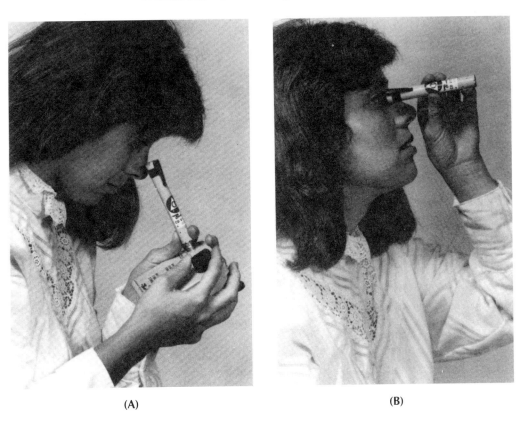

FIGURE 38.6 (A) Pencil dosimeter being charged using the charging unit. The dosimeter must be pushed down to engage the charging unit contacts. (B) Reading the pencil dosimeter by looking toward a light.

materials are very sensitive to radiation and yet they are very stable. TLDs are able to store the information without being read for days or months. They are also reusable, since after heating or annealing, they are again ready to accumulate information. TLDs are able to record absorbed doses accurately in the range of 2.5×10^{-4} to 2.5×10 C/kg (10 to 1,000,000 mR). Unfortunately, the

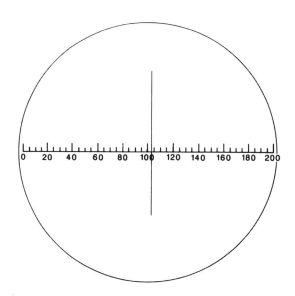

FIGURE 38.7 Example of pencil dosimeter scale reading of 2.5×10^{-5} C/kg (103 mR).

TLD is unable to provide information concerning the energy of the incident radiation. Another disadvantage is that only one reading of the crystalline material is possible, and if a mistake is made while processing, it is not possible to retrieve the information.

FILM BADGES

In contrast to a TLD, the film badge is able to provide a permanent record. Film badges are not as sensitive to radiation as TLDs; however, they are able (through placement of shielding outside the film) to give some estimate of the incident radiation energy as well as the absorbed dose. Technical problems have limited the use of film badges in some accident situations, such as stapling the film badge to a piece of paper prior to processing and allowing light to leak onto the film through the staple hole. Additionally, leaving a film badge in an area that is hot (in excess of 130°F.) will cause the emulsion to be darkened when processing occurs. Film badges tend to be somewhat less inexpensive than TLDs. Both TLDs and film badges must be replaced periodically as they will record accumulated natural background radiation prior to, during, and after an accident; thus, a TLD or film badge that has been in storage for 6 months will already have a baseline reading of between 1.25×10^{-5} C/kg and 3.75×10^{-5} C/kg (50 and 150 mR).

It is important during management of a radioactively contaminated patient to have the film badge or TLD in a protected environment. If contamination from the patient were to get on the film badge, it would continue to expose the film badge or TLD even after it was taken off and thus give an erroneously high reading. In most radiation accident management situations, it is prudent to wear both a pocket or pencil dosimeter and either a TLD or film badge. This allows one to have an instantaneous and accessible estimate of radiation dose (from the pencil dosimeter) as well as a slightly more accurate method (TLD or film badge) that can be processed after the accident.

There is always a great discussion regarding the proper placement of personnel dosimeters. Generally, they are worn either on the collar or at the belt level. At present, no regulations exist that require placement in a certain anatomical location. Most of these devices also have a serial number, which should ultimately be placed on a dosimeter log and recorded with the wearer's name and social security number. The reading of the pen dosimeter should also be recorded on the same sheet of paper.

PHYSICAL ASSESSMENT OF ABSORBED DOSE

At absorbed doses in excess of 0.25 Gy to the whole body and in excess of 1.0 Gy to the extremities, ultimate patient management depends on biological dosimetry and tissue response. In such instances, film badges and TLDs are only of supporting value. With lower absorbed doses, however, there are few if any biological findings, and in these circumstances, personnel dosimeters, accident reconstruction, and history are the most important factors in dose assessment. The methods of biological assessment are discussed in Chapters 4, 5, 14, and 40.

Personal Dosimeters

Some of the limitations of these devices have been discussed earlier in this chapter. Of course, their use for dose estimation purposes is only helpful in an accidental situation where an occupationally exposed person who was already wearing such a dosimeter was involved in the accident. In over half the accidents that are evaluated each year, no dosimeters have been worn. Another limitation is that dosimeters only will measure the dose to the single point on the body where the dosimeter was worn. Several graphic examples have been given in other chapters, which indicate that in accidental situations there may be extreme dose gradients over very short distances and thus a film badge or TLD worn on the waist may not accurately reflect midline body dose or maximal dose to the patient, both of which are much more clinically relevant. Another difficulty with personal dosimeters is the limitation imposed by the beam direction and possible shielding of the dosimeter by the body. For example, if a personal dosimeter has a reading of 0.2 Gy, this will not be clinically significant if, in fact, it was an entrance dose. If, however, this represents the exit dose from the patient and the radiation was not very penetrating, then the entrance dose on the side of the patient opposite the film badge could have been several gray. Probably the most common type of serious radiation accident involves handling of an unsuspected but highly intense radioactive source. In these circumstances, the fingers of the hand may have absorbed doses in excess of 100 Gy, but due to the inverse-square law and rapid dropoff of radiation exposure with distance, a film badge worn on the belt may only have recorded 0.5 Gy. One could easily imagine similar problems with dosimeter interpretation when a radioactive source was inadvertently placed in a pocket and the dosimeter was worn on the collar. Although there are significant limitations to use of data from such dosimeters, they do at least provide a single data point in time and space, which is better than nothing.

History

The importance of early, detailed, and accurate recording of the accident history cannot be overemphasized. The following will present at least a partial list of data that should be obtained to have a useful history:

Name of patient
Employer
Company
Physical injuries and treatment
Skin surface contamination, including location, dose rate, and decontamination procedures utilized, if applicable
Internal contamination, including radionuclide chemistry, particle size, and suspected route of contamination (other useful information in this regard would include nasal counts, wound counts, whole-body counts, and bioassay samples already collected)
Evaluation of exposure to penetrating radiation, including precise location and position of patient relative to the radiation source at the time of exposure
Exact time and duration of exposure

Was dosimeter worn? Where? What type?

Where is the current location of the dosimeter?

Symptoms such as nausea, vomiting, anorexia, or diarrhea and the exact time of occurrence of each

Have blood counts or cytogenetic samples been obtained for biologic dosimetry purposes?

Home phone number of individual as well as contact at work

Were any other individuals present during the accidental exposure, and if so who were they and where are they?

Has source of exposure been terminated or does a possibility for continuing exposure of other persons still exist?

Such a history will quickly identify whether one is dealing with a significant radiation accident, an incident, or essentially a nonaccident or imaginary event.

ACCIDENT RECONSTRUCTION

Often the history will be sufficient to give a fairly reasonable dose estimate, provided the nature of the radiation source is accurately identified. In circumstances in which there has been a very steep gradient of exposure or in which several people are involved and there may have been shielding, reconstruction of the accident situation may be useful. In such circumstances, a phantom of soft tissue equivalent that has a skeleton within it can be utilized. Such Rando-type phantoms are made with horizontal sections, each about 1 cm thick. There are holes in which TLDs can be placed while the accident is reconstructed. If the source of exposure is then activated again, one may determine with a reasonable degree of accuracy what the dose distribution was within the body. Such reconstruction may be useful to determine prognosis and therapy of the patient. As one example, it is often difficult for clinicians to determine the best spot to look for surviving bone marrow, and phantom reconstructions can give dose estimates to the bone marrow in different portions of the skeleton.

RADIATION ACCIDENTS, INCIDENTS, AND NONACCIDENTS

Significant accidents usually have whole-body absorbed doses over 0.25 Gy and doses to extremities over several grays. At absorbed-dose levels less than these, biological damage is minimal and biological changes are difficult, if not impossible, to detect. The authors prefer to classify exposures from this range down to acute exposures in the range of 10 mGy as radiation *incidents*. In this dose range there would be no detectable nonstochastic effect, although there may be a slightly increased risk for stochastic effects such as cancer.

Events in which acute doses approach the range of the natural background that one might receive in a year or lower (<2 mGy) essentially represent *nonaccidents*. Unfortunately, the potentially exposed person may not see it this way and future legal problems are certainly a possibility. Thus, even in situations where absorbed dose is likely to be nonexistent or negligible, it is still useful to document incidents and nonaccidents in a file. Such files should contain at least some elements of the history, allegations, and how the conclusion was reached that the exposure was negligible. It is also important to meet with the individual, discuss the event, and reassure him or her. Of course, every radiation safety officer has at least one story of the amount of time and effort taken to deal with an individual who is convinced that he or she is a victim of alien death rays, a malfunctioning television set, or a microwave oven that is influencing his or her personality and vital energies. There is no easy solution to such problems other than reassurance, although in most cases this is of little avail, and the person will leave unhappy and attempt to seek another source of consultation.

USE OF PERSONAL MONITORS TO ESTIMATE EFFECTIVE DOSE

Personal monitors only measure the dose at the point where they were worn. Unless there was a very rare accidental condition in which the radiation dose was extremely uniform, these values are of limited use in medical treatment. There are issues related to the recommended or regulatory occupational dose limits. These are expressed in effective dose or equivalent dose to the skin, eye, thyroid, or extremity. For strongly penetrating radiation (above 40 keV) using the recorded dose usually will not overestimate the effective dose by more than a factor of 3. Regardless of the geometry, if the energy of the incident radiation is below 30 keV, the effective dose is extremely difficult to calculate as a result of a single personal dosimeter measurement.[4]

ISSUES RELATED TO RADIATION EXPOSURE RECORDS

Instruments, detectors, and personal dosimeters will generate values that need to be recorded, analyzed, and maintained. These will not only relate to the potential radiation field but also may include data on air concentration, time in an environment, internal contamination, bioassay data, and even committed dose. Other uses of the records include evidence of regulatory compliance, data for epidemiological studies, and information for making or contesting claims.[5]

Accident records are likely to be kept in a number of places. The most obvious one is in the radiation protection program of a facility handling radiation sources or radionuclides. Records are also likely to be in the emergency room of the hospital where the patient(s) were treated, in various medical records at the hospital, clinics, and in physicians' offices. Records may also exist in occupational or facility clinics of the employer, records of investigating authorities, and accident registries.

All of these records will vary in terms of accuracy, completeness, format, quality control, access, and definitions. For optimal medical treatment of an accident patient, all the information will be useful. For medical purposes the most useful item is the equivalent dose to specific organs. Although this information is necessary to calculate an effective dose, the organ doses are often then discarded since they may not be needed for regulatory purposes. In accidental exposure situations organ doses should always be maintained. These records should be made available to the individual and their significance should be explained. The records also need to be maintained in a way that protects individual privacy.

SUMMARY

In summary, a wide variety of survey instruments can be utilized both in accident management and in estimation of absorbed dose. Personal dosimeters also may be used, but have some limitations that must be recognized. In cases in which there has been a significant radiation accident, use of biological indicators should take precedence over physical assessment of dosimetry. Accident reconstruction can be useful in patient management to give an idea of the absorbed dose distribution throughout the body. Physical dosimetry becomes particularly important in estimation of lower absorbed doses where no biological damage is evident. Probably the most important aspect of dose estimation is obtaining an accurate and detailed history.

REFERENCES

1. NCRP, Calibration of Survey Instruments Used in Radiation Protection for the Assessment of Ionizing Radiation Fields and Radioactive Surface Contamination, Rep. 112, National Council on Radiation Protection and Measurements, Bethesda, MD, 1991.

2. Brodsky, A., Ed., *Handbook of Radiation Measurement and Protection*, 2nd ed., CRC Press, Boca Raton, FL, 1982.
3. Shleien, B. and Terpilak, M., *The Health Physics and Radiological Health Handbook,* Nuclear Lectern Associates, Olney, MD, 1984.
4. NCRP, Use of Personal Monitors to Estimate Effective Dose Equivalent and Effective Dose to Workers for External Exposure to Low-LET Radiation, Rep. 122, National Council on Radiation Protection and Measurements, Bethesda, MD, 1995.
5. NCRP, Maintaining Radiation Protection Records, Rep. 114, National Council on Radiation Protection and Measurements, Bethesda, MD, 1992.

39 Evaluation of Neutron Exposure

Fred A. Mettler, Jr. and George Voelz

CONTENTS

Introduction 501
Sodium-24 Activation 501
Phosphorus-32 502
References 505

INTRODUCTION

Neutron exposure is an element of criticality accidents (see Chapter 11). Evaluation of radiation dose from neutrons can be done by one of four methods. These are (1) blood analysis for sodium-24 (^{24}Na), (2) a quick-sort method, (3) hair analysis for phosphorus-32 (^{32}P), and (4) activation of metal objects such as jewelry. Each method has some limitations.

SODIUM-24 ACTIVATION

Whole-body neutron doses on the order of 10 rad (0.1 Gy) can be identified by determining the amount of ^{24}Na in blood in the first week postexposure. Sodium-24 is produced by the neutron interaction with ^{23}Na. With a 30-min count of a 10-ml blood sample, activity as low as 3.9×10^{-5} μCi/cc of ^{24}Na (physical half-life, 15 h) can be identified. The conversion factor is 1.6 times 0.1 Gy of fission spectrum neutrons per microcurie per cubic centimeter. Of course, the time elapsed since exposure needs to be included to correct for the physical decay of ^{24}Na. The formula thus becomes:

$$D = 1.6 \times 10^3 \, C \times e^{0.0462t}$$

where D equals dose in Gy, C equals the concentration of ^{24}Na in blood in μCi/cc at time t, and t equals time in hours between accident and analysis.

The quick-sort method can be utilized in cases in which there is no internal or external contamination and only external gamma or neutron exposure. This involves a direct survey of the body with a simple Geiger-type survey instrument held against the abdominal area. Immediately after an accident there will be an error factor in the estimate of dose of as much as 50% caused by activated ^{38}Cl (37-min half-life); however, this decays quickly and decreases to a 1% error 4 h after the accident. The formula, $D = 1.1^{K/M}$, calculates the first collision neutron dose in rads. K is the count rate in counts per minute (cpm) for a Geiger tube instrument (calibrated to indicate a response of 3200 cpm in a 1 mR/h radiation field from a gamma source) and M is the body weight of the exposed person in kilograms. Typical sensitivity shows about 65 cpm for 0.01 Gy in a standard man.[1,2] Note should be made that sodium equilibrates rapidly in the body (less than 20 min) and information regarding dose obtained from induced ^{24}Na is essentially an average whole-body dose. This is of limited clinical value because people seriously exposed in criticality accidents usually are close to the source and have a very steep gradient of nonuniform exposure across their bodies.

The conversion factors have been estimated from phantom and animal experiments. Actual measurements of ^{24}Na in various criticality accidents in the literature are presented in Table 39.1. The results are somewhat variable probably because assorted conversion factors were used to estimate the neutron doses reported and because the accidents differed in the gamma/neutron ratios.

In the 1999 Tokaimura (Japan) criticality accident, the Geiger counter readings over the three patients at about 3 h postexposure were about 26,000, 15,000, and 4000 cpm. By utilizing the quick-sort conversion factors from above, this would suggest an average neutron dose of 4.0, 2.3, and 0.6 Gy. This is probably the correct order of magnitude and gave an early picture of the general relationship between the patients who were ultimately estimated to have total (gamma and neutron) doses of about 17, 8, and 2 to 3 Gy.

PHOSPHORUS-32

Neutron dose to localized areas on critical organs of the body can be estimated by determining the ^{32}P activity in hair and by knowing the neutron spectrum. The reaction ^{32}S (n,p) ^{32}P in body hair produces the activity. Hair samples are often the only samples that can be used to indicate the extent of exposure to different parts of the body and the orientation of the patient to the neutron source. Fortunately, hair has essentially no phosphorus in it normally and the concentration of sulfur in hair is independent of ethnicity. Different 1-g hair samples can be obtained from the head, chest, pubic area, legs, and sometimes even the back area. These should all be carefully labeled. Following chemical separation and evaporation to dryness, the ^{32}P activity can be measured with a low background proportional counter or similar device. Dose in Gy = $5.5 \times 10^2 A$, where A equals activity per gram of hair. This formula holds for time = 0 and needs to be corrected for physical decay of the ^{32}P (half-life, 15 days) since the time of the accident.[3]

Neutron activation of other materials such as film badge inserts, belt buckles, metal buttons, shoe nails, pocket change, rings, eyeglasses, watchbands, and pens as well assorted tools can all be examined for neutron activation. To translate the activation data to personal exposure one needs to determine the neutron energy range, the activation cross section for that energy, and the neutron flux.

In many respects, neutron dosimetry suffers from the same problems that are inherent in other forms of dosimetry. Ultimately, medical management is based upon the patient's clinical findings regardless of the estimated dose. Similar to all dosimetry related to accidents, the error range is probably at least ± 20%. The clinical presentation, course, and therapy will depend upon specific injury to specific tissues. With the inhomogeneity of exposure present in many accidents, few physical methods other than electron spin resonance (see Chapter 40) and ^{32}P activation that will be able to provide the required information. Clinical findings such as location and timing of skin erythema are probably the best current method of assessing inhomogeneous dose distribution. Computer programs have been recently developed using Monte Carlo programs that also are quite useful.

TABLE 39.1
Induced ^{24}Na Results in Various Criticality Accidents

Accident	Total Body, µCi/kg	Total in Body, µCi	Blood, nCi/gm	Serum, nCi/mg Na (specific activity)	Serum ^{24}Na T = 0	Meter Reading	Est. Neutron Dose	
LASL III								
Pt. K	4.1	293	5.31	3.8	12.3 nCi/g	15 mR/h (60 rad/mR/h) (213 cpm/rad)	835–970 rad neutrons 3000–4000 rad gamma 3900–4900 rad total	Fatal
Pt. D	0.014	1.1		0.01			2.8 neutron, total 130 rad	
Pt. R.	0.007	0.60					1.4 neutron, total 35 rad	
L		0.15						
M		0.14						
Z		0.14						
Mayak 68								
Shift Sup.			5000 decays/min/ml				24,500 rad total	Fatal
Operator			15,800 decays/min/ml				700 rad total	
Mol 65		315					50 rad neutron 550 rad gamma	
Argonne 52								
A			110 dpm/ml				2 reps, total 159	
B			76 dpm/ml				4.2 reps, total 126	
C			25 dpm/ml				1.0 rep. total 61	
D			23 dpm/ml				0.15 rep. total 11	
LASL								
Case 1		1.1		0.49	900 cpm/5 ml		200 rad neutron 110 rad gamma	Fatal, 24 days
Case 2				0.03 (1.1 dps/mg Na)	56 cpm/5 ml		8 rad neutron 0.1 rad gamma	Died age 62, AML
Case 3				1.99 (73.6 dps/mg Na)	10,240 cpm/5 ml		1000 rad neutron 114 rad gamma	Fatal, 9 days

TABLE 39.1 (CONTINUED)
Induced ^{24}Na Results in Various Criticality Accidents

Accident	Total Body, µCi/kg	Total in Body, µCi	Blood, nCi/gm	Serum, nCi/mg Na (specific activity)	Serum ^{24}Na $T = 0$	Meter Reading	Est. Neutron Dose	
Case 4				0.36 (12.8 dps/mg Na)	1800 cpm/5 ml		166 rad neutron 114 rad gamma	Died age 54, MI
Case 6				0.19 (7.1 dps/mg Na)	620 cpm/3 ml		51 rad neutron 11 rad neutron	Died age 83, aplastic anemia
Case 7				0.10 (3.0 dps/mg/Na)	260 cpm/3 ml		33 rad neutron 9 rad gamma	Died, Korean War age 27
Case 8				0.05 (2 dps/mg Na)	180 cpm/3 ml		12 rad neutron 4 rad gamma	Died age 42, AML
Case 9				0.04 (1.5 dps/mg Na)	135 cpm/3 ml		9 rad neutron 3 rad gamma	Alive age 67
Case 10				0.03 (1.2 dps/mg Na)	110 cpm/3 ml		7 rad neutron 2 rad gamma	Alive age 55
Sarov 1997			275 Bq/ml 7.4 nCi/ml			8 mR/h at surface 0.5 mR/h at 0.5 m They indicate this = 14 Gy neutrons whole body	4500 rad neutron 350 rad gamma (from gamma neutron shoulder dosimeter)	Fatal (6h)
Tokaimura								
O			178 Bq/ml			15 µSv/h	4.0 Gy	Fatal (83 days)
S			98 Bq/ml			8 µSv/h	2.3 Gy	Fatal (211 days)
Y			23 Bq/ml			1.5 µSv/h	0.6 Gy	

REFERENCES

1. Saunder, F.W. and Auxier, J.A., Neutron activation of sodium and anthropomorphous phantoms, *Health Phys.*, 8, 371–379, 1962.
2. Parker, H.M. and Newton, C.E., Jr., The Hanford criticality accident: dosimeter techniques, interpretations and problems in personal dosimetry for radiation accidents, *IAEA Symp. Proc.*, STI/PUB/99, International Atomic Energy Agency, Vienna, 1965, 567.
3. Peterson, D.F. and Langham, W.H., Neutron activation of sulphur and hair, *Health Phys.*, 12, 381–384, 1966.
4. Bottollier-Depois, J.F., Gaillard-Lecanu, E., Roux, A. et. al., New approach for dose reconstruction: application to one case of localized irradiation with radiological burns, *Health Phys.*, 79 (3), 251–256, 2000.

40 The Current Status of Biological Dosimeters

Douglas B. Chambers and Harriet A. Phillips

CONTENTS

Introduction 507
Cell Death 508
    General 508
    Apoptosis 508
Forms of Nuclear Alterations in Irradiated Cells 510
    Chromosomal Aberrations 510
    Premature Chromosome Condensation (PCC) 510
    Fluorescence *in Situ* Hybridization 510
    Micronucleated Cells 511
Gene Mutations 512
    The Hypoxanthine-Guanine Phosphoribosyl Transferase (HGPRT) Gene 512
    The Glycophorin A Gene 512
Biochemical Markers 513
Physical Dosimeters 513
    Electron Spin Resonance 513
    Optically Stimulated Luminescence 514
Concluding Remarks 514
References 516

INTRODUCTION

Ionizing radiation damages DNA as the result of either a direct interaction between the radiation and the DNA or an indirect interaction through the formation of free radicals or chemical intermediates that can damage the DNA.[1] Ionizing radiation can also damage other cellular components. The response of cells and cell organelles can occur immediately or be delayed by hours, days, or longer following radiation exposure. The cellular responses are structural and functional changes to cells and cell organelles (especially DNA). In addition, there are also several reversible alterations in the structure of different cell organelles. The radiation-induced changes in the supramolecular organization of the membranes, including plasma membrane, as well as different cell organelle membranes, can play a significant role in the development of acute radiation injury.

Somosy[2] lists various morphological alterations of nuclear chromatin (for example, changes of fine structure, development of chromosomal aberrations, etc.), which are thought to originate from the radiation-induced damage to the supramolecular organization of DNA and/or nucleus-specific proteins. He also notes that these effects may not be specific to radiation in itself but may be considered general stress responses to the application of various injurious agents or treatments to cells. Nonetheless, qualitative and/or quantitative evaluation of any changes in chromosomes by various techniques such as morphological analysis of metaphase chromosomes, fluorescence *in situ* hybridization (FISH), development of micronuclei, and other assays are considered as useful biological indicators or "biological dosimeters" of radiation injury.

In addition to its use in the medical application of radiation, biological dosimetry is very often required in cases of radiation accidents, especially when there may be a lack of physical dosimetry or after partial-body exposure with the physical dosimeter outside the field of radiation.[3,4] Biological dosimetric methods have the advantage that, unlike physical dosimetry, they take into account interindividual variations in radiation sensitivity. For example, a dose of 2.5 Gy can be lethal to some people, whereas a dose of 5 Gy can be nonlethal to a few people. Thus, biological dosimetry can be a complement to physical dosimeters.

For biological dosimetry to be practical, the tests need to be relatively rapid, simple to perform, reliable, reproducible, sensitive, and specific so that accurate results can be obtained. No currently available technique satisfies all of these (ideal) requirements and, very often, combinations of several dosimetric methods are required. Requirements for biological dose monitoring in occupational and accidental exposure have been summarized by Trivedi[5] and Trivedi and Greenstock.[6] A recent literature review on the current status of biodosimeters was conducted by SENES.[7] This chapter discusses currently available biological dosimeters in the context of the various morphological and or chemical changes that result after exposure to radiation.

The available techniques can be divided based either on physical assays or on assays that assess cell damage as follows:

1. Biophysical techniques, which can give data about the dose distribution in the organism, e.g., electron spin resonance and optically stimulated luminescence.
2. New biochemical parameters, which are stimulated as part of a repair mechanism when the cells are damaged by radiation.
3. New cytogenic techniques, which assess damage or changes to chromosomes in the cell.

It is important to remember that some of the damage arising from exposure to ionizing radiation is similar to that arising from other causes "spontaneously" or that arising from exposure to other exogenous stimuli. This observation combined with the observations that there is considerable interindividual variability, that various biological indicators decrease with time since exposure, and that ionizing radiation is ubiquitous presents some limitations to the application of biological dosimeters.

CELL DEATH

General

Cell death may be the ultimate consequence of cellular radiation injury.[8-10] Cell death caused by ionizing radiation can be broken down into two main categories depending upon the time of disintegration of cells after exposure. The two categories are interphase death and reproductive or mitotic death.[2] Interphase death can be defined as the breakdown of cellular structures before entering into the first mitotic division after irradiation. Reproductive or mitotic death occurs during mitosis and one or even several divisions after irradiation. Both interphase and reproductive death may be manifested as either apoptosis or necrosis.[8,11-13]

Apoptosis

Apoptosis is expressed as an active, intrinsic mechanism based on the concerted action of specific proteases and endonucleases.[14] Necrosis follows irreversible destruction of cell membranes, followed by collapse of cellular metabolism resulting from extrinsic damage to the cell.

It is generally thought that apoptosis is the main form of ionizing radiation-induced cell death in lymphocytes, thymocytes, and lymphoid and myeloid cell lines. The process starts within minutes following irradiation and can last for several hours. Fibroblasts (V79, L-929), Chinese hamster ovary (CHO) cells, and several human tumor cell lines seem in practice unable to undergo apoptosis *in vitro* and generally die via necrosis. The dose of irradiation also plays a role in the determination of the type of cell death. For example, high doses may cause cell destruction by necrosis, whereas lower doses may induce apoptosis.[15] There are a number of biochemical assays that have emerged for sensitive and rapid detection of apoptotic cells in human lymphocytes.[16–19]

Boreham et al.[20] used two assays to measure radiation-induced apoptosis in isolated peripheral blood lymphocytes: the *in situ* terminal deoxyneucleotidyl transferase (TdT) assay and fluorescence analysis of DNA unwinding (FADU). They investigated the induction of apoptosis at low doses in blood samples to assess the sensitivity of the assays and to determine the variability of the responses. Induction of apoptosis in lymphocytes irradiated *in vitro* was proportional to dose and was detected at doses as low as 0.05 Gy. This is sensitive in comparison to other cytogenic tests (which are discussed in more detail in subsequent sections). Lymphocytes from individuals had reproducible dose responses; however, there was variation between different individuals. The induction kinetics of apoptosis in lymphocytes *in vitro* indicated that the maximum response was reached approximately 72 h after irradiation. This provides an opportunity to collect samples for analysis after radiation exposure. The results also indicate that radiation-induced apoptosis in human lymphocytes has the kinetics, sensitivity, and reproducibility to be a potential biological dosimeter.

Minimal expertise is needed to run apoptosis tests in comparison to other cytogenic tests and results can be available in 1 to 2 days. Since apoptotic cells are naturally removed from circulation, this end point may have a "self-reset" process. A problem with some of the current biological dosimeters, such as chromosomal aberration and micronucleus frequencies, is the large intraindividual variability. Also, these end points cannot be corrected for high background levels. In the case of the FADU assay used by Boreham et al.,[20] intraindividual variation may be minimal. Background levels can be accounted for by comparison to an *in vitro* calibration dose–response curve generated for the individual after the effects of the exposure have disappeared. One of the limitations of using apoptosis as a biological dosimeter is that, if the kinetics of radiation-induced apoptosis are similar *in vitro* and *in vivo*, it becomes essential to collect blood samples as soon as possible after exposure.

Menz et al.[21] proposed flow cytometry to assay for radiation-induced cell apoptosis-associated DNA condensation using CD4 and CD8 T lymphocytes. Apoptosis was quantified as the fraction of CD4-positive or CD8-positive cells with a characteristic reduction of cell size and DNA content. The authors found that the optimal time for analysis was 4 days after exposure, at which time the dose–response curves were linear. The lowest dose level that could be distinguished was 0.05 Gy. However, due to interdonor variation, unless dose–response curves are established for each donor, the sensitivity of this test is 0.1 Gy. This compares well with the sensitivities of established assays, such as scoring dicentrics or micronuclei.

The single cell gel (SCG) or "comet" assay has been determined to be a sensitive technique for the direct visualization of DNA damage in individual cells.[22] This test involves the sandwiching of a small number of cells between thin layers of agarose, lysing at neutral pH, electrophoresis, staining with fluorimetric dye, then visualization using a fluorescence microscope. The intensity of the fluorescence is related to the amount of DNA damage produced in the cell. At neutral pH, damaged cells in apoptosis or necrosis and less damaged cells have distinct shapes or "signatures." The proportion of cells undergoing apoptosis is directly related to the radiation dose, whereas the necrotic cells are an indicator of the conditions at which the cells were isolated or incubated. This technique was evaluated against the dicentric chromosome assay, which is widely used as a biological dosimeter. Preliminary results suggest that the rate of apoptosis at a specified time after apoptosis is reproducible and can be measured using the "comet" assay. The level of detection was

0.3 Gy. However, the apparent variability in the apoptotic response of individuals to ionizing radiation results in this test not being practical for biodosimetry at this time.

The major problem with the assays for apoptosis is that they are performed *in vitro*; research and studies are continuing to examine whether the cells *in vivo* react in the same manner. It cannot be used a long period after exposure since the apoptotic cells will have been absorbed by the body.

In summary, apoptosis seems to offer the possibility of providing a quick indicator of exposure to radiation; however, the various test methods need more research and comparisons and validation before they can be used as a reliable biodosimeter.

FORMS OF NUCLEAR ALTERATIONS IN IRRADIATED CELLS

CHROMOSOMAL ABERRATIONS

Ionizing radiation produces different types of DNA lesions, which include DNA base alterations, DNA–DNA cross-links, and single- and double-strand breaks.[23,24] The various lesions can be caused either directly by the radiation energy or they can develop as a consequence of radiation-induced genomic instability in the surviving cells.[25–27] Statistical issues associated with the use of chromosomal aberrations as biological dosimeters have been discussed by Cologne et al.[28] The measurement of chromosomal aberrations provides an informative, useful, and widely used technique for indicating radiation exposure.

PREMATURE CHROMOSOME CONDENSATION (PCC)

In this method, peripheral blood lymphocytes are collected and fused with mitotic cells from another source (for example, CHO cells). After fusion, the hybrids contain both the human G_0 interphase and hamster metaphase chromosomes. The G_0 lymphocytes then undergo chromatin condensation followed by disaggregation of their nuclear membrane and further condensation of chromatin into 46 single chromatids. Therefore, after exposure to radiation, either *in vivo* or *in vitro*, chromosome damage can be visualized and quantified as the number of chromatid segments in excess of 46. In theory, PCC can be carried out with any cell type (dividing or nondividing) or any stage of the cell cycle.[3] The test has been reported to assess doses as low as 0.05 Gy; however, blood must be obtained within hours of radiation exposure since a longer delay will result in cellular repair mechanisms being initiated.

Durante and colleagues[29] used a protocol based on the use of calyculin A to induce PCC in different phases of the cell cycle. Chromosome exchanges were measured by FISH. This is an example of combining two protocols for use as a biological dosimeter. They determined that this method is a powerful method to be used in biodosimetry because it overcomes problems related to poor *in vitro* growth or cell cycle aberrations.

As discussed above, the main advantage of this technique over the micronucleus test described below or any conventional chromosomal aberration is the rapidity of the process (1 vs. 72 h for the micronucleus assay) and the higher sensitivity due to reduced repair mechanisms and interphase death. However, very few studies are available that validate this test and investigate confounding factors, and a highly trained technician is needed to carry out the fusion process. In addition, this test is limited by the fact that it only analyses chromosome fragments since Giemsa staining does not allow visualization of the centromeric regions and, therefore, the identification of dicentrics, centric rings, and acentric fragments.[30]

FLUORESCENCE *IN SITU* HYBRIDIZATION

The established method for detection of these chromosomal aberrations involves the use of blocked stained preparations, which detect unstable aberrations such as dicentrics, rings, acentric fragments, and other asymmetrical rearrangements. FISH with whole chromosome libraries (chromosome "painting") offers a potentially faster and more accurate method of identifying chromosomal aberrations and thus is currently the assay of choice for biodosimetry.[31] A minimum of 4 days is needed for the painting procedure and analysis. Individual external doses of about 0.1 Gy can be reliably measured using this technique.[32] To assess low-dose levels reliably, a large number of metaphases need to be scored.[33] The background incidence of dicentric aberrations observed at metaphase is about 1 in 1000 cells. Since radiation-induced aberrations arise at the rate of about 4/100 cells/Gy, then the ability to detect a dose of 0.1 Gy would require about 1000 lymphocytes to be scored, which would take approximately 3 days. Another disadvantage that makes FISH inaccessible to some laboratories is the high cost of the probes and the highly sensitive fluorescence microscope with optics and an ultraviolet light.

Recently, a number of authors have compared FISH to other assays for assessing exposure such as the conventional metaphase analysis, G-banding.[31–37] Plummer et al.[31] found that FISH offered a sensitive method for assessing radiation exposure and compared favorably with G-banding. In addition, they as well as Bauchinger[35] purport that FISH with chromosome painting has a potential for use in long-term retrospective studies if it can be used to score stable aberrations. Schmidt et al.[34] found that the accuracy of dicentric and translocation scoring could be improved using FISH in comparison to conventional assay techniques using Giesma staining. In comparison, Roy et al.[36] and Lindholm et al.[37] found that there was no statistically significant difference between scoring dicentrics using FISH or the conventional staining technique.

Durm et al.[38] have proposed a fast-FISH technique, which utilizes hybridization with a buffer that does not contain the denaturing agent, formamide. The use of formamide results in hybridization taking several days and also involves several time-consuming washing steps to remove it. They were able to demonstrate that the fast-FISH technique involved ten fewer working steps than the standard FISH procedure. However, once hybridization occurred, there was no decrease in the time required for specimen preparation and analysis. They suggest that this fast-FISH methodology can be adapted to be useful in chromosome painting so that stable chromosomes can be scored for retrospective dosimetry and that the technique has application for use in biological dosimetry.

At present, FISH seems to be the biological dosimeter of choice since it has been demonstrated to be specific for radiation. In conjunction with chromosome painting, FISH can be a useful tool for retrospective biological dosimetry. The biggest drawbacks of the technique are the large cost of the materials and equipment, and the need for a skilled technician to perform the assay. Further development of the fast-FISH technique may alleviate some of these concerns.

MICRONUCLEATED CELLS

Micronuclei are formed from chromosomal fragments and whole chromosomes and are located in the cytoplasm of irradiated cells.[2] These chromosomal fragments do not possess centromeres and are not incorporated into the nucleus of the dividing cell. Thus, they form a small satellite structure that resembles but is definitely different from the main nucleus.[39] This smaller "secondary nucleus" is called a micronucleus. An increase in the number of micronucleated cells is generally observed in cell cultures exposed to ionizing radiation.[40,41] Micronuclei are reported to last only for a short time.[42]

Counting the frequency or number of micronuclei can be used as a biological dosimeter. The assaying of micronuclei is a simple and useful technique for quantitative analysis of chromosomal lesions induced by ionizing radiation.[41,43]

The lymphocytes need to be cultured for more than 2 days including incubation for 24 to 32 h with cytochalasin B, which blocks the separation of the cytoplasm and leads to the formation of the characteristic large binucleated lymphocytes. In general, micronuclei are counted in at least 1000 cells. The rate of counting is very rapid and can be completed within an hour. Some attempt has been made to automate the counting of the micronuclei.[44] It is important to generate dose–response curves for different conditions of radiation exposure and radiation quality.[3] Radiation doses of 0.2 Gy can accurately be detected. For lower doses (0.05 Gy), control data prior to the individual being exposed to radiation are necessary. The test is relatively cheap and does not require a highly trained technician.

Micronuclei disappear rapidly after exposure so that they can only be used as a short-term dosimeter. Cells also need to be cultivated for at least 72 h. In addition, like apoptosis, this indicator is not radiation specific. Thus, the establishment of control data for each individual is important. The rate of formation of micronuclei is thought to increase with age, alcohol and tobacco use, and is reported to be higher in women.[42]

The micronucleus assay, although relatively cheap and easy to use, is not a practical biodosimeter at this time since it is not specific for radiation and detection limits of the test restrict it from being used to assess low doses of exposure. However, it may be a useful test for prescreening multiple individuals since a qualified technician is not necessary.

GENE MUTATIONS

In general, radiation randomly changes the genome base sequence as a result of free-radical-mediated chemical alterations to individual nucleotides. The various point mutations occur on different chromosomes and, in addition, in different genes. Therefore, if the function of a particular gene is known or an assay is available, these can serve as biological indicators of exposure to radiation. Two such assays have been used extensively in the literature: the hypoxanthine-guanine phosphoribosyl transferase (HPRT) gene assay and the glycophorin A gene assay.

THE HYPOXANTHINE-GUANINE PHOSPHORIBOSYL TRANSFERASE (HGPRT) GENE

HGPRT is an enzyme that incorporates hypoxanthine or guanine into the purine monophosphate pool for nucleic acid synthesis. Mutation at the HPRT locus is one of the best-characterized assays in cultured mammalian cells.[45] However, this test is limited since it can only be used a short time after exposure since the signal rapidly fades. The HPRT mutation assay measures the HPRT mutations in T lymphocytes. In the past it was only possible to culture lymphocytes for a short time; the discovery of the T-cell growth factor (interleukin-2, or IL-2) has allowed for the longer-term growth of these lymphocytes in culture and allows for the measurement of mutant frequencies.

Seifert and colleagues[46] found that there was a positive relationship between age of the individual and mutant frequencies. Smoking also resulted in increased mutant frequencies. Thus, this test is not specific to radiation exposure. Hiari and colleagues[45] also found that smoking and age resulted in higher mutant frequencies. They also found a large variation in mutant frequencies between individuals and a weak dose–response relationship.

Albertini et al.[47] investigated how the quality of the radiation affects the efficiency of induction of HPRT mutations. Their data showed that radiation quality did indeed affect the efficiency of induction of mutations both *in vivo* and *in vitro*. They surmise that the HPRT assay could be used to determine more precisely the induction of mutations resulting from individual exposures to radiation.

THE GLYCOPHORIN A GENE

Glycophorin A (GPA) is the major glycoprotein expressed on the surface of human erythrocytes.. The GPA assay involves the use of a fluorescent-labeled monoclonal antibody against the glycophorin protein to measure the loss of a red blood cell allele (alternative form of a gene) in individuals exposed to radiation.[48,49] GPA is purported to be a very stable indicator with lifelong persistence. The assay involves flow cytometry and as such enables examination of a large number of people within a short time.

Saenko et al.[50] investigated the use of GPA to assess variant frequencies in individuals exposed to radiation for a long period of time. They found that although the GPA assay had previously been used to assess acute radiation exposure, the test had limited potential to be used as a biodosimeter of prolonged irradiation especially in the dose interval up to 2.0 Gy. This was due to the large variability in the results.

The test is simple to run and relatively cheap. The disadvantage of GPA as a biodosimeter lies in the fact that the test does not seem to be very reproducible within the same individual. Additionally, there seems to be a large intraindividual variability and there has not yet been a careful calibration using persons with known exposure.

In general, gene mutant assays are not specific to exposure to radiation only. In particular, the HPRT assay is influenced by a number of confounding factors such as age and smoking. In addition, there are indications that both the GPA and HPRT assays still need to be calibrated and validated. Based on all these findings, it is unlikely that gene mutation assays would be appropriate biodosimeters for assessing the effects of radiation exposure.

BIOCHEMICAL MARKERS

Barret et al.[51] have reported an early increase in serum amylase levels in humans after the parotid gland or pancreas has been irradiated. The dose threshold for this test is around 1 Gy. The difficulties with assaying for serum amylase arise from the lack of a dose–response relationship in humans, large interindividual variability, and the large number of confounding factors such as infection, inflammation, etc.[42] This was also discussed in Trivedi and Greenstock.[6]

Recent biochemical investigations have identified several parameters that could be useful. Studies have shown that the radioinduced inflammatory mediator IL-6 can be considered as a good indicator in the first day after radiation exposure. After the first day, serum iron, which occurs as a result of extravascular hyperhemolysis and of inflammation, can be examined. Finally, 3 to 8 days after exposure, cholesterol and apolipoproteins may be appropriate indicators.[52]

The presence of biochemical proteins in the blood has not been demonstrated to be dose dependent. In addition, the presence of confounding factors indicate that these analytes may not be the most appropriate indicators for determining radiation dose; however, they may be useful as a quick screening procedure for determining high dose exposure to radiation.

PHYSICAL DOSIMETERS

ELECTRON SPIN RESONANCE

A major consequence of the action of ionizing radiation on organic polymers is the creation of free radicals, of which the mass density is proportional to the dose. Electron spin resonance (ESR) can detect these free radicals, which have a long life in polymers. The surface under the absorption spectrum is proportional to the number of spins present in the resonance cavity and as a consequence the dose.[53] The detection limit is around 0.05 Gy and the signal exponentially decreases with time. Therefore, ESR is a rapid methodology for the evaluation of dose with good accuracy. The only practical biological material that is currently used is teeth. Bones can be used; however, these are only available after autopsies and thus are unsuitable as a general population dosimeter.

ESR tooth enamel signals can avoid some of the problems associated with chromosomal aberration methods. The dose evaluation data provided by ESR do not depend on the time after exposure. In addition, the limit of detection is about 0.1 Gy.[54,55] Haskell and colleagues[56] have reported detection limits of 0.05 Gy after the removal of the organic component in dentine.

ESR in dental enamel is a good measure of absorbed dose; however, it does not provide a direct measure of whole-body dose and has problems with intersample variability in sensitivity to radiation. Additionally, ESR is limited in sensitivity and requires a large array of laboratory equipment and extracted teeth if dental enamel is to be used.[57]

ESR was applied to whole deciduous teeth of children by Haskell and co-workers.[58] This test allows the feasibility of making direct measurement of absorbed gamma ray dose in the days and weeks following exposure. They presented a technique, which required little sample preparation and under conditions of rapid screening resulted in a detection limit of 0.5 Gy. The largest error in the process was the determination of an appropriate background signal. This test would have to be adapted for use with adults or may in fact be inappropriate for the extrapolation.

The main drawback of the ESR method stems from the lack of biological material other than teeth and the necessity for very specialized people to carry out the test. In addition, detection limits seem to vary.

OPTICALLY STIMULATED LUMINESCENCE

Optical technology holds the promise of being sensitive, amenable to miniaturization, and noninvasive. The underlying phenomenon surrounding optically stimulated luminescence (OSL) is similar to ESR; however, in OSL the only trapped electrons detected are those that can be freed by absorption of near-visible or visible photons. The first successful detection of time-dependent OSL from gamma-irradiated enamel was recently reported by Godfrey-Smith and Pass.[59]

Godfrey-Smith and Pass[59] developed a dose–response curve for infrared-stimulated luminescence (IRSL) for dental enamel following gamma irradiation ranging from 0 to 480 Gy. Since the IRSL signals were proportional to the absorbed radiation doses, they demonstrate the feasibility of using OSL as a dosimeter. The task at hand now is to decrease the detection limit by two to three orders of magnitude (to at least that of ESR) and to establish a dose–response relationship.

The ESR and OSL techniques still seem to be in the earliest stages of development for use as biodosimeters. Detection limits have to be decreased and the methods need much more validation before they can be useful as biodosimeters. However, with the perfection of OSL in dental enamel, the development of a noninvasive, integrating biodosimetric technique that is sufficiently sensitive, reliable, specific, convenient, and inexpensive will be closer to realization.

CONCLUDING REMARKS

There continues to be efforts to increase the ease, rapidity, and reliability of assays for use as biological dosimeters. Even though the requirements of a biodosimeter can be enumerated,[5,6] the concept of a successful dosimeter is still a continuously evolving process and thus it still does not appear that a single efficient assay for use as a biological dosimeter is yet available.

Over the past decade, it seems that a major emphasis by researchers has been focused on FISH. Improvements have been suggested to allow a more rapid analysis (less than 4 days) of radiation exposure using this technique; however, the cost of probes and the equipment necessary to conduct this test is quite high.

Confounding factors such as age, smoking status, and gender also seem to play a role in some of the assays that are not specific to radiation and thus these tests, such as GPA and HPRT assays, may only be appropriate for use as screening tools. In the authors' view, it is unlikely that these assays will find any widespread use. There have also been reports of a so-called adaptive response for a number of indicators of cell damage. This means that a small radiation dose can reduce the amount of cellular damage caused by a later higher dose. In such cases, the use of a biological dosimeter may in fact not be able to give an accurate dose estimate based on this response.

From the recent literature, it is apparent that most of the assays under investigation can only accurately detect doses with detection limits in the range of 0.1 to 0.5 Gy. Table 40.1 provides a summary of the lowest detection limits reported for each of the discussed dosimeters. Further refinement of these detection limits is yet to be achieved.

TABLE 40.1
Summary of Detection Limits for Test Methods

Test Method	Detection Limit (Gy)
Apoptosis	0.1–0.3
FISH	0.1
Premature chromosome condensation	0.05
Micronucleated cells	0.2
Gene mutations	2
Biochemical indicators	1
Physical biodosimeters	0.1

It is important to determine the level of confidence that can be placed in the detection limits that are shown in Table 40.1. In general, the scatter of data at the low dose level is quite high such that a dose of 0.1 Sv can be estimated to be as low as 0 Sv or as high as 1.5 Sv.[28] Thus, there are still challenges in obtaining reliable dose estimates from biological dosimeters in the low dose range.

Cell death (apoptosis) is becoming one of the new emerging fields for use as a biological indicator. Several tests have been presented to measure apoptosis as a consequence of exposure to radiation in cells. Apoptosis cannot be used as a retrospective dosimeter because apoptotic cells are removed from circulation quickly. The use of cell death as a biological dosimeter is only in its infancy. To date, only *in vitro* testing has been carried out. Thus, more validation is necessary before apoptosis test methods can be uses for biological dosimetry.

Currently, ESR or OSL are the only available techniques for measuring physical dose and these tests are the only tests that may be able to assess accurately long-term retrospective dosimetry in biological tissue such as bone, teeth, fingernails, and hair. However, FISH or fast-FISH in conjunction with chromosome painting may also be useful in retrospective dosimetry. A disadvantage of all of these techniques is the high cost for equipment and supplies and the need for trained technicians to carry out measurements.

At present, one particular assay cannot be applied in every situation to assess radiation dose. Therefore, it becomes a decision-making process regarding which assay or combination of assays is most appropriate to assess a particular situation. Table 40.2 provides suggested areas where it may be advantageous to use the various test methods. For example, in retrospective dosimetry at long times after exposure, FISH or biophysical techniques (ESR/OSL) are the only currently

TABLE 40.2
Suggested Uses for the Various Available Biodosimeters

Screening	Medical/Occupational Exposure	Retrospective Dosimetry
Apoptosis	Apoptosis	
	Premature chromosome condensation	
	FISH	FISH
Micronucleated cells	Micronucleated cells	
Gene mutations		
Biochemical markers		
		Biophysical techniques

Note: Research is still ongoing in the area of biodosimetry, and it is still possible that a single biodosimeter may emerge from these studies.

available techniques to be used. For screening applications involving a large number of individuals, less costly techniques such as apoptosis, micronucleated cells, or other techniques might be more appropriate for the first level of determining exposure before graduating to a more sophisticated and expensive technique.

REFERENCES

1. Burkart, W., Jung, T., and Frasch, G., Damage pattern as a function of radiation quality and other factors, *C.R. Acad. Sci.*, Ser. III, 322(2–3), 89–101, 1999.
2. Somosy, Z., Radiation response of cell organelles, *Micron*, 31(2), 165–181, 2000.
3. Verschaeve, L., Comparison of cytogenetic methods for biological dosimetry of radiation exposure, *Nucleus*, 36(1–2), 1–12, 1993.
4. Goldman, M., Integrated retrospective radiation dose assessment, *Stem Cells*, 15(Suppl. 2), 157–161, 1997.
5. Trivedi, A., Bio-indicators for radiation dose assessment, AECL Rep. AECL-10245, Atomic Energy of Canada Limited, Chalk River, Canada, 1990.
6. Trivedi, A. and Greenstock, C.L., Recent Developments in Biodosimetry, A report prepared for the Atomic Energy Control Board, AECB Project No. 7.176.1, 1995.
7. SENES Consultants Limited, Literature Review of the Current Status of Biological Dosimeters, April, Prepared for the Atomic Energy Control Board, Ottawa, Canada, 2000.
8. Harms-Ringdahl, M., Nicotera, P., and Radford, J.R., Radiation-induced apoptosis, *Mutat. Res.*, 366, 171–179, 1996.
9. Blank, K.R., Rudoltz, M.S., Kao, G.D., Muschel, R.J., and McKenna, W.G., Review: the molecular regulation of apoptosis and implication for radiation oncology, *Int. J. Radiat. Biol.*, 71, 455–466, 1997.
10. Hendry, J.H. and West, C.M.L., Apoptosis and mitotic cell death: their relative contributions to normal-tissue and tumour radiation response, *Int. J. Radiat. Biol.*, 71, 709–719, 1997.
11. Akagi, Y., Ito, K., and Sawanda, S., Radiation-induced apoptosis in Molt-4 cells: a study of dose effect relationships and their modification, *Int. J. Radiat. Biol.*, 64, 47–56, 1993.
12. Nakano, H. and Shinohara, K., X-ray induced cell death: apoptosis and necrosis, *Radiat. Res.*, 140, 1–9, 1994.
13. Szumiel, I., Review: ionizing radiation-induced cell death, *Int. J. Radiat. Biol.*, 6, 329–341, 1994.
14. Khodarev, N.N., Sokolova, I.A., and Vaughan, A.T.M., Mechanisms of induction of apoptotic DNA fragmentation, *Int. J. Radiat. Biol.*, 73, 455–467, 1998.
15. Payne, C.M., Bjore, G.C., and Schultz, D.A., Changes in the frequency of apoptosis after low- and high-dose X-irradiation of human lymphocytes, *J. Leukocyte Biol.*, 52, 433–440, 1992.
16. Collins, R.J., Harmon, B.V., Gobe, G.C., and Kerr, J.F.R., Internucleosomal DNA cleavage should not be the sole criterion for identifying apoptosis, *Int. J. Radiat. Biol.*, 61, 451–453, 1992.
17. Darzynkiewicz, Z., Bruno, S., Del Bino, G., Gorczyca, W., Holtz, M.A., Lassota, P., and Traganos, F., Features of apoptotic cells measured by flow cytometry, *Cytometry*, 13, 795–808, 1992.
18. Omerod, M.G., Sun, X-M., Brown, D., Snowden, R.T., and Cohen, G.C., Quantification of apoptosis and necrosis by flow cytometry, *Acta Oncol.*, 32, 417–424, 1993.
19. Basnakian, A.G. and James, S.J., A rapid and sensitive assay for the detection of DNA fragmentation during early phases of apoptosis, *Nucl. Acids Res.*, 22, 2714–2715, 1994.
20. Boreham, D.R., Gale, K.L., Maves, S.R., Walker, J.-A., and Morrison, D.P., Radiation-induced apoptosis in human lymphocytes: potential as a biological dosimeter, *Health Phys.*, 71(5), 685–691, 1996.
21. Menz, R., Andres, R., Larsson, B., Ozsahin, M., Trott, K., and Crompton, N.E., Biological dosimetry: the potential use of radiation-induced apoptosis in human T-lymphocytes, *Radiat. Environ. Biophys.*, 36, 175–181, 1997.
22. Wilkins, R.C., Kizilian, N., McLean, J.R., Wilkinson, D., Reinhardt-Poulin, P., Johnson, F., and Gibbons, D., The "single cell 'comet' assay" as a biological dosimeter, August 1998.
23. Schulte-Fronhlinde, D. and Bothe, E., The development of chemical damage of DNA in aqueous solution, in *The Early Effects of Radiation in DNA*, Fielden, E.M. and O'Neils, Eds., NATO ASI Series II: Cell Biology, 54, Springer-Verlag, Berlin, 1991, 317–332. Cited in Somosky.[2]

24. Lett, J.T., Damage to cellular radiation from particulate radiation, the efficacy of its processing and the radiosensitivity of mammalian cells. Emphasis on DNA strand breaks and chromatin break, *Radiat. Environ. Biophys.*, 31, 257–277, 1992.
25. Kadhim, M.A., Lorimore, S.A., Townsend, K.M., Godhead, D.T., Buckle, V.J., and Wright, E.G., Radiation-induced genomic instability: delayed cytogenic aberrations and apoptosis in primary human bone marrow cells, *J. Radiat. Biol.*, 67, 287–293, 1995.
26. Morgan, W.F., Day, J.P., Kaplan, M.I., McGhee, E.M., and Limoli, C.L., Genomic instability induced by ionizing radiation, *Radiat. Res.*, 146, 247–258, 1996.
27. Lloyd, D.C., Chromosomal analysis to assess radiation dose, *Stem Cells*, 15(Suppl. 2), 195–201, 1997.
28. Cologne, J.B., Pawel, D.J., and Preston, D.L., Statistical issues in biological radiation dosimetry for risk assessment using stable chromosome aberrations, *Health Phys.*, 75(5), 518–529, 1998.
29. Durante, M., Furusawa, Y., and Gotoh, E., A simple method for simultaneous interphase-metaphase chromosome analysis in biodosimetry, *Int. J. Radiat. Biol.*, 74(4), 457–462, 1998.
30. Pantelias, G.E., Iliakis, G.E., Sambani, C.D., and Politis, G., Biological dosimetry of absorbed radiation by C-banding of interphase chromosomes in peripheral blood lymphocytes, *Int. J. Radiat. Biol.*, 63(3), 349–354, 1993.
31. Plummer, S.M., Pheasant, A.E., Johnson, R., Faux, S.P., Chipman, J.K., and Hulten, M.A., Evaluation of the relative sensitivity of chromosome painting (FISH) as an indicator of radiation-induced damage in human lymphocytes, *Hereditas*, 121, 139–145, 1994.
32. Bauchinger, M., Quantification of low-level radiation exposure by conventional chromosome aberration analysis, *Mutat. Res.*, 339(3), 177–189, 1995.
33. Granath, F., Grigoreva, M., and Natarajan, A.T., DNA content proportionality and persistence of radiation-induced chromosomal aberrations studied by FISH, *Mutat. Res.*, 366(2), 145–152, 1996.
34. Schmidt, E., Braselmann, H., and Nahrstedt, U., Comparison of gamma-ray induced dicentric yields in human lymphocytes measured by conventional analysis and FISH, *Mutat. Res.*, 348, 125–130, 1995.
35. Bauchinger, M., Cytogenetic research after accidental radiation exposure, *Stem Cells*, 13(Suppl. 1), 182–190, 1995.
36. Roy, L., Sorokine-Durm, I., and Voisin, P., Comparison between fluorescence in situ hybridization and conventional cytogenetics for dicentric scoring: a first-step validation for the use of FISH in biological dosimetry, *Int. J. Radiat. Biol.*, 70(6), 665–669, 1996.
37. Lindholm, C., Salomaa, S., Tekkel, M., Paile, W., Koivistoinen, A., Ilus, T., and Veidebaum, T., Biodosimetry after accidental radiation exposure by conventional chromosome analysis and FISH, *Int. J. Radiat. Biol.*, 70(6), 647–656, 1996.
38. Durm, M., Sorokine-Durm, I., Haar, F.M., Hausmann, M., Ludwig, H., Voisin, P., and Cremer, C., Fast-FISH technique for rapid, simultaneous labeling of all human centromeres, *Cytometry*, 31, 153–162, 1998.
39. Fenech, M., The cytokinesis-block micronucleus technique: a detailed description of the method and its application to genotoxicity studies in human populations, *Mutat. Res.*, 285, 35–44, 1993.
40. Cornforth, M.N. and Goodwin, E.H., Transmission of radiation-induced acentric chromosomal fragments to micronuclei in normal human fribroblasts, *Radiat. Res.*, 126, 210–217, 1991.
41. Müller, W.-U., Streffer, C., and Wuttke, K., Micronucleus determination as a means to assess radiation, *Stem Cells*, 13, 199–206, 1995.
42. Fatôme, M., Agay, D., Martin, S., Mestries, J.C., and Multon, E., Biological dosimetry after a criticality accident, *Radiat. Prot. Dosimetry*, 70(1–4), 455–459, 1997.
43. Almássy, Z., Krepinsky, A.B., Bianco, A., and Köteles, G.L., The present state and perspectives of micronucleus assay in radiation protection. A review, *Appl. Radiat. Isotopes*, 38, 241–249, 1987.
44. Tates, A.D., Van Welie, M.T., and Ploem, J.S., The present state of the automated micronucleus test for lymphocytes, *Int. J. Radiat Biol.*, 58, 813–825, 1990.
45. Hirai, Y., Kusunoki, Y., Kyoizumi, S., Awa, A.A., Pawel, D.J., Nakamura, N., and Akiyama, M., Mutant frequency at the HPRT locus in peripheral blood T-lymphocytes of atomic bomb survivors, *Mutat. Res.*, 329(2), 183–196, 1995.
46. Seifert, A.M., Demers, C., Dubeau, H., and Messing, K., HPRT-mutant frequency and lymphocyte characteristics of workers exposed to ionizing radiation on a sporadic basis: a comparison of two exposure indicators, job title and dose, *Mutat. Res.*, 319, 61–70, 1993.

47. Albertini, R.J., Clark, L.S., Nicklas, J.A., O'Neill, J.P., Hui, T.E., and Jostes, R., Radiation quality affects the efficiency of induction and the molecular spectrum of HPRT mutations in human T cells, *Radiat. Res.*, 148(5 Suppl.), S76–S86, 1997.
48. Langois, R., Bigbee, W.L., and Gensen, R.H., Measurements of the frequency of human erythrocytes with gene expression loss phenotypes at the glycophorin A locus, *Hum. Genet.*, 74, 353–362, 1986.
49. Akiyama, M., Kusunoki, Y., Umeki, S., Hirai, Y., Nakamura, N., and Kyoizumi, S., Evaluation of four somatic mutation assays as biological dosimeters in humans, in *Radiation Research: A Twentieth-Century Perspective Vol II: Congress Proceedings*, Dewey, W.C. et al., Eds., Academic Press, New York, 1992, 177–182. Cited in Saenko et al.[50]
50. Saenko, A.S., Zamulaeva, I.A., Smirnova, S.G., Orlova, N.V., Selivanova, E.I., Saenko, V.A., Matveeva, N.P., Kaplan, M.A., Nugis, V.Y., Nadezhina, N.M., and Tsyb, A.F., Determination of somatic mutant frequencies at glycophorin A and T-cell receptor loci for biodosimetry of prolonged irradiation, *Int. J. Radiat. Biol.*, 73(6), 613–618, 1998.
51. Barrett, A., Jacobs, A., Kohn, J., Raymond, J., and Powles, R.L., Changes in serum amylase and its isoenzymes after whole body irradiation, *Br. Med. J.*, 285, 170–171, 1982.
52. Martin, S., Dosimetrie biologique appliquee aux rayonnements gamma et neutron-gamma. Rapport de synthesis finale. Comande DRET 91/1006, July, 1995. Cited in Fatôme et al.[42]
53. Sagstuen, H., Theysen, H., and Henriksen, T., Dosimetry by ESR spectroscopy following a radiation accident, *Health Phys.*, 45, 961–968, 1982.
54. Ceve, P., Shara, M., and Ravnik, C., Electron paramagnetic resonance of irradiated tooth enamel, *Radiat. Res.*, 51, 581–589, 1972.
55. Aldrich, J.E. and Pass, B., Dental enamel as an in vivo radiation dosimeter: separation diagnostic X-ray dose from dose due to natural sources, *Radiat. Prot. Dosimetry*, 17, 175–179, 1986.
56. Haskell, E.H., Kenner, G.H., and Hayes, R.B., Electronic paramagnetic resonance dosimetry of dentine following removal of organic material, *Health Phys.*, 68(4), 579–584, 1995.
57. Pass, B., Collective radiation biodosimetry for dose reconstruction of acute accidental exposures: a review, *Environ. Health Perspect.*, 105(Suppl. 6), 1397–1401, 1997.
58. Haskell, E.H., Hayes, R.B., and Kenner, G.H., An EPR dosimetry method for rapid scanning of children following a radiation accident using deciduous teeth, *Health Phys.*, 76(2), 137–144, 1999.
59. Godfrey-Smith, D.I. and Pass, B., A new method of retrospective radiation dosimetry: optically stimulated luminescence in dental enamel, *Health Phys.*, 72(5), 744–749, 1997.

41 Psychosocial Effects of Radiation Accidents

Steven M. Becker

CONTENTS

Introduction 519
Key Features of Radiation Accidents 519
Psychological Effects 520
High-Risk Groups 521
Social Impacts 522
Psychosocial Effects — Implications for Radiation Accident Preparedness and Response 522
Conclusion..524
References 524

INTRODUCTION

Accidents involving radiation can have profound psychosocial effects on individuals, families, and communities. Indeed, it is evident from recent experience and research that psychosocial impacts can be among the most significant and challenging consequences of radiation accidents. It is crucial, therefore, for radiation accident emergency plans and training to include a robust psychosocial component. Similarly, emergency and postemergency response efforts need to include provisions for addressing a full range of psychosocial impacts. This chapter briefly reviews the current understanding of psychosocial issues and highlights several implications for radiation accident management.

KEY FEATURES OF RADIATION ACCIDENTS

Radiation and other toxic hazards have the capacity to "unnerve human beings in new and special ways."[1] People find such agents "a good deal more threatening than both natural hazards of even the most dangerous kind and mechanical mishaps of considerable power." For one thing, situations involving radiation (or hazardous chemicals) involve risks that are seen as involuntary and unfamiliar. Both of these features are believed to trigger more concern than other sorts of risks.[2,3] Then, too, toxic agents are generally invisible: they are "without substance and cannot be apprehended by the use of the unaided senses, and for that reason they seem especially terrifying."[1] Frightening historical associations (e.g., Hiroshima and Nagasaki) and the generally negative images that people tend to associate with nuclear technology may contribute further to the sense of dread.

Radiation is also viewed as having the potential to cause hidden and irreversible damage and as having the capacity to produce forms of illness and death that arouse particular dread. In addition, such situations are seen to represent special dangers to children and pregnant women. Again, all of these factors are thought to be connected with a greater sense of alarm.[2] Furthermore, invisible contaminants are seen as posing an unbounded or open-ended threat. Because long-term health consequences may take years to develop, the danger is seen as having no end. There is a continuing sense of vulnerability and concern, and people can remain in a "permanent state of alarm and anxiety."[1] Also playing a role is the fact that radiation accidents and other situations involving toxic hazards are a result of human activities; that is, they are man-made in origin. People who are victimized by such events "feel a special measure of distress when they come to think that their affliction was caused by other human beings."[1]

Taken together, these features and perceptions make radiation and radiation accidents a remarkably powerful stressor. "The insidious and lethal nature of radiation," writes Mickley,[4] "makes it especially feared." Similarly, Rosa and Freudenberg,[5] drawing on the work of Slovic and colleagues,[6] note that "nuclear risks are perceived to be the riskiest — and are the most dreaded."

PSYCHOLOGICAL EFFECTS

A wide range of psychological effects can result from radiation accidents. At one end of the spectrum are common stress reactions that are typically associated with both natural and human-made disasters. The effects can be emotional, physical, cognitive, or interpersonal in nature, ranging, for example, from fatigue, insomnia, or impaired concentration to emotional numbing or social withdrawal.[7] As is the case with other types of disaster, many mild to moderate stress reactions are transient in nature. Such reactions represent a normal reaction to a highly abnormal situation.[8] "Relief from stress and the passage of time usually lead to the reestablishment of equilibrium, but information about normal reactions, education about ways to handle them, and early attention to symptoms can speed recovery and prevent long-term problems."[9]

What complicates the picture considerably, however, it that exposure to invisible contaminants has also been shown to produce a chronic state of alarm. In the aftermath of a radiation accident, many people are left with a continuing sense of vulnerability and a pervasive feeling of uncertainty. Whether the source of the danger is removed from the community or, alternatively, whether the survivors are relocated away from the danger zone, people continue to have serious concerns about the longer-term health implications of the incident. Thus, although the immediate emergency may be over, and although considerable time may have passed, the incident continues to act as a powerful and persistent stressor. As Ursano, McCaughey, and Fullerton[10] have written, contamination incidents "produce long-term anticipatory stress of the possible, the probable and the imagined risks to health and family."

Studies carried out more than 6 years after the Chernobyl disaster found a high prevalence of psychological distress and psychiatric disorders (mainly milder psychiatric syndromes) in the severely contaminated Gomel region.[11] A comparison of this area with a control region found significantly higher levels of psychopathology among the exposed population. While the effects in the overall population in the exposed area were mainly at a subclinical level, a significantly higher risk of psychiatric disorders was found among mothers with children under 18 years of age. The researchers speculate that "psychiatric symptoms among these women are fostered by genuine concern about the health of their children...."[12] The Chernobyl studies reinforce earlier findings about the effects of the Three Mile Island nuclear accident. Research conducted by Baum and colleagues[13] found evidence of long-term emotional, behavioral, and physiological stress after TMI. Similarly, studies carried out by Bromet and colleagues[14] found that the accident had a long-term adverse effect on the mental health of mothers of young children years after the accident.

Persistent stress can produce a marked deterioration in people's quality of life. At a minimum, having long-term health concerns about one's loved ones as a more or less permanent feature of day-to-day existence affects someone's attitude toward the present and hopes for the future. Further, it is now widely accepted that long-term stress is deleterious to health (e.g., high blood pressure, cardiovascular problems, digestive disorders). In a situation where large numbers of people are suffering from chronic, unremitting stress related to a radiation accident, this can translate into substantial problems of physical illness and significantly increased utilization of health care facilities.[15]

It is also important to note that concern about potential exposure can be enough to produce chronic stress reactions. In research carried out 3½ years after the Goiânia radiological accident in Brazil, Collins and de Carvalho[16] found that people who had been exposed to radiation, and others who had not been exposed but were concerned about potential exposure, showed similar psychological, behavioral, and cardiovascular-neuroendocrine effects. Both groups reported more fear than controls, both exhibited decrements in performance on speed and accuracy tests, and both had significantly higher blood pressure than controls. Concluded the authors: "Anticipatory stress associated with potential exposure to ionizing radiation resulted in a level of stress similar to that from actual exposure to ionizing radiation." Clearly, then, the psychosocial effects of a radiation accident can extend far beyond the immediate area of impact.

Meanwhile, for a smaller portion of the population, there is the risk that serious and persistent mental health problems may develop as a result of exposure to the trauma of a radiation accident. Problems can include depression, anxiety disorders, substance abuse, and post-traumatic stress disorder (PTSD). PTSD is a "a prolonged post-traumatic stress response."[7] Among the features associated with PTSD are a persistent reexperiencing of a traumatic event; persistent avoidance of stimuli associated with the trauma and a numbing of general responsiveness; and persistent symptoms of increased arousal such as irritability, outbursts of anger, or exaggerated startle response.[17]

In sum, a radiation accident is a highly stressful event with the potential to cause substantial short- and long-term psychological effects. In the aftermath of large-scale accidents, the numbers of people affected by chronic stress and other problems can be quite large.[18] This has certainly been the case with respect to Chernobyl, where one of the principal effects has been psychosocial. (The other has been a sharp increase in childhood thyroid cancer.) In the words of the World Health Organization, psychosocial effects have been "an important health consequence of the Chernobyl accident in view of the size of the population affected and the burden on the health care system."[19]

HIGH-RISK GROUPS

In the general literature on disaster, several subpopulations are usually identified as being at greater risk of psychosocial impacts or as having special needs. One such group is emergency/disaster workers. These personnel can encounter extraordinary stresses and highly traumatic situations in the line of duty, including threats to their own health and safety, seeing gruesome injuries, having to handle bodies, etc.[20] This can put such workers at higher risk for psychological effects. Having to operate in a radiologically contaminated environment would likely add further to the stresses faced by emergency workers.

Children can be "a particularly vulnerable group,"[21] and assistance efforts need to be informed by a current understanding of children's postdisaster reactions, relevant techniques for the assessment of children, and strategies of intervention.[22] Other groups that have been identified in the general disaster literature include people with preexisting mental illness or psychiatric disabilities[23] and older people, since they may have limited support networks, mobility impairment, illnesses, etc.[7]

In addition to the general disaster literature, studies specifically focused on radiation accidents have identified mothers with young children as being at significantly greater risk for psychosocial effects. As noted earlier, studies carried out after both Three Mile Island and Chernobyl identified women with young children as being at significantly greater risk for psychological effects than the general population. Another group that has been identified as being at higher risk of psychological effects is cleanup workers. People who were involved in cleaning up the Chernobyl nuclear accident, for example, have been reported to be at greater risk for a range of social and psychological problems.[24] Last, the Chernobyl experience also suggests that evacuees may be at greater risk.[11]

SOCIAL IMPACTS

Along with their potential to cause psychological effects, radiation accidents can also produce a wide range of social impacts. A widespread loss of trust can be one such effect; so, too, can a sense of betrayal, resentment, outrage, and anger. As Erikson[1] has observed: "Technological disasters ... being of human manufacture, are at least in principle preventable, so there is always a story to be told about them, always a moral to be drawn from them, always a share of blame to be assigned."[1]

The disruption of community networks that can follow in the wake of evacuation represents another important social impact. Clearly, when a situation requires large numbers of people to be moved, especially when they have to be permanently relocated, there can be enormous social adjustment problems. Children's education may be interrupted and adults may have to find new sources of employment. In addition, people who are relocated from a contaminated area may not be fully accepted by long-time residents of the communities where resettlement takes place. Certainly, many social problems were evident in the aftermath of the Chernobyl relocations, which involved the evacuation and resettlement of more than a quarter of a million people.[25,26] Accidents involving toxic agents can also produce community division over such matters as compensation.

One of the most troubling and persistent impacts of incidents involving radiation is the problem of stigma. Residents of affected communities may be seen by others as "tainted" and as "people to be avoided."[27,28] Social stigma can be powerful and pervasive. Following the radiological accident in Goiânia (Brazil), people from the city found themselves the focus of fears and the targets of discrimination. As Kasperson and Kasperson[29] have noted: "Hotels in other parts of Brazil refused to allow Goiânia residents to register. Some airline pilots refused to fly airplanes that had Goiânia residents aboard. Cars with Goiânia license plates were stoned in other parts of Brazil."[29]

Social stigma has also been observed after more recent accidents, including the 1999 criticality incident in Tokaimura (Japan). One manifestation has been economic. Even though government tests indicated that fields and agricultural products from Tokai and surrounding areas were not radioactively contaminated, it became difficult to sell one of the main crops — dried potatoes — under the Tokai name. As one resident explained, in the aftermath of the accident, the name "Tokaimura" is "not popular." There is also evidence that some people from Tokai have experienced others kinds of stigma. For example, a number of residents have reported that when they or their family members visited resorts, springs, or hotels in other parts of Japan, they were asked not to go into the public baths.

Thus, along with the wide range of psychological impacts noted earlier, social effects such as disruption, dislocation, and stigma are now recognized to be important consequences of radiation accidents.

PSYCHOSOCIAL EFFECTS — IMPLICATIONS FOR RADIATION ACCIDENT PREPAREDNESS AND RESPONSE

Given the importance of psychosocial effects after radiation accidents, it is crucial for local, state, national, and international emergency plans to include a well-developed psychosocial component. It is also vital for hospitals and other health care facilities that may be called upon to deal with radiation accidents to have provisions for dealing with psychosocial effects. Among other things, emergency plans need to take into account the fact that very large numbers of people may request assistance after an accident.

The Goiânia accident provides a dramatic illustration of this point. Following the radiological incident, over 112,000 people sought medical examinations.[30] Significant numbers of those who arrived were experiencing psychosomatic symptoms similar to symptoms of radiation exposure. According to de Carvalho, "the fear was so intense that some people fainted in the queues as they approached their moment of monitoring. Many complained of vomiting and diarrhea...."[31]

After a major radiation accident, then, extraordinary demands can be placed on the health and human service system. Facilities may be deluged with very large numbers of people seeking assistance, including many who are experiencing psychosocial effects. An inadequately prepared health and human service system could easily be overwhelmed. Plans should also anticipate large numbers of concerned family members, members of the press, and interested members of the public appearing at the hospital, telephoning with questions, etc. Finally, hospital and other emergency plans should ensure that adequate mental health support is available for health care personnel, since the stress of working long hours in a contamination situation may take a toll on them as well.

If the incorporation of a well-developed psychosocial component is essential in radiation accident emergency planning, it is also important in training. Exercises are a crucial means of improving preparedness, and the inclusion of psychosocial issues can greatly enhance the degree of realism and robustness. For example, decontamination or medical management exercises can benefit from having to deal not only with mock physical casualties, but also with a mix of mock physical and mock psychological casualties — some with injuries, some with radiation exposure, some contaminated, and many others with stress-related symptoms (headaches, nausea, rashes). Exercises can also play an important role in familiarizing medical staff with the psychosocial effects that are likely to arise after a radiation accident. Similarly, well-designed training exercises can help to acquaint social and behavioral staff with the unique challenges posed by contamination situations.[32]

In the aftermath of an accident, information that is as accurate and complete as possible should be provided as early as possible. Research suggests that an early lack of accurate information can contribute to both anger and fear.[33] Attempts to limit or suppress information only serve to undermine trust and destroy public confidence.

The medical and psychosocial components of a radiation accident response effort should be well integrated, both in terms of approach and personnel.[34] A medical response that lacks an adequate psychosocial component may leave important impacts of an incident unaddressed, while a mental health component that is totally divorced from the medical response is likely to be unsuccessful. Information centers, toll-free hotlines, etc. should also endeavor to use an integrated approach. It might be useful, for example, to have a single point of contact for people to telephone or visit, and to have a multi-profession team on duty. Such a team might include information officers, health physicists, doctors and nurses, psychologists, social workers, counselors, etc. Finally, epidemiological follow-up after a radiation accident should include a well-developed psychosocial component. This will help in obtaining a picture of overall public health impacts (including psychosocial effects), and may also assist in the identification of high-risk groups.

Terms such as *radiophobia* should be avoided when discussing people's concerns about radiation. Aside from the fact that the clinical value of such terms is debatable, words like *radiophobia* could easily be seen as dismissive of people's health concerns or as suggesting that people are behaving in a manner that is somehow "irrational." People should never be sent away or "dismissed"; rather, individuals should be treated with respect, and their symptoms — regardless of cause — should be taken seriously.

In cases where people have been exposed to radiation, "the best method available for preventing the development of ... adverse psychological effects" is to "provide exposed patients with health care that will enable them to maintain a sense of control over their health."[35] Doctors and patients will need to collaborate in matching vigilance programs to patient needs. Among other things, strategies for reducing overall risk through lifestyle change may be useful.

Efforts to restore social support are crucial after a radiation accident. As Figley[36] notes, "the family, plus the social support system in general, is the single most important resource to emotional recovery from catastrophe." Augmentation of social support is particularly important where evacuation and relocation have affected community networks. Outreach is also vital. People do not generally seek out psychosocial assistance services, and contamination-related stigma can make them even less likely to do so. Particular efforts may also need to be devoted to high-risk groups such as children and mothers with young children.

Because there is a strong likelihood that stigma will be a significant problem in the aftermath of any radiation accident, and because it could hamper recovery efforts, it is important that officials have in place a plan for addressing it. Such a plan should be informed by current social and behavioral science research on stigma after contamination episodes, and should include a multidimensional approach that incorporates education programs, media campaigns, community forums, and other measures.

Finally, to enhance public trust and confidence in the aftermath of a radiation accident, it is valuable for service development, delivery, and evaluation to involve key stakeholders through such mechanisms as advisory boards. Similarly, decisions that affect the community need to be grounded in an approach that is open, participatory, and inclusive.

CONCLUSION

Psychosocial effects can be both widespread and long lasting, constituting some of the most significant and challenging consequences of a radiation accident. Consideration of psychosocial factors, therefore, needs to be an integral part of radiation accident training, preparedness, and response.

REFERENCES

1. Erikson, K., *A New Species of Trouble: The Human Experience of Modern Disasters*, W.W. Norton, New York, 1995.
2. Bennett, P., Understanding responses to risk: some basic findings, in *Risk Communication and Public Health*, Bennett, P. and Calman, K., Eds., Oxford University Press, Oxford, U.K., 1999.
3. Stokes, J.W. and Banderet, L.E., Psychological aspects of chemical defense and warfare, *Mil. Psychol.*, 9(4):395–415, 1997.
4. Mickley, G.A., Psychological factors in nuclear warfare, in Medical Consequences of Nuclear Warfare, Textbook of Military Medicine Series, Part I, Warfare, Weaponry, and the Casualty, Walker, R.I. and Cerveny, T.J., Eds., TMM Publications, Office of the Surgeon General, Walter Reed Army Medical Center, Washington, D.C., 1989.
5. Rosa, E.A. and Freudenberg, W.R., The historical development of public reactions to nuclear power: implications for nuclear waste policy, in *Public Reactions to Nuclear Waste: Citizens' Views of Repository Siting*, Dunlap, R.E., Kraft, M.E., and Rosa, E.A., Eds., Duke University Press, Durham, NC, 1993.
6. Slovic, P., Layman, M., and Flynn, J.H., Perceived risk, trust and nuclear waste: lessons from Yucca Mountain, in *Public Reactions to Nuclear Waste: Citizens' Views of Repository Siting*, Dunlap, R.E., Kraft, M.E., and Rosa, E.A., Eds., Duke University Press, Durham, NC, 1993.
7. Young, B.H., Ford, J.D., Ruzek, J.I., Friedman, M.J., and Gusman, F.D., *Disaster Mental Health Services: A Guidebook for Clinicians and Administrators*, National Center for Post-Traumatic Stress Disorder, Menlo Park, CA, 1998.
8. Myers, D., *Disaster Response and Recovery: A Handbook for Mental Health Professionals*, Center for Mental Health Services, Rockville, MD, 1994.
9. Hartsough, D.M. and Myers, D.G., Disaster Work and Mental Health: Prevention and Control of Stress among Workers, Center for Mental Health Services, Substance Abuse and Mental Health Services Administration, U.S. Public Health Service, Washington, D.C., 1985.
10. Ursano, R.J., Fullerton, C.S., and McCaughey, B.G., Trauma and disaster, in *Individual and Community Responses to Trauma and Disaster: The Structure of Human Chaos*, Ursano, R.J., McCaughey, B.G., and Fullerton, C.S., Eds., Cambridge University Press, Cambridge, MA, 1994, 3–27.
11. Havenaar, J.M., van den Brink, W., Kasyanenko, A.P., van den Bout, J., Meijler-Iljina, L., Poelijoe, N.W., and Wohlfarth, T., Mental health problems in the Gomel region (Belarus): an analysis of risk factors in an area affected by the Chernobyl disaster, *Psychol. Med.*, 26:845–855, 1996.
12. Haavenaar, J.M., Rumyantzeva, G.M., van den Brink, W., Poelijoe, N.W., van den Bout, J., van Engeland, H., and Koeter, M.W.J., Long-term mental health effects of the Chernobyl disaster: an epidemiologic survey of two former Soviet regions, *Am. J. Psychiatr.*, 154:1605–1607, 1997.

13. Baum, A., Fleming, R., and Davidson, L.M., Natural disaster and technological catastrophe, *Environ. Behav.*, 15:333–354, 1983.
14. Bromet, E.J., Parkinson, D.K., and Dunn, L.O., Long-term mental health consequences of the accident at Three Mile Island, *Int. J. Mental Health*, 19:48–60, 1990.
15. Baum, A. and Fleming, I., Implications of psychological research on stress and technological accidents, *Am. Psychol.*, 48:665–672, 1993.
16. Collins, D.L. and de Carvalho, A.B., Chronic stress from the Goiânia Cs-137 Radiation Accident, *Behav. Med.*, 18:149–157, 1993.
17. American Psychiatric Association, 1994. *Diagnostic and Statistical Manual of Mental Disorders*, 4th ed. (DSM-IV), American Psychiatric Association, Washington, D.C., 1994.
18. Lee, T.R., Environmental stress reactions following the Chernobyl accident, in *One Decade After Chernobyl*, International Atomic Energy Agency, Vienna, 1996, 283–310.
19. WHO, Health Consequences of the Chernobyl Accident: Results of the IPHECA Pilot Projects and Related National Programmes, Summary Report, World Health Organization, Geneva, 1995.
20. Ursano, R.J., McCaughey, B.G., and Fullerton, C.S., The structure of human chaos, in *Individual and Community Responses to Trauma and Disaster: The Structure of Human Chaos*, Ursano, R.J., McCaughey, B.G., and Fullerton, C.S., Eds., Cambridge University Press, Cambridge, MA, 1994, 403–410.
21. Farberow, N.L. and Gordon, N.S., Manual for Child Health Workers in Major Disasters, Center for Mental Health Services, Substance Abuse and Mental Health Services Administration, U.S. Public Health Service, Washington, D.C., 1981.
22. Pynoos, R.S., Goenjian, A.K., and Steinberg, A.M., A public mental health approach to the postdisaster treatment of children and adolescents, *Child Adolescent Psychiatr. Clin. North Am.*, 7:195–210, 1998.
23. Responding to the Needs of People with Serious and Persistent Mental Illness in Times of Disaster, Emergency Services and Disaster Relief Branch, Center for Mental Health Services, Substance Abuse and Mental Health Services Administration, Washington, D.C., 1996.
24. Koscheyev, V.S., Leon, G.R., and Greaves, I.A., Lessons learned and unsolved public health problems after large-scale disasters, *Prehosp. Disaster Med.*, 12(2):120–131.24, 1997.
25. Page, G.W., Environmental health policy in Ukraine after the Chernobyl accident, *Policy Stud. J.*, 23:141–151, 1995.
26. UNESCO, Community Development Centres for Social and Psychological Rehabilitation in Belarus, Russia and Ukraine: Achievements and Prospects, UNESCO Chernobyl Programme, Paris, 1996.
27. Edelstein, M.R., *Contaminated Communities: The Social and Psychosocial Impacts of Residential Toxic Exposure*, Westview, Boulder, CO, 1988.
28. Kroll-Smith, J.S., Couch, S.R., Technological hazards: social responses as traumatic stressors, in *The International Handbook of Traumatic Stress Syndromes*, Wilson, J.P. and Raphael, B., Eds., Plenum Press, New York, 1991, 79–91.
29. Kasperson, R.E. and Kasperson, J.X., The social amplification and attenuation of risk, *Ann. Am. Acad. Political Social Sci.*, 545:95–105, 1996.
30. IAEA, *The Radiological Accident in Goiânia*, International Atomic Energy Agency, Vienna, 1988.
31. de Carvalho, A.B., Psychological aspects of a radiological accident, paper presented at the Ninth Annual National Radiological Preparedness Conference, Baton Rouge, LA, March 29–31, 1999.
32. Becker, S.M., Psychosocial assistance after environmental accidents: a policy perspective, *Environ. Health Perspect.*, (National Institutes of Health), 105(S6), 1557–1563, 1997.
33. Bowler, R.M., Mergler, D., Huel, G., and Cone, J.E., Psychological, psychosocial, and psychophysiological seqeulae in a community affected by a railroad chemical disaster, *J. Traum. Stress*, 7(4):601–624, 1994.
34. Becker, S.M., Environmental disaster education at the university level: an integrative approach, *Saf. Sci.*, 35(1):95–104, 2000.
35. Vyner, H.M., The psychological dimensions of health care for patients exposed to radiation and other invisible environmental contaminants, *Soc. Sci. Med.*, 27(10):1097–1103, 1988.
36. Figley, C.R., Traumatic stress: the role of the family and social support system, in *Trauma and Its Wake: Traumatic Stress Theory, Research, and Intervention*, Figley, C.R., Ed., Brunner/Mazel, New York, 1986.

42 Accidental Radiation Exposure during Pregnancy

Fred A. Mettler, Jr.

CONTENTS

Introduction 527
Effects of *in Utero* Irradiation 528
    General 528
    Effects of the Central Nervous System 528
    Risk of Leukemia and Childhood Cancer 529
Accidental Exposures in Diagnostic Radiology and Other Low-Dose Situations 530
    General 530
    Diagnostic Radiology 530
Accidental Internal Exposure 532
    General 532
    Exposure to Radioiodine 532
    Breast-Feeding 534
    Other Specific Radionuclides 534
        Tritium (^{3}H) 534
        Strontium 534
        Iron 534
        Cobalt 534
        Inert Gases 535
        Gallium 535
        Technetium 535
        Cesium 535
        Cerium and Rare Earths of the Lanthanide Group 535
Accidental Exposure during Radiotherapy and Other External High-Dose Situations 535
    General 535
    Radiotherapy 536
Becoming Pregnant after Accidental Radiation Exposure 536
Counseling and Possible Termination of Pregnancy 537
References 538

INTRODUCTION

Accidental radiation exposure of a pregnant female is always a source of great concern and anxiety. Usually accidental exposure of pregnant women has occurred when there are public releases of radionuclides (e.g., Chernobyl) and during medical procedures. There are probably thousands of women each year who do not know they are pregnant and receive X-ray examinations, nuclear medicine procedures, radiation therapy, or occupational exposure. All of these are in some way accidental. The International Commission on Radiological Protection (ICRP) has published a wide variety of recommendations in the past,[1-6] including information on pregnancy and radiation. There is a recent ICRP Report on Pregnancy and Medical Radiation, which contains much of the material presented here as well as considerations regarding nonaccidental exposure.[7]

EFFECTS OF *IN UTERO* IRRADIATION

GENERAL

Radiation effects on the fetus have the same general mechanisms as radiation effects on adults. They are either due to cell killing (deterministic effects) or due to unrepaired or misrepaired DNA damage (stochastic effects). With deterministic effects (such as mental retardation) there is a practical threshold, and the higher the dose, the more severe the effect. Stochastic effects (such as induction of leukemia) do not have a known threshold, and the higher the dose, the more probable the effect. The severity of stochastic effects is independent of dose. When radiation doses are protracted they typically have less biological effect.

Deterministic effects from ionizing radiation during pregnancy include a wide range of effects, including lethality, central nervous system abnormalities, cataracts, growth retardation, malformations, and even behavioral disorders. Since the fetal neural system is most sensitive and has the longest period of development, radiation-induced abnormalities are rarely seen in humans without neuropathology. This syndrome is recognizable but can be produced by other noxious agents. The effects of exposure to radiation on the conceptus depend on the time of exposure relative to conception and the amount of absorbed dose. When the number of cells in the conceptus is small and their nature is not yet specialized, the effect of damage to these cells is most likely to take the form of failure to implant or of an undetectable death of the conceptus; malformations are unlikely or very rare. Exposure of the embryo in the first 2 weeks following conception is not likely to result in malformation or fetal death, despite the fact that the central nervous system and the heart are beginning to develop in the third week. During the rest of the period of major organogenesis, conventionally taken to be from the third week after conception, malformations may be caused, especially in the organs under development at the time of exposure.[8-10] These effects have a threshold of 100 to 200 mGy or higher. This dose is higher than is reached in most diagnostic radiology or diagnostic nuclear medicine procedures, but it is possible from radiation therapy and high-dose accidental exposure (either occupational or public).

EFFECTS ON THE CENTRAL NERVOUS SYSTEM

During the period of 8 to 25 weeks postconception, the central nervous system (CNS) is very sensitive to radiation.[11,12] Fetal doses in excess of 100 mGy may result in a decrease of intelligence quotient (IQ). During this same time, fetal doses in the range of 1000 mGy (1 Gy) result in a high probability of severe mental retardation. The CNS is less sensitive to these effects at 16 to 25 weeks of gestational age and rather resistant after that. Radiation effects on the developing CNS are probably the result of cell killing and of changes in cellular differentiation and neuronal migration. Lower than expected IQ values have been reported in some children exposed *in utero* at Hiroshima and Nagasaki. There have been two principal quantitative findings. The first is reduction of IQ with increasing dose. This effect is very dependent on fetal age. Regardless of the time of gestation, IQ reduction cannot be clinically identified at fetal doses of less than 100 mGy. In the period from 8 to 15 weeks after conception a fetal dose of 1000 mGy reduces IQ by about 30 points. A similar, but smaller, shift is detectable following exposure in the period from 16 to 25 weeks.

In addition to a reduction in IQ there have also been scientific reports from Hiroshima and Nagasaki of a dose-related increase in the frequency of children classified as "severely retarded."

This is not unexpected. If the fetal radiation dose is high and there is a large reduction in IQ, there will be more children born who are severely mentally retarded. At fetal doses of 1000 mGy during 8 to 15 weeks gestational age, the probability of this effect is about 40%. The effects of all levels of dose are less marked following exposure in the period from 16 to 25 weeks after conception and have not been observed for other periods. Severe mental retardation has not been reported at fetal doses of less than 500 mGy.

It is important to relate the magnitude of radiation effects to those abnormalities that occur spontaneously in the population in the absence of radiation exposure. The normal incidence of mental retardation in the population depends on the definition of mental retardation that is used. At the present time, most organizations define an IQ below 70 as mental retardation. Current prevalence figures indicate that the "normal" incidence of persons with an IQ below 70 is approximately 3%. In other words, in the absence of radiation exposure, 3 of 100 pregnancies will result in delivery of a child with mental retardation. Severe mental retardation (in which an individual is incapable of self-care) occurs spontaneously in about 1 in 200 (0.5%) births. As can be seen from the above data, at fetal doses of 100 mGy, the spontaneous incidence of mental retardation is much larger than a potential radiation effect on IQ reduction. On the other hand, at fetal doses of 1000 mGy during 8 to 15 weeks postconception, the probability of a radiation-induced significant decrease in IQ and resultant mental retardation rises to about 40%, which is much higher than the spontaneous rate of about 3%. Note should be made that radiation-induced mental retardation may sometimes be distinguished from other forms of retardation. Heterotopic gray matter and microcephaly suggest radiation or maternal alcoholism as a potential cause, whereas a child with cerebral palsy, normal head size, and a documented hypoxic episode during delivery would not have irradiation as a likely etiology.

RISK OF LEUKEMIA AND CHILDHOOD CANCER

Radiation has been shown to cause leukemia and many types of cancer in both adults and children. Throughout most of pregnancy, the embryo/fetus is assumed to be at about the same risk for potential carcinogenic effects of radiation as are children. As a result of radiation exposure, after conception and until delivery there is felt to be an increased risk of childhood cancer and leukemia.[13-17] The spontaneous incidence of childhood cancer and leukemia from ages 0 to 18, without radiation exposure, is about 2 to 3/1000. The magnitude of risk following radiation exposure and whether the risk changes throughout pregnancy have been the subject of many publications, yet interpretation of the data remains open to debate. One type of epidemiological study (case-control) has shown raised risks associated with obstetric X-ray examinations of pregnant women. Similar results have not been found in cohort studies.

There is some evidence of possibly raised leukemia in the atomic bomb survivors who were irradiated *in utero*, but there is no increasing leukemia trend with dose and the cases did not occur during childhood. Risk can be expressed either as relative or absolute risk. Relative risk indicates the risk as a function of the "background" cancer risk. A relative risk of 1.0 indicates that there is no effect of irradiation, whereas a relative risk of 1.5 for a given dose indicates that the radiation will cause a 50% increase in cancer above background rates. Absolute risk estimates simply indicate the excess number of cancer cases expected in a population due to a certain radiation dose. A recent analysis of many of the epidemiological studies conducted on prenatal X-ray and childhood cancer are consistent with a relative risk of 1.4 (a 40% increase over the background risk) following a fetal dose of 10 mGy. The best methodological studies, however, suggest that the risk is probably lower than this. Even if the relative risk were as high as 1.4, the individual probability of childhood cancer after *in utero* irradiation is very low since the background incidence of childhood cancer is so low. Recent absolute risk estimates for cancer risk from ages 0 to 15 after *in utero* irradiation from ages 0 to 15 has been estimated to be in the range of 600/10,000 persons each exposed to 1000 mGy (or 0.6%/100 mGy). This is essentially equivalent to a risk of 1/170 per 100 mGy of exposure. Estimates of excess lifetime cancer risk as a result of *in utero* exposure have not clearly been demonstrated among Japanese atomic bomb survivor studies even though the population has been followed for about 50 years.

ACCIDENTAL EXPOSURES IN DIAGNOSTIC RADIOLOGY AND OTHER LOW-DOSE SITUATIONS

General

Probably the most common situation in which there is accidental low-dose exposure of a pregnant female occurs during diagnostic radiology. The fetal doses are usually low with a few exceptions noted below. The rationale applied in diagnostic radiology also applies to other accidental situations in which there is accidental external gamma- or X-ray exposure.

Diagnostic Radiology

Radiation doses resulting from most diagnostic procedures present no substantial risk of causing fetal death, malformation, or impairment of mental development. For diagnostic radiology, fetal dose estimation is usually not necessary unless the fetus is in the direct beam. Evaluation of fetal doses from pelvic fluoroscopy is subject to more uncertainty than doses from plain radiography or computed tomography (CT).

Diagnostic irradiation of the pregnant patient can lead to apprehension about possible fetal effects. Even though the absorbed doses to the conceptus are generally small for most diagnostic radiography, such concern may lead to inappropriate suggestions that the pregnancy should be terminated. Because fetal dose from such procedures is almost always less than 100 mGy (the minimum threshold level where radiogenic malformations might occur and the individual probability of radiogenic cancer is very low), accidental fetal irradiation from diagnostic procedures almost never justifies terminating a pregnancy.

After low-dose examinations (such as a maternal chest radiograph) in which the conceptus is not in the X-ray beam, there is no real need to do individual fetal dose estimations. However, after high-dose abdominal or pelvic CT or fluoroscopy, an estimate of the absorbed dose and the associated risk to the fetus should be made by a qualified expert. With such an expert and carefully worded advice, the patient and husband or other appropriate persons should then be in a position to reach their own conclusions. This is discussed later in the chapter.

Determination of the absorbed dose to the embryo or fetus from plain film abdominal or pelvic radiography examinations is difficult but usually can be estimated within a 50% error. For diagnostic radiographic examinations, one can utilize the mean skin exposure/film (for a given examination) and then estimate the absorbed dose at a certain depth if the technical factors concerning the beam energy are known. If the technical factors are not well known, the mean dose to the ovaries often gives an approximation of fetal dose. Table 42.1 gives typical uterine or fetal doses for some common routine examinations in the United Kingdom. It should be noted that when dosimetry surveys have been performed within a particular country for diagnostic radiology examinations, there could be a variation by factor of 30 or more for the same examination. This is a function of variations in kVp, waveform, filtration, presence of a grid, film and screen combinations, film processing, and a number of other factors. There is a general expectation that doses from digital fluoroscopy equipment may be lower than with conventional equipment, but this is not often the case. As a result, facility-specific measurements and calculations of fetal doses may be necessary if fetal doses are suspected of exceeding 10 mGy.

In diagnostic radiology, fetal dose is also significantly affected by patient anatomy including the thickness of the patient, whether the uterus is anteverted or retroverted, and even the distension

TABLE 42.1
Approximate Fetal Doses from Common Diagnostic Procedures in the United Kingdom

Examination	Mean (mGy)	Maximum (mGy)
Conventional X-ray		
Abdomen	1.4	4.2
Chest	<0.01	<0.01
Intravenous urogram	1.7	10
Lumbar spine	1.7	1.0
Pelvis	1.1	4
Skull	<0.01	<0.01
Thoracic spine	<0.01	<0.01
Fluoroscopic		
Barium meal (UGI)	1.1	5.8
Barium enema	6.8	24
Computed Tomography		
Abdomen	8.0	49
Chest	0.06	0.96
Head	<0.005	<0.005
Lumbar spine	2.4	8.6
Pelvis	25	79

Source: Adapted from Diagnostic Medical Exposures: Advice on Exposure to Ionising Radiation during Pregnancy, National Radiological Protection Board, Oxon, U.K., 1998.

of the bladder. The "fetal dose" is often mentioned and it is often assumed that this dose is uniform; but this is only the case early in pregnancy. As the fetus grows larger, the absorbed dose becomes less uniform. Finally, it is rare for a patient to only have one diagnostic examination, and it is useful to see if other examinations were also performed during the gestation. The estimation of fetal dose after fluoroscopy is more difficult and the range of uncertainty is greater than for routine radiographic examinations. It is extremely difficult to estimate the dose without knowing the fluoroscopy time and the location of the beam. Unfortunately, the fluoroscopy time or other useful parameters are often not recorded. Even if these factors are known, one still cannot be sure how long the conceptus was in the primary beam since the radiologist is usually moving the fluoroscopic beam. Other factors that affect fluoroscopy dose are whether conventional or pulsed fluoroscopy was used, the magnification mode, and whether a grid was used. Usually these factors are not recorded and can only be estimated based upon the usual practice at that medical facility. In most fluoroscopy cases, a "best-guess" estimate and sometimes a "worst-case" estimate of fetal dose is made. Usually, the best estimate and the uncertainty are expressed to the patient and the referring physician.

There are other potential accidental low-dose exposure situations. These might occur in an occupational setting and in these circumstances a female may have been wearing a personal dosimeter. In such circumstances it will be necessary to evaluate the nature of the ambient radiation and then make some estimate of the fetal dose. One can envisage other situations in which a member of the public is inadvertently and transiently exposed (such as to an unrecognized industrial radiography source). In these circumstances fetal dose can only be estimated by the reconstruction of the events that occurred with particular emphasis on time and distance relative to the source.

ACCIDENTAL INTERNAL EXPOSURE

GENERAL

Most accidental exposures of pregnant females involving internal exposure are the result of nuclear medicine procedures.[18–21] As a result, most of this section is devoted to nuclear medicine. There have been rare situations (such as Chernobyl) in which pregnant females have been exposed to internal contamination by radionuclides. One of the predominant radionuclides in reactor accidents with environmental releases is radioiodine and the comments below relative to use of radioiodine in nuclear medicine are applicable.

Irradiation of the embryo or fetus from maternal internal contamination with radionuclides may be divided into two major categories. The first are those radionuclides that do not cross the placenta to the fetus, remaining on the maternal side of the circulation and structure. These radionuclides may irradiate the fetus if the radiation emitted is relatively penetrating (i.e., energetic beta, gamma, and X rays). Medical radionuclides are often included in this group because most emit energetic gamma rays. Early in pregnancy, when the embryo or fetus is quite small, its irradiation is quite uniform and may be approximated by the dose to the ovary or uterus.

A second major category of radionuclides causing radiation exposure of the embryo and fetus are those that cross the placenta into the fetal circulation. Many of them are ionic in chemical form. After they cross the placenta, they may be distributed in the body of the embryo or fetus or may concentrate locally if the fetal target organ is mature enough to have a physiological function. An example of such a radionuclide is radioiodine. Many of the data concerning placental transfer of radionuclides come from animal experimentation.

Most diagnostic nuclear medicine procedures in developed countries are done with short-lived radionuclides (such as technetium-99m) and these do not cause large fetal doses. There are, however, some radiopharmaceuticals (such as iodine-131) that do cross the placenta and that can pose significant fetal risks.

As with diagnostic radiology procedures, the pregnant patient can be apprehensive after a procedure has been performed. In the case of nuclear medicine, the patient may be even more apprehensive realizing that an administered radioactive material has been incorporated into her, that it will be there for some time, and that it potentially may cross the placenta to the fetus. As a result of this, more careful explanation to the patient and her husband or other appropriate persons may be needed to put the potential radiation risks into perspective. Careful estimation of fetal doses is not usually necessary after diagnostic nuclear medicine studies involving technetium-99m radiopharmaceuticals. If there has been inadvertent administration of other radiopharmaceuticals (such as radioiodine or gallium), more attention should be given to calculation of the fetal dose and explanation of potential risks.

Typical uterine/fetal doses for common radiopharmaceuticals are presented in Table 42.2. The activity for most radiopharmaceuticals is usually measured just prior to administration and recorded. While there may be some individual differences of metabolism and localization of radiopharmaceuticals in very ill patients, in most cases pregnant women have essentially normal distribution of radiopharmaceuticals and the estimated fetal doses will be reasonably accurate.

EXPOSURE TO RADIOIODINE

Radioiodine easily crosses the placenta and therapeutic or large accidental intakes can pose significant issues for the fetus particularly permanent hypothyroidism and the risk of thyroid cancer. Because certain radiopharmaceuticals, including iodine-131 as iodide and phosphorus-32 as phosphate, can rapidly cross the placenta, the possibility of pregnancy should be very carefully considered before such radionuclides are given for therapy or for a whole-body iodine-131 scan for thyroid carcinoma. The fetal thyroid begins to accumulate iodine at about 10 weeks of gestational age.

TABLE 42.2
Fetal Whole-Body Dose[a] from Common Nuclear Medicine Examinations in Early Pregnancy and at Term

Procedure, Radiopharmaceutical, and Administered Activity	Early (mGy)	9 Months (mGy)
^{99m}Tc bone scan (phosphate), 750 MBq	4.6–4.7	1.8
^{99m}Tc lung perfusion (MAA), 200 MBq	0.4–0.6	0.8
^{99m}Tc lung ventilation (aerosol), 40 MBq	0.1–0.3	0.1
^{99m}Tc thyroid scan (pertechnetate), 400 MBq	3.2–4.4	3.7
^{99m}Tc red blood cell, 930 MBq	3.6–6.0	2.5
^{99m}Tc liver colloid, 300 MBq	0.5–0.6	1.1
^{99m}Tc renal DTPA, 750 MBq	5.9–9.0	3.5
^{67}Ga abscess/tumor, 190 MBq	14–18	25
^{123}I thyroid uptake, 30 MBq[b]	0.4–0.6	0.3
^{131}I thyroid uptake, 0.55 MBq[b]	0.03–0.04	0.15
^{131}I metastates imaging, 40 MBq[b]	2.0–2.9	11.0

[a] Includes maternal and fetal self-dose contributions.
[b] Fetal thyroid doses are much higher than fetal whole-body dose. Fetal thyroid doses are 5 to 15 mGy/MBq for iodine-123 and 0.5 to 1.1 Gy/MBq for iodine-131.

Source: Adapted from Russell, J.R., et al., *Health Phys.*, 73(5):756–769, 1997; and from ICRP Publications 53 and 80.

Radioiodine therapy is essentially contraindicated in patients who are known to be pregnant. If radioiodine treatment of thyroid carcinoma is to be performed, it should be delayed until after delivery. If this is done, the physician should also be aware that radioiodine is excreted in breast milk and breast-feeding should be stopped completely after a therapeutic dose.

A major problem occurs when a female, who is not thought to be pregnant, is treated for thyroid carcinoma and is discovered to be pregnant after administration of the radioiodine. Most commonly, the pregnancy is early and the major problem is fetal whole-body dose due to gamma emissions from radioiodine in the maternal bladder. During pregnancy, the whole-body dose to the conceptus is in the range of 50 to 100 µGy/MBq of administered activity. This dose can be reduced by hydrating the patient and by encouraging frequent voiding. If the conceptus is more than 8 weeks postconception (and the fetal thyroid may accumulate iodine) and the pregnancy is discovered within 12 h of iodine administration, giving the mother 60 to 130 mg of stable potassium iodide (KI) will partially block the fetal thyroid and reduce thyroid dose. After 12 h postradioiodine administration, this intervention is not very effective. If a patient is discovered to be pregnant shortly after a therapeutic radioiodine administration, maternal hydration and frequent voiding should be encouraged to help eliminate maternal radioactivity and to reduce radioiodine residence time in the bladder. If the pregnancy is discovered later, the placental transfer of radioiodine can result in very high absorbed doses to the fetal thyroid that may cause significant fetal thyroid damage. Since the fetal whole-body dose is usually below 100 mGy, there is no reason to terminate the pregnancy; however, the mother should be given usual levels of replacement thyroid hormone.

Patients treated with radioiodine can be a significant radiation source to pregnant family members. The dose to a family member staying at a distance of 0.5 m from the patient until the radioactivity totally decays (about 10 weeks) is about 1.3 mGy from a hyperthyroid patient and 6.8 mGy from a thyroid cancer patient. Perhaps more important, these patients can transfer radioiodine contamination to family members by direct contact or through indirect means.

BREAST-FEEDING

Many radionuclides and radiopharmaceuticals can be transferred to a baby via breast milk. Cessation of breast-feeding for at least some period is recommended for most nuclear medicine studies. Breast-feeding is usually stopped for 3 weeks after all iodine-131 and iodine-125 radiopharmaceuticals, except labeled hippurate, and after sodium-22, gallium-67, and thallium-201. It is stopped for 12 h after iodine-labeled hippurates and all technetium-99m compounds, except labeled red blood cells, -phosphonates, and -DTPA and for at least 4 h after the latter compounds.[22]

OTHER SPECIFIC RADIONUCLIDES

In situations in which there is accidental exposure of a pregnant female to an unusual radionuclide, the reader is referred to reports of the ICRP and the National Council on Radiation Protection and Measurements (NCRP), which provide detailed information.[18-21] Here, a few radionuclides that have been present in accidents are considered.

Tritium (^{3}H)

Tritium may be present either as tritiated water (HTO) or labeled organic compounds. HTO rapidly crosses the placenta. Since the fetus has a higher water concentration than an adult, the dose to the fetus is about 40 to 70% higher than to the mother. Organically bound tritium may break down, forming tritiated water, and fetal doses are probably about 40% higher than doses to the mother.

Strontium

Several studies have been performed on placental transfer of strontium during gestation. Few available human data indicate the percentage of strontium transferred across the placenta, but there does appear to be some discrimination with a ratio of 0.3 early in pregnancy and about 0.45 in the second and third trimesters.

Iron

Iron metabolism has been studied since the 1940s in attempts to evaluate nutritional requirements of pregnant women. The mother's body is the largest contributor to the fetal dose of iron-59, accounting for approximately 70% of the dose early in pregnancy and decreasing to 50% of the dose later in pregnancy. Total-body dose to the fetus from internal deposition ranges between 10 and 20% of the total dose, increasing slightly during pregnancy. The dose from iron 59 in the fetal liver as a contributor to the fetal dose accounts for less than 10% at 10 weeks of gestational age, but rises rapidly to approximately 30% at 15 weeks. The critical organ in the fetus is the liver, which receives 3 to 6 Gy/37 MBq administered intravenously to the mother. The dosimetry of iron is complicated because iron is involved in many complex metabolic roles in formation of hemoglobin and in composition of enzymes; it also occurs in the form of free iron.

Cobalt

In accidental exposure, cobalt is usually present in a metallic or inorganic form. Since cobalt has energetic gamma rays, there would be substantial irradiation of the fetus from maternal content. Up until 8 weeks of pregnancy, the dose to the embryo is essentially the same as that to the uterus. Cobalt chloride does cross the placenta and the concentration in the fetus is close to that in the mother.

Inert Gases

There is very little experimental evidence concerning the placental transfer of either xenon or krypton, and placental transfer is assumed to be free in both directions. Thus, the dose to the fetus should be quite similar to the maternal dose. The major exception to this may be krypton-81m, which is utilized for some pulmonary function tests and has a half-life of only 13 s. In this instance, fetal dose is substantially less than that of the mother.

Gallium

Gallium-67 is used widely in nuclear medicine for detection of tumors and abscesses. The fetal dose from gallium may be higher than expected as a result of its active transport across the placenta. The whole-body dose to the fetus is 0.4 mGy/MBq, with five times this dose to the fetal spleen.

Technetium

Technetium-99m is the most widely used radionuclide in nuclear medicine. As a pertechnetate, it rapidly crosses the placenta and localizes in the stomach, colon, and thyroid. Absorbed doses to the fetal thyroid are about 1 mGy/MBq, with about a third of this dose to the stomach and colon. Other technetium-99m-labeled radiopharmaceuticals may or may not cross the placenta, depending upon the radiopharmaceutical or cell type that has been labeled.

Cesium

Cesium-137 appears to have a metabolic pathway similar to, but not dependent on, that of potassium or rubidium. Excretion of potassium (and possibly cesium) depends to a large extent on hormones; this dependence may result in decreased fetal concentration during pregnancy. The data indicate that extrapolation from guinea pigs and observations in humans appear to give comparable results. For cesium-137, the fetal-to-maternal plasma ratio appears to be about 0.13, although the ICRP suggests a ratio of 1.0 be used. Interestingly, pregnant women appear to have about one half the retention time of cesium compared to with nonpregnant females.

Cerium and Rare Earths of the Lanthanide Group

Radionuclides in the lanthanide group have little clinical importance to the fetus. The target tissue is the maternal reticuloendothelial system, because rare earths precipitate at the pH of body fluids and are then collected by the reticuloendothelial cells. In addition, rare earths are practically insoluble and do not cross the digestive tract. An exception is yttrium-90, which enters the body as strontium-90, subsequently decays to yttrium-90 after absorption, and then becomes concentrated in the skeleton.

ACCIDENTAL EXPOSURE DURING RADIOTHERAPY AND OTHER EXTERNAL HIGH-DOSE SITUATIONS

GENERAL

External high doses to the fetus can be very problematical and can result in significant adverse outcomes. These can occur during radiotherapy but also in accidental situations. As an example, Chapter 15 describes two accidents in which pregnant females were inadvertently exposed to an industrial radiography source. The exposure resulted in fetal death.

RADIOTHERAPY

In pregnant patients, cancers that are remote from the pelvis usually can be treated with radiotherapy. This, however, requires careful planning. Cancers in the pelvis cannot be adequately treated during pregnancy without severe or lethal consequences for the fetus. For treatment of tumors in the pelvis, the fetus either can be in or very close to the primary beam and effects on the fetus are typically severe (usually fetal death). When external radiotherapy is utilized for treatment of tumors at some distance from the fetus, the most important factor in fetal dose is the distance from the edge of the radiation field. The dose decreases approximately exponentially with distance. Fetal doses for a typical photon treatment regimen for brain cancer are in the range of 30 mGy.[23] For anterior and posterior mantle treatments of the chest for Hodgkin's disease, the dose to portions of an unshielded fetus can be 400 to 500 mGy.[24]

With cobalt-60, at distances greater than 10 cm from the field, the dose is higher because of leakage from the machine head. The dose distribution outside of the primary radiation beam may vary among machines of the same nominal type and energy, as well as with field and phantom size. As a result, machine-specific measurements should be made. For cobalt-60 (10 × 10 cm fields) as a crude estimate the off-axis dose as a percent of dose at D_{max} on central axis is as follows:

Distance from Field Edge (cm)	Percent
10	1.7
20	0.7
30	0.4
40	0.3
50	0.15

With photons from an accelerator, the percentage of off-axis dose is lower by a factor of about 2 to 5 (depending upon the photon energy).

A brachytherapy patient is often kept in the hospital until the sources are removed. Such patients can occasionally be a source of radiation to a visiting pregnant family member, the potential dose to the family member's fetus is very low, irrespective of the type of brachytherapy. Prostate brachytherapy can be done with permanent implantation of radioactive gold-198 or iodine-125 "seeds" and the patient is discharged from the hospital with these in place. The short range of the emissions from these radionuclides is the reason that the patient can be discharged and is the reason that these patients present no danger to pregnant family members.

When there is a suspicion of potentially high accidental doses to the mother or fetus, the final estimates of the fetal dose should be calculated and documented. This should include details about the technical factors. An appropriately trained medical physicist should do such calculations and convey the potential risks to the mother. Although local regulations vary, it is often necessary to keep these records for many years and usually until the child becomes an adult.

BECOMING PREGNANT AFTER ACCIDENTAL RADIATION EXPOSURE

Females often are concerned about becoming pregnant after accidental radiation exposure. The patients fall into several categories: those who have had radiotherapy for a malignancy, those who have internal radionuclides (such as radioiodine), and a final group including both men and women who have been accidentally exposed occupationally or as members of the public. Most are worried about the potential effect of the radiation exposure on future offspring.

Most radiation oncologists request that their patients not become pregnant for 1 to 2 years after completion of therapy. This is not primarily related to concerns about potential radiation effects, but rather about the risk of relapse of the tumor that would require more radiation, surgery, or chemotherapy. Most female patients are advised not to become pregnant for at least 6 months after radiotherapy with radioiodine. This is not based upon potential heritable radiation effects, but rather upon the need to be sure (1) that the hyperthyroidism or cancer is controlled and (2) that another treatment with radioiodine will not be needed when the patient is pregnant.

The ICRP has recommended that enough radionuclide be cleared to ensure that the unborn child not receive a dose in excess of 1 mSv unless it is medically necessary for the health of the mother. There are occasional circumstances in which phosphorus-32, strontium-89, or iodine-131 metaiodobenzylguanidine are used for therapy. To keep the dose to the fetus below 1 mGy, pregnancy should be avoided for 3, 24, and 3 months, respectively.

Preconception irradiation of either parent's gonads has not been shown to result in increased cancer or malformations in the children. Over the last three decades, it has become clear that risks of transmitting radiation-acquired abnormalities to offspring from irradiation of the parents gonads prior to conception have not been identified. Comprehensive studies of the children and grandchildren of the atomic bomb survivors have not identified any heritable effects that would be linked to parental radiation exposure. New studies of the survivors of childhood cancer treated with radiation therapy also have not shown genetic effects in their offspring. Despite this, there have been recommendations that women should refrain from becoming pregnant for several months after radiation therapy. Such recommendations were based upon experiments in mice that demonstrated that mature oocytes were more radiosensitive than immature oocytes. The use of a particular number of months for humans to refrain from getting pregnancy is arbitrary. To be conservative, in the absence of a significant amount of human data with doses in excess of 500 mGy, some authors still recommend that if a female receives preconception ovarian doses of over 500 mGy, that pregnancy be delayed for at least 2 months.

COUNSELING AND POSSIBLE TERMINATION OF PREGNANCY

Even though one may attempt to identify pregnant patients, to avoid unnecessary radiation exposure, and prevent accident, some pregnant females need medical treatment using radiation or accidentally receive radiation exposure. Despite attempts to keep occupationally exposed pregnant women from exceeding recommended limits, they will still receive some radiation exposure.

The issue of pregnancy termination is undoubtedly managed differently around the world. It is complicated by individual ethical, moral, and religious beliefs, as well as perhaps subject to laws or regulations at a local or national level. This complicated issue involves much more than radiation protection issues. Counseling can be done after attempting to estimate the dose to the conceptus from the procedure and comparing radiogenic risk with the other risks of pregnancy. Women exposed to even low levels of ionizing radiation often believe that they have a much higher risk of malformations than the naturally occurring risk, but appropriate counseling can be beneficial. One useful approach is to indicate to the patient the probability of *not* having a child with either a malformation or cancer (Table 42.3).[25]

With the exception of radiotherapy of the abdomen or pelvis and major accidents, the magnitude of effects that may occur from medical radiation is generally small compared with the normal incidence of other problems during pregnancy. In a nonexposed population, approximate risks during pregnancy include a 15% or greater spontaneous abortion rate, a 2 to 4% major malformation incidence from causes other than radiation, a 4% intrauterine growth retardation rate (mostly due to hypertension), and an 8 to 10% incidence of genetic diseases.

For fetal doses less than 100 mGy, there is no medical justification for terminating a pregnancy because of radiation exposure. A conservative lifetime radiogenic risk factor for induction of

TABLE 42.3
Probability of Birthing Healthy Children

Dose[a] to Conceptus (mGy)	Probability of Child with No Malformation, %	Probability Child Will Not Develop Cancer (age 0–19), %
0	97	99.70[c]
0.5	97	99.70
1.0	97	99.69
2.5	97	99.69
5	97	99.67
10	97	99.50
50	97	99.40
100	—[b]	99.10

[a] Refers to absorbed dose above natural background. This table assumes a conservative radiation risk for fatal and nonfatal cancer of 1/17,000/mGy fetal dose and a linear dose–response relationship or a 40% increase above background cancer at 10 mGy. Many epidemiological studies suggest that the risk may be lower than that shown in this table.

[b] Although the exact risk in humans is uncertain, animal data suggest that malformations due to radiation are not likely at doses less than 100 to 200 mGy. Above this, malformations would only occur if exposure were between 3 and 8 weeks. The risk of malformation is low at 100 to 200 mGy but will increase with increasing dose. Decreased IQ and possible retardation are only detectable when fetal doses exceed 100 mGy during week 8 to 25 gestation.

[c] Values in the third column have been rounded. Background risk of childhood cancer calculated from U.S. National Cancer Institute Surveillance, Epidemiology and End Results Report, 1994.

childhood cancer or leukemia at 100 mGy is about 1 in 170. Without radiation exposure, the lifetime risk of cancer is about 1 in 3 and for fatal cancer the risk is about 1 in 5. As pointed out earlier, malformations due to radiation probably do not occur at fetal doses less than 100 to 200 mGy.

When the dose to the fetus exceeds 100 to 200 mGy, the approach to the problem is slightly different. This situation may involve high accidental exposure, and the estimates of absorbed fetal dose will have a larger factor of uncertainty. If the fetal absorbed dose is high, e.g., in excess of 500 mGy, and it was incurred during the first 3 to 16 weeks of conception, there is a substantial chance of growth retardation and CNS damage. Although it is possible that the fetus may survive doses in this range, the parents should be informed of the high risks involved. In the intermediate dose range 100 to 500 mGy, the situation is less clear-cut, although such circumstances arise relatively infrequently. In this absorbed dose range the risk of a measurable reduction in IQ must be seriously considered if the fetus was exposed between 8 and 15 weeks of gestational age. In such instances, a qualified biomedical or health physicist should calculate the absorbed fetal dose as closely as possible, and the physician should ascertain the individual and personal situation of the parents. For example, if the dose to the fetus was estimated to be just above 100 mGy and the parents had been trying to have a child for several years, they may not wish to terminate the pregnancy. This should be a personal decision made by the parents after they are appropriately informed.

REFERENCES

1. International Commission on Radiological Protection, 1990 Recommendations of the International Commission on Radiological Protection, *Ann. ICRP*, 21(1–3), 1991.
2. International Commission on Radiological Protection, Radiological Protection in Biomedical Research, ICRP Publ. 62, *Ann. ICRP*, 22(3), 1991.
3. International Commission on Radiological Protection, Summary of the Protection of the Patient in Diagnostic Radiology, *Ann. ICRP*, 22(3), 1993.

4. International Commission on Radiological Protection, Summary of Protection of the Patient in Nuclear Medicine, *Ann. ICRP*, 1993.
5. International Commission on Radiological Protection, Radiological Protection and Safety in Medicine, ICRP Publ. 73, *Ann. ICRP*, 26(2), 1996.
6. International Commission on Radiological Protection, General Principles for the Radiation Protection of Workers, ICRP Publ. 75.
7. International Commission on Radiological Protection, *Pregnancy and Medical Radiation*, Pergamon Press, Oxford, U.K., 2000.
8. International Commission on Radiological Protection, Dose coefficients for the offspring after intakes of radionuclides by the mother before and during pregnancy, Pergamon Press, Oxford, U.K. (in press).
9. Brent, R.L., The effect of embryonic and fetal exposure to x-ray, microwaves, ultrasound, magnetic resonance and isotopes, in *Medical Disorders during Pregnancy*, 2nd ed., Barron and Lindheimer, Eds., Mosby Yearbook, St. Louis, MO, 1994, 487–518.
10. Brent, R.L. and Beckman, D.A., Developmental effects following radiation of embryonic and fetal exposure to x-ray and isotopes: counseling the pregnant and nonpregnant patient about these risks, in *Health Effects of Low Level Exposure to Ionizing Radiation*, Hendee, W.K. and Edwards, F.M., Eds., Institute of Physics Publishing, Philadelphia, 1996, Chap. 6, 169–213.
11. United Nations Scientific Committee on the Effects of Atomic Radiation (UNSCEAR), 1993 Report to the General Assembly, Annex H, Radiation Effects on the Developing Human Brain, United Nations, New York, 1993.
12. International Commission on Radiological Protection, Developmental Effects of Irradiation on the Brain of the Embryo and Fetus, ICRP Publ. 49, *Ann. ICRP*, 16(4), 1986.
13. Boice, J.D., Jr. and Miller, R.W., Childhood and adult cancer after intrauterine exposure to ionizing radiation, *Teratology*, 59:227–233, 1999.
14. Doll, R. and Wakeford, R., Risk of childhood cancer from fetal irradiation, *Br. J. Radiol.*, 70:130–139, 1997.
15. Delongchamp, R.R., Mabuchi, K., Yoshimoto, Y., and Preston, D., Cancer mortality among atomic bomb survivors exposed in utero or as young children. October 1950–May 1992, *Radiat. Res.*, 147: 385–395, 1997.
16. Yoshimoto, Y., Delongchamp, R., and Mabuchi, K., In utero exposed atomic bomb survivors: cancer risk update, *Lancet*, 344:345–346, 1994.
17. Miller, R.W. and Boice, J.D., Jr., Cancer after intrauterine exposure to the atomic bomb, *Radiat. Res.*, 147:396–397, 1997.
18. National Council on Radiation Protection and Measurements, Radionuclide Exposure of the Embryo/Fetus, Rep. 128, National Council on Radiation Protection and Measurements, Bethesda, MD, 1998.
19. Sinclair, V.T.K., Adelstein, S.J., Brent, R.L. et al., Considerations regarding the unintended exposure of the embryo, fetus or nursing child, NCRP Commentary 9, National Council on Radiation Protection and Measurements, Bethesda, MD, 1994, 1–21.
20. Russell, J.R., Stabin, M.G., and Sparks, R.B., Placental transfer of radiopharmaceuticals and dosimetry in pregnancy, *Health Phys.*, 73(5):747–755, 1997.
21. European Commission, Radiation Protection, Guidance for Protection of Unborn Children and Infants Irradiated Due to Parental Medical Exposures, Luxembourg, 1998.
22. Sneed, P., Albright, N., Wara, W. et. al., Fetal dose estimates for radiotherapy of brain tumors during pregnancy, *J. Radiat. Oncol. Biol. Phys.*, 32(3):823–830, 1995.
23. Stovall, M., Blackwell, C., Cundiff, J. et al., Fetal dose from radiotherapy with photon beams: report of the AAPM Radiation Therapy Task Group No. 36, *Med. Phys.*, 22(1):63–82, 1995.
24. Wagner, L., Lester, R., and Saldana, L., Eds., *Exposure of the Pregnant Patient to Diagnostic Radiations: A Guide to Medical Management*, 2nd ed., Medical Physics Publishing, Madison, WI, 1997.

Glossary

Absolute risk: *See* Risk, absolute.

Absorbed dose: When ionizing radiation passes through matter, some of its energy is imparted to the matter. The amount absorbed per unit mass of irradiated material is called the absorbed dose, and it is measured in Gy or rad. *See* Threshold dose.

Absorbed dose equivalent: *See* Dose equivalent.

Accelerator: Device imparting high kinetic energy to a charged particle.

Accident: An unintentional or unexpected happening that is undesirable or unfortunate, especially one resulting in injury, damage, harm, or loss.

Actinide series: The series of elements beginning with number 89 and continuing through number 105, which together occupy one position in the periodic table. The series includes uranium, element number 92, and all the man-made transuranic elements. The group is also referred to as the *Actinides*. *Compare* Lanthanide series.

Activation: The process of making a material radioactive by bombardment with neutrons, protons, or other nuclear particles.

Activity: *See* Radioactivity, Specific activity.

Acute radiation exposure: Radiation exposure received during a short time period (e.g., 24 h).

Acute radiation syndrome (ARS): The collective term for the hematopoietic, gastrointestinal, and cardiovascular/central nervous system forms of response to whole-body acute or subacute exposure to radiation. Usually requires absorbed doses in excess of 2 Gy (200 rad). The syndrome is a clinical manifestation of the responses of the individual body systems and their relative sensitivity to radiation. The clinical course is predictable and is divided into prodromal, latent, and manifest periods of illness. If recovery occurs, it usually comes 5 to 10 weeks after the radiation exposure.

ALARA: Acronym for "as low as is reasonably achievable;" operating philosophy for maintaining occupational radiation exposures.

Alpha particle: Nucleus of a helium atom emitted by certain radioisotopes upon disintegration. Contains two protons and two neutrons.

Annihilation: Reaction between a pair of particles resulting in their disintegration and the production of an equivalent amount of energy in the form of photons.

Annual dose limits: Any of the annual dose equivalent limits for individual members of the public or workers recommended by the International Commission on Radiologic Protection as part of its system of dose limitation.

Annual limit on intake (ALI): The activity of a radionuclide which, when taken alone, would irradiate a person to the limit set for each year of occupational exposure.

Anticontamination clothing (Anti-C's): Clothing usually consisting of coveralls, shoe covers, gloves, and hood or cap. These provide protection for the user from skin contamination. Sometimes referred to as *protective clothing* although it does not provide protection from gamma rays or X rays and only moderate protection from beta particles.

Atom: Smallest unit of an element that can exist and still maintain the properties of the element.

Atomic mass: Mass of a neutral atom, usually expressed in atomic mass units.

Atomic number: Number of protons in an atom, the symbol of which is Z.

Atomic weight: Average weight of the neutral atoms of an element.

Attenuation: The reduction in the intensity of radiation as it passes through any material, e.g., through lead shielding or body tissues.

Auger electron: An orbital electron ejected by a characteristic X ray. The characteristic X ray is usually emitted following electron capture or internal conversion.

Average life: The mean time during which an atom exists in a particular form. The average life is 1.44 times the physical half-life.

Background: Detected disintegration events not emanating from the sample. Natural background is that radiation which is a natural part of a person's environment, primarily natural radioactivity and cosmic rays.

Battery check: A check to determine that the batteries of a radiation survey meter are charged enough. Generally, a battery check position is present on the range knob and if the knob is placed in this position and the batteries are strong enough, the needle will be deflected upward into the "batt OK" range.

Becquerel (Bq): The SI unit of radioactivity; 1 becquerel is one disintegration per second (dps); 1 becquerel equals 2.7×10^{-11} Curie(Ci) or 27 picocuries (pCi).

BEIR: Biological Effects of Ionizing Radiation. A series of reports by a Committee of the U.S. National Academy of Sciences.

Beta particle: An electron of positive or negative charge.

Bioassays: Methods used for determining the amount of internal radioactive contamination.

Biohazards: Micro-organisms or viruses that cause disease, or substances such as toxins or venoms produced by living organisms.

Body burden: The amount of radioactive material present in a human or animal.

Boiling water reactor: A reactor system that utilizes a boiling water system to cool the reactor core. The steam generated by the water passing over the core is sent directly to turn the turbines and generate electricity.

Bremsstrahlung X rays: Photonic emissions caused by the slowing down of beta particles in matter.

Buffer zone: A zone set up in the hospital radiation emergency area that acts as a buffer between the room in which the patient is being decontaminated and the clean area of the hospital emergency room. The buffer zone is within the controlled area.

By-product material: Radioactive material arising from controlled fission.

Carcinogen: An agent or substance capable of causing induction of a cancer. A complete carcinogen may contain both initiating and promoting capabilities. Other terms involved in the process of carcinogenesis may be as follows:

Co-carcinogen: An agent that can cause cancer by itself but which, when combined with another carcinogen, produces an effect greater than the sum of either individually (i.e., it is synergistic).

Initiator: A substance or agent that primes a cell to the development of a tumor. Usually, it will not cause a tumor by itself.

Promotor: A substance or agent that will not cause a tumor by itself, but will once an initiator has acted on the cell of interest.

Carcinogenesis: The process of induction of cancer in a cell.

Carrier: Quantity of stable isotopes of an element mixed with radioactive isotopes of that element.

Carrier-free: Adjective describing a radionuclide that is free of its stable isotopes.

Cell cycle: The cycle undergone by the nuclear DNA from one cell division to the next. It consists of G_1, a period of growth; S, a period of chromosomal DNA replication; G_2, period of further growth; and mitosis (M) (G stands for "gap" in DNA replication activity and S stands for "synthesis").

Central nervous system syndrome: Part of the acute radiation syndrome. Results when there are acute exposures involving the upper portion of the body in excess of 50 Gy. Usually fatal within 48 to 72 h regardless of treatment methods. Manifested by confusion, ataxia, hypotension, and coma.

Centromere: The small constricted region on a chromosome at which identical chromatids are joined and by which the chromosome is attached to a spindle fiber. The position of the centromere determines the length of the arms of the chromosome and, for any particular chromosome, is constant in location.

Chain reaction: A self-sustaining reaction. In a fission nuclear chain reaction a fissionable nucleus absorbs a neutron, then fissions and releases enough more neutrons to enter other fissionable nuclei and keep the reaction going.

Charged particle: An ion or elementary atomic particle that carries a positive or negative electrical charge.

Chromosome aberration: Alteration from normal structure or number.

Chromosomes: Various-sized structural elements in the cell nucleus, composed of DNA and proteins, which carry the genes that convey the genetic information. Chromosomes have a species-specific morphology and number.

Cladding: The outer metallic jacket about nuclear fuel elements. Prevents corrosion of the fuel as well as the release of radioactive fission products into the coolant of the reactor core.

Collective dose equivalent: The collective dose equivalent to a population in units of man-sievert (man-Sv) or man-rem that is the sum of the products of the individual (or *per capita* dose equivalents) and the number of individuals in each exposed group in a population.

Committed dose equivalent: The dose equivalent to any tissue in the body that will be accumulated over a period of 50 years after the intake of a radionuclide.

Congenital: Present at birth. Does not imply either genetic or nongenetic causation.

Containment vessel: The heavy metallic receptacle that surrounds and contains the core of a reactor. Also may refer to a receptacle used during transport of radioactive material.

Contamination (radioactive): A radioactive substance in a material or place where it is undesirable.

Controlled area: An area where entry, activities, and exit are controlled to assure radiation protection and to prevent the spread of radioactive contamination.

Cosmic rays: Radiation of many sorts, but mostly atomic nuclei (protons) with very high energies originating outside Earth's atmosphere. Cosmic radiation is part of the natural background radiation. Some cosmic rays are more energetic than any anthropogenic forms of radiation.

Counts per minute (cpm): The number of counts or nuclear events detected by a radiation survey device such as a Geiger counter. Since not all events that occur are detected, cpm are always less than actual disintegrations per minute (dpm) emanating from a radioactive material.

Critical mass: The smallest mass of fissionable material that will support a self-sustaining chain reaction under stated conditions.

Critical organ: (1) Organ of interest; (2) organ most radiobiologically affected by a technique.

Criticality: The state of a nuclear reactor liquid or experimental assembly when it is sustaining a chain reaction.

Curie (Ci): Standard measure of rate or radioactive decay; based on the disintegration of 1 g radium or 3.7×10^{10} disintegrations per second; 1 curie expressed in SI units is 3.7×10^{11} becquerels (Bq).

Cyclotron: A device consisting of two hollow D-shaped chambers for accelerating charged particles to energies up to 15 MeV or more by periodic accelerations through a potential difference.

Daughter radionuclide: Decay product produced by a radionuclide. The element from which the daughter was produced is called the "parent."

Decay: Radioactive disintegration of a nucleus of an unstable nuclide.

Decay constant (lambda): The probability per unit of time that a given radionuclide atom will undergo a radioactive transformation.

Decay, radioactive: The spontaneous transformation of one nuclide into a different nuclide or into a different energy state of the same nuclide. The process results in a decrease, with time, of the original radioactive atoms in sample. Radioactive decay involves (1) the emission from the nucleus of alpha particle, beta particles (electrons), or gamma rays; (2) the nuclear capture or ejection of orbital electrons; or (3) fission. Also called radioactive disintegration. *See* Half-life.

Decay schemes: Diagram showing the decay mode or modes of a radionuclide.

Decontamination: The removal or reduction of radioactive contaminants from surface or equipment, for example, by cleaning and washing.

Delayed neutrons: Neutrons emitted by radioactive fission products in a nuclear reactor over a period of seconds or minutes after a fission takes place. Fewer than 1% of the neutrons are delayed; more than 99% are prompt neutrons. Delayed neutrons are important considerations in reactor design and control. *Compare* Fast neutrons.

Delayed radiation effects: Manifestations of radiation damage that become evident months or years after irradiation. Examples include atrophy, fibrosis, ulceration, cancer, and genetic effects.

De minimus: An expression derived from the Latin "de minimus non jurate lex" (the law is not concerned with trivialities). A *de minimus* level is one that is so low as to be trivial.

Deoxyribonucleic acid (DNA): The nucleic acid primarily contained within the cell nucleus, which carries the genetic information.

Detector: A material or device that is sensitive to radiation and can produce a response signal suitable for measurement or analysis.

Deuterium (symbol: ^{2}H or D): An isotope of hydrogen whose nucleus contains one neutron and one proton and, therefore, is about twice as heavy as the nucleus of normal hydrogen, which is only a single proton. Deuterium is often referred to as heavy hydrogen; it occurs in nature as 1 atom to every 6500 atoms of normal hydrogen. It is nonradioactive. *Compare* Tritium.

Diploid: Possessing a paired set of chromosomes, one set from the father and one set from the mother (2n). Characteristic of all somatic cells.

Disintegration: General process of radioactive decay, usually measured per unit time: disintegrations per second (dps).

Dose: A term denoting the amount of energy absorbed. Absorbed dose is the energy imparted to matter by ionizing radiation per unit mass of irradiated material at the point of interest. Usually expressed in rads (conventional unit) or grays (SI unit). Cumulative dose is the total dose resulting from repeated exposures to radiation.

Dose equivalent (H): A unit of biologically effective dose, defined as the absorbed dose in rads multiplied by the quality factor (Q). (For all X rays, gamma rays, beta particles, and positrons likely to be used in nuclear medicine, the quality factor is 1.) The dose equivalent (H) is given by the equation $HDQN$, where D is absorbed dose, Q is the quality factor, and N is the product of modifying factors (N is usually 1 also).

Dose equivalent commitment: For any specified decision, practice, or operation, the infinite time integral of the *per capita* dose equivalent rate for a specified population. In other words, the dose committed over a certain time period resulting from an action.

Dose ranges: Arbitrary designations of dose. Low dose range is roughly 0 to 0.2 Gy in a single dose or 10 mGy/year of uniform whole-body radiation; intermediate dose, roughly 0.2 to 2.5 Gy; high dose, above 2.5 Gy.

Dose rate: The radiation dose delivered per unit time and measured, e.g., in Gy or Sv/h. *See* Absorbed dose.

Dose rate contour line: A line on a map or a diagram joining all points at which the radiation dose rate is the same at a given time.

Dosimeter: A device that measures radiation dose, such as a film badge.

Dosimeter, pocket: A device used to determine the radiation dose a person has received by utilization of a small air-filled ionization chamber (about the size and shape of a pen). Dose can be read by holding it up to the light and looking through it. Not as sensitive or as accurate as either a film badge or a thermoluminescent dosimeter (TLD).

Dosimeter, thermoluminescent (TLD): A dosimeter worn by a person to measure radiation dose. Contains a radiation-sensitive crystal that gives off light when heated. Amount of light emitted is proportional to radiation dose. About the size and shape of a film badge.

Dosimetry: The measurement of radiation doses.

Doubling dose (genetic): That radiation dose estimated to double the spontaneous or natural incidence of any given effect.

Effective half-life: *See* Half-life, effective.

Electromagnetic radiation: Radiation consisting of associated and interacting electric and magnetic waves that travel at the speed of light, such as light, radio waves, gamma rays, and X rays. All electromagnetic radiation can be transmitted through a vacuum. *Compare* Ionizing radiation.

Electron: An elementary particle with a negative electrical charge. Electrons surround the positively charged nucleus of the atom.

Electron capture: Method of radioactive decay in which the nucleus captures an orbital electron, which then interacts with a proton, effectively negating the proton and transmuting the nucleus to that of another element.

Electron volt (eV): A unit of energy equal to the kinetic energy required by an electron when accelerated through a potential difference of 1 volt (1 eV = 1.6×10^{-19} J).

Element: Pure substance consisting of atoms of the same atomic number that cannot be decomposed by ordinary chemical means.

Embryo: The organism in the first stages of development. In humans, this is generally considered to be the period from the end of the second week through the eighth week of gestation.

Emergency: A sudden, urgent, usually unforeseen occurrence or occasion requiring immediate action.

Emergency coordinator: The individual within an institution or facility who is assigned the responsibility for developing an emergency plan, as well as maintaining the plan and its distribution lists.

Emergency director: The individual designated in the emergency plan to exercise command and control over all emergency response personnel for the duration of the emergency.

Enriched uranium: Uranium in which the percentage of the fissionable isotope (uranium-235, or ^{235}U) has been increased above the 0.7% normally found in natural uranium.

Erythema: A medical term for reddening of the skin. May occur following high doses of radiation received over a short period of time.

Epilation: Loss of hair. May occur transiently or permanently after large exposures to radiation.

Exposure: A term relating to the amount of ionizing radiation that is incident upon living or inanimate material.

Exposure rate: Increment of exposure to expressed per unit time may be expressed in units of C/kg/min or R/min.

Fast neutrons: Neutrons with energy greater than approximately 100,000 eV. *Compare* Delayed neutrons, Thermal neutrons.

Fertile material: A material, not itself fissionable by thermal neutrons, that can be converted into a fissile material by irradiation in a nuclear reactor. There are two basic fertile materials, the uranium isotope ^{238}U and the thorium isotope ^{232}Th. When these fertile materials capture neutrons, they are partially converted into the fissile plutonium isotope ^{239}Pu and the fissile uranium isotope, respectively.

Fetus: Unborn offspring in humans, refers to the period from 8 weeks after fertilization until birth.

Film badge: Photographic film shielded from light; worn by an individual to measure radiation exposure.

Fissile material: Although used as a synonym for fissionable material, this term has acquired a more restricted meaning; namely, any material fissionable by neutrons of all energies, especially thermal, or slow, neutrons, as well as fast neutrons. The uranium isotope ^{235}U and the plutonium isotope ^{239}Pu are examples of fissile material.

Fission: The splitting of a heavy nucleus into two approximately equal parts (which are nuclei of lighter elements), accompanied by the release of a relatively large amount of energy and generally one or more neutrons. Fission can occur spontaneously, but usually is caused by nuclear absorption of gamma rays, neutrons, or other particles. *Compare* Fusion.

Fission products: The nuclei (fission fragments) formed by the fission of heavy elements plus the nuclides formed by the radioactive decay of the fission fragments. *See* Decay, radioactive.

Fuel cycle: The series of steps involved in supplying fuel for nuclear power reactors. It includes mining, refining, fabricating the fuel elements, using them in a nuclear reactor, chemical processing to recover the fissionable materials remaining in the spent fuel (not done in the United States as of 1984), reenriching the fuel material, and refabricating it into new fuel elements.

Fuel element: A rod, a tube, a plat, or other mechanical shape or form into which nuclear fuel is fabricated.

Fusion: The formation of a heavier nucleus from two lighter ones, such as hydrogen isotopes, with the attendant release of energy. It takes energy input to cause fusion fuel to fuse, but once fused, it releases much more energy than that put in. *Compare* Fission.

Fusion fuel: Commonly used fusion fuels for laboratory experiments are isotopes of hydrogen, namely, deuterium and tritium. Hydrogen itself is the fusion fuel of the sun. Other "futuristic" fusion fuels include helium and lithium.

Gamma emission: Nuclear process in which an excited nuclide deexcites by emission of a nuclear photon.

Gamma radiation: Electromagnetic radiation emitted by an atomic nucleus as a result of a nuclear transformation.

Gamma ray: Radiation emitted from the nucleus having a wavelength range from 10^{-9} to 10^{-12} cm.

Gastrointestinal syndrome: Part of the acute radiation syndrome. Usually occurs following whole-body acute absorbed doses in excess of 5 Gy (500 rad). Manifested in 1 to 4 weeks after exposure by diarrhea, fluid loss, electrolyte imbalance, and sepsis.

Geiger–Mueller counter (tube): A high-voltage (>1000 V) gas tube used to detect ionizing particles. It is based upon the avalanche effect observed when ions are accelerated by an electric field under appropriate conditions. Can be used to detect gamma and X rays as well as energetic beta particles. Cannot detect alpha particles. Generally this instrument is used to detect low radiation levels and should not be used in radiation fields >500 mR/h.

Genetic effects of radiation: Radiation effects that can be transferred from parent to offspring. Any radiation-caused changes in the genetic material of germ cells. *Compare* Somatic effects of radiation.

GeV: One billion electron volts. Also written BeV. *See* Electron volt.

Giga (G): A prefix that multiplies a basic unit by one billion (10^9).

Glove box: A sealed box in which workers, remaining outside and using gloves attached to and passing through openings in the box, can safely handle and work with radioactive materials that emit poorly penetrating radiation (e.g., plutonium).

GM tube: *See* Geiger–Mueller counter.

Gray (Gy): The SI unit of radiation absorbed dose; 1 gray is equal to an energy deposition of 1/kg (100 rad). *See also* rad.

Ground state: The state of lowest energy of a system.

Half-life: *Radioactive:* For a single radioactive decay process, the time required for the activity of a given sample to decrease to half its initial value by that process. *Biological:* The time required for the amount of a particular substance in a biological system to be reduced to half of its initial value by biological processes when the rate of removal is approximately exponential. *Effective:* The time required for the amount of a particular specimen of a radionuclide in a system to be reduced to half its initial value as a consequence of both radioactive decay and other processes, such as biological elimination.

Half-value layer (HVL): Thickness of absorbing material necessary to reduce the intensity of radiation by one half.

Haploid: Having a single set of unpaired chromosomes (N23 in humans) characteristic of the gametes.

Health physicist: A person qualified by training and experience to be professionally engaged in the practice of health physics.

Health physics: The science concerned with the recognition, evaluation, and control of health hazards from ionizing radiation.

Hematopoietic syndrome: Part of the acute radiation syndrome. Usually presents following acute whole-body doses >1 Gy and occurs 1 to 4 weeks after exposure. Major manifestations are decreases in circulating platelets, lymphocytes, and granulocytes.

High radiation area: An area where the radiation dose to a person could exceed 1 mSv in 1 h. There are special requirements for controlling access to such areas.

HVL: *See* Half-value layer.

ICRP: International Commission on Radiological Protection.

ICRU: International Commission on Radiation Units and Measurements.

Incident: An occurrence or situation of seemingly minor importance.

Intermediate neutrons: Neutrons having energy greater than thermal neutrons but less than fast neutrons. The range is between 0.5 and 100,000 eV. Also called epithermal neutrons. *Compare* Thermal neutrons.

Internal contamination: Radioactive contamination within a person's body caused by radioactive material that has been inhaled, ingested, or absorbed through the skin or wounds.

Inverse-square law: The radiation intensity of any source decreases inversely as the square of the distance between the source and the detector (e.g., doubling the distance from a source decreases the intensity by one fourth).

Inversion: A chromosomal abnormality in which a segment of the chromosome recombines in an inverted relationship following breakage.

Ion pair: A closely associated positive ion and negative ion (usually an electron) having charges of the same magnitude and formed from a neutral atom or molecule by radiation.

Ionization: The process whereby a charged portion (usually an electron) of an atom or molecule is given enough kinetic energy to dissociate.

Ionization chamber: A closed vessel used for the detection of radiation energy and containing a gas and two electrodes maintained at a potential difference. Any radiation incident upon this container forms ions that move to the appropriate electrode, producing a current that can be measured.

Ionizing radiation: Radiation that produces ion pairs along its path through a substance. *Compare* Electromagnetic radiation.

Irradiation: Exposure to radiation.

Isobar: Nuclides that have the same total number of neutrons and protons but are different elements.

Isomer: One of two or more nuclides having the same number of neutrons and protons in their nuclei, but having different energies. A nuclide in the excited state and a similar nuclide in the ground state are isomers.

Isotones: Nuclides having the same number of neutrons but a different number of protons.

Isotopes: Nuclides having the same number of protons but a different number of neutrons.

Karyotype: A systemized array of chromosomes from a single cell, prepared by photography, that demonstrates the number and morphology of the chromosome complement.

Kerma: Kinetic energy released in material. A unit of quantity that represents the kinetic energy transferred to charged particles by the uncharged particles per unit mass of medium. Expressed in rads or grays.

keV: Thousand electron volts = 10^3 eV.

Lanthanide series: The series of elements beginning with lanthanum, element number 57, and continuing through lutetium, element number 71, which together occupy one position in the periodic table of the elements. These are the "rare earths" — all having chemical properties similar to lanthanum. They also are called the *lanthanides*. *Compare* Actinide series.

Latent period: Usually refers to the time elapsed between radiation exposure and the clinical appearance of an effect (such as appearance of a cancer or cataracts).

LET: *See* Linear energy transfer.

Lethal dose: A dose of ionizing radiation sufficient to cause death. Median lethal dose (MLD or LD) is the dose required to kill, within a specified period of time (usually 30 days), half the individuals in a large group of organisms similarly exposed. The $LD_{50/60}$ for humans is about 3 to 4.5 Gy (300 to 450 rad).

Light water reactor (LWR): May be either a boiling or pressurized water reactor. Uses as coolant ordinary water (H_2O) instead of heavy water (D_2O). LWRs are the most common reactor type in the United States.

Linear energy transfer (LET): Amount of energy lost by ionizing radiation by way of interaction with matter per centimeter of path length through the absorbing material.

Low specific activity (LSA): Radioactive material in which the activity is essentially uniformly distributed and in which the amount of activity is low. Will not present a serious public health hazard if released.

Lugol's solution: A saturated iodine solution.

man-rem: *See* Person rem.

Mass number (A): The sum of neutrons and protons in a nucleus.

Maximum permissible body burden (MPBB): The maximum quantity or concentration for activities or radionuclides inside the body, set by requiring that it does not result in doses to critical organs in excess of those specified for external radiation. Note should be made that this level often does not represent a significant medical problem nor should it be used to require intervention or treatment.

Maximum permissible concentration (MPC): An obsolescent term for the amount of radioactive material in the air, water, or food that might cause a maximum permissible dose at a standard rate of intake.

Maximum permissible dose (MPD): The maximum amount of radiation that may be received by an individual within a specified time period with the expectation of no significantly harmful result to the individual. The permissible limits of occupational exposures of persons younger than 18 years of age are considerably reduced. MPD is a regulatory concept.

Metaphase: The stage of mitosis or meiosis when the centromeres of the contracted chromosomes are arranged on the equatorial plate.

Metastable state: An excited nuclear state of a particular isotope that has a finite half-life and decays by gamma emission. Examples: ^{99m}Tc, Tc(6h), ^{38m}Cr, ^{38}Cl(07s).

MeV: One million (10^6) electron volts.

Micro (μ): A prefix that divides a basic unit by one million (10^{-6}).

Microcurie (μCi): That quantity of radioactive material having 3.7×10^4 disintegrations per second. One millionth part of a curie.

Micrometer (μm): One millionth of a meter; formerly micron.

Milli (m): A prefix that divides a basic unit by one thousand (10^{-3}).

Millicurie (mCi): That quantity of radioactive material having 3.7×10^{-7} disintegrations per second. One thousandth part of a curie.

Mitosis: Somatic cell division by which the mother cell produces two daughter cells, each with the identical chromosome complement as the original cell.

Monitoring: Periodic or continuous determination of the amount of ionizing radiation or radioactive contamination present. Also referred to as *surveying*.

MPC: *See* Maximum permissible concentration.

MPD: *See* Maximum permissible dose.

N: *See* Neutron number. Also used as the abbreviation for the haploid number of chromosomes in the human.

NCRP: National Council on Radiation Protection and Measurements.

Neutron number (N): Number of neutrons in a nucleus.

Glossary

Nonstochastic effect: Describes effects whose severity is a function of dose. Some may have an apparent clinical threshold. Examples of nonstochastic effects include skin erythema, cataracts, and bone marrow depression.

Nuclear Regulatory Commission (NRC): U.S. government agency regulating by-product material.

Nucleon: Any particle commonly contained in the nucleus of an atom.

Nucleus: The small, positively charged core of an atom. It is only about 1/10,000 the diameter of the atom but contains nearly all the mass of the atom. All nuclei contain both protons and neutrons, except the nucleus of ordinary hydrogen, which consists of a single proton.

Nuclide: A general term applicable to all atomic forms of the element. The term is often used incorrectly as a synonym for isotope, which properly has a more limited definition. Whereas isotopes are the various forms of a single element (hence, a family of nuclides) and all have the same atomic number and number of protons, nuclides comprise all the isotopic forms of all the elements. Nuclides are distinguished by their atomic number, atomic mass, and energy state.

Parent radionuclide: Radionuclide that decays to a specific daughter nuclide either directly or as a member of a radioactive series.

Person rem: A unit of collective population dose calculated by multiplying the number of persons exposed times their average individual whole-body dose in Sv.

Personal monitor: *See* Thermoluminescent dosimeter and Film badge.

Photon: An energy quantum of electromagnetic radiation. *See* gamma radiation.

Photopeak: The peak (maximum intensity) in a gamma spectrum as measured by a scintillation detector.

Pico (p): A prefix that divides a basic unit of one trillion (10^{-12}). Same as *micromicro*.

Point source: Any radiation source measured from a distance that is much greater than the linear size of the source. A source whose linear dimensions are less than 10% of the measurement distance may be considered a point source.

Positron: A particle equal in mass to the electron, but with a positive electric charge.

Promotor: *See* Carcinogen.

Protective clothing: Special clothing worn to prevent radioactive contamination from getting on the skin. Actually a misnomer for anticontamination clothing.

Proton: An elementary particle with a mass 1873 times that of an electron and a positive charge equal to the basic electronic charge.

Quality factor (QF): Linear energy transfer-dependent factor by which absorbed doses are to be multiplied to account for the varying effectiveness of different radiations. The QF for 250 kVp X rays is equal to 1.

rad: Radiation absorbed dose. The unit of absorbed dose of ionizating radiation; 1 rad is equal to 100 erg/g. *See also* Gray.

Radiation: Energy propagated through space or matter as waves (gamma rays, ultraviolet light) or as particles (such as alpha or beta rays). External radiation comes from a source outside the body, whereas internal radiation is from a source inside the body (such as radionuclides deposited in tissues).

Radiation accident: An accident in which there is an unintended exposure to radiation or radioactive contamination.

Radiation area: Any accessible area in which the level of radiation is such that a major portion of an individual's body could receive in any 1 h a dose in excess of 50 μSv or in any five consecutive days a dose in excess of 1.5 μSv.

Radiation emergency area (REA): A term used by hospitals to refer to the area (usually in or near the emergency room) that has been designated to treat injured and radioactively contaminated patients. This area has access and egress controlled to avoid spread of radioactive contamination.

Radiation, ionizing: Any radiation that has high enough energy to break apart chemical bonds and cause atoms to form ions (charged particles), e.g., gamma and X rays.

Radiation, nonionizing: Radiation from other portions of the electromagnetic spectrum that do not have enough energy to create ions, e.g., microwaves, radar, visible light.

Radiation, penetrating: Radiation that can penetrate deeply into tissues, e.g., gamma, X rays, beta particles. This term usually only refers to ionizing radiation.

Radiation safety officer (RSO): A person (often a health physicist or physician) who has the responsibility for overseeing radiation safety in an organization.

Radiation sickness: The prodromal manifestations of acute radiation injury, varying in severity, scope, and etiology, depending upon the conditions of exposures. *See* Acute radiation syndrome.

Radioactive: *See* Radioactivity.

Radioactive contamination: Deposition of radioactive material in any place where it may harm persons, spoil experiments, or make products or equipment unsuitable or unsafe for some specific use. The presence of unwanted radioactive matter. Also, radioactive material found on the walls of vessels in spent-fuel processing plants or radioactive material that has leaked into a reactor coolant. Often called *contamination*.

Radioactivity: The property of certain nuclides of emitting radiation by spontaneous transformation of their nuclei.

Radionuclide: Unstable nucleus that transmutes by way of nuclear decay.

Radionuclidic purity: Amount of total radioactive species in a sample that is the desired radionuclide.

Radiopharmaceutical: Radioactive drug used for therapy or diagnosis.

Radioprotector: Compound that inhibits the radiation response of biological systems.

Radioresistance: A relative resistance of cells, tissues, organs, or organisms to the harmful action of radiation.

Radiosensitivity: A relative susceptibility of cells, tissues, organs, or organisms to the harmful action of radiation.

Radiosensitizer: Substance that enhances the radiation response of biological systems.

Radium (Ra): A radioactive metallic element with atomic number 88. As found in nature, the most common isotope has an atomic weight of 226. It occurs in minute quantities associated with uranium in pitchblende, carnotite, and other minerals. Uranium decays to radium in a series of alpha and beta emissions. By virtue of being an alpha and gamma emitter, radium is used as a source of luminescence and as a radiation source in medicine and radiography.

Glossary

Radon (Rn): A radioactive element and the heaviest gas known. Its atomic number is 86 and its atomic weight varies from 200 to 226. It is a daughter of radium in the uranium radioactive series.

Range switch: A switch on a radiation survey meter that changes the scale of the meter, e.g., from 0 to 10 mR/h to 0 to 100 mR/h.

Rare earths: A group of 15 chemically similar metallic elements, numbers 57 through 71 in the periodic table; also known as the lanthanide series.

Rate meter: Device, used in conjunction with a detector, that measures the rate of activity of a radioisotope; usually in units of counts per minute or counts per second.

RBE: *See* Relative biological effectiveness.

Reactor (nuclear): A device in which a fission chain reaction can be initiated, maintained, and (preferably) controlled.

Reference man: An "ideal man" utilized for radiation protection purposes. Has defined anatomical and physiological specifications. Defined in ICRP Rep. 23.

Relative biological effectiveness (RBE): Ratio of the biological response derived from a particular radiation as compared with another radiation exposure.

Relative risk: *See* Risk, relative.

rem: *See* Roentgen equivalent man.

Reprocessing: The process by which spent fuel from a nuclear reactor is separated into waste material, uranium, and plutonium to be reused as a nuclear fuel.

Restricted area: When used in the context of radiation, refers to a controlled-access area in which the dose to a person could exceed 20 µSv in any 1 h or 1 mSv in any 1 week.

Ring dosimeter: A thermoluminescent dosimeter worn on the finger in order to be able to measure absorbed dose to the hands.

Risk, absolute: The excess risk attributed to irradiation and usually expressed as the numerical difference between irradiated and nonirradiated populations (e.g., one case of cancer per million people irradiated per year per rad). Absolute risk may be given on an annual basis or lifetime (50-year) basis.

Risk, relative: The ratio between the number of cancer cases in the irradiated population to the number of cases expected in the unexposed population. A relative risk of 1.1. indicates a 10% increase in cancer due to radiation, compared to the "normal" incidence. Relative risk is more appropriate to use when considering selected population groups.

Roentgen (R): Quantity of gamma or X radiation per cubic centimeter of air that produces one electrostatic unit of charge.

Roentgen equivalent man (rem): The unit of dose equivalent. The absorbed dose in rads multiplied by the quality factor of the type of radiation. *See* Sievert.

RSO: *See* Radiation safety officer.

Scattered radiation: Radiation that, during its passage through a substance, has been deviated in direction and perhaps with an energy loss.

Scenario: An account or synopsis of a projected course of action or events.

Scintillation counter: An instrument that detects radiation by counting the small flashes of light produced when the radiation interacts with the detector crystal.

Sealed source: A radioactive source sealed in an impervious container, which has sufficient mechanical strength to prevent contact with or dispersion of the radioactive material under conditions of use for which it was designed. Such sources are generally used for radiation therapy and industrial radiography.

Shield (shielding): A body of material used to reduce the intensity of radiation.

Shielding: Any material used to absorb beta-, X-, and gamma-ray radiation.

SI units: International system of units. SI refers to Système International d'Unités. Radiation units include J/kg, Gy, Sv, and Bq.

Sievert (Sv): The SI unit of dose equivalent. The absorbed dose in Gy multiplied by the quality factor of the type of radiation; 1 sievert equals 100 rem.

Somatic effects of radiation: Effects of radiation limited to the exposed individual, as distinguished from genetic effects, which also affect subsequent unexposed generations. Large radiation doses can cause somatic effects that are fatal. Smaller doses may make the individual noticeably ill, may produce temporary changes in blood-cell levels detectable only in the laboratory, or may produce no detectable effects. Also called physiological effects of radiation. *Compare* Genetic effects of radiation.

Specific activity: Unit pertaining to the disintegrations per gram of a radioisotope.

Spent fuel: Nuclear reactor fuel that has been irradiated (used) to the extent that it can no longer effectively sustain a chain reaction.

Stochastic effect: An effect whose probability of occurrence in an irradiated population or individual is a function of dose. Commonly regarded as not having a threshold dose. An example is radiation carcinogenesis.

Survey meter: Meter that measures rate of radioactive exposure, usually in units of mR/h.

Thermal neutrons: Neutrons in thermal equilibrium with their surrounding medium. Thermal neutrons are those that have been slowed down by a moderator to an average speed of about 220 m/s at room temperature from the much higher initial speeds they had when expelled by fission. *Compare* Fast neutrons, Intermediate neutrons.

Thermoluminescent dosimeter (TLD): Type of crystal used to monitor radiation exposure by emitting light; often used in a body, wrist, or ring badge. Must be processed in order to be read.

Thorium (Th): A naturally radioactive element with atomic number 90 and, as found in nature, an atomic weight of approximately 232. The fertile thorium isotope ^{232}Th is abundant and can be transmuted to the fissionable uranium isotope ^{233}U by neutron irradiation. *See* Fertile material.

Threshold dose: The minimum dose of radiation that will reproduce a detectable biological effect.

Transient equilibrium: Equilibrium reached by a parent–daughter radioisotope pair in which the half-life of the parent is longer than the half-life of the daughter.

Transuranic nuclide: A nuclide having an atomic number greater than that of uranium (>92). Includes neptunium, plutonium, americium, and curium.

Tritium (^{3}H or T): A radioactive isotope of hydrogen with two neutrons and one proton in the nucleus. It is anthropogenic and heavier than deuterium (heavy hydrogen). Tritium is used as a label in chemical and biological experiments. Its nucleus is a triton. *Compare* Deuterium.

UF conversion: The process of converting the solid uranium oxide (commonly called *yellow cake*) that comes from uranium mining and milling into a uranium fluoride gas.

UNSCEAR: United Nations Scientific Committee on the Effects of Atomic Radiation. A committee of the U.N. General Assembly.

Uranium (U): The basic raw material of nuclear energy. A radioactive element with atomic number 92 and, as found in natural ores, an average atomic weight of approximately 238. The two principal natural isotopes are ^{235}U (0.7% of natural uranium), which is fissionable, and ^{238}U (99.3% of natural uranium), which is fertile. Natural uranium also includes a minute amount of ^{234}U.

Warning labels: *See* Radioactive White, Radioactive Yellow labels.

Weighting factor (W_T): The ratio of the stochastic risk arising from a tissue T to the total risk when the whole body is irradiated uniformly. Concept derived for use by the International Commission on Radiologic Protection.

Whole-body counter: A device used to identify and measure radionuclides in the body (body burden) of humans and animals. It uses heavy shielding (to keep out background radiation), ultrasensitive scintillation detectors, and electronic equipment.

Whole-body (total) exposure: An exposure of the body to external radiation, in which the entire body rather than an isolated part is irradiated. Also may occur when a radioactive material is uniformly distributed throughout the tissues of the body.

Wipe test: A test for radioactive contamination by wiping the surface with a filter paper–like material and then measuring the paper with an appropriate radiation detector. Results are often reported in cpm/100 cm^2 of the area wiped.

Yellow cake: The semirefined product from uranium mining and milling operations that is sent to conversion plants.

Z number: *See* atomic number.

Appendix 1
Sample Radiation Emergency Plan for a Medical Facility

This sample plan was developed by the U.S. National Council on Radiation Protection and Measurements and is published in Developing Radiation Emergency Plans for Academic, Medical or Industrial Facilities, NCRP Rep. 111, Bethesda, MD, 1991. Copies of the full report may be obtained by writing to the National Council on Radiation Protection and Measurements, 7910 Woodmont Avenue, Bethesda, MD, U.S.A. 20814.

The following text contains a sample emergency plan for a large medical facility and several associated Emergency Plan Implementing Procedures (EPIPS) for individuals involved in the plan. This plan is for demonstration purposes only, and should not be applied directly to other facilities without careful consideration and considerable revision. It is intended as a guide to the reader to be used in constructing such a plan for another facility. Assumptions and designated responsibilities may be significantly different for actual facilities.

BACKGROUND INFORMATION

The XYZ Medical Facility is a large medical center serving a sizable metropolitan area. It consists of a medical school, biomedical research facilities, and a teaching hospital with a full range of diagnostic and therapy clinics. The facility has a broad research license and a broad human use license for the use of radionuclides issued by the appropriate regulatory agency. The medical facility is fully staffed with security, plant maintenance, legal and public relations personnel.

XYZ MEDICAL FACILITY EMERGENCY PLAN

1 INTRODUCTION

The XYZ Medical Facility is an institution committed to the health care and treatment of humans and the conduct of medical research. The XYZ Medical Facility is located at [give complete address of primary management offices, e.g., 100 College Street, State Capitol, Any State] with auxiliary facilities located at [give exact addresses of each facility as applicable, e.g., 101 Medical Science Park, Capitol Annex, Any State]. The purpose of the XYZ Medical Facility Emergency Plan is to provide the organization with an adequate and timely response for employees and associated support agencies designed to cope with radiation emergencies.

The objectives of the emergency plan are to prevent or mitigate the harmful effects resulting from those events classified as radiation emergencies, which occur within this institution's facilities, or those occurring elsewhere, which impact on this institution or its services.

The management of XYZ Medical Facility approves the radiation emergency plan and pertinent procedures, and is committed to the support of those individuals named in the plan as being responsible for its development, implementation, and maintenance. This emergency plan is designed to provide a framework to respond effectively to an emergency involving radiation whether the event occurs within the facility or at another location. All reports of emergencies received by the XYZ Medical Facility involving radiation will be routed to the Emergency Director or a designated alternate. Based on the initially reported information, the Emergency Director will classify and declare an emergency in accord with the approved emergency plan radiation classification system.

2 INSTRUCTIONS AND RESPONSIBILITIES

2.1 General Instructions for All Employees in the Event of a Radiation Emergency

In the event of a radiation emergency, the following instructions are applicable to all employees.

An employee at the scene of the emergency should provide general first aid, warn other people to leave the area, and isolate the area. The employee should:

- Report the event to appropriate emergency response contact.
- Take actions designed to minimize radiation exposure and radioactive contamination.
- Not use telephone or elevators except for emergency needs or activity related to emergency.
- Follow emergency plan guidance.
- Be cognizant of assigned emergency plan duties.
- Have available pertinent portions of emergency plan for ready reference, such as call lists, Emergency Plan Implementing Procedures (EPIPs), reference data (radiation handbooks).
- Direct all requests from media representatives to the designated Emergency Public Information Manager.
- Keep the Functional Area Manager or Emergency Director apprised of his or her location, actions and the conditions affecting the assigned area of response.
- Use sound radiation protective measures, proper radiation monitoring equipment, and be alert at all times for any hazards, such as physical, chemical, biological, fire, or explosion.

2.2 Organization and Responsibilities

The following duties are applicable to designated emergency personnel.

2.2.1 Emergency Coordinator (EC)

[Name], Vice President for Research, is assigned the position of XYZ Medical Facility Emergency Coordinator in accordance with Job Description # [...]. The EC is responsible for the overall coordination of the total XYZ Medical Facilities Emergency Program to include: the development and maintenance of the emergency plan, positions, implementing procedures, and advising management on the selection and training of individuals assigned to key emergency plan positions. The EC shall be responsible for the conduct of training, drills, and exercises as required for both employees and outside agency personnel. The EC shall report to and provide assistance to the Emergency Director in the event of a declared emergency.

2.2.2 Emergency Director (ED)

[Name], Vice President for Research Support, is assigned the position of XYZ Medical Facility Emergency Director in accord with Job Description # […]. The ED is responsible for directing the emergency response upon activation of the emergency plan. The ED has the authority and responsibility to initiate any emergency actions within the provisions of the emergency plan to include the classification, upgrading, downgrading, and termination of the emergency and the exchange of information with authorities responsible for coordinating and implementing off-site emergency measures. The following individuals are also assigned to the position of ED (as alternates) with the same responsibility and authority as described above in order to assure the immediate availability of an individual to respond as ED in the event the individual named above is not available.

Radiation Safety Officer alternate: [Name]
Deputy Radiation Safety Officer alternate: [Name]

2.3 EMERGENCY MANAGERS OF FUNCTIONAL AREAS

The Chief [Department or Service Head or overall Supervisor] of each of the functional areas listed in the emergency plan is designated as emergency manager of that functional area upon activation of the emergency plan. The manager of each functional area, upon activation of the emergency plan, shall report to the Emergency Director at the designated location and be available to provide advice and consultation on all aspects of the emergency having impact on the functional area. Each emergency functional area manager has the authority and responsibility for providing all the services of the pertinent department contained in the provisions of the emergency plan.

In the absence of the chief of the functional area, the individual on-site who is exercising the highest level of supervision of the pertinent department or service shall assume the duties and responsibilities of emergency manager of that functional area until relieved properly. [If the above broad statement approach for defining the authority and responsibility of emergency functional area managers is inappropriate, the following are examples describing individual emergency functional area manager positions.]

2.3.1 Emergency Medical Manager (EMM)

[Name], Chief of Emergency Medicine, is assigned the position of XYZ Medical Facility Emergency Manager in conjunction with Job Description # […]. The EMM is responsible for providing advice and consultation to the Emergency Director on all medical aspects of the emergency upon activation of the emergency plan. The EMM has the authority and is responsible for the provision of medical services within the provisions of the emergency plan. The following individual is also assigned to the position of EMM with the same responsibility and authority as described above in order to ensure immediate availability of an individual to respond as EMM in the event the individual named above is not available.

Chief Resident, Emergency Medicine: [Name]

2.3.2 Emergency Radiation Protection Manager (ERPM)

[Name], Radiation Safety Officer, is assigned the position of Emergency Radiation Protection Manager in accord with Job Description # […]. The ERPM is responsible for the initial assessment of the radiological aspects of the emergency (actual or potential) and to be available to provide advice and consultation to the ED on all radiation protection aspects of the emergency prior to and upon activation of the plan. The ERPM has the authority and responsibility for provision of all radiation protection services within the provisions of the emergency plan. The following individual is also assigned the position of ERPM with the same authorities and responsibilities as described above in order to ensure immediate availability of an ERPM in the event the individual named above is not available.

Radiation Safety Officer: [Name]

2.3.3 Emergency Safety and Security Manager (ESSM)

[Name], Chief of Security, is assigned the position of Emergency Safety and Security Manager (ESSM) in accord with Job Description # [...]. The ESSM is responsible for assessment of actual or potential general safety and security aspects of all emergencies, and shall be available to provide advice and consultation to the ED on all matters relating to general safety, security, and traffic control upon activation of the Emergency Plan. The ESSM shall provide personnel and/or supervision to accomplish the following: rescue of injured individuals, conduct of personnel accountability, orderly evacuation of affected areas, control of access to the emergency site, as well as within the affected areas of the facility. The ESSM shall provide for control of vehicular traffic on hospital property and coordinate the activities of activated off-site agencies having similar responsibilities. The following individual is assigned the position of ESSM with the same authority and responsibility as described above in order to ensure immediate availability of an ESSM in the event the individual named above is not available.

Assistant Chief of Security: [Name]

2.3.4 Emergency Plant Services Manager (EPSM)

[Name], Manager of Plant Services, is assigned the position of the Emergency Plant Services Manager (EPSM) in accord with Job Description # [...]. The EPSM shall provide the Emergency Director with advice and assistance on those aspects of any emergency situation directly involving or having impact on those services and utilities supplied and/or maintained by the Plant Services Department. The following emergency response functions are among those provided by the EPSM: damage assessment and control, repair and/or corrective action, technical support, liaison with utilities suppliers. The following individual is also assigned the position of EPSM with the same authority and responsibilities as described above in order to ensure immediate availability of an EPSM in the event the individual named above is not available.

Assistant Manager, Plant Services: [Name]

2.3.5 Emergency Fire Protection Manager (EFPM)

[Name], Fire Chief, is assigned the position of Emergency Fire Protection Manager (EFPM) in accord with Job Description # [...]. The EFPM shall be available to provide the Emergency Director advice and assistance on those aspects of any emergency situation directly involving or having impact on those services or equipment supplied or maintained by the fire protection department. The following emergency response functions are among those provided by the EFPM: fire control, damage assessment, rescue and first aid, liaison with off-site fire protection organizations. The following individual is also assigned the position of EFPM with the same authority and responsibilities as described above in order to ensure immediate availability of an EFPM in the event the individual named above is not available.

Assistant Chief, Fire Protection: [Name]

2.3.6 Emergency Public Information Manager (EPIM)

[Name], Public Information Officer, is assigned the position of Emergency Public Information Manager (EPIM) in accord with Job Description # [...]. The EPIM shall be available to provide the Emergency Director with advice and assistance in development, preparation, and timely dissemination of factual information pertaining to the emergency situation directly involving the institution and its impact on the institution and the general public. The following emergency response functions are among those provided by the EPIM: act as the primary spokesman for the Emergency Director in the development, preparation, and release of information regarding the emergency to all outside news media representatives; respond to media and public inquiries pertaining to the emergency; and maintain active rumor control. The following individual is also named to the position of EPIM with the same authority and responsibilities as described above to ensure immediate availability of an EPIM in the event the individual named above is not immediately available.

Assistant Manager, Public Information: [Name]

2.3.7 Communications Manager (ECM)

[Name], Communications Manager, is assigned the position of Emergency Communications Manager (ECM) in accord with Job Description # [...]. The ECM shall be available to provide advice and assistance in the provision of communication equipment and service required for use by emergency response personnel. The following emergency response functions are among those provided by the ECM: make available appropriate operating communication equipment in areas designated by the Emergency Director, provide a means of maintaining a record of communications, provide and maintain status boards in the Emergency Control Center. The following individual is assigned to the position of ECM with the same authorities and responsibilities as described above in order to ensure immediate availability of an ECM in the event the individual named above is not available.

Assistant Manager, Communications: [Name]

2.3.8 Off-Site Agencies

The following off-site agencies have agreed to respond and supply support in specified emergency situations occurring at the XYZ Medical Facility. The decision to use such agencies and the extent of support provided by off-site organizations will be in accord with provisions of this emergency plan and the letters of agreement currently in effect.

- Municipal Fire and Rescue Service (Chief)
- Municipal Police (Chief)
- State Police (Commander)
- City Hospital (Chief Administrator)

EMERGENCY PLAN ORGANIZATIONAL CHART

XYZ Medical Facility
Director

| **Emergency Coordinator** | **Emergency Director** |
Telephone Ext.	**Telephone Ext.**
Emergency Functional Area Manager Ext.	**Off-Site Agencies** *(Support)* Municipal Fire & Rescue Service Telephone No.
Emergency Radiation Protection Manager Ext.	Municipal Police Telephone No.
Emergency Safety and Security Manager Ext.	State or Province Police Telephone No.
Emergency Fire Protection Manager Ext.	*(Regulatory)* Local, State, or Province Regulatory Agency Telephone No.
Emergency Public Information Manager Ext.	State Health Department Telephone No.
	National Regulatory Agency, Regional Regulatory Office Telephone No.
Emergency Communications Manager Ext.	*(Sample Others)* Radioactive Materials Users Telephone No.
	Consultants Telephone No.

3 NOTIFICATION

3.1 INDIVIDUAL EMPLOYEE RESPONSIBILITY

To report an emergency:

   By Phone, Dial #: 999
   Radio, Use Call Letters: XYZ

Sample Radiation Emergency Plan for a Medical Facility

An emergency is considered to be any condition that exists or appears to be imminent, which would result in a threat to the health and safety of employees, patrons, or the general public or cause serious damage to the facilities and/or equipment of this organization. Any employee recognizing an emergency should report it immediately.

3.2 Emergency Operator Responsibilities

The Emergency Operator is the person who answers all calls to the designated emergency number. Upon receiving a call reporting an emergency, the Emergency Operator shall obtain from the caller and record on an initial notification form (See example on page 4 in attached EPIP #NE-1) as much information as possible pertaining to the emergency. Following receipt of the initial report of the emergency the Emergency Operator will complete the notification of the XYZ Medical Facility in accord with EPIP entitled: Notification of Emergency.

4 Emergency Control Center (ECC)

The ECC is located in Room # […]. of the XYZ Medical Facility. This room is commonly known as the Trauma Center Conference Room. The ECC is the room to which the Emergency Director and pertinent emergency functional area managers report upon the declaration of a Level-One or Level-Two Emergency. It is in the ECC that the ED and emergency functional area managers conduct their operations designed to control the emergency. The ECC is equipped with the quantities and types of equipment and materials as listed in EPIP # […]. entitled ECC Equipment. Activation of the ECC is initiated by the first member of the emergency response organization to arrive. That individual will act as ED until the ED arrives.

5 Emergency Support Centers (ESC)

Emergency Support Center (ESC) is the designation given to each of the primary operational offices of those functional area managers designated to respond to the ECC.

These areas or facilities are designated as ESC to ensure their ready access in the event of a declared emergency. Upon declaration of an emergency, the entire staff of the designated ESC for a functional area will be made aware of the emergency classification and will prepare to respond to the emergency at the direction of the ED or their functional area manager.

6 Training

All individuals assigned to primary, alternate, and/or backup emergency response positions by name shall be trained in accord with the position training requirements outlined in the XYZ Medical Facility Training Manual.

Individuals assigned position in the emergency response organization (ERO) must have satisfactorily completed the specified training for the positions to which they are, or may be, assigned prior to being allowed to respond in a declared emergency. Training and retraining of ERO position personnel will be accomplished approximately annually, but not to exceed 15 months. All general employees must receive the basic emergency response training outlined in the XYZ Medical Facility Training Manual during their initial employee orientation.

Records of all training provided will be maintained by the XYZ Medical Training Department. Individual training documentation shall include as a minimum:

- Name of attendee
- Date of training
- Lesson title

- Instructor's name
- Results of any tests or evaluations

7 EMERGENCY PLAN EXERCISES

Emergency exercises shall be conducted by the following Emergency Functional Area Managers in accord with the following schedule:

Medical—annually
Public Information—annually
Radiation Protection—semiannually
Plant Services—semiannually
Fire Protection—semiannually
Safety and Security—semiannually
Communications—quarterly

Exercises shall be accomplished at periods that provide for training and evaluation of all shifts of the affected functional groups at least annually.

8 RECOVERY

The recovery phase begins when the conditions leading to or resulting from the emergency have been reduced to a level manageable by normal operational personnel and procedures. The recovery phase will end at the direction of the Emergency Director when: (1) operation of the facility is returned to the normal operational organization and (2) the equipment, facilities, and supplies required by the XYZ Facility Emergency Plan have been reconstituted.

8.1 Responsibilities

The Emergency Director will be responsible for the initiation of the recovery phase activities. The Emergency Director will be responsible for the thorough transfer of information from the emergency response organization to normal operational personnel regarding conditions leading to, during, and existing at the termination of the emergency.

8.2 Concept of Operation

The Emergency Director will, at the initiation of the recovery phase, arrange for smooth transfer of information and control from the emergency response organization to normal operational personnel.

Special emphasis will be placed on the provision of information and records of unusual conditions resulting from the emergency, such as radiation levels, contamination, chemical hazards, physical hazards, biological hazards, fire hazards, and ventilation changes.

8.3 Reestablishment of Emergency Facilities

The Emergency Control Center will be returned to its normal operational use. Emergency functional area managers will be assigned the tasks of ensuring that all equipment, supplies, forms, and documents used during the emergency at the Emergency Control Center and the Emergency Support Centers are returned and are restored to the required preemergency level.

8.4 Reports

The Emergency Director assisted by the Emergency Coordinator will determine the documentation and reports required by the XYZ Medical Facility management and the regulatory agencies. Following the determination of such documentation and reports, the Emergency Director will assign subtasks to the pertinent emergency response personnel, setting deadlines appropriate to meet management and regulatory requirements.

9 REVIEW, REVISION, AND DISTRIBUTION OF THE EMERGENCY PLAN

The XYZ Medical Facility Emergency Plan with all applicable EPIPs and appendices to include letters of agreement with support agencies shall be reviewed and revised as needed. Revised portions of the plan and appendices will be distributed immediately. The Emergency Coordinator is responsible for review, revision, and distribution of the plan and appendices. The Emergency Coordinator shall be assisted in this review and revision by affected functional area managers.

9.1 Revisions

All required revisions of the plan, EPIPs, and appendices shall be entitled:

Revision of

and be conducted in conjunction with EPIP Emergency Plan Documents.

9.2 Distribution

Following approval, all revisions will be distributed to all official recipients of the plan in accord with EPIP entitled:

Distribution of Emergency Plan Documents

SAMPLE EMERGENCY PLAN IMPLEMENTING PROCEDURES (EPIPS)

The following contains sample EPIPs. The sample EPIPs provided here cover *only* a limited number of tasks or functions that may be required to support a specific emergency plan. Each emergency plan will require the development of those EPIPs necessary to accomplish the desired response. The following EPIPs are provided as examples of form and content. The XYZ Medical Facility is continued as an example institution.

XYZ MEDICAL FACILITY
Notification of Emergency

1. Purpose
   1.1 This procedure provides instruction for notifying the emergency response organization and off-site agencies of the declaration of an emergency condition at the XYZ Medical Facility.
2. Applicability
   2.1 This procedure applies to the Emergency Operator, the Emergency Director, and other specifically designated members of the emergency response organization upon declaration of an emergency condition.
3. Responsibilities

3.1 The Emergency Operator
    3.1.1 Receives and records initial report of emergency.
    3.1.2 Directs all reports of events (actual or suspected) to the Emergency Director.
    3.1.3 Accomplishes notification of emergency response organization for emergencies as directed by Emergency Director.

3.2 Emergency Director
    3.2.1 Based on initial information obtained from pertinent functional area managers or others classifies the emergency in an expeditious manner in accord with EPIP # […] entitled: Classification of Emergency.
    3.2.2 Directs that the notification of emergency response organization be accomplished by the Emergency Operator.
    3.2.3 Directs that the notification of off-site support and regulatory agencies be accomplished as appropriate by the Emergency Coordinator.

3.3 Emergency Coordinator
    3.3.1 Accomplishes notification of off-site agencies as directed by the Emergency Director.
    3.3.2 Provides assistance in ensuring complete notification by contacting and verifying notification calls as necessary.

3.4 Emergency Functional Area Managers
    3.4.1 Emergency functional area managers who are contacted shall accomplish notification of pertinent groups within their respective departments.

4. Instructions
    4.1 Emergency Director and Emergency Coordinator shall report to the predesignated Emergency Center.
    4.2 All emergency functional area managers shall report to the predesignated Emergency Control Center.

5. References
    Facility Emergency Plan
    EPIP # [ ], Classification
    Facility License Conditions

6. Attachments
    6.1 XYZ Notification Form
    6.2 XYZ Medical Facility Emergency Organization Call List, for emergencies outside the hospital that impact on the hospital

Approved by	
Emergency Coordinator	Date
Approved by	
Facility Director	Date
Approved by	
Emergency Director	Date

XYZ NOTIFICATION FORM

Notification received by
Reported: Date   Time   AM/PM
Occurred: Date   Time   AM/PM
Reported by: Title
  Phone Number:
  Address:

Incident Location:
Building: Room No. or Other Area:
Town: County (if known):
Exact Location:

Type of Incident
Fire, Explosion, Injury, Auto Collision, Other

Injuries Involved
Number: Type:

Description of Materials Involved
What type of material is involved?
  Chemical: [Name]
  Form: Liquid — Solid — Powder   Other:
  Volume:
  Radioactive Material: [Name]
  Isotope: [Designation] Contamination, Exposure — internal or external
  Form: Liquid — Powder — Sealed Source
  Quantity: Curies, Millicuries, Other

Incident Mode
Motor Carrier, Railroad, Pipeline, Storage
Aircraft, Manufacturing, Other
Elaborate here and on back of this form if necessary:

Local Officials on Scene
Fire, Sheriff, Police
Highway Patrol, Other

Emergency Operator Signature:

XYZ MEDICAL FACILITY
FOR EMERGENCIES WITHIN HOSPITAL

Emergency Call Tree
Emergency Report Typically Received
By Designated Emergency Operator Who Notifies

Emergency Director
   Classifies Emergency and Directs

Emergency Coordinator #
                  Notifies Pertinent Off-Site Assistance
                  as Designated by Emergency Director
                      (See Attached Phone List)

Emergency Operator Call	
Functional Area Managers	Hospital Director
Medical #	Administrator on Call
Radiation Protection	Medical Departments
Fire Protection	Nursing Supervisor #
Security #	Senior Emergency Medicine Resident
Emergency Coordinator	Senior Surgical Resident #
Communication	Anesthesia Resident on Call
Public Information	Internal Medicine Resident on Call
Plant Service #	Orthopedic Resident on Call
Special Hazard	Radiology Resident on Call
Others, as appropriate	Pediatric Resident on Call
	Blood Bank Technologist
	Pharmacy Director

RADIOLOGICAL MONITORING

1. Purpose
   1.1 This procedure provides instructions for performing radiological monitoring activities during an emergency to include determination of habitable areas, facility radiological monitoring, and postemergency monitoring.
2. Applicability
   2.1 This procedure is applicable to the Emergency Director, Emergency Radiation Protection Manager, radiation protection personnel, and other individuals involved in on-site radiological monitoring.
   2.2 This procedure should be implemented for emergencies classified as a Level-One Emergency or Level-Two Emergency; however, it may be implemented at the discretion of the Emergency Director for an "Incident."
3. Responsibilities
   3.1 Emergency Radiation Protection Manager (ERPM)
      3.1.1 Provide advice and direction to the Emergency Director regarding radiological monitoring activities to be conducted and protective measures to be implemented for facility personnel.
      3.1.2 Keep the Emergency Director informed of radiological conditions, protective measures to be implemented during evacuation of assembly areas or the facility as required, and provide the results of the postemergency sampling.
      3.1.3 Determine the need for postemergency sampling, identify the samples obtained and to be obtained, and evaluate the results of such sampling activities.
      3.1.4 Organize and dispatch the on-site (facility) radiological monitoring personnel/teams, direct the activities to be accomplished, and evaluate the results of monitoring activities.
   3.2 Emergency Director
      3.2.1 Based upon radiological conditions, authorize reclassification of the emergency.
      3.2.2 If recommended by the ERPM authorize evacuation of selected buildings or areas or total facility.
      3.2.3 Based upon recommendations of the Emergency Radiation Protection Manager, authorize increased personnel exposure limits, as required.
4. Radiological Monitoring
   4.1 Radiological monitoring inside the facility shall be conducted to support required response actions.
   4.2 At least one radiation protection representative should accompany each rescue, repair and reentry team upon initial entry into an area where an actual or potential radiological hazard exists.
   4.3 Prior to dispatch of personnel into an actual or potential radiological hazard area.
      4.3.1 The ERPM shall ensure that required protective apparel and devices are used properly.
      4.3.2 Respiratory protection equipment, if required, should be checked and determined to be operable, and the user should be aware of equipment limitations.
      4.3.3 Dosimetry of sufficient range should be worn to monitor adequately whole-body and extremity doses where applicable.
      4.3.4 Equipment and supplies anticipated to be required for the tasks should be available and checked to ensure operability as necessary.
      4.3.5 Appropriate primary and backup communications means should be assigned and checked prior to departure.

4.3.6 Briefings of team members should be conducted to the extent necessary to ensure team personnel are aware of the task assigned as well as methods and special precautions to be observed.

4.4 After dispatch of the team the radiation protection representative assigned to the team should in addition to monitoring dose rates and total exposures:

4.4.1 Provide guidance to team members pertaining to exposure control.

4.4.2 Inform and advise the ERPM or ED of unanticipated radiological conditions encountered.

4.4.3 Upon completion of team assignment and return from radiation areas, the radiation protection representative should provide guidance in removal of protective clothing and equipment and monitoring and decontamination of personnel exiting the emergency area.

4.4.4 Upon completion of assignment, the radiation protection representative will provide all pertinent radiological information during a debriefing of the team.

4.5 The ERPM shall advise the ED of necessity for accomplishment of and results of analysis of postemergency sampling.

4.6 Documentation of on-site radiological monitoring activities and postemergency sampling results should be recorded appropriately with copies being made and supplied to:

4.6.1 Incident log

4.6.2 Emergency Director

4.6.3 Emergency Radiation Protection Manager

4.6.4 Appropriate control points or agencies

Approved by
Emergency Coordinator   Date

Approved by
Emergency Director   Date

Approved by
Emergency Radiation Protection Manager   Date

Appendix 2

World Health Organization Radiation Accident Coordinating Centers

Argentina	Department of Health Physics POB 3268 Buenos Aires, Argentina Fax:+541 382 5680 or +541 381 0971 Tel:+541 382 5680
Armenia	Research Centre of Radiation Medicine and Burns 375078 Davidasben Yerevan, Armenia Fax:+3742 340 800 Tel:+3742 341 144
Australia	Radiation Protection and Radiation Emergency Yallambia, Victoria 3093 Australia Fax:+613 9432 1835 Tel:+613 9433 2211
Brazil	Radiation Protection and Medical Preparedness for Radiological Accidents Avenida Salvador Allende (vio9) Jocorepogu, CP 37750, CEP 22780 Rio de Janeiro, Brazil Fax:+5521 442 2539 or +5521 442 1950 Tel:+5521 442 1927 or +5521 442 9614
China	Institute of Radiation Medicine 27, Tai Ping Road, 100850 Beijing, China Fax:+8610 821 4653 Tel:+8610 821 3044 or 821 4653
France	Centre International de Radiopathologie BP No. 34, Batiment 01, F-92269 Fontenay-aux-Roses, France Fax:+331 4638 2445 Tel:+331 4554 7266

Germany	Institute for Occupational Health University of Ulm, Pf. 2060 D-89069 Ulm, Germany Fax:+49 731 502 3415 Tel:+49 731 502 3400
India	Bhabha Atomic Research Centre 400085 Mumbai, India Fax:+9122 556 0750 Tel:+9122 551 1677
Japan	Radiation Effects Research Foundation 5-2 Hijiyama Park Minami-Ku, J-732 Hiroshima, Japan Fax:+11 8182 263 7279 Tel:+11 8182 261 3131
Russian Federation	State Research Centre, Institute of Biophysics 46, Zhivopisnaya 123182 Moscow, Russia Fax:+7095 190 3590 Tel:+7095 190 5156
	Central Research Institute of Roentgenology and Radiology Pesochnij 2 189646 St. Petersburg, Russia Fax:+7812 437 8787 Tel:+7812 437 8781
	All-Russian Centre on Ecological Medicine 17, Botkinskaya 194175 St. Petersburg, Russia Fax:+7812 541 8805 Tel:+7812 248 3419
	Medical Radiological Research Centre 4, Koroliev 249020 Obninsk, Russia Fax:+7095 956 1440 Tel:+7095 956 1439
	Urals Research Centre for Radiation Medicine Medgorodok, FIB 454076 Chelyabinsk, Russia Fax: +73512 344 321
United Kingdom	National Radiological Protection Board (NRPB) Chilton Didcot Oxfordshire OX1 1 ORQ United Kingdom Fax:+441235 822 630 Tel:+441235 822 612

World Health Organization Radiation Accident Coordinating Centers

United States
: Radiation Emergency Assistance
REAC/TS
Oak Ridge, TN 37831-0117
United States
Fax: 001 865 576 9522
Tel: 001 865 576 3131

World Health Organization (WHO)
: Headquarters
CH-1211 Geneva 27, Switzerland
Fax: 0041 22 791 0746
Tel: 0041 22 791 3763

International Atomic Energy Agency (IAEA)
: Headquarters
Wagramer Strasse 5, RO.
Box 100
A-1400 Vienna, Austria
Tel: 431 2060 29309 (for emergency service during office hours)
Tel: 431 239270 (for emergency service 24 hours)
Fax: 431 20607

Appendix 3

Conversion Tables for SI and Conventional Units

TABLE A3.1
Conventional and International (SI) Unit Conversions

Factor	Prefix	Symbol	Factor	Prefix	Symbol
10^{18}	exa	E	10^{-1}	deci	d
10^{15}	peta	P	10^{-2}	centi	c
10^{12}	tera	T	10^{-3}	milli	m
10^{9}	giga	G	10^{-6}	micro	µ
10^{6}	mega	M	10^{-9}	nano	n
10^{3}	kilo	k	10^{-12}	pico	p
10^{2}	hecto	h	10^{-15}	femto	f
10^{1}	deka	da	10^{-18}	atto	a

TABLE A3.2
Conversion of Exposure Units

Coulomb/kilogram (C/kg)	Roentgen (R)
10	38,000
1	3,880
10^{-1}	388
10^{-2}	38.8
10^{-3}	3.88
10^{-4}	0.388 (388 mR)
10^{-5}	3.88×10^{-3} (38.8 mR)
10^{-6}	3.88×10^{-3} (3.88 mR)
10^{-7}	3.88×10^{-4} (388 µR)
10^{-8}	3.88×10^{-5} (38.8 µR)
10^{-9}	3.88×10^{-6} (3.8 µR)
10^{-10}	3.88×10^{-7} (388 nR)
10^{-11}	3.88×10^{-8} (38.8 nR)

TABLE A3.3
Conversion of Absorbed Dose Units

SI Units		Conventional Units	
100 Gy	(10^2 Gy)	10,000 rad	(10^4 rad)
10 Gy	(10^1 Gy)	1,000 rad	(10^3 rad)
1 Gy	(10^0 Gy)	100 rad	(10^2 rad)
100 mGy	(10^{-1} Gy)	10 rad	(10^1 rad)
10 mGy	(10^{-2} Gy)	1 rad	(10^0 rad)
1 mGy	(10^{-3} Gy)	100 mrad	(10^{-1} rad)
100 µGy	(10^{-4} Gy)	10 mrad	(10^{-2} rad)
10 µGy	(10^{-5} Gy)	1 mrad	(10^{-3} rad)
1 µGy	(10^{-6} Gy)	100 µrad	(10^{-4} rad)
100 nGy	(10^{-7} Gy)	10 µrad	(10^{-5} rad)
10 nGy	(10^{-8} Gy)	1 µrad	(10^{-6} rad)
1 nGy	(10^{-9} Gy)	100 nrad	(10^{-7} rad)

TABLE A3.4
Conversion of Dose Equivalent Units

100 Sv	(10^2 Sv)	=	10,000 rem	(10^4 rem)
10 Sv	(10^1 Sv)	=	1,000 rem	(10^3 rem)
1 Sv	(10^0 Sv)	=	100 rem	(10^2 rem)
100 mSv	(10^{-1} Sv)	=	10 rem	(10^1 rem)
10 mSv	(10^{-2} Sv)	=	1 rem	(10^0 rem)
1 mSv	(10^{-3} Sv)	=	100 mrem	(10^{-1} rem)
100 µSv	(10^{-4} Sv)	=	10 mrem	(10^{-2} rem)
10 µSv	(10^{-5} Sv)	=	1 mrem	(10^{-3} rem)
1 µSv	(10^{-6} Sv)	=	100 µrem	(10^{-4} rem)
100 nS	(10^{-7} Sv)	=	10 µrem	(10^{-5} rem)
10 nSv	(10^{-8} Sv)	=	1 µrem	(10^{-6} rem)
1 nSv	(10^{-9} Sv)	=	100 nrem	(10^{-7} rem)

TABLE A3.5
Conversion of Radioactivity Units

100 TBq	(10^{14} Bq)	2.7 kCi	(2.7×10^3 Ci)
10 TBq	(10^{13} Bq)	270 Ci	(2.7×10^2 Ci)
1 TBq	(10^{12} Bq)	27 Ci	(2.7×10^1 Ci)
100 GBq	(10^{11} Bq)	2.7 Ci	(2.7×10^0 Ci)
10 GBq	(10^{10} Bq)	270 mCi	(2.7×10^{-1} Ci)
1 GBq	(10^9 Bq)	27 mCi	(2.7×10^{-2} Ci)
100 MBq	(10^8 Bq)	2.7 mCi	(2.7×10^{-3} Ci)
10 MBq	(10^7 Bq)	270 µCi	(2.7×10^{-4} Ci)
1 MBq	(10^6 Bq)	27 µCi	(2.7×10^{-5} Ci)
100 kBq	(10^5 Bq)	2.7 µCi	(2.7×10^{-6} Ci)
10 kBq	(10^4 Bq)	270 nCi	(2.7×10^{-7} Ci)
1 kBq	(10^3 Bq)	27 nCi	(2.7×10^{-8} Ci)
100 Bq	(10^2 Bq)	2.7 nCi	(2.7×10^{-9} Ci)
10 Bq	(10^1 Bq)	270 pCi	(2.7×10^{-10} Ci)
1 Bq	(10^0 Bq)	27 pCi	(2.7×10^{-11} Ci)
100 mBq	(10^{-1} Bq)	2.7 pCi	(2.7×10^{-12} Ci)
10 mBq	(10^{-2} Bq)	270 fCi	(2.7×10^{-13} Ci)
1 mBq	(10^{-3} Bq)	27 fCi	(2.7×10^{-14} Ci)

Appendix 4
Absorbed Dose Estimates from Radionuclides

These charts can be used to estimate absorbed dose from a variety of accidental situations involving radionuclides. Table A4.1 is derived from data in ICRP Rep. 68, Dose Coefficients for Intakes of Radionuclides by Workers, International Commission on Radiological Protection, Pergamon Press, Oxford, U.K., 1995. For age-dependent doses to members of the public from intake of radionuclides, the reader is referred to ICRP Reps. 67, 69, 71, and 72

Tables A4.2 to A4.6 contain corrected data from NCRP Rep. 111, National Council on Radiation Protection and Measurements, Bethesda, MD, 1991. These latter tables do not use the new ICRP models.

TABLE A4.1
Effective Dose Coefficients for Intakes of Radionuclides by Workers (Sv/Bq)

Nuclide	Physical $t_{1/2}$	Type[a]	Inhalation[b] 1 μm AMAD	Inhalation[b] 5 μm AMAD	Ingestion[b]
Americium-241	4.32E+02y	M	3.9E-05	2.7E-05	2.0E-07
Americium-243	7.38E+03y	M	3.9E-05	2.7E-05	2.0E-07
Arsenic-74	17.8d	M	2.1E-09	1.8E-09	1.3E-09
Arsenic-77	1.62d	M	3.8E-10	4.2E-10	4.0E-10
Barium-140	12.7d	F	1.0E-09	1.6E-09	2.5E-09
Cadmium-109	1.27y	F	8.1E-09	9.6E-09	2.0E-09
		M	6.2E-09	5.1E-09	
		S	5.8E-09	4.4E-09	
Calcium-45	163d	M	2.7E-09	2.3E-09	7.6E-10
Calcium-47	4.53d	M	1.8E-09	2.1E-09	1.6E-09
Californium-252	2.63y	M	1.8E-05	1.3E-05	9.0E-08
Carbon-14	5.7E+03y				5.8E-10
Cerium-141	32.5d	M	3.1E-09	2.7E-09	7.1E-10
		S	3.6E-09	3.1E-09	
Cerium-144	284d	M	3.4E-08	2.3E-08	5.2E-09
		S	4.9E-08	2.9E-08	
Cesium-134	2.06y	F	6.8E-09	9.6E-09	1.9E-08
Cesium-137	30.0y	F	4.8E-09	6.7E-09	1.3E-08
Chromium-51	27.7d	F	2.1E-11	3.0E-11	3.8E-11
		M	3.1E-11	3.4E-11	3.7E-11
		S	3.6E-11	3.6E-11	
Cobalt-57	271d	M	5.2E-10	3.9E-10	2.1E-10
		S	9.4E-10	6.0E-10	1.9E-10
Cobalt-58	70.8d	M	1.5E-09	1.4E-09	7.4E-10
		S	2.0E-09	1.7E-09	7.0E-10
Cobalt-60	5.27y	M	9.6E-09	7.1E-09	3.4E-09
		S	2.9E-08	1.7E-08	2.5E-09

TABLE A4.1 (CONTINUED)
Effective Dose Coefficients for Intakes of Radionuclides by Workers (Sv/Bq)

Nuclide	Physical $t_{1/2}$	Type[a]	Inhalation[b] 1 μm AMAD	Inhalation[b] 5 μm AMAD	Ingestion[b]
Curium-242	163d	M	4.8E-06	3.7E-06	1.2E-08
Curium-243	28.5y	M	2.9E-05	2.0E-05	1.5E-07
Curium-244	18.1y	M	2.5E-05	1.7E-05	1.2E-07
Europium-152	13.3y	M	3.9E-08	2.7E-08	1.4E-09
Europium-154	8.8y	M	5.0E-08	3.5E-08	2.0E-09
Europium-155	4.96y	M	6.5E-09	4.7E-09	3.2E-10
Fluorine-18	1.83h	F	3.0E-11	5.4E-11	4.9E-11
		M	5.7E-11	8.9E-11	
		S	6.0E-11	9.3E-11	1.9E-10
Gallium-67	3.26 d	F	6.8E-11	1.1E-10	
		M	2.3E-10	2.8E-10	
Gallium-72	14.1h	F	3.1E-10	5.6E-10	1.1E-09
		M	5.5E-10	8.4E-10	
Gold-198	2.69d	F	2.3E-10	3.9E-10	1.0E-09
		M	7.6E-10	9.8E-10	
		S	8.4E-10	1.1E-09	
Hydrogen-3	12.3y				1.8E-11
Indium-114m	49.5d	F	9.3E-09	1.1E-08	4.1E-09
		M	5.9E-09	5.9E-09	
Iridium-192	74.0d	F	1.8E-09	2.2E-09	1.4E-09
		M	4.9E-09	4.1E-09	
Iridium-192		S	6.2E-09	4.9E-09	
Iodine-123	13.2h	F	7.6E-11	1.1E-10	2.1E-10
Iodine-125	60.1d	F	5.3E-09	7.3E-09	1.5E-08
Iodine-131	8.04d	F	7.6E-09	1.1E-08	2.2E-08
Iron-52	8.3h	F	4.1E-10	6.9E-10	1.4E-09
		M	6.3E-10	9.5E-10	
Iron-55	2.7y	F	7.7E-10	9.2E-10	3.3E-10
		M	3.7E-10	3.3E-10	
Iron-59	44.5d	F	2.2E-09	3.0E-09	1.8E-09
		M	3.5E-09	3.2E-09	
Lead-210	22.3y	F	8.9E-07	1.1E-06	6.8E-07
Mercury-197 (inorganic)	2.67d	F	6.0E-11	1.0E-10	2.3E-10
		M	2.9E-10	2.8E-10	
Mercury-203 (inorganic)	46.6d	F	4.7E-10	5.9E-10	5.4E-10
		M	2.3E-09	1.9E-10	
Molybdenum-99	2.75d	F	2.3E-10	3.6E-10	7.4E-10
		S	9.7E-10	1.1E-09	1.2E-09
Neptunium-237	2.14E+06y	M	2.1E-05	1.5E-05	1.1E-07
Neptunium-239	22.36d	M	9.0E-10	1.1E-09	8.0E-10
Phosphorus-32	14.3d	F	8.0E-10	1.1E-09	2.4E-09
		M	3.2E-09	2.9E-09	
Plutonium-238	87.7 y	M	4.3E-05	3.0E-05	2.3E-07
		S	1.5E-05	1.1E-05	8.8E-09
Plutonium-239	2.41E+04y	M	4.7E-05	3.2E-05	2.5E-07
		S	1.5E-05	8.3E-06	9.0E-09
Polonium-210	138d	F	6.0E-07	7.1E-07	2.4E-07
		M	3.0E-06	2.2E-06	

TABLE A4.1 (CONTINUED)
Effective Dose Coefficients for Intakes of Radionuclides by Workers (Sv/Bq)

Nuclide	Physical $t_{1/2}$	Type[a]	Inhalation[b] 1 μm AMAD	Inhalation[b] 5 μm AMAD	Ingestion[b]
Potassium-42	12.4h	F	1.3E-10	2.0E-10	4.3E-10
Promethium-147	2.62y	M	4.7E-09	3.5E-09	2.6E-10
		S	4.6E-09	3.2E-09	
Promethium-149	2.21d	M	6.6E-10	7.6E-10	9.9E-10
		S	7.2E-10	8.2E-10	
Radium-224	3.66d	M	2.9E-06	2.6E-06	6.5E-08
Radium-226	1.60E+03y	M	1.6E-05	1.2E-05	2.8E-07
Rubidium-86	18.6d	F	9.6E-10	1.3E-09	2.8E-09
Ruthenium-106	1.01y	F	8.0E-09	9.8E-09	7.0E-09
		M	2.6E-08	1.7E-08	
		S	6.2E-08	3.5E-08	
Scandium-46	83.8d	S	6.4E-09	4.8E-09	1.5E-09
Silver-110m	250d	F	5.5E-09	6.7E-09	2.8E-09
		M	7.2E-09	5.9E-09	
		S	1.2E-08	7.3E-09	
Sodium-22	2.6 y	F	1.3E-09	2.0E-09	3.2E-09
Sodium-24	15.0h	F	2.9E-10	5.3E-10	4.3E-10
Strontium-85	64.8d	F	3.9E-10	5.6E-10	5.6E-10
		S	7.7E-10	6.4E-10	3.3E-10
Strontium-90	29.1y	F	2.4E-08	3.0E-08	2.8E-08
		S	1.5E-07	7.7E-08	2.7E-09
Sulfur-35 (inorganic)	87.4d	F	5.3E-11	8.0E-11	1.4E-10
		M	1.1E-09	1.1E-09	1.9E-10
Technetium-99m	6.02h	F	1.2E-11	2.0E-11	2.2E-11
		M	1.9E-11	2.9E-11	
Technetium-99	2.13E+05y	F	2.9E-10	4.0E-10	7.8E-10
		M	3.9E-09	3.2E-09	
Thallium-201	3.04d	F	4.7E-11	7.6E-11	9.5E-11
Thorium-230	7.7E+04y	M	4.0E-05	2.8E-05	2.1E-07
		S	1.3E-05	7.2E-06	8.7E-08
Thorium-232	1.4E+10y	M	4.2E-05	2.9E-05	2.2E-07
		S	2.3E-05	1.2E-05	9.2E-08
Uranium-235	7.04E+08y	F	5.1E-07	6.0E-07	4.6E-08
		M	2.8E-06	1.8E-06	8.3E-09
		S	7.7E-06	6.1E-06	
Uranium-238	4.47E+09y	F	4.9E-09	5.8E-07	4.4E-08
		M	2.6E-06	1.6E-06	7.6E-09
		S	7.3E-06	5.7E-06	
Yttrium-90	2.67d	M	1.4E-09	1.6E-09	2.7E-09
		S	1.5E-09	1.7E-09	
Zinc-65	244d	S	2.9E-09	2.8E-09	3.9E-09
Zirconium-95	64.0d	F	2.5E-09	3.0E-09	8.8E-10
		M	4.5E-09	3.6E-09	
		S	5.5E-09	4.2E-09	

[a] Type F (fast lung clearance), Type M (moderate), Type S (slow).
[b] Expressed as 50-year committed effective dose.

TABLE A4.2
Skin Contamination Dose Equivalent Rate Factors at a Depth of 7 mg/cm^2

Radionuclide	Infinite Area Source[a,b] (mSv-cm/MBq-h)	Point Source[c] (mSv/MBq-h)
^{14}C	305	2.45×10^6
^{22}Na	1870	3.3×10^6
^{24}Na	2357	2.3×10^6
^{32}P	2397	2.2×10^6
^{35}S	332	2.4×10^6
^{36}Cl	2178	2.8×10^6
^{45}Ca	884	3.6×10^6
^{57}Co[d]	78	nv[f]
^{59}Fe	1283	3.6×10^6
^{60}Co	1146	3.7×10^6
^{67}Ga[d]	322	nv[f]
^{90}Sr-^{90}Y (equilibrium)	4272	5.4×10^6
^{99m}Tc[d]	243	nv[f]
^{111}In[d]	367	nv[f]
^{123}I[d]	360	nv[f]
^{125}I[e]	417	nv[f]
^{131}I	1694	3.3×10^6
^{137}Cs-^{137}Ba (equilibrium)	1941	3.5×10^6
^{147}Pm	612	3.0×10^6
^{192}Ir	1592	3.2×10^6
^{201}Tl	343	nv[f]
^{204}Tl	1803	3.0×10^6

[a] Appropriate for sources with average radii larger than the range of the radiation in water.
[b] Multiply by 3.7 to obtain the dose equivalent rate in rad-cm^2/mCi-h.
[c] Multiply by 3.7 to obtain the dose equivalent rate in rad/mCi-h.
[d] See text for application of table. Values from McGuire, E.L. and Dalrymple, G.V., Beta and electron dose calculations to skin due to contamination by common nuclear medicine radionuclides, *Health Physics*, 58:399–403, 1990.
[e] Recommended value from Johnson, J.R. and Lamothe, E.S., Dose to the basal layer of the skin from iodine-125 contamination, *J. Radiation Protection and Dosimetry*, 20:253–256, 1987.
[f] No value provided.

Source: From Cross, W.G. et al., Tables of beta-ray dose distributions in water, air, and other media, Report of AECL-7617, Atomic Energy of Canada, Ltd., 1982. With permission.

TABLE A4.3
Maximum External Photon and Electron Dose Equivalent Factors for Any Organ for Selected Radionuclides for Point and Infinite Area Sources[a,b]

Radionuclide	Point Sources[a,b] (mSv-cm²/Bq-h)	Area Source[b,c] at 1 m[d]-Photon (mSv-cm²/Bq-h)	Area Source[b,c] at 1 m[d]-Electrons (mSv-cm²/Bq-h)
^{22}Na	3.1×10^{-6}	8.5×10^{-5}	$5.1 \times 10^{-6,e}$
^{24}Na	4.8×10^{-6}	1.4×10^{-4}	2.1×10^{-4}
^{32}P	nv[f]	nv	2.7×10^{-4}
^{51}Cr	4.2×10^{-8}	1.7×10^{-6}	0
^{57}Co	2.3×10^{-7}	8.7×10^{-6}	0
^{59}Fe	1.7×10^{-6}	4.5×10^{-5}	5.3×10^{-7}
^{60}Co	3.4×10^{-6}	9.3×10^{-5}	7.5×10^{-8}
^{67}Ga	2.9×10^{-7}	nv	nv
^{90}Sr-^{90}Y (equilibrium)	nv	2.4×10^{-10}	3.8×10^{-4}
^{99m}Tc	1.5×10^{-7}	8.7×10^{-6}	0
^{111}In	5.1×10^{-7}	nv	nv
^{123}I	1.9×10^{-7}	nv	nv
^{131}I	5.8×10^{-7}	1.9×10^{-5}	6.2×10^{-6}
^{137}Cs-^{137}Ba (equilibrium)	8.6×10^{-7}	2.5×10^{-5}	3.9×10^{-5}
^{192}Ir	1.3×10^{-6}	nv	nv
^{201}Tl	2.1×10^{-8}	nv	nv

[a] Point source factors from Jaeger, R.G. et al., Engineering Compendium on Radiation Shielding, Vol. 1, Shielding Fundamentals and Methods, International Energy Agency, Springer-Verlag, New York, 1968.

[b] Area source factors from Kocher, D.C., Dose rate conversion factors for external exposure to photon and electron radiation from radionuclides occurring in routine releases from nuclear fuel cycle activities, *Health Physics*, 38:543–622, 1980.

[c] Specific gamma factors were multiplied by the factors for converting from roentgens to rads in water given in NCRP Rep. 69 (NCRP, 1981) and assuming a Q of 1. To obtain mSv/h, multiply by activity in Bq and divide by the square of the distance in cm.

[d] Value is maximum at 1 m above contaminated surface. To obtain mSv/h, multiply by the surface contamination in Bq/cm².

[e] Value is at 70 μm. Dose calculated to basal layer. Assume bare source dispersed on ground.

[f] nv indicates no value has been provided.

TABLE A4.4
Maximum Photon Dose Equivalent Rate Conversion Factors for Any Organ and Electron Dose Equivalent Rate Conversion Factors for Skin for Submersion in Contaminated Air

Radionuclide	Photon Dose Equivalent Rate[a] (mSv-cm³/Bq-h)	Electron Dose Equivalent Rate[b]
^{14}C	0	7.8×10^{-4}
^{22}Na	4.5×10^{-1}	4.0×10^{-2}
^{24}Na	9.2×10^{-1}	1.2×10^{-1}
^{32}P	0	1.6×10^{-1}
^{35}S	0	9.5×10^{-4}
^{57}Co	3.9×10^{-2}	9.8×10^{-3}
^{59}Fe	2.4×10^{-1}	2.0×10^{-2}
^{60}Co	0.5×10^{-2}	1.5×10^{-6}
^{85}Kr	4.8×10^{-4}	4.4×10^{-2}
^{90}Sr-^{90}Y (equilibrium)	1.4×10^{-8}	2.5×10^{-1}
^{99m}Tc	3.9×10^{-2}	3.2×10^{-4}
^{131}I	9.0×10^{-2}	3.0×10^{-2}
^{133}Xe	1.2×10^{-2}	9.6×10^{-3}
^{137}Cs-^{137}Ba (equilibrium)	1.2×10^{-1}	4.3×10^{-2}
^{147}Pm	1.1×10^{-6}	6.0×10^{-3}

[a] Value is the maximum over all organs, excluding skin, semi-infinite cloud.

[b] Value is for infinite medium dose to basal layer, 70 μm depth and does not include the photon skin dose. Photon skin dose is approximately equal to the value in the photon dose column.

Sources: From Berger, M.J., Beta ray dose in tissue equivalent material immersed in a radioactive cloud, *Health Physics*, 26:1–12, 1974. And from Kocher, D.C. and Eckerman, K.F., Electron dose rate conversion factors for external exposure of the skin, *Health Physics*, 40:467–476, 1981.

TABLE A4.5
Absorbed Dose Estimates (mSv/MBq) from Various Radionuclides in Critical Organs or Lungs (50-Year Commitment)

Radionuclide	Critical Organ	Dose in Organ Critical Organ	Lung
Americium-241	Bone	8.1×10^6	5.7×10^5
Americium-243	Bone	8.1×10^6	5.4×10^5
Arsenic-74	Total body	2.7	97.3
Arsenic-77	Total body	0.11	7.57
Barium-140	Bone	132	351
Cadmium-109	Liver	143	405
Calcium-45	Bone	200	64.8
Calcium-47	Bone	32.4	67.5
Californium-252	Bone	3.0×10^6	1.37×10^6
Carbon-14	Total body	0.162	54
Cerium-141	Liver	89.1	111
Cerium-144	Bone	4320	4590
Cesium-137	Total body	8.1	405
Chromium-51	Total body	0.189	7.29
Cobalt-57	Total body	0.243	43.2
Cobalt-58	Total body	1.35	167.4
Cobalt-60	Total body	4.05	702
Curium-242	Liver	1.45×10^5	1.57×10^5
Curium-243	Liver	4.05×10^6	5.67×10^5
Curium-244	Liver	2.97×10^6	5.67×10^5
Europium-152	Kidney	1.86×10^4	2970
Europium-154	Bone	9180	7.83×10^4
Europium-155	Kidney	2511	513
Fluorine-18	Total body	0.019	0.81
Gallium-72	Liver	6.48	12.7
Gold-198	Total body	0.27	23.5
Hydrogen-3	Total body	0.54	—
Indium-114m	Kidney, spleen	1674	459
Iodine-125	Thyroid	1458	—
Iodine-131	Thyroid	1755	—
Iron-55	Spleen	324	6.21
Iron-59	Spleen	1890	200
Lead-210	Kidney	3.24×10^5	2.48×10^4
Mercury-197	Kidney	5.94	2.43
Mercury-203	Kidney	81	83.7
Molybdenum-99	Kidney	46	2.54
Neptunium-237	Bone	7.56×10^6	4.86×10^5
Neptunium-239	Colon	6.21	7.29
Phosphorus-32	Bone	27	151
Plutonium-238	Bone	7.02×10^6	5.67×10^5
Plutonium-239	Bone	8.10×10^6	5.4×10^5
Polonium-210	Spleen	2.97×10^5	4.05×10^4
Potassium-42	Total body	0.22	15.1
Promethium-147	Bone	594	459
Promethium-149	Bone	11.9	19.2
Radium-224	Bone	2970	1.89×10^4
Radium-226	Bone	2.7×10^6	1.11×10^5

TABLE A4.5 (CONTINUED)
Absorbed Dose Estimates (mSv/MBq) from Various Radionuclides in Critical Organs or Lungs (50-Year Commitment)

Radionuclide	Critical Organ	Dose in Organ Critical Organ	Lung
Rubidium-86	Total body	2.43	178
Ruthenium-106	Kidney	216	5940
Scandium-46	Liver	189	405
Silver-110m	Total body	2.16	891
Sodium-22	Total body	4.86	0.32
Sodium-24	Total body	0.46	0.62
Strontium-85	Total body	5.94	89.1
Strontium-90	Bone	8.6×10^4	1107
Sulfur-35	Testis	1.1×10^4	0.02
Technetium-99m	Total body	0.0027	0.17
Technetium-99	Kidney	35.1	35.1
Thorium-230	Bone	7.83×10^6	4.86×10^5
Thorium-232	Bone	7.83×10^6	4.86×10^5
Uranium-235	Kidney	4.6×10^4	4.6×10^5
Uranium-238	Kidney	4.32×10^4	4.32×10^5
Uranium natural	Kidney	4.6×10^4	4.6×10^5
Yttrium-90	Bone	32.4	46
Zinc-65	Total body	17.8	74.5
Zirconium-95	Total body	0.81	294

Note: To obtain values in rems/mCi of radionuclide in organ, multiply values in table by 3.7.

Source: From *Medical Effects of Ionizing Radiation*, Mettler, F.A. and Moseley, R.D., Eds., Grune & Stratton, New York, 1985. With permission.

Appendix 5

Specific Gamma Ray Constants

Nuclide	Gamma Constant	Nuclide	Gamma Constant
Actinium-227	~2.2	Lanthanum-140	11.3
Antimony-122	2.4	Lutecium-177	0.09
Antimony-124	9.8	Magnesium-28	15.7
Antimony-125	~2.7	Manganese-52	18.6
Arsenic-72	10.1	Manganese-54	4.7
Arsenic-74	4.4	Manganese-56	8.3
Arsenic-76	2.4	Mercury-197	~0.4
Barium-131	~3.0	Mercury-203	1.3
Barium-133	~2.4	Molybdenum-99	0.9
Barium-140	12.4	Neodymium-147	0.8
Beryllium-7	~0.3	Nickel-65	~3.1
Bromine-82	14.6	Niobium-95	4.2
Cadmium-115m	~0.2	Osmium-191	~0.6
Calcium-47	5.7	Palladium-109	0.03
Carbon-11	5.9	Platinum-197	~0.5
Cerium-141	0.35	Potassium-42	1.4
Cerium-144	~0.4	Potassium-43	5.6
Cesium-134	8.7	Radium-226	8.25
Cesium-137	3.3	Radium-228	~5.1
Chlorine-38	8.8	Rhenium-186	~0.2
Chromium-51	0.16	Rubidium-86	0.5
Cobalt-56	17.6	Ruthenium-106	1.7
Cobalt-57	0.9	Scandium-46	10.9
Cobalt-58	5.5	Scandium-47	0.56
Cobalt-60	13.2	Selenium-75	2.0
Copper-64	1.2	Silver-110m	14.3
Europium-152	5.8	Silver-111	~0.2
Europium-154	~6.2	Sodium-22	12.0
Europium-155	~0.3	Sodium-24	18.4
Gallium-67	~1.1	Strontium-85	3.0
Gallium-72	11.6	Tantalum-182	6.8
Gold-198	2.3	Technetium-99m	0.60
Gold-199	~0.9	Tellurium-121	3.3
Hafnium-175	~2.1	Tellurium-132	2.2
Hafnium-181	~3.1	Thulium-170	0.025
Indium-114m	~0.2	Tin-113	~1.7
Iodine-124	7.2	Tungsten-185	~0.5
Iodine-125	~0.7	Tungsten-187	3.0
Iodine-126	2.5	Uranium-234	~0.1
Iodine-130	12.2	Vanadium-48	15.6

Nuclide	Gamma Constant	Nuclide	Gamma Constant
Iodine-131	2.2	Xenon-133	0.1
Iodine-132	11.8	Ytterbium-175	0.4
Iridium-192	4.8	Yttrium-88	14.1
Iridium-194	1.5	Yttrium-91	0.01
Iron-59	6.4	Zinc-65	2.7
Krypton-85	~0.04	Zirconium-95	4.1

Note: The gamma ray constant/10 = R/h at 1 mCi. The following gives examples of the use of specific gamma ray constants The conventional constant gives the exposure in R/mCi/h at 1 cm or the constant divided by 10 gives exposure in R/h at 1 m from 1 Ci. The specific gamma ray constant can be used to find the exposure rate (R/h) for a source of activity A (mCi) at any distance d (cm) by using the following formula:

$$\text{Exposure rate} = \frac{\text{Gamma ray constant} \times A}{d^2}$$

As an example, to calculate the exposure rate at 92 cm (3 ft) from a 1 Ci (1000 mCi) source of cobalt-60, the calculation would be as follows:

$$\text{Exposure rate} = \frac{13.2 \times 1000}{(92)^2} = \frac{13,200}{8464} = 1.56 \text{ R/h}$$

The gamma constant can be multiplied by 3×10^{-5} to give dose in mSv/h/MBq.

Appendix 6

Radionuclides Listed Alphabetically

Radionuclide	Physical Half-Life	Effective Half-Life	Radiation
Americium-241	458 years	139 years	α,e⁻,γ
Americium-243	7950 years	194 years	α,γ
Antimony-122	67 h	—	β⁻,β⁺,γ
Antimony-124	60 days	—	β⁻,γ
Antimony-125	2.7 years	—	β⁻,e⁻,γ
Argon-37	35 days	—	γ
Arsenic-74	18 days	17 days	β⁻,β⁺,γ
Arsenic-76	26.5 h	—	β⁻,γ
Arsenic-77	39 h	24 h	β⁻,γ
Barium-131	12 days	—	γ,e⁻
Barium-133	7.2 years	—	γ,e⁺
Barium-137m	2.55 min	—	γ,e⁻
Barium-140	13 days	11 days	β⁻,γ,e⁻
Beryllium	53 days	—	γ
Bismuth-207	30 years	—	e⁻,γ
Bismuth-210	5.01 days	—	α,β⁻,γ
Bromine-82	35.34 h	—	β⁻,γ
Cadmium-109	453 days	140 days	γ,e⁻
Cadmium-115	53.5 h	—	β⁻,γ
Cadmium-115	43 days	—	β⁻,γ
Calcium-45	165 days	162 days	β⁻
Calcium-47	4.5 days	4.5 days	β⁻,γ
Califomium-242	2.6 years	2.2 years	γ,α,N
Carbon-11	20.3 min	—	β⁺,γ
Carbon-14	5730 years	12 days	β⁻
Cerium-141	33 days	30 days	β⁻,e⁻,γ
Cerium-144	284 days	280 days	β⁻,e⁻,γ
Cesium-131	9.70 days	—	γ
Cesium-134	2.05 years	—	β⁻,γ
Cesium-137	30.0 years	70 days	β⁻,e⁻,γ
Chlorine-36	3.1×10^5 years	—	β⁻,γ
Chromium-51	27.8 days	27 days	e⁻,γ
Cobalt-57	270 days	9 days	e⁻,γ
Cobalt-58	71.3 days	8 days	β⁺,γ
Cobalt-60	5.26 years	10 days	β⁻,γ
Copper-64	12.8 h	—	β⁻,e⁻,β⁺,γ
Curium-242	163 days	155 days	α,N,γ
Curium-243	32 years	27.5 days	α,γ
Curium-244	17.6 years	16.7 years	α,N,γ
Dysprosium-159	144 days	—	e⁻,γ

Radionuclide	Physical Half-Life	Effective Half-Life	Radiation
Erbium-169	9.4 days	—	β^-,e^-,γ
Europium-152	13 years	3 years	$\beta^+,\beta^-,e^-,\gamma$
Europium-154	16 years	3 years	β^-,e^-,γ
Europium-155	2 years	1.3 years	β^-,e^-,γ
Fluorine-18	2 h	2 h	β,γ
Gadolinium-153	242 days	—	e^-,γ
Gallium-67	78.1 h	—	γ
Gallium-68	68.3 min	—	γ,β^+
Gallium-72	14.1 h	12 h	γ,β
Germanium-71	11.4 days	—	γ
Gold-195	183 days	—	e^-,γ
Gold-198	2.7 days	2.6 days	β^-,e^-,γ
Gold-199	75.6 h	—	β^-,e^-,γ
Hafnium-181	42.5 days	—	β^-,e^-,γ
Holmium-166	26.9 h	—	β^-,e^-,γ
Hydrogen-3	12 years	12 days	β^-
Indium-111	2.8 days	—	γ
Indium-113m	100 min	—	e^-,γ
Indium-114	72 s	—	β^+,γ,β^-
Indium-114m	49 days	27 days	$e^-,\gamma(DR)$
Iodine-123	13 h	—	γ
Iodine-125	60 days	42 days	e^-,γ
Iodine-129	1.7×10^7 years	—	β^-,e^-,γ
Iodine-130	12.4 h	—	γ,β^-
Iodine-131	8.05 days	8 days	β^-,e^-,γ
Iridium-192	74 days	—	e^-,β^-
Iridium-194	17.4 h	—	β,X
Iron-52	8.3 h	—	β^-
Iron-55	2.6 years	1 year	
Iron-59	45 days	42 days	β^-
Krypton-81m	13.0 s	—	β^-
Krypton-85	10.76 years	—	
Lanthanum-140	40.22 h	—	β^-
Lead-210	2 years	1.3 years	α,e^-,β^-
Lutetium-177	6.7 days	—	e^-,β^-
Magnesium-28	21 h	—	e^-,β^-
Manganese-54	303 days	—	e^-
Mercury-197	2.7 days	2.3 days	e^-
Mercury-197m	24 h	—	e^-
Mercury-203	4 days	11 days	e^-,β^-
Molybdenum-99	67 b	1.5 days	β^-
Neodymium-147	11.1 days	—	e^-,β^-
Neptunium-237	2×10^6 years	200 years	α
Neptunium-239	2.3 days	2.3 days	β
Nickel-63	92 years	—	β^-
Niobium-95	35 days	—	β^-
Nitrogen-13	10 min	—	β^+
Osmium-191	15 days	—	β^-,e^-,γ
Oxygen-15	124 s	—	γ,β^+
Palladium-103	17 days	—	γ
Palladium-109	13.47 h	—	β^-,e^-,γ
Phosphorus-32	14 days	14 days	β^-
Plutonium-238	88 years	63 years	γ,α
Plutonium-239	2.4×10^4 years	197 years	γ,α

Radionuclides Listed Alphabetically

Radionuclide	Physical Half-Life	Effective Half-Life	Radiation
Polonium-210	138 days	46 days	α,γ
Potassium-42	12 h	12 h	β^-,γ
Praseodymium-142	19.2 h	—	β^-,γ
Praseodymium-143	13.6 days	—	β^-
Praseodymium-144	17.3 min	—	β^-,γ
Promethium-147	2.6 years	1.6 years	β^-
Promethium-149	2.2 days	2.2 days	β^-,γ
Protactinium-233	27.0 days	—	β^-,e^-,γ
Protactinium-234	6.75 h	—	β^-,e^-,γ
Radium-224	3.6 days	3.6 days	$\gamma,\alpha(DR)$
Radium-226	160 years	44 years	$\alpha,e^-,\gamma(DR)$
Rhenium-186	90 h	—	β^-,e^-,γ
Rhodium-106	30 s	—	β^-,γ
Rubidium-82	1.3 min	—	γ,β^+
Rubidium-86	19.0 days	13.2 days	β^-,γ
Ruthenium-97	2.9 days	—	e^-,γ
Ruthenium-103	39.6 days	—	β^-,γ
Ruthenium-106	367 days	2.5 days	$\beta^-(DR)$
Samarium-151	87 years	—	β^-,e^-,γ
Samarium-153	47 h	—	β^-,e^-,γ
Scandium-46	84 days	40 days	β^-,γ
Selenium-75	120.4 days	—	e^-,γ
Selenium-77m	17.5 s	—	γ
Silver-110	24.4 s	—	β^-,γ
Silver-110m	253 days	5 days	β^-,e^-,γ
Silver-111	7.5 days	—	β^-,γ
Sodium-22	2.60 years	11 days	γ,β^+
Sodium-24	15 h	14 h	β^-,γ
Strontium-85	64 days	64 days	e^-,γ
Strontium-87m	2.83 h	—	e^-,γ
Strontium-89	52 days	—	β^-,γ
Strontium-90	28 years	15 years	$\beta^-(DR)$
Sulfur-35	88 days	44 days	β^-
Tantalum-182	115 days	—	β^-,e^-,γ
Technetium-99	2.12×10^9 years	20 days	β^-
Technetium-99m	6.0 h	—	e^-,γ
Tellurium-132	78 h	—	β^-,e^-,γ
Terbium-160	72.1 days	—	β^-,e^-,γ
Thallium-201	73 h	—	γ
Thallium-204	3.8 years	—	β^-,γ
Thorium-230	8×10^4 years	200 years	α,γ
Thorium-232	1.4×10^{10} years	200 years	$\alpha,\gamma(DR)$
Thulium-170	130 days	—	β^-,e^-,γ
Tin-113	115 days	—	γ
Tin-119m	250 days	—	e^-,γ
Titanium-44	48 h	—	$e^-,\gamma(DR)$
Tungsten-185	75 days	—	β^-
Tungsten-187	23.9 h	—	β^-,e^-,γ
Uranium-235	7.1×10^8 years	15 days	$\alpha,\gamma(DR)$
Uranium-238	4.51×10^9 years	—	$\alpha,e^-,\gamma(DR)$
Xenon-127	36.4 days	—	e^-,γ
Xenon-133	5.27 days	—	β^-,e^-,γ
Ytterbium-169	32 days	—	e^-,γ
Yttrium-90	64 h	64 h	β^-

Radionuclide	Physical Half-Life	Effective Half-Life	Radiation
Yttrium-91	58.8 days	—	β^-,γ
Zinc-65	245 days	194 days	β^-,e^-,γ
Zinc-69	57 min	—	β^-
Zirconium-95	66 days	56 days	$\beta^-,\gamma(DR)$

Note: DR = daughter radiation, N = neutron.

Source: Mettler, F.A. and Moseley, R.D., Eds., *Medical Effects of Ionizing Radiation,* Grune & Stratton, New York, 1985. With permission.

Index

A

Abdominal discomfort, 28
Absorbed dose
  physical assessment of, 497
  summary of accumulated, 341
  units, conversion of, 576
Accelerators, accidents involving, 225
Accident(s)
  characteristics of involving small geographic areas, 19
  classification of radiation, 21
  investigation form, 48
  localized, 19
  major radiation, 138–141
  nuclear submarine, 157
  number of in registry by state, 170
  reconstruction, 261, 498
  registration and management, 153
  Therac-25, 295
Accident management, application of radiation protection principles to, 449–452
  accidental exposure, 449
  dose limits and overexposure, 450–452
  intervention, 450
  limitation of occupational exposure in emergencies, 450
Acetaminophen, 282
Acid burns, 422
Acneform skin eruptions, 331
Actovegin, 231
Acute effects, 72
Acute lymphoblastic leukemia, 84
Acute myeloblastic leukemia, 174
Acute–phase proteins, 463
Acute radiation nephritis, 107
Acute radiation pneumonitis (ARP), 92
Acute radiation sickness (ARS), 24, 28, 33–51, 198, 223
  acute radiation effects from internal contamination, 42–48
  cerebral syndrome of, 42
  change of lymphocyte counts in initial days of, 39
  criteria for diagnosis and prognosis, 34–41
  early identification and management of ARS patients, 48–49
  effect of local radiation injury on, 41–42
  forms of, 35
  latent phase of, 39
  patients, early identification and management of, 48
  prodromal phase of, 38
  survivors
    follow-up of, 203
    long-term risks of, 208
Acute radiation sickness (ARS), treatment of, 53–67
  bone marrow depression, 61–64
    bone marrow transplantation, 61–62
    transfusions, 61
    use of cytokines, 62–64
  early treatment, 57–58
    early neurological or severe hypotensive effects, 57–58
    initial management, 57
  gastrointestinal complications, 58–61
    nausea, vomiting, and diarrhea, 58–60
    prevention and treatment of infections, 60–61
  lethal dose, 54–55
  prognostic categories, 55–57
  research, 64–65
Acute radiation syndrome, 15, 18, 22, 33, 54, 58
Acute radiological syndrome, accidents leading to, 150
Acyclovir, 61, 202
Adenocarcinoma, lung, 481
Adult respiratory distress syndrome, 106
AERC, see Automatic exposure rate controls
Agranulocytosis, 41
ALARA doses, see As low as reasonably achievable doses
Alarm systems, 211
Albuquerque, New Mexico, U.S.A., iridium-192 acid skin burn in, 421–423
Algeria, accident in, 248
ALI, see Annual limit on intake
Alkaline phosphatase, 92, 463
Alloimmunization, 61
Alpha emitters, 321, 322, 412
Alpha particles, range of, 5
Aluminum-containing antacids, 331
Alycon II radiotherapy unit, 299
Americium, 325, 347
  -241, 382, 386
  application of to burn surface, 379
Americium accident victim, lifetime follow-up of 1976, 337–343
  case management, 338
  effectiveness of DTPA therapy, 341–342
  initial medical care and findings, 337–338
  medical course, 1977 to 1987, 339–340
  medical course, September 1976 to January 1977, 338–339
  radiation dosimetry evaluation, 340–341
Amicacin, 202

Amifostine, 65
Aminoglycosides, 202
Ammonium chloride, 333
Amputation
   defects, 229
   of distal aspects of digits, 289
   leg, 180, 201, 273
AMU, *see* Atomic mass units
Androgen, injection of, 361
Ankle, localized skin lesions on, 263
Ankylosing spondylitis, 108, 112
Annual limit on intake (ALI), 421
Antacids, aluminum-containing, 331
Antibiotics, 393
Anticoagulation, direct, 203
Anti-infectious agents, 232
Antinecrotic drug, 190
Antioxidants, 317
Antithymocyte globulin (ATG), 192
Antithyroid drugs, 332
Aorta
   calcification, radiography for, 463
   pulse wave velocity, 463
Apoptosis, 508, 515
Aprotinine, 190
ARP, *see* Acute radiation pneumonitis
ARS, *see* Acute radiation sickness
Arteriole, radiation injury involving, 71
As low as reasonably achievable (ALARA) doses, 449
Aspartate oxoglutarate aminotransferase, 468
Ataxia-telangiectasia, 464
ATG, *see* Antithymocyte globulin
Atherosclerosis, 98
   in ARS survivors, 204
   premature, 302
Atomic bomb data, uncertainties in, 54
Atomic bomb survivors, 34
   circulatory diseases in, 98
   mortality analysis, 486
   test items for long-term follow-up of, 463
   under 30 years of age, 79
Atomic mass units (AMU), 3
ATSDR, *see* U.S. Agency for Toxic Substances and Disease Registry
Automatic exposure rate controls (AERC), 316
Autopsy, 254
   data, 305
   records, 300
   U.S. Transuranium Registry-sponsored, 340
Azoospermia, 267

B

Bacteriological examination, 262
Bacteriological tests, 201
Baker explosion, underwater, 471
Barium sulfate, 331
Becquerel, Henri, 73
BED, *see* Biologically effective dose
Beta aminoisobutyric acid, 185

Beta burns, 77, 204, 475
Beta emitters, 473
Beta-gamma emitter, 321
Beta radiation, 4, 72
Beta ray-induced skin injuries, 150
Biochemical markers, 513, 515
Biodosimeters, suggested uses for available, 515
Biokinetic models, 324
Biological dosimeters, current status of, 507–518
   biochemical markers, 513
   cell death, 508–510
      apoptosis, 508–510
      general, 508
   forms of nuclear alterations in irradiated cells, 510–512
      chromosomal aberrations, 510
      micronucleated cells, 511–512
      premature chromosome condensation, 510–511
   gene mutations, 512–513
      glycophorin A gene, 512–513
      hypoxanthine-guanine phosphoribosyl transferase gene, 512
   physical dosimeters, 513–514
      electron spin resonance, 513–514
      optically stimulated luminescence, 514
Biological dosimetry, 463
Biological half-life, 359
Biologically effective dose (BED), 301
Biological response, 7
Bladder injury, 107
Blast cells, 114
Blood
   cell counts, 476
   counts, serial, 199
   pool images, 284
   studies, 445
   urea nitrogen (BUN), 106, 468
   vessels, radiation effects on large peripheral, 96
Bloom syndrome, 464
BMT, *see* Bone marrow transplantation
Body burden
   americium-241, 382
   radionuclide, 380
Bone
   mineral densitometer, 463
   radiation effects on, 110
   radiography, 463
   tumor, 482
Bone marrow
   allogenic transplantation, 200
   cell cultures, 256
   depression, 61, 174, 244, 272, 276
   distribution, age-related, 255
   doses, 255
   examination, 192
   failure, 191
   radiosensitivity of, 328
   recovery, 215
   scintigraphies, 256
   suppression, 63
   syndrome, 27, 94, 115
   transplantation (BMT), 61, 188, 203, 250

Index

Bovine spongiform encephalitis (BSE), 318
Bowel perforation and necrosis, 309
Brachytherapy, 294, 536
Bragg effect, 230
Brain necrosis, 82, 307
Bravo, 471
Breast cancer, 456
Breast-feeding, 534
Brescia
    fatal accidents in, 211
    irradiation at commercial irradiation facility in, 214
Bronchial necrosis, 308
Brown–Sequard syndrome, 86
BSE, *see* Bovine spongiform encephalitis
Budd–Chiari syndrome, 105
Buffer zone, 427
BUN, *see* Blood urea nitrogen
Burn(s), 379
    acid, 422
    beta, from fallout, 475
    chemical, 384
    common, 394
    contaminated by radioactive substances, 399
    nitric acid, 338
    radioactive contamination of, 406
    radioactivity monitoring of contaminated, 412
    radionuclide metabolism in contaminated, 384
    site, decontamination at, 368
    thermal, 380, 384, 425
Buttocks, local radiation injury to, 230, 237

C

Calcium, 332, 463
Camera, 241, 278
Cancer(s), 466
    after Chernobyl accident, 206
    breast, 456
    cervical, 107, 454, 457
    colon, 454
    detection tests, 463
    G-CSF therapy and, 63
    hyperkeratosis into, 30
    liver, 454
    mortality rates, solid, 487
    ovarian, 454
    in pelvis, 536
    pancreatic, 454
    prostate, 454
    radiogenic, 457
    risk, 205
        background, 529
        childhood, 529
    on scars, 30
    screening, 454, 457
    skin, 481
    thyroid, 29, 207, 208, 456, 521
    uterine, 454
Candida, 188, 192
Capillary, radiation injury involving, 71

Carbenicillin, 202
Cardiovascular diseases, 463, 465
Cardiovascular shock, 58
Carotid disease, 98
Cartilage
    radiation effects on, 110
    radioresistance of, 111
Case management, 338
Cataract(s), 27, 34, 183
    formation, 89, 90, 474
    identification of, 89
Causal protection, classification of principles and
        techniques of, 365
Cefamizin, 202
Cefobid, 202
Cell
    death, 7, 8, 23, 508
    proliferation, dyshematopoeitic, 264
Cellulitis, 284
Central nervous system (CNS), 35, 308, 528
    complications, 308
    damage, 538
    radiation-induced changes in, 82
Cephazolin sodium, 216
Cerebrospinal fluid pressure, elevation of, 82
Cerium, 535
Cerium-144, 386
Cervical cancer, 107, 296, 454, 457
Cesium, 355
    -137, 197, 241
    application of to burn surface, 379
    rate of elimination of, 360
    volatile radionuclides of, 196
CFU-GEMM cloning ability, 256
Chelation
    agents, 333, 365
    therapy, 335, 342, 350, 351
Chemical burns, 384
Chernobyl
    accident
        cancer after, 206
        exposure of lungs and thyroid of patients who died
            after, 200
        lessons, 208
    ARS survivors, late lethality of, 205
    disaster, psychiatric symptoms appearing after, 520
    distribution of gamma energy at, 34
    incidence rate of malignancies in decade after, 18
    patients, patterns of dose distribution in, 37
Chernobyl, medical aspects of accident at, 195–210
    acute radiation sickness, 198–201
    cancer after Chernobyl accident, 206
    Chernobyl accident lessons, 208–209
    evaluation of people without ARS, 205–206
    expected clinical symptoms as function of dose, 198
    follow-up of ARS survivors, 203–205
    initial accident details, 196–197
    initial medical response, 198
    principles of organizational decisions, 206–208
    therapy and outcomes of patients with ARS,
        201–203

Chest
    burn, from industrial radiography source, 244
    counters, 347
    dosimeter, 188
    radiograph, 217, 248
Cheyne–Stokes rhythm, 214
Child abuse, 244
Childhood cancer
    risk of, 529
    studies of survivors of, 537
    thyroid cancer, 521
China Institute for Radiation Protection, 153
Chinese hamster ovary (CHO) cells, 509
Chinese nuclear accidents, 149–155
    accident registration and management, 153–154
    accidents leading to acute radiological syndrome and deaths, 150–153
        Sanli'an accident, 150–152
        Shanghai 6.25 cobalt-60 source accident, 152–153
        Xinzhou accident, 153
    application of radioisotopes and nuclear technology, 150
    status of radiation protection and accidents in nuclear industry, 149–150
CHO cells, see Chinese hamster ovary cells
Cholinesterase, 468
Chondrocalcinosis, 111
Chondrosarcomas, 116
Chordomas, 116
ChRD, see Chronic radiation disease
Chromosome
    aberration(s), 35, 463, 466
        analysis, 152
        stable, 462
        unstable, 266
    analysis, 214, 216, 250
    exchanges, 510
    painting, 510–511
Chronic clinical period, 72
Chronic obstructive pulmonary disease (COPD), 95
Chronic radiation disease (ChRD), 486
Chronic radiation nephritis, 107
Chronic radiation sickness, 24, 28, 29
Chronic radiation syndrome, 15
Chronic roentgen ulcers, 73
CIDI, see Composite International Diagnostic Interview
Cigarette smoking, 481
Ciprofloxazin, 270
Circulatory system disease, 481
Cirrhosis, 106
Citrates, 373
Civil defense training, 259
Clindamycin, 270
Clonazepam, 217
Cloning ability, CFU-GEMM, 256
CMI, see Cornell Medical Index
CNS, see Central nervous system
Cobalt, 534
    -58 experiments, 383
    -60, 241
        radiation sources with, 20
        source accident, 152
        X-rays, 72

teletherapy, 293
Cockayne's syndrome, 464
Colitis, 307
Colon
    cancer of, 454
    radiation-induced changes in, 102
Colorado plateau miners, 96
Comet assay, 509
Commercial irradiation facilities, medical data for patients involved in fatal accidents at, 212
Committed dose, 452
Common burns, 394
Composite International Diagnostic Interview (CIDI), 464
Computed tomography (CT), 83, 94, 313, 530
Computer phantom, doses calculated using, 275
Confidentiality, 460
Congestive heart failure, 340
Connective tissue, mature, 9
Contaminated injuries, anatomic localization of, 366
Contaminated room, 427
Contamination
    acute radiation effects from internal, 42
    definition of, 10
    environmental, 133
    indices, microbial, 202
    internal, 438
    measurements of internal, 209
    plutonium oxide, 405
    wound, 385
COPD, see Chronic obstructive pulmonary disease
Cornea
    transplant sutures, 340
    ulceration of, 88
Cornell Medical Index (CMI), 463, 464
Coronary artery disease, chronic, 337
Corticosteroids, 361
Costa Rica, 2-year medical follow-up of radiotherapy accident in, 299–311
    dose reconstruction, 301
    records and examinations, 300–301
    results, 301–309
        deceased patients, 305–307
        number of fractions, 301
        sites of irradiation and catastrophic complications, 307–309
        treatment dose, 302–304
Cranial radiation, 303
C-reactive protein, 463, 464, 468
Creatinine clearance, reduced, 107
Criticality accidents, 173–194
    Argonne, Illinois, U.S.A., (June 1952), 176
    Chelyabinsk-70 (April 1968), 188–189
    Constituyente, Argentina (September 1983), 190
    Hanford, Washington, U.S.A. (April 1962), 187
    Idaho Chemical Processing Plant, U.S.A. (October 1959), 186–187
    induced ^{24}Na results in various, 503–504
    Kurchatov Institute, Moscow, Russia (February 1971), 189
    Kurchatov Institute, Moscow, Russia (May 1971), 189
    Los Alamos, New Mexico, U.S.A. (August 1945), 174

Index

Los Alamos, New Mexico, U.S.A. (December 1958), 186
Los Alamos, New Mexico, U.S.A. (May 1946), 175–176
Mayak production Facility, Russia (December 1968), 189
Mayak, Russia (April 1957), 181–182
Mayak, Russia (January 1958), 183
Mayak, Russia (March 1953), 176–181
Mol, Belgium (December 1965), 188
Oak Ridge, Tennessee, U.S.A. (June 1958), 183–185
Sarov (Arzimas-16) Vniief, Russia (June 1997), 190–191
Sarov Vniief, Russia (March 1963), 187
with serious exposures, 175
Siberian Chemical Combine, Russia (December 1978), 190
Siberian Chemical Combine, Russia (July 1961), 187
Tokaimura, Japan (September 1999), 191–192
Vinca, Yugoslavia (October 1958), 185–186
Wood River Junction, Rhode Island, U.S.A. (July 1964), 187
Crypts of Lieberkühn, 101
Crystallography accidents, 229
CT, *see* Computed tomography
Curie, Marie, 73
Curie Institute, 262, 265, 266
Curium, 325
Cutaneous laser Doppler, 227
Cutaneous syndrome, 223
Cyclosporin-A, 217
Cyclotron workers, exposure of to neutrons, 90
Cystitis, acute, 107
Cytogenetics, 248, 255
Cytogenic dosimetry, 199
Cytokines, 57, 62, 64, 463
Cytomegalovirus, 61, 92, 218

D

Dark current, exposure to, 225
Deaths, radiation related, 307
Debridement procedures, 351
Decontamination
  ability, 388
  effectiveness, 387
  efforts, effective, 423
  patient, 431
  procedures, 337
  skin, 22, 320
  supplies, 428
  tabletops, 431
Decorporation therapy, 410
Defense in depth, 143
Depigmentation, 75
Depression, 84
Dermatitis, toxic, 260
Desquamation, 74, 226, 273
  moist, 285, 356
  overexposure of pelvis resulting in, 306

Dexamethasone, 270, 274
Diabetes mellitus, 315
Diagnostic film, 280
Diagnostic imaging results, 283
Diagnostic tests, 445
Dialysis, renal failure requiring, 106
Diethylenetriaminepentaacetic acid (DTPA), 334
  administration of by inhalation, 354
  application efficiency, 397
  chelation decision, 346
  finger wound processed with, 403
  inhalation administration, 396
  therapy, effectiveness of, 341, 353, 406
  treatment efficiency, multivariant study of, 396
Dijon Conference, 135, 145
Dimercaprol, 335
Direct radiation effects, 70
Displacement therapy, 331
Diuretics, 333
DNA
  bond, radiation breaking of, 8
  damage to, 7
  –DNA cross-links, 510
  ionizing radiation damage to, 507
  irradiation of structural elements of, 27
  -level mutation, 466
  regeneration of, 231
Dose(s), 6
  absorbed, physical assessment of, 497
  as low as reasonably achievable, 449
  assessment, 265, *see also* Instrumentation and physical dose assessment, in radiation accidents
  biological effectiveness of, 35
  bone marrow, 255
  calculation of using computer phantom, 275
  clinical symptoms as function of, 198
  committed, 452
  distribution, patterns of in Chernobyl patients, 37
  effect of distance on radiation, 11
  effective, use of personal monitors to estimate, 499
  –effect relationship, 15
  equivalent stem cell, 47
  equivalent units, conversion of, 576
  estimated radiation, in exposed populations, 476
  estimates, 41, 270
  factors influencing patient and staff, 316
  fetal, estimates of, 531
  levels, 207
  limits, 12, 450
    misconceptions about, 452
    recommended annual, 12
  mean, 250, 266
  methods for assessing personal absorbed, 489
  rate characteristics, 223
  reconstruction, 152, 301
  reduction, principles of, 10
  ways of reducing radiation, 11
Dosimeter(s)
  pencil, 491, 492, 495
  personal, 492, 497
  physical, 513

pocket, 492
thermoluminescent, 279
Dosimetry, 324
  biological, 463
  cytogenetic, 248
  electron spin resonance, 266
Down syndrome, 488
DTPA, see Diethylenetriaminepentaacetic acid
Dyshematopoeitic cell proliferation, 264

E

EB virus, see Epstein–Barr virus
EC, see Emergency Coordinator
ECC, see Emergency Control Center
ECG, see Electrocardiogram
ECM, see Emergency Communications Manager
ED, see Effective dose
Edema, soft-tissue, 284
EDF, see Emergency Decontamination Facility
Effective dose (ED), 6, 499
EFPM, see Emergency Fire Protection Manager
Electrocardiogram (ECG), 445
Electrolyte
  imbalance, 59, 101
  loss, 400
Electromagnetic radiations, 2
Electron
  accelerators, 164
  beam machine, local irradiation injury of hands with, 289–290
  spin resonance (ESR), 41, 100, 266, 462, 513
Element, seizures by, 144
Emergency
  personnel, 441
  plan exercises, 564
Emergency Communications Manager (ECM), 561
Emergency Control Center (ECC), 563, 564
Emergency Coordinator (EC), 558
Emergency Decontamination Facility (EDF), 337, 342
Emergency Director, 559
Emergency Fire Protection Manager (EFPM), 560
Emergency Medical Manager (EMM), 559
Emergency operator responsibilities, 563
Emergency Plan Implementing Procedures (EPIPs), 557, 558, 565
Emergency Public Information Manager (EPIM), 561
Emergency Radiation Protection Manager (ERPM), 559
Emergency room management, of radiation accidents, 49, 437–447
  decontamination, 438–439
  radiation accident management example, 440–445
  radiation emergency team duties, 439–440
  specific problems, 445–446
    blood and other laboratory studies, 445
    electrocardiograms, 445
    high-activity source or metal fragments in patient, 446
    psychological, 445
    radiographs, 445–446
    surgical emergencies, 446

Emergency Safety and Security Manager (ESSM), 560
Emergency Support Centers (ESC), 563
Emetics, 329
EMM, see Emergency Medical Manager
Emphysema, 96
Endoscopy, 101, 313
Enraf-Nonius X-ray Diffraction Unit, 278
Eosinophilia, 63
Eosinophil count, 257
Epidemiological research, planning and implementation of, 458
Epilation, 177, 178, 179, 212
EPIM, see Emergency Public Information Manager
EPIPs, see Emergency Plan Implementing Procedures
EPO, see Erythropoietin
Epstein–Barr (EB) virus, 465
Equivalent stem cell dose, 47
Erbium-169 citrate, 112
ERPM, see Emergency Radiation Protection Manager
Erythema, 74, 227
Erythrocytes sedimentation rate, 463
Erythropoietin (EPO), 65, 192, 220
ESC, see Emergency Support Centers
Esophagus
  motility, impairment of, 100
  radiosensitivity of, 100
ESR, see Electron spin resonance
ESSM, see Emergency Safety and Security Manager
Ethiofos, 65
Expectorants, 333
Explosions, nuclear, 157
Exposure(s)
  definition, 472
  inhalation, 345
  occupational
    guidance for emergency, 451
    limitation of in emergencies, 450
  –outcome relationship, 459
  potential, 449
  radioiodine, 532
  units, conversion of, 575
  whole-body, 27
Eye, effects of radiation on, 87

F

FADU, see Fluorescence analysis of DNA unwinding
Fallout
  beta burns from, 475
  from nuclear explosion, 157
Fanconi's anemia, 464
Fast-FISH technique, 511
Feces
  excretion, of radioactive material, 325
  samples, 348
  -to-urine ratios, 358
Ferric ferrocyanide, 357
Ferrocyne, 399, 409
Ferrokinetics studies, 256
Fertility, among ARS survivors, 204

Index

Fetal dose, estimates of, 531
Fibroblasts, 9, 113
Fibrosis, 96, 232
Field of view (FOV), 316
Filagrastim, 62
Film
  badge, 491, 492, 494, 496
  diagnostic, 280
  radiography, 313
Finger
  lesions, 290
  wound, dissection of, 400
First aid, 409, 425, 438
FISH, *see* Fluorescence *in situ* hybridization
Fission
  products, 195, 388
  yield, 187
Fissionable materials, 173
Flow cytometry, 509
Fluid imbalance, 59
Fluorescence
  analysis of DNA unwinding (FADU), 509
  in situ hybridization (FISH), 462, 463, 508, 510, 515
Fluoroscopy, medical accidents with local injury from use of medical, 313–318
  accident reports, 314–315
  contribution of operational and equipment factors, 316–317
    equipment factors, 316
    operational factors, 316–317
  postaccident treatment of skin injuries, 317–318
    early treatments, 317–318
    later treatments, 318
  specific cases, 315–316
Follicle–stimulating hormone (FSH), 264
Follow-up, *see* Long-term follow-up, of people after radiation exposure; Marshall Islands, long-term follow-up after accidental exposure to radioactive fallout in; Monitoring and epidemiological follow-up, of people accidentally exposed
Forced fluids, 332
Formamide, 511
FOV, *see* Field of view
Fractionation scheme, 291
Free-radical scavengers, 8, 317
French Radiation Protection Institute (ISPN), 272
Fresh skin microtraumas, 384
FSH, *see* Follicle–stimulating hormone
Fuel cladding, defects in, 78
Fukuryu Maru, 473
Fundamentals, of radiation accidents, 1–13
  biological response, 7–9
  dose limits, 12
  electromagnetic and particle radiations, 2–4
    particle radiations, 3–4
    X rays and gamma rays, 2
  principles of dose reduction, 10–12
    distance, 11
    shielding, 11–12
    time, 10–11

quantities and units, 4–7
  dose, 6
  effective dose, 6–7
  equivalent dose, 6
  exposure, 5
radioactivity, 7
  general, 7
  nuclear transformations, 7
types of radiation accidents, 9–10
Funduscopy, 463

G

Gallium, 535
Gamma camera scintillation, 421
Gamma dose rates, 485
Gamma globulin, 202
Gamma glutamine transpeptidase, 217
Gamma radiation alarm, 216
Gamma ray constants, 587–588
Gamma spectroscopy, 323
Ganglion cells, 9
Gastrointestinal absorption, reduction of, 329
Gastrointestinal complications, treatment of, 58
Gastrointestinal manifestations, 221
Gastrointestinal symptoms, 184
Gastrointestinal syndrome, 60, 99
Gastrointestinal tract
  neutron radiation of, 103
  radiation effects on, 99
G banding, 463
G-CSF, *see* Granulocyte colony–stimulating factor
Geiger counter, 57, 242, 443, 493
Geiger–Mueller counters, 490
Gene mutations, 512, 515
General Health Questionnaire (GHQ), 464
General Safety Protocol, 286
Genetic polymorphism, 463
Gentamicin, 202
Georgia (1997), accident involving abandoned radioactive sources in, 259–268
  circumstances of accident, 259–260
  clinical course after accident recognition, 262–265
    clinical evolution, 1998 to 1999
    clinical findings, 262–264
    surgical treatment, 264–265
  dose assessment, 265–266
    local exposures, 265–266
    whole-body exposure, 266
  initial response, 260–261
GFR, *see* Glomerular filtration rate
GHQ, *see* General Health Questionnaire
Giemsa staining, 510
Glial cells, 9, 82
Glomerular filtration rate (GFR), 106
Glossary, 541–555
Glove box operations, 410
Glucocorticoids, 219
L-Glutamine, 217
Glycophorin A (GPA), 462, 463, 512

Glycoprotein products, 63
GM-CSF, *see* Granulocyte/macrophage colony–stimulating factor
Goiânia accident, Brazil (1987), internal contamination in, 355–360
    description of accident, 355–356
    efficacy of Prussian Blue therapy, 357–360
    internal contamination, 357
Goiter, toxic multinodular, 81
Gold
    -198, 361
        colloid, 112
        misadministration of, 53
    fatal accidental overdose with radioactive, 361–362
Good engineering practice, 143, 144
Governmental infrastructures, of radiation safety, 137
GPA, *see* Glycophorin A
Graft-vs.-host disease, 62, 192, 203, 217, 218
Grafting, 237
Graft procedure, three-step, 273
Granisetron, 59
Granulocyte(s), 113
    Chernobyl schematic data for, 44
    colony–stimulating factor (G-CSF), 60, 113, 191, 248, 270, 276
    /macrophage colony–stimulating factor (GM-CSF), 60, 113
Granulocytosis, 56
Graves' disease, 81
Ground nuclear explosion, 393
Growth retardation, 538
Guinier camera, 278

H

Hair loss, 185
Half-value layer (HVL), 2
Halogens, 373
Haloperidol, 217
Hand(s)
    late effect of LRI to, 234, 236
    local irradiation injury of with electron beam machine, 289–290
    long-term radiation effects on, 245
Hashimoto's thyroiditis, 79
Head, proton beam irradiation through, 238
Heart
    disease, radiation-induced, 97
    radiation effects on, 96
Hematological evolution, 271
Hematology, 463, 464
Hematopoietic syndrome, 114
Hematopoietic systems, radiation effects on, 112
Hematuria, 107
Hemipelvectomy, 276
Hemorrhage, 307
Heparin, 203, 339
Hepatic cells, radiation-induced changes in, 103
Hepatic injury, clinical signs of, 105
Hepatitis

B virus antigen, 463
    radiation, 105, 106
Hepatocytes
    hyperchromic, 361
    necrosis, 103
Hexametaphosphate (HMP), 388
High-LET radiation, 80
Hiroshima, 53
    atomic bomb radiation in, 23
    autopsies of victims at, 80
    laboratory tests conducted at Radiation Effects Research Foundation in, 468
    neutron exposure at, 89
    studies on A-bomb survivors in, 461
Histoautoradiography tests, 380, 382
Historical associations, frightening, 519
HMP, *see* Hexametaphosphate
Hodgkin's disease, 79, 97, 102, 110, 536
Hospitals, treatment of exposed patients at, 22
Hospital preparation, for radiation accidents, 425–435
    area
        designation, 427–428
        setup, 429–430
    communications, 426
    drills, 434
    floor covering, 430
    instrumentation, 432–433
    patient decontamination, 431
    procedures, 433
    protective clothing, 432
    security, 434
    shielding, 431–432
    supplies, 428
    ventilation, 431
HPRT, *see* Hypoxanthine-guanine phosphoribosyl transferase
5-HT3, *see* 5-Hydroxytryptamine
HTO, *see* Tritiated water
HVL, *see* Half-value layer
Hybridoma growth factor, 65
Hydrocodone, 282
5-Hydroxytryptamine (5-HT3), 58
Hyperkeratosis into cancer, 30
Hypermotility, 102
Hyperpigmentation, 305, 306
Hyperproteinemia, 101
Hypertension, 107, 204
Hyperthyroidism, 76, 78
Hypoalbuminemia, 217
Hypotension, transient incapacitation syndrome with enurological findings due to, 193
Hypotensive effects, treatment of severe, 57
Hypothyroidism, 331, 476
    laboratory, 79
    subclinical, 79
Hypovolemia, 28
Hypovolemic shock, 295
Hypoxanthine-guanine phosphoribosyl transferase (HPRT), 512
    assay, 513
    gene, 512

Index

I

IAEA, *see* International Atomic Energy Agency
IARC, *see* International Agency for Research on Cancer
ICRP, *see* International Commission on Radiological Protection
IL-3, *see* Interleukin 3
Illicit Trafficking Radiation Monitoring Assessment Program (ITRAP), 146
IND, *see* Investigational new drug
Indomethacin, 59
Inert gases, 535
Infectious diseases, 463, 465
Information exchange, dynamics of, 199
Infrared-stimulated luminescence (IRSL), 514
Inhalants, 333
Inhalation
    DTPA administration by, 354
    exposure, 345
Injury(ies)
    anatomic localization of contaminated, 366
    radiological and nuclear accidents resulting in radiation, 16
Insect bite, 269
Institute Curie, 249
Instrumentation and physical dose assessment, in radiation accidents, 489–500
    personal dosimeters, 492–496
        film badges, 496
        pencil or pocket dosimeters, 492–493
        thermoluminescent dosimeters, 494–496
    physical assessment of absorbed dose, 497
        accident reconstruction, 498
        history, 497–498
        issues related to radiation exposure records, 499
        personal dosimeters, 497
    radiation accidents, incidents, and nonaccidents, 498
    radiation detection instruments, 490–492
        Geiger–Mueller counters, 490–492
        ionization chamber survey meters, 490
        scintillation detectors, 492
    use of personal monitors to estimate effective dose, 499
Intake, 324
Intelligence quotient (IQ), 85, 528
Interferon, low-dose, 204
Interleukin 3 (IL-3), 64, 65
Internal contamination, 438
    acute radiation effects from, 42
    measurements of, 209
Internal contamination, assessment and treatment of, 319–336, *see also* Goiânia accident, Brazil (1987), internal contamination in
    basis for treatment decisions, 328–329
    biokinetic models and dosimetry, 324–328
    blocking and diluting agents, 331–335
        chelating agents, 333–335
        lung lavage, 335
        mobilizing agents, 332–333
    initial evaluation, 321–324
    initial priorities, 320–321
    treatment, 329–331
        aluminum-containing antacids, 331
        barium sulfate, 331
        emetics, 329
        ion-exchange resins, 330
        Prussian Blue, 330–331
        purgatives, 329–330
        stomach lavage, 329
Internal irradiation, 115
Internal radiation, 80
International Agency for Research on Cancer (IARC), 17
International Atomic Energy Agency (IAEA), 34, 133, 168, 299
    Emergency Response Centre, 147
    intervention levels recommended by, 450, 451
International Chernobyl Project, 81
International Commission on Radiological Protection (ICRP), 17, 136, 324
    intervention levels recommended by, 450, 451
    model, 327
    radiation, 6
    recommendations, 145
International Criminal Police Organization (INTERPOL), 135, 146
INTERPOL, *see* International Criminal Police Organization
Interstitial myocardial fibrosis, 97
Intestinal syndrome, 27
Intramuscular injection, ^{239}Pu resorption and distribution after, 374–375
In utero irradiation, 528
Inversion, 463
Investigational new drug (IND), 334
In vivo measurements, 352
Iodide goiter, 331
Iodine, 325
    -125, 171
    -131, 171
    period, 205
    volatile radionuclides of, 196
Ion-exchange
    fabrics, 385
    resins, 330
Ionization chamber survey meters, 490, 491, 492
Ionizing radiation(s), 8, 27, 459
    cell cultures exposed to, 511
    characteristics of, 5
    exposures, accidental, 169
    sources of, 133
    thresholds for skin effects, 315
IQ, *see* Intelligence quotient
Iridium-192, 241, 246, 421–423
Iron, 534
Irradiation
    diagnostic, of pregnant patient, 530
    internal, 115
    in utero, 528
    large intestine mucosa before, 104
    pathogenesis of whole-body, 437
    pelvic, 114
    radionuclide, 91, 105, 108
    through head, 238

Irradiation facility(ies)
  in China, 218
  irradiation at commercial, in Brescia, 214
  medical data for patients involved in fatal accidents at commercial, 212
  Nesvizh, 220
  in San Salvador, 214
Irradiation facilities, accidents at industrial, 211–222
  Brescia, Italy, 214
  China, 218–220
  Kjeller, Norway, 214
  Nesvizh, Belarus, 220–222
  San Salvador, El Salvador, 214–216
  Soreq, Israel, 216–218
IRSL, see Infrared-stimulated luminescence
Ischemic disease, 204
Isodose curves, 54
ISPN, see French Radiation Protection Institute
ITRAP, see Illicit Trafficking Radiation Monitoring Assessment Program

J

Jaundice, 105

K

Karnovski index, 254
Kefzol, 202
Kidney, radiosensitivity of, 106
Kurchatov Institute, 189

L

Laboratory test accuracy, 462
Lacrimal glands, 88
Lactate dehydrogenase (LDH), 92
Laryngeal necrosis, 308
Laser Doppler, cutaneous, 227
Last image hold, 316
Late clinical period, 72
LDH, see Lactate dehydrogenase
Leg amputation, 180, 201, 273
Lens opacities, 89
Leoxasol, 231
Lesion(s)
  finger, 290
  ulcerated, 273
LET, see Linear energy transfer
Lethal dose, mean, 54
Leukemia, 34, 40, 174, 208, 488
  acute lymphobastic, 84
  radiation-induced, 257
  risk of, 529
Leukine®, 63
Leukoencephalopathy, 83
Lhermitte's sign, 86
Linear accelerator, accident at in Zaragoza, Spain, 294
Linear energy transfer (LET), 2, 74

Lithium deuteride reflector, around plutonium core, 187
Liver
  alcoholic, 315
  cancer, 454
  disease
    nonmalignant, 106
    veno-occlusive, 103, 218
  function, 217
Localized radiation, first phase of, 227
Local radiation injury (LRI), 33, 157, 223–240
  clinical course and classification of, 226–227
  conditions of accidental localized exposure, 223–225
  local radiation injury of hand, 228–230
  local radiation injury to other parts of the body, 230–231
  misdiagnosis of, 246
  radiobiology of local radiation injuries, 225–226
  role of physical dosimetry, 226
  treatment of, 231–239
Long-term follow-up, of people after radiation exposure, 461–469
  biological dosimetry, 462
  epidemiological methods, 461–462
  follow-up over generation, 466
    examination of second generation, 466
    storage of biological materials, 466
  tests for cancer, 464
    hematology, 464
    molecular biology, 464
    tumor markers, 464
    ultrasound examination, 464
  tests for noncancer diseases, 464–466
    cardiovascular disease, 465
    immunological abnormality, 466
    infectious diseases, 465
    ophthalmological diseases, 465
    parathyroid diseases, 465
    psychological problems, 464–465
    subclinical inflammation, 466
  time and human factors, 462–464
Los Alamos, see Manhattan Project plutonium workers, at Los Alamos
Los Alamos National Laboratory, 175, 182, 340, 366
LRI, see Local radiation injury
Lucky Dragon, 473
Lung
  adenocarcinoma of, 481
  counts, 347
  dose, relationship between protraction of and mortality, 93
  lavage, 335
  nonuniform radiation doses in, 326
  radiosensitivity of, 92
Lymphatic systems, radiation effects on, 112
Lymphatic vessel damage, 370
Lymphocyte(s), 9, 177, 179, 247
  Chernobyl schematic data for, 44
  count, 38, 39
  peripheral blood, 200
Lymphoid exhaustion, 27
Lymphopenia, 40

Index

M

Macrophage colony–stimulating factor (M-CSF), 65
Mad cow disease, 318
Magnetic resonance imaging (MRI), 83, 262, 313
Malfunction 54 message, 296
Malignant neoplasms, 41
Manganese-54 experiments, 383
Manhattan Project plutonium workers, at Los Alamos, 477–483
    clinical data, 481–482
    dosimetry, 478–480
    history of Manhattan Project workers, 477–478
    mortality data, 480
Marrow depression, 116
Marshall Islands
    distribution of gamma energy at, 34
    long-term follow-up after accidental exposure to radioactive fallout in, 471–476
        evaluation of Marshall Island population, 473–476
        study of U.S. servicemen, 471–473
    population, evaluation of, 473
    thermonuclear explosion at, 80
Mass attenuation coefficient, 280
Maternal radioactivity, 533
Mayak Production Facility, 189
Mayak Radiochemical Association workers, 366
M-CSF, *see* Macrophage colony–stimulating factor
MDA, *see* Minimum detectable activity
Mean dose, 250, 266
Mean physical dose, 47
Medical characteristics, of radiation accidents, 15–22
    accidents involving small geographic areas, 19–21
    large accidents, 17–19
Medical data, for patients involved in fatal accident at commercial irradiation facilities, 212–213
Medical examination form, 49
Medical facility, sample radiation emergency plan for, 557–570
    background information, 557
    radiological monitoring, 569–570
    sample emergency plan implementing procedures, 565
    XYZ Medical Facility, for emergencies within hospital, 568
    XYZ Medical Facility emergency plan, 557–565
        Emergency Control Center, 563
        emergency plan exercises, 564
        Emergency Support Center, 563
        instructions and responsibilities, 558–562
        notification, 562–563
        recovery, 564–565
        review, revision, and distribution of emergency plan, 565
        training, 563–564
    XYZ Medical Facility notification of emergency, 565–566
    XYZ notification form, 567
Medical information checklist, 440
Medical monitoring, 454, 456
Medical treatment, of radiation therapy accidents, 292
Megakaryocytes, mature, 113
Memorandum of understanding (MOU), 146
Mental retardation, 85, 488, 529
Mercury, 325
Metal objects, activation of, 501
Metamyelocytes, 252
Methicillin-resistant *staphylococcus aureus* (MRSA), 60
Methotrexate, 84, 85
Microbial contamination indices, 202
Micronucleated cells, 511
Micronucleus assay, 512
Microsurgery techniques, 232
Midline tissue dose (MTD), 55
Minimum detectable activity (MDA), 357
Mobilizing agents, 332
Model Project in Radiation Protection, 137
Moist desquamation, 285, 356
Monitoring and epidemiological follow-up, of people accidentally exposed, 453–460
    epidemiological follow-up, 457–459
        choice of population and outcome to be studied, 458
        data sources and quality, 458–459
        issues of study design, 458
    medical monitoring, 454–457
        assessment of benefit of medical monitoring, 456
        costs of medical monitoring, 456
        effects of accuracy of monitoring and disease prevalence, 455
        medical monitoring considerations, 457
        monitoring of sensitive populations, 456
        screening for specific cancers, 457
Monte Carlo programs, 502
Mood alteration, 302
Morocco, accident in, 253
Mortality
    ascertainment, 472
    data, 480
MOU, *see* Memorandum of understanding
MRI, *see* Magnetic resonance imaging
MRSA, *see* Methicillin-resistant *staphylococcus aureus*
MTD, *see* Midline tissue dose
Mucositis, 99
Multiple myeloma, 454
Muscle
    cells, 9
    radiation effects on, 110
    wounds, 371, 388
Myelocytes, 252
Myelodepression, evaluation of, 203
Myelodysplastic syndrome, 24, 340
Myeloleukemia, chronic, 487
Myelopathy, 295
Myeloproliferative syndrome, 339
Myocardial infarction, 176, 425
Myocarditis, diagnosis of, 97
Myofibroblasts, 318

N

Nagasaki, 53
    atomic bomb radiation in, 23
    laboratory tests conducted at Radiation Effects Research Foundation in, 468

neutron exposure at, 89
   studies on A-bomb survivors in, 461
Naprosyn, 270
Nasal herpes, 255
Nasal smear, 411
Nasal swabs, 322
Nasogastric suction, 443
National Radiation Protection Board (NRPB), 422
Neck, X-ray therapy of, 79
Necrosis, 27
Neogemodez, 203
Nervous system, resistance of to radiation effects, 81
Neupogen®, 62
Neurodermatitis, 245
Neuropsychological abnormalities, 85
Neutron(s)
   exposure, 501–505
      cyclotron workers, 90
      Hiroshima, 89
      Nagasaki, 89
      phosphorus-32, 502
      sodium-24 activation, 501–502
   irradiation, 77
   radiation, 100, 103
   thermal, 173
Neutrophil
   dysfunction, 60
   recovery, 63
News media, 434
Nitric acid burns, 338
Nitrogen-acidic plutonium, 373
Nitrogen-acidic polonium-210, 372
Noble gases, 17
Non-Hodgkin's lymphoma, 454
Nonsteroidal anti-inflammatory (NSAI) medications, 285
Nose swipes, 346
Novocain, 393
NRC, see Nuclear Regulatory Commission
NRPB, see National Radiation Protection Board
NSAI medications, see Nonsteroidal anti-inflammatory medications
Nuclear accidents
   large-scale, 17
   resulting in radiation injury, 16
Nuclear explosion(s)
   fallout from, 157
   ground, 393
Nuclear fuel
   chemical processing of, 20
   cycle systems, Chinese, 149
Nuclear industry
   development of, 149
   status of radiation protection in, 149
Nuclear medicine therapy, 167
Nuclear power plant accident, factors influencing potential health effects in, 195
Nuclear Regulatory Commission (NRC), 135, 168
Nuclear submarine accidents, 157
Nuclear technology, 150
Nuclear transformations, 7
Nuclear weapon detonation, 77

Nurses, visiting home, 285
Nursing personnel, 439

O

Oak Ridge Institute for Science and Education (ORISE), 168
Occupational exposure
   guidance for emergency, 451
   limitation of in emergencies, 450
Off-site agencies, 561
Oncology, radiation, 300
Ondansetron, 59
Ophthalmological diseases, 463, 465
Optically stimulated luminescence (OSL), 514
Optic neuropathy, radiation-induced, 88
Oral cavity, radiation effects on, 99
Organ
   damage, 28
   injury, radiation-induced, 285
   radionuclide incorporation, 392
   weighting factors, 6
Organizational decisions, 206
ORISE, see Oak Ridge Institute for Science and Education
Oropharyngeal syndrome, 198
Orphan sources, 136
OSL, see Optically stimulated luminescence
Osteogenic sarcoma, 481, 483
Osteoporosis, 229, 230
Osteosarcoma, 112, 257
Ovary
   cancer of, 454
   follicular cells, 9
Oxalates, 373
Oxygen effect, 8

P

Paget's disease, 111
Pain control, 285
Pancreatic cancer, 454
Pap smear, 457
Paralysis, 302
Paraplegia, 302
Parathyroid
   diseases, 465
   extract, 333
Particle radiations, 2, 3
Patient decontamination, 431
PB, see Prussian Blue
PCC, see Premature chromosome condensation
Pelvis
   cancer in, 108, 536
   irradiation of, 114
   radiotherapy, 101, 108
Pencil dosimeter, 491, 492, 495
Penicillamine, 330
Pentoxyfylline, 282
Perineum, necrosis of, 305

Peripheral blood lymphocytes, 200
Peripheral lymphocyte count, 339, 474
Peripheral nerves, resistance of to radiation damage, 87
Peripheral vasodilator, 289
Peritonitis, 307
Personal dosimeters, 492, 497
Personal monitors, use of to estimate effective dose, 499
PET, see Positron emission scanning
Peyer's patches, 60
Pharynx, radiation effects on, 99
Phlebosclerosis, 98
Phosphate, 332
Phosphorus, 325
Phosphorus-32, 112, 116, 502
Photon energies, half value layers for, 4
Physical dosimeters, 513
Physics neutron pile, 188
Pigmentation, of linear treatment fields, 304
Pipracil, 202
Piroxicam, 282
Platelet(s), 113
   Chernobyl schematic data for, 44
   counts, 183
   transfusions, 219, 220, 257
Plutonium, 42, 175, 322, 378
   -239, 348, 349
   compound(s)
      behavior of different, 376
      contaminants, wound decontamination experiment results for, 391
   -contaminated wound care, 354
   depositions, estimated, 479
   excretion, after CaDTPA chelation, 348
   facilities, 365
   nitrogen-acidic, 373
   oxide
      contamination, 405
      resorption, for skin injuries of white rats, 377
   particles, inhalation of, 478
   pentacarbonate resorption, 376
   recovery of from irradiated uranium rods, 176
   urinalysis for, 478
   wound dissemination, 379
Plutonium accidents, two Los Alamos, 345–354
   inhalation exposures, 345–350
      DTPA chelation decision, 346–347
      fecal samples, 348–349
      lung counts, 347
      nose swipes, 346
      urine bioassays, 348
   plutonium-contaminated wound, 350–354
      chelation therapy, 351
      initial wound counts and excision, 351
      in vivo measurements, 352
      second tissue excision, 351
      urine bioassay results, 353
Pneumocystis carinii, 92
Pneumonia, 34, 215
Pneumonitis, radiation, 93, 221
Pneumothorax, 215
Pocket dosimeter, 492

Poisson's law, 266
Polonium
   -210, 386
   application of to burn surface, 379
Polyform exudative erythema, 260
Positron emission scanning (PET), 83
Post-radiation, 24
Post-traumatic stress disorder (PTSD), 521
Potential exposures, 449
Prednisone administration, 95
Pregnancy, accidental radiation exposure during, 527–539
   accidental exposures in diagnostic radiology and other low-dose situations, 530–531
      diagnostic radiology, 530–531
      general, 530
   accidental exposure during radiotherapy and other external high-dose situations, 535–536
      general, 535
      radiotherapy, 536
   accidental internal exposure, 532–535
      breast-feeding, 534
      exposure to radioiodine, 532–533
      general, 532
      other specific radionuclides, 534–535
   becoming pregnant after accidental radiation exposure, 536–537
   counseling and possible termination of pregnancy, 537–538
   effects of *in utero* irradiation, 528–530
      effects on central nervous system, 528–529
      general, 528
      risk of leukemia and childhood cancer, 529–530
Pregnancy termination, 537
Pregnant patient, diagnostic irradiation of, 530
Premature chromosome condensation (PCC), 510, 515
Prochlorperazine dimaleate, 184
Proctosigmoiditis, radiation, 103
Prognostic categories, 55
Proportional counter, 413
Prostaglandins, 65, 101
Prostate cancer, 454
Protective clothing, 432
Protein(s)
   acute-phase, 463, 466
   C-reactive, 463
   electrophoresis, 463, 468
   variants, 466
Proteolysis inhibitors, 231
Proton accelerators, 164
Prussian Blue (PB), 330, 357, 399
Pseudomonas aeroginosa, 264
Psychological effects, 206
Psychological problems, 445, 463
Psychosocial effects, of radiation accidents, 519–525
   high-risk groups, 521
   implications for radiation accident preparedness and response, 522–524
   key features of radiation accidents, 519–520
   psychological effects, 520–521
   social impacts, 522
PTSD, see Post-traumatic stress disorder

Public relations, 440
Pulsed fluoroscopy, 316
Purgatives, 329
Pyknosis, 101

Q

Quadriplegia, 302
Quinidine preparation, 340

R

RADEV, 146
Radiation(s)
  accident(s), 498
    classification of, 21
    consequences of, 1
    key features of, 519
    major, 138–141, 171
    management example, 440
    procedure for handling, 433
    types of, 9, 10
  beta, 72
  cranial, 303
  dermatitis, 73
  detection instruments, 490
  disaster drill, 434
  edema, 82
  effects, direct, 70
  electromagnetic, 2
  emergency area (REA), 427, 428, 429, 439
  exposure
    records, 499
    units of, 5
  handbooks, 558
  hepatitis, 105, 106
  high-LET, 80
  ICRP, 6
  incidents, 498
    major types on in territory of former U.S.S.R., 164
    in territory of former U.S.S.R., 158–163
  -induced diarrhea, 59
  -induced heart disease (RIHD), 97
  injury(ies)
    animal data regarding, 25
    local, 30
    mechanisms involved in expression of, 25
    most common type of in United States, 171
    radiological and nuclear accidents resulting in, 16
  instrumentation, 432
  internal, 80
  ionizing, 5, 8, 27, 459
    accidental exposures, 169
    cell cultures exposed to, 511
    sources of, 133
    thresholds for skin effects, 315
  necrosis, imaging of, 83
  neutron, 100, 103
  nonaccidents, 498

oncology, 300
particle, 2, 3
pneumonitis, 93, 94, 221
protection
  principles, see Accident management, application of radiation protection principles to
  statis of, 149
retinopathy, 88
safety personnel, 429
sickness
  acute, 24, see Acute radiation sickness
  chronic, 24, 28, 29
  development of, 25
  pathogenetic classification of in humans, 26
  severity grade of, 25
sickness classification, 23–31
  local radiation injury, 30
  schemes, 24–27
  whole-body exposure, 27–29
sources, 16
  with cobalt-60, 20
  human factors and, 145
  out of control, 152
  safety of, 134
stress, 25
survey and monitoring instruments, 491
syndromes, 23
total-body, 53
ulcer, transformation of, 30
whole-body, 53
Radiation Emergency Assistance Center/Training Site (REAC/TS), 167
Radiation Effects Research Foundation (RERF), 466
Radiation Protection Advisory Team (RAPAT), 137
Radiation Safety Officer, 279
Radiation therapy, accidents in, 291–297
  overdose from malfunction of high-dose-rate brachytherapy equipment in United States, 1992, 294–295
  Riverside, Ohio, U.S.A., 1974 to 1976, 293
  Therac-25 accidents, 295–297
  underexposure during radiotherapy accident in United Kingdom, 1982 to 1990, 293–294
  Zaragoza, Spain, 1990, 294
Radioactive isotope resorption, 369
Radioactive material(s)
  fecal excretion of, 325
  internal deposition of, 320
  meltings of, 142–143
  products contaminated with imported into United States, 143
  safety of, see Safety of radiation sources, security of radioactive materials and
  security of, 134
Radioactive source(s)
  dangerous, 269
  highly intense, 224
Radioactive wastes, 16
Radioactivity, 7
  burdens, 398
  induced, 183

Index

maternal, 533
units, conversion of, 577
Radiocesiums, 323
Radiocolloids, 373
Radiogardase, 358
Radiogenic cancers, 457
Radiographs, 445
Radiography accidents, causes and characteristics of industrial, 243
Radiography sources, accidental radiation injury from industrial, 241–258
  accident in Texas, U.S.A., 246
  case of child abuse, 244–245
  causes and characteristics of industrial radiography accidents, 243–244
  local exposure, 244–246
  local and whole-body exposure, 246–253
    accident in Algeria, 1978, 248–253
    accident in Iran, 1996, 246–248
  whole-body exposure, 253–257
    accident in Morocco, 1984, 253–257
    accident in Ukraine, 1988 to 1991, 257
Radioiodine
  exposure to, 532
  uptake of, 323
Radioisotopes, application of, 150
Radiological Accident in Goiânia, 355
Radiological accidents, 224
Radiological monitoring, 569–570
Radiology, interventional, 314
Radionuclide(s)
  administration, models of intramuscular, 376
  alpha-emitting, 326, 366
  availability of, 389
  beta-emitting, 490
  body burdens, 380
  cesium, 196
  distribution, in organs and tissues, 383
  estimating internal deposition of, 322
  excretion of absorbed, 329
  gamma-emitting, 490
  imaging, 285
  importance of in accidental situations, 18
  incorporation, organ, 392
  inhalation, 22, 96, 195, 198
  on intact skin, 438
  internal deposition of long-lived, 64
  iodine, 196
  irradiation, 91, 105, 108
  listed alphabetically, 589–592
  metabolism, 368
  modes of intake of, 364
  multiorgan deposition of in body, 43
  penetration capability in lead of, 12
  removal of from injured area, 385
  resorption, 369, 381
  transportation of, 406
Radionuclides, absorbed dose estimates from, 579–586
  absorbed dose estimates from radionuclides in critical organs or lungs, 585–586
  effective dose coefficients for intakes of radionuclides by workers, 579–581
  maximum external photon and electron dose equivalent factors, 583
  maximum photon dose equivalent rate conversion factors, 584
  skin contamination dose equivalent rate factors, 582
Radiopharmaceuticals, accidents occurring with use of, 170
Radiophobia, 523
Radiosensitivity, 9
Radiostrontium, 369
Radiotherapy
  accidents, examples of, 293
  patients, major reported accidents involving, 292
  pelvic, 101
  protocols, 310
  whole-lung, 95
Radium, 42, 73, 325
RAPAT, see Radiation Protection Advisory Team
Rare earth elements (REE), 373
RBE, see Relative biological effectiveness
REA, see Radiation emergency area
REAC/TS, see Radiation Emergency Assistance Center/Training Site
Recovery workers, 206
Rectum, radiation-induced changes in, 102
Red cell transfusions, 203
REE, see Rare earth elements
Reepithelialization, 226
Regulatory Authority Information System, 145
Relative biological effectiveness (RBE), 77
Renal failure, 332
Renal insufficiency, 108, 192
Repoliglukin, 203
Reproductive organs, 108
RERF, see Radiation Effects Research Foundation
RES, see Reticular endothelial system
Resorption rates, differences in, 372
Respiratory infection, 340
Respiratory insufficiency, 222
Respiratory tract, radiosensitivity of, 92
Reticular endothelial system (RES), 378
Reticulocytes, 252
Retinopathy, radiation, 88
Rhabdomyosarcoma, 89
Rhenium-186 sulfide, 112
Rhinotracheitis, acute, 198
RIHD, see Radiation-induced heart disease
Road-mapping, 316
Russian Federal Nuclear Center (VNITF), 188

S

Safety
  audit modifications, 287
  culture, 144
  requirements for, 137
  service personnel, 408
Safety of radiation sources, security of radioactive materials and, 133–147

agency's current program, 145–147
current issues, 135–137
quantifying of problem, 134–135
requirements for safety, 137–145
yardstick for safety and security, 137
Salivary glands, 91
Sandoglobulin, 202
San Juan de Dios Hospital, accident at, 310
San Ramon, Peru, localized irradiation from industrial radiography source in, 269–276
dose estimates, 270–272
later medical care, 273
medical care during first 30 days, 270
San Salvador
fatal accidents in, 211
radiation injury at industrial irradiation facility in, 214
Sargramostim, 63
SCG, see Single cell gel
Schwann cells, 82
Scintillation
counter, 491
detectors, 413
Sealed radiation source, 16, 151
Sebaceous gland activity, suppression of, 75
Secondary nucleus, 511
Security, of radioactive materials, see Safety of radiation sources, security of radioactive materials and
Seizures
by element, 144
of radioactive sources, 144
Self-inflicted injury, 167
Self-reset process, 509
Serial blood counts, 199
Serum
calcium, 463
disease, 260
glutamic-oxaloacetic transaminase (SGOT), 91
glutamic-pyruvic transaminase (SGPT), 91–92
Sex ratio imbalances, 463, 466
Sexual behavior, among ARS survivors, 204
SGOT, see Serum glutamic-oxaloacetic transaminase
SGPT, see Serum glutamic-pyruvic transaminase
Shielding, 11, 431, 449
Sialic acid, 463, 466
Siberian Chemical Combine, 187, 190
Sievert (Sv), 6
Silicosis, 96
Single cell gel (SCG), 509
Skin
atrophy, 77, 226
burn, 295, 421–423
cancer, 481
decontamination, 22, 320, 395
eruptions, acneform, 331
grafting, full-thickness, 285
injury(ies)
beta ray–induced, 150
depth and character of mechanical, 367
postaccident treatment of, 317
time of onset of clinical signs of, 73
lesions, on ankle, 263

microtraumas, fresh, 384
radionuclide(s)
contamination of, 380
on intact, 438
reaction, 76
tolerance, to radiation, 76
ulceration, 74, 297
Skin wounds and burns, contaminated by radioactive substances, 363–419
general characteristics of radioactive contamination of wounds and burns, 365–368
methods and techniques of control of radioactive contamination of wounds and burns, 385–407
acceleration of body excretion of radioactive substances resorbed in wounds, 394–399
background, 385
control of radioactive contamination of wounds and burns, 406–407
decontamination of burns contaminated by radioactive substances, 393–394
experience with human wounds and burns contaminated by radioactive substances, 399–406
prevention of radionuclide body absorption and removal of radionuclides from injured area, 385–393
practice and procedures of medical care of skin wounds and burns contaminated by radioactive substances, 407–414
background, 407–408
care at accident site, 408–409
medical care at local medical facility, 409–410
radioactivity monitoring of contaminated wounds and burns, 412–414
specialized hospital care, 410–411
unique aspects of radionuclide metabolism in contaminated skin wounds and burns, 368–384
burns, 379–384
radionuclide metabolism in contaminated wounds and burns, 384
wounds, 369–378
Slit-lamp examination, 463
Small artery, radiation injury involving, 71
Small intestine, radiation effects on, 101
SMR, see Standardized mortality ratios
Social stigma, observation of after recent accidents, 522
Sodium
-24 activation, 501
bicarbonate, 333
Soft-tissue edema, 284
Solcoseril, 203, 231
Solid cancer mortality rates, 487
SOMA/LENT grading system, 310
Somnolence, 84
Soreq accident, 218
Sor-Van Facility, fatal accidents in, 211
Source–victim geometry, 250
Specific tissues, direct effects of radiation on, 69–131
bone, cartilage, and muscle, 110–112

low-LET radiation, 110–112
neutron or high-LET radiation, 112
radionuclide irradiation, 112
eye, 87–91
high-LET radiation, 90
low-LET radiation, 88–90
radionuclide irradiation, 91
gastrointestinal tract, 99–103
colon, sigmoid, and rectum, 102–103
esophagus, 100
liver, 103–106
oral cavity and pharynx, 99–100
small intestine, 101–102
stomach, 101
heart and vessels, 96–98
general, 96
low-LET radiation, 96–98
hematopoietic and lymphatic systems, 112–116
high-LET radiation, 115
internal irradiation, 115–116
low-LET radiation, 114
nervous system, 81–87
brain, 82–85
peripheral nerves, 87
spinal cord, 86–87
reproductive organs, 108–110
low-LET radiation, 109–110
high-LET radiation, 110
radionuclide irradiation, 110
respiratory tract, 92–96
lung, 92–96
trachea, 92
salivary glands, 91–92
general, 91
low-LET radiation, 91–92
skin and mucosa, 72–78
low-LET radiation, 74–77
neutron irradiation, 77
radiation of skin by radionuclides, 77–78
thyroid, 78–81
high-LET radiation, 80
internal irradiation, 80–81
low-LET radiation, 79–80
urinary system, 106–108
high-LET radiation, 108
low-LET radiation, 106–108
radionuclide irradiation, 108
Spectroscopy, 229
Spermatogonia, 9
Spinal cord, direct injury to, 86
Spontaneous abortion, 537
Sputum cytology, 482
Stab wounds, 370, 378, 401
Standardized mortality ratios, 480 (SMR), 480
Staphylococcus
  aureus, 264
  methicillin-resistant, 273
Stem cell transplantation, 57, 62
Sterility, 109
Steroid administration, 95
Stochastic effects, identification of, 15

Stomach
lavage, 329
radiation effects on, 101
Strontium, 42, 325, 332, 534
-89, 115, 386
application of to burn surface, 379
Suicide, 225, 231
Surface seekers, 112
Surrounding injection, of tissues, 390
Sv, *see* Sievert
Synthroid, 476
Systemic deposition, 324

T

Taurine excretion, 185
TBP, *see* Tributylphosphate
T-cell surface markers, 463
TD, *see* Tolerance dose
TdT assay, *see* Terminal deoxynucleotidyl transferase assay
Techa River, epidemiological evaluation of population accidentally exposed near, 485–488
Technetium-99m, 283, 532, 535
Technological disasters, 522
Telangiectasia, 75, 76, 102, 226
Teletherapy, cobalt, 293
Telethermography, 262
Terminal deoxynucleotidyl transferase (TdT) assay, 509
Testes, radiosensitivity of, 109
Test methods, detection limits for, 515
Therac-25 accidents, 295
Thermal burns, 380, 384, 425
Thermoluminescent dosimeter (TLD), 279, 433, 444, 492
Thigh, local radiation injury to, 230
Thorium, 42
Three Mile Island, 426
Thrombocytes, 177, 178, 179, 247
Thrombocytopenia, 105, 361
Thrombopoietin (TPO), 192
Tymol turbidity test, 468
Thyroid, 78
acute effects of external radiation on, 80
cancer, 207, 208, 456
childhood, 521
metastatic, 115
radiation-induced, 29
function studies, 19
radiosensitivity of, 328
storm, 81
Thyrotoxicosis, 79
Tinea capitus, 84
TIPS, *see* Transjugular intrahepatic portosystemic shunt
Tissue excision, 351
TLD, *see* Thermoluminescent dosimeter
T leukocytes, 222
T lymphocytes, elimination of, 203
TNF, *see* Tumor necrosis factor
Tokaimura accident, 94
Tolerance dose (TD), 77
Toluene, 421

Tonsillitis, 184
Total bilirubin, 468
Total-body radiation, 53
Toxemia, 33
Toxic dermatitis, 260
TPO, see Thrombopoietin
Tracheal necrosis, 308
Transformation of radiation ulcer, 30
Transfusion therapy, 201
Transient incapacitation syndrome, with neurological findings due to hypotension, 193
Transjugular intrahepatic portosystemic shunt (TIPS), 315
Translocation, 463
Transplants, use of in recent radiation accidents, 63
Traumatologists, 314
Trauma treatment room, 430, 442
Treatment decisions, basis for, 328
Tributylphosphate (TBP), 384
Tritiated water (HTO), 534
Tritium, 46, 323, 325
Tropisetron, 59
Troxevasin, 203
Tuberculosis, 108
Tumor(s)
  eradicating, 291
  markers, 464
  necrosis factor (TNF), 65
  rate of after Chernobyl accident, 18
  Wilms', 95, 105

U

Ulcers, recurrent, 265
Ultrasound, 262, 313, 463, 464
United Nations Scientific Committee on the Effects of Atomic Radiation (UNSCEAR), 17
United States
  major radiation accidents in, 171
  most common type of radiation injury in, 171
  radiations accidents in, 167–172
    background, 168
    registries, 168–169
    U.S. Registry, 169–171
Units, 575–577
  conventional and international unit conversions, 575
  conversion of absorbed dose units, 576
  conversion of dose equivalent units, 576
  conversion of exposure units, 575
  conversion of radioactivity units, 577
UNSCEAR, see United Nations Scientific Committee on the Effects of Atomic Radiation
Uptake, 324
Uranium, 325
  accumulation of during filtration of uranyl oxalate precipitate, 181
  fission products, 43
  rods, recovery of plutonium from irradiated, 176
Uranyl oxalate precipitate, accumulation of uranium during filtration of, 181
Uric acid, 468

Urinalysis, 468
Urinary bladder epithelium, 9
Urinary excretion curve, plutonium-239, 349
Urinary system, radiosensitivity of, 106
Urine bioassays, 348
U.S. Agency for Toxic Substances and Disease Registry (ATSDR), 455
U.S. Argonne National Laboratory, 176
U.S. Department of Defense, 474
U.S. Department of the Interior, 474
U.S. Food and Drug Administration, 338
U.S. Institute of Medicine, 453, 471
U.S. Oak Ridge National Laboratories, 183, 281
U.S. Registry, 169
U.S.S.R., radiation accidents in former, 157–165
U.S. Transuranium Registry, 340
Uterine cancer, 454

V

Vascular compromise, 285
Vascular endothelitis, 75
Vasoconstrictive agents, 365
Vasopressor amines, 186
Veno-occlusive disease, 103, 105
Ventilation, 431, 449
Very seriously exposed patients, summary of, 177–179
Victim treatment, summary data on, 400–404
Vinca reactor criticality accident, 185
Vincristine, 84
Visiting home nurses, 285
VNITF, see Russian Federal Nuclear Center
Vocacite, 387
Volume seekers, 112

W

Wastes, radioactive, 16
Weapon detonation, 78
White blood cell counts, 184
WHO, see World Health Organization
Whole-body dose
  estimated acute, 56
  maximum survivable, 55
Whole-body exposure, 27
Whole-body radiation, 53, 70
Whole-lung radiotherapy, 95
Wilms' tumor, 95, 105
Wisconsin, U.S.A., fatal accidental overdose with radioactive gold in, 361–362
World Health Organization (WHO), 168, 261, 426, 571–573
Wound(s), 369
  care, plutonium-contaminated, 354
  contamination, radioactive, 385
  counts, 351
  decontamination experiment results, 391
  detection of alpha emitters in, 412
  dissemination, plutonium, 379

Index

healing, influence of radiation on, 407
muscle, 371, 388
plutonium citrate-contaminated, 390
radioactive contamination of, 406
radioactivity monitoring of contaminated, 412
radionuclide metabolism in contaminated, 384
stab, 370, 378, 401
treatment, surgical, 398

X

Xenograft, 264
Xeroderma pigmentosum, 464
Xerostomia, 91
Xinzhou accident, 153
X-ray(s), 2
   cobalt-60, 72
   devices, 157
   diffraction
      safety course, 286
      units, 277
   -generating devices, 169
   vision, 313

X-ray diffraction accident, exposure analysis and medical evaluation of low-energy, 277–287
   clinical evaluation, 281–285
      days 1 through 7, 281
      days 8 through 14, 282
      diagnostic imaging results, 283–285
      months 5 through 12, 282
      weeks 2 through 12, 282
      years 2 through 4, 283
   description of accident, 278–279
   exposure assessment, 279–281
   key findings and recommendations, 286–287
      procedural changes, 286
      safety audit modifications, 287
      training enhancements, 286
   recommendations for evaluation and treatment of extremity radiation exposure, 285–286

Y

Yttrium-90 silicate citrate, 112